The Complete Textbook of Animal Health and W...

Commissioning Editors: *Joyce Rodenhuis, Robert Edwards*
Development Editors: *Louisa Welch, Sally Davies*
Project Manager: Jane Dingwall
Designer/Design Direction: George Ajayi
Illustration Manager: Gillian Richards
Illustrators: Samantha Elmhurst, Deborah Maizels

The Complete Textbook of Animal Health and Welfare

Edited by

Jane Williams RCVS CertEd VN

Section Head for Environment and Land-based Studies, South Devon College, Paignton, Devon, UK

Foreword by

Dr R Scott Keller DVM

Coordinator of Veterinary Medical Technology, Joliet Junior College, Joliet, Illinois, USA

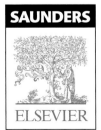

SAUNDERS

ELSEVIER

Edinburgh   London   New York   Oxford   Philadelphia   St Louis   Sydney   Toronto 2009

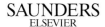

SAUNDERS
ELSEVIER

First published 2009, © Elsevier Limited. All rights reserved.

ISBN 978 0 7020 2944 8

British Library Cataloguing in Publication Data
A catalogue record for this book is available from the British Library

Library of Congress Cataloging in Publication Data
A catalog record for this book is available from the Library of Congress

Notice
Knowledge and best practice in this field are constantly changing. As new research and experience broaden our knowledge, changes in practice, treatment and drug therapy may become necessary or appropriate. Readers are advised to check the most current information provided (i) on procedures featured or (ii) by the manufacturer of each product to be administered, to verify the recommended dose or formula, the method and duration of administration, and contraindications. It is the responsibility of the practitioner, relying on their own experience and knowledge of the patient, to make diagnoses, to determine dosages and the best treatment for each individual patient, and to take all appropriate safety precautions. To the fullest extent of the law, neither the Publisher nor the Editor assumes any liability for any injury and/or damage to persons or property arising out of or related to any use of the material contained in this book.

The Publisher

your source for books, journals and multimedia in the health sciences
www.elsevierhealth.com

Working together to grow libraries in developing countries
www.elsevier.com | www.bookaid.org | www.sabre.org

ELSEVIER   BOOK AID International   Sabre Foundation

The publisher's policy is to use **paper manufactured from sustainable forests**

Printed in China

Contents

Contents

vi

Contributors

Julian Chapman
Senior Head Keeper of Mammals
Paignton Zoo Environmental Park
Paignton
Devon, UK

Donna de Haan MBA
Senior Lecturer
University of Worcester
Worcester, UK

Debbie Duke BSc(Hons)
Lecturer and Course Manager
Duchy College
Callington
Cornwall, UK

Lucy Dumbell MSc
Senior Lecturer – Equine Science
Hartpury College
Gloucester, UK

John Dutton BSc(Hons) PhD FRGS
Senior Lecturer
Institute of Science and the Environment
University of Worcester
Worcester, UK

Hayley Randle BSc(Hons) PhD
Senior Lecturer
Duchy College
Department of Animal Science
Callington
Cornwall, UK

Rachel Rayers BSc
Lecturer
Animal Management, Environment and Land-based Studies
South Devon College
Paignton
Devon, UK

Jane Williams RCVS CertEd VN
Section Head for Environment and Land-based Studies
South Devon College
Paignton
Devon, UK

Lisa Yates BSc(Hons)
Lecturer in Animal and Horse Care
Environment and Land-based Studies
South Devon College
Paignton
Devon, UK

Foreword

Most people I know or meet have an interest or desire to learn more about animals, their care, their welfare, and their health. I would even say that many of these people are passionate about animal care. And, why not? Animals affect every part of our lives. They provide companionship. Many animal species develop bonds with humans and vice-versa. The human-animal bond with companion animals like dogs, cats, and horses can positively affect our health, and emotional wellbeing. Livestock provide us with clothing and food. Laboratory animals have given us medicines, surgical procedures and continue to help medical advancement for both humans and other animals. Wildlife are an integral part of our ecosystems and the delicate balance we have with them affects our world. Animals have played a large part in the development of agriculture and transportation. We are affected by animals in every part of our lives, and it is not hard to see why people need to care for their health and welfare.

With animals playing such a large part in our lives it makes sense that people would want to learn more about animal health and welfare. I have spent over three decades learning about and caring for animals. I still continue to learn and search for material that is concise, accurate, and easy to reference. That is why I like this book. *The Complete Textbook of Animal Health and Welfare* is a comprehensive resource with a logical progression chapter by chapter. It is formatted so that specific topics can be easily found. While no one book can tackle all species and their care *The Complete Textbook of Animal Health and Welfare* does a remarkable job. For people who work with animals and those who want to learn more about animal health and welfare this book is a concise, accurate and comprehensive resource.

You would be hard-pressed to find an animal care topic not covered in this book. It includes detailed coverage of a wide array of animal care topics. Animal science or biology students might particularly find interesting sections on anatomy and physiology, research methods, nutrition, husbandry and ecology. A veterinary or veterinary technician student might find particularly interesting sections on pharmacology, fluid therapy, radiology, anaesthesia, first aid and animal diseases. Animal breeders might find interesting sections on genetics and behaviour. Others, such as groomers, researchers and wildlife rehabilitators will also find this book invaluable. Animal enthusiasts of all kinds will find new knowledge in sections that cover cutting-edge and complementary therapies. Do you know what chickweed is used for? As you read *The Complete Textbook of Animal Health and Welfare* you will learn fun facts that you didn't know. Do you know about illegal cricket fighting? Do you know what lamppost disease is? If not, they can be found in this book.

As a veterinarian and a veterinary technician educator I particularly like how easy it is for me to find what I am looking for in this book. The format is consistent throughout each chapter. Even though different experts have written different parts of this book it reads as if one person wrote the entire thing. Take, for example, chapter 9: I particularly like the logical progression from choosing a pet to keeping it healthy from infectious disease. I think one of the most difficult things to learn when it comes to animal care is about all the infectious diseases. This book does a great job of concisely covering most of the prominent infectious diseases, and it does so for many different species. For each infectious disease we can easily find what the cause is, what the pathogenesis is, what the relevant clinical signs are, what treatment includes and how to prevent the disease. I don't know of any other source that does it so well because it is concise, consistent, and covers so much. This is one reason this book is truly 'Complete'.

Being 'Complete' is a hard thing to live up to in any field. However, in the animal kingdom it can be especially hard because of all its diversity. The editor and authors of *The Complete Textbook of Animal Health and Welfare* have done an admirable job of living up to a 'Complete' book. This book covers topics on dogs, cats, horses, livestock, birds, reptiles, fish, exotic animals and even more, such as marine mammals. Take a look at the table of contents and you will see a 'Complete' list of animal health and welfare topics. Select and turn to a chapter that interests you. Take a look at the chapter contents that are highlighted at the start of each chapter. I think that those of us who are passionate about animal care will find a lot in this book that will expand our knowledge.

So whether you select and read your favourite chapter, search and locate a particular topic, or read the book cover to cover, I think you will agree that *The Complete Textbook of Animal Health and Welfare* is a concise, accurate, and comprehensive resource for those who have an interest or desire to learn more about animal care.

Dr. R. Scott Keller DVM
Coordinator of Veterinary Medical Technology, Joliet Junior College, Joliet, Illinois USA
2009

Preface

The original idea for this text was formulated as a result of my own teaching practice as I continually observed animal care, animal management and animal science students struggle to find a book which encompassed the range of disciplines that mirrored their programmes of study.

The modern animal professional must obtain a varied knowledge base, including anatomy and physiology, husbandry and management, veterinary knowledge and much more. This text aims to be a starting point for the undergraduate or college student, providing core knowledge.

I have used a range of awarding body syllabi to plan the contents and have been fortunate that a variety of educational and vocational experts have contributed to the text. I am extremely grateful for the work they have put into their chapters.

My aim was to produce a modern text that provides clear information on all aspects of animal health and welfare for companion, farm and zoo animals. I hope this has been achieved and you, the reader, will gain an insight and apply the principles discussed to promote good practice in all aspects of animal management.

Jane Williams
April 2008

Acknowledgements

I would like to thank all the contributors for their dedication to the production of this work, despite busy workloads and I would also like to thank their friends and family for their patience during this venture.

I also wish to acknowledge the contribution of South Devon College, Hartpury College, Hartpury Equine Therapy Centre and Paignton Zoo, which allowed free access to their facilities and graciously permitted me to reproduce photographs within the text. Equally I must thank the team at Elsevier, particularly Joyce Rodenhuis, Robert Edwards, Sally Davies and Louisa Welch, who have proved a great help during this, my first publication.

Finally I would like to dedicate this book to the two- and four-legged friends who maintain my sanity: Abbey and Harvey were an inspiration whilst Phoebe, Tilly, Ellie, H, Kubu, Kavangy and Stan have been willing photographic models, providing many amusing moments during the process! My husband, Karl, has been thoroughly supportive during my neglect and kept me fed and watered, walked the dogs and helped with the horses – all of which I am more than grateful for. My mum and dad always had an encouraging word when I became frustrated and I will be eternally grateful to my Uncle Stanley who first instilled a passion in me for all things animal and pointed me down this path – thank you all.

Chapter | **1** | *Jane Williams*

Introduction to the animal body

This chapter introduces the chemical composition of the body and the distribution of body water and discusses cytology and the processes of cell division – mitosis and meiosis. The types of body tissues are identified and their main properties stated.

BODY CHEMISTRY

The mammalian body is a complex unit comprising billions of cells structured into tissue types which combine to form organ systems, all working together to maintain life. The body is made up of organic (carbon-based molecules) and inorganic materials.

Inorganic content of the body

Water and minerals make up the inorganic content of the body. Minerals include:

- Calcium
- Phosphorus
- Iron
- Copper
- Manganese
- Iodine.

These minerals do not exist in the body in their pure form but are present as ions. Ions are positively or negatively charged particles that may be made up of one element or of two or more in combination. For example,

- H^+ is a hydrogen ion
- OH^- is a hydroxide ion.

An electrolyte is a substance that will split up into ions when it is dissolved in water. For example, sodium chloride (salt) will split into Na^+ and Cl^- ions.

- Ions that carry one or more positive charges are called *cations*
- Ions that carry one or more negative charges are called *anions*.

The most important inorganic substances are:

- Water
- Minerals:
  - Calcium
  - Phosphorus
  - Magnesium.

These minerals are stored in the body within the bones and the teeth, giving rigidity and structure. They are also essential for muscle and nerve function and play a part in blood clotting and lactation. It is important that the correct amount of these minerals is present in the body. It is also important that certain of these minerals, e.g. phosphorus and calcium, are present in the correct proportion to each other. Sodium, potassium and calcium are important in the regulation of fluid balance within the body between intracellular and extracellular fluid. Iron and copper are found in all tissues and have an important role in haemoglobin production (oxygen transport around the body).

Body water content and distribution

Approximately 60–70% of the body's weight is water. This water can be divided into two types:

1. Extracellular fluid: all body fluid outside the cells: 20% of body weight
2. Intracellular fluid: all fluid inside cells: 40% or body weight.

Extracellular fluid can be divided into:

- Plasma – fluid part of the blood
- Interstitial – surrounds the cells of the body outside the blood vascular system
- Cerebrospinal fluid
- Lymph.

In extracellular fluid, the main cation is sodium and the main anion is chloride. The main functions of extracellular fluid are to bathe the cells and to provide a medium for molecules to be transported in and out of cells.

In intracellular fluid the main cation is potassium; intracellular fluid is found within the cells but its function is also to facilitate transportation of molecules in and out of the cell.

Acidity and alkalinity

The body needs to maintain the correct degree of acidity and alkalinity. An acid is a substance that liberates hydrogen ions in solution. An alkali or base is a substance that accepts hydrogen ions. For example, $HCO_3 \rightarrow H^+ + HCO^{3-}$. This means that carbonic acid (H_2CO_3) in solution gives hydrogen ions and bicarbonate ions. Carbonic acid is an acid because it gives up or produces a hydrogen ion in solution. The bicarbonate ion is an alkali or base because if the chemical reaction is reversed, the bicarbonate ion will accept the hydrogen ion to form carbonic acid.

The acidity of a solution is measured by its hydrogen ion concentration ranging from 1 to 14 on the pH scale. As pH value decreases acidity increases, 7 is neutral pH, and as pH value increases alkalinity increases. Body fluids are at a pH of 7.35 and it is important that this level is maintained.

Homeostasis is the process by which the body regulates the acid–base balance, temperature control and fluid balance.

Organic compounds of the body

These are chemicals that are built on a carbon molecule base. There are three important types of organic body components:

1. Amino acids and proteins
2. Sugars and carbohydrates
3. Fatty acids and glycerol (lipids).

Amino acids and proteins

- Amino acids are the building blocks of proteins
- Two amino acids join to form a dipeptide link
- Lots of amino acids join to form a polypeptide link
- Several hundred amino acids join to form a protein
- Polymerisation is the process of joining simple units together
- Amino acids contain carbon, hydrogen, oxygen and nitrogen
- They can also contain sulphur and amino acids
- There are 20 amino acids.

Proteins in the body are either:

- Structural – collagen or keratin
- Functional – enzymes or hormones.

Dietary proteins need to be broken down to amino acids before they can be absorbed by the body.

Sugars and carbohydrates

- Sugar and carbohydrates are made of carbon, hydrogen and oxygen
- They comprise different types of simple sugars to complex sugars
- Simple sugars join to form chains of polysaccharides or carbohydrates
- They are an energy source
- They can be stored as glycogen (in liver)
- Dietary carbohydrates need to be broken down to simple sugars before they can be absorbed by the body.

Fatty acids and glycerol (lipids)

- Fatty acids and glycerol are made of carbon, hydrogen and oxygen
- Lipids form cell membranes and steroids, insulate nerves and act as a food store and body insulation
- Lipids need to be broken down to fatty acids and glycerol to be utilised by the body.

Enzymes

- Enzymes are organic catalysts
- A catalyst is a substance that speeds up a chemical reaction without altering itself
- They are involved in chemical reactions throughout the body, e.g. food breakdown, cell reactions, oxygen transport.

CYTOLOGY

The study of cells is known as cytology. All living organisms are made up of cells: some consist of one cell whereas others consist of billions. The cell is the smallest unit of living material capable of carrying out all the activities required for life.

Cell theory

Cell theory puts forward the idea that cells are the fundamental units of life and that new cells are formed only by the division of pre-existing cells. In 1838 and 1839, two German scientists, Matthias Schlieden and Theodor Schwann, voiced the opinion that plants and animals are composed of groups of cells and that the cell is the basic unit of life. This was expanded in 1855 by Rudolph Virchow, who stated that new cells are formed by the division of previously existing cells.

Cells are studied using microscopes. There are two types: light and electron microscopes. Using a light microscope in stained tissues, cell organelles can be viewed, with the exception of the endoplasmic reticulum, which must be viewed using an electron microscope.

Cell structure

Prokaryotic cells (pro – before, karyo – nucleus)

- Prokaryotic cells were probably the first form of life on earth
- Their DNA is not surrounded by a nuclear membrane
- They contain *no* membrane-bound organelles
- There are only two types: bacteria and blue-green algae
- They can have cell walls
- The cell membrane can become invaginated (folded in on itself) to form a sac in which metabolic processes occur.

Eukaryotic cells (eu – true, karyo – nucleus)

- Eukaryotic cells evolved many years after prokaryotes
- There are lots of differences between prokaryotes and eukaryotes
- Eukaryotic cells have membrane-bound organelles within the outer plasma membrane of the cell
- They are generally larger than prokaryotic cells.

Membrane-bound organelles can be an advantage because:

- They increase the proportion of cell membrane area to cell volume: the presence of organelle membranes gives a greater surface area for metabolic processes to take place
- The rate of a metabolic pathway can be controlled inside membrane-bound organelle by regulating the rate at which the first reactant is allowed to enter the cell through the organelle membrane
- If the enzymes for one metabolic reaction are together within an organelle, their close proximity to each other will increase the metabolic rate
- Harmful reactants/enzymes can be isolated inside an organelle, preventing damage to the rest of the cell.

There are two main types of eukaryotic cells: plant and animal cells.

Inside the eukaryotic cell

Cytoplasm

- Cytoplasm is the fluid component of cell
- It can be a solution or colloidal suspension of vital suspension
- It contains protein, salts, glucose, nucleus and organelles
- Metabolic processes can occur due to the presence of cytoplasm
- Cytoplasm is able to flow: this is known as cytoplasmic streaming – a wave-like motion allowing movement within the cell
- Cell organelles are suspended within the cytoplasm.

Cell membrane

- Cell membrane acts as a boundary between the cell and its environment
- It surrounds the entire cell
- It is selectively permeable, i.e. it has the ability to 'choose' which molecules are allowed in and out
- Selective permeability:
  - allows small molecules to enter the cell
  - prevents large molecules entering the cell
  - provides the hydrophobic inner core to prevent ionic transfer

- It is constructed of a double phospholipid layer interspersed with protein molecules
- Structures in the membrane are able to move, hence the name 'fluid mosaic model' – the lipid and protein molecules effectively float in a fluid base with some protein molecules anchoring the membrane to the cytoskeleton:
  ○ The membrane has the same consistency as salad oil
  ○ It allows active transport of materials into the cell
  ○ The embedded protein molecules give support, allow individual cells to be recognised as targets for chemical reactions, e.g. hormone action, and play a role in active transport
- Two types of proteins are found in the cell membrane:
  ○ Integral proteins are located through the entire width of the membrane
  ○ Peripheral proteins are only loosely bound to the membrane surface.

Functions of the cell membrane include:

- Transport:
  ○ Active transport
  ○ Diffusion
  ○ Osmosis
  ○ Passive transport
  ○ Endocytosis and exocytosis
- Enzymatic activity: recognition of 'key and lock' mechanisms for specific chemical reactions
- Signal transduction: recognition of a specific molecule entering the cell, which activates transducer molecules which in turn trigger the next stage of a chemical reaction, e.g. glycogen to glucose
- Intercellular joining: two cells that join together, e.g. cell and antibody
- Cell-to-cell recognition: recognition of the target cell by another
- Point of attachment for the cytoskeleton and cellular matrix.

Nucleus

- This can be thought of as the 'brain' of the cell
- It is usually spherical or oval in shape
- It is often the largest structure in the cell (approximately 5 μm wide)
- It is located near the centre of the cell
- It controls the cell's activity and stores the hereditary material or deoxyribonucleic acid (DNA) in chromosomes
- It is bound by a nuclear envelope – a double membrane containing large pores to allow molecules to pass between the nucleus and the cytoplasm, e.g. ribonucleic acid (RNA), in cell division.

Nucleoplasm

- The nucleoplasm is the cytoplasm component of the nucleus
- Nucleoplasm contains strands of chromatin organised into the chromosomes, which have a role in cell division.

Nucleolus

- The nucleolus is a dark body within the nucleus: it is thought to manufacture ribosomal RNA
- Nuclear DNA makes up genes which carry the chemically coded instructions for protein synthesis
- Messenger RNA molecules pass from the nucleus into the cytoplasm and to the ribosomes to stimulate the production of proteins in the cell
- The genome is the sum of a cell's genetic material.

Centrosome

- The centrosome lies near the nucleus within the cytoplasm
- It consists of two centrioles
- It has a role in cell division during the formation of the spindle apparatus.

Mitochondria (plural)

- These are considered to be the 'powerhouses' of the cell
- They range in shape from spherical to highly elongated and range in size from 1 to 10 μm
- They are sites of chemical reactions to convert food substances to stored energy in the cell
- The mitochondrion is bound by a double membrane
- The inner membrane is folded repeatedly into projections called cristae which increase the surface area in which reactions can take place
- The outer membrane acts like a sieve and allows small molecules to pass through to the inside
- The inner membrane is 'tight' and contains enzymes and protein molecules which are required to convert food products into energy (adenosine diphosphate (ADP) is converted to adenosine triphosphate (ATP)).

Ribosomes

- These are sites of protein synthesis in the cell
- They present as free ribosomes in the cytoplasm
- Bound ribosomes are also found attached to the rough endoplasmic reticulum.

Endoplasmic reticulum

- This comprises a network of fine channels running throughout the cytoplasm

- There are two distinct but connected types – rough and smooth endoplasmic reticulum.

Smooth endoplasmic reticulum

- Smooth endoplasmic reticulum contains no ribosomes (hence its name)
- It is a site of lipid synthesis
- It is a site of carbohydrate metabolism
- It is a site of detoxification of certain drugs and poisons.

Rough endoplasmic reticulum

- This form has ribosomes attached or embedded on to it
- These provide sites of protein synthesis
- It plays a role in protein transportation in the cell
- Proteins synthesised by rough endoplasmic reticulum are sent to the Golgi body in small vesicles formed from the invaginations of the endoplasmic reticulum membrane.

Golgi body (Golgi apparatus)

- This can be considered as a protein-packaging and processing plant
- Proteins produced by rough endoplasmic reticulum are modified, stored and dispatched by Golgi apparatus
- It is formed of stacks of flattened membrane sacs or vesicles.

Lysosomes

- These are sacs containing digestive enzymes surrounded by a membrane to prevent leakage into the cytoplasm
- Around 40 different types of enzymes have been identified
- Lysosomes digest fats, proteins and carbohydrates
- The enzymes originate from the Golgi apparatus, where they are identified and packaged to lysosomes by unique carbohydrate signals attached to proteins
- Lysosomes can break down cell organelles in times of deficiency to utilise energy to preserve the cell
- They also digest foreign antigens (proteins) that enter the cell by fusing with the vesicle in which the antigen is contained or encompassing the antigen within itself
- If the cell dies, the lysosome initiates a self-destruct mechanism for the cell, the membrane breaks down and the enzymes contained within the lysosome are released to digest the cell. This is known as autolysis.

Vacuoles and vesicles

- These are membrane-surrounded sacs within the cell
- Vacuoles are larger than vesicles
- They act as storage sites
- Protozoa can have projectile vacuoles which remove excess water from the cell like a pump.

Cytoskeleton

- Cells from different animal tissues have vastly different sizes and shapes
- Cell shape and size are determined by the cell's cytoskeleton
- The cytoskeleton is a highly dynamic and constantly changing framework of protein filaments that form an invisible tubular skeleton within the cytoplasm.

CELL TRANSPORT

Cells exchange various materials by a number of chemical processes. These include:

- Active transport
- Diffusion
- Osmosis
- Endocytosis
- Exocytosis.

Active transport

Active transport involves the movement of molecules into the cell against a concentration gradient, i.e. from an area of low concentration to an area of high concentration. This often occurs because, although the substance is present in a higher concentration inside the cytoplasm. the cell still requires more of it. Active transport requires energy from the cell to complete the process. Cells can use electrical potential derived from the high concentration of ions in their proximity. Active transport is achieved by utilising *protein pumps*. Protein pumps are present in the plasma membrane and draw molecules into the cell using the energy from ATP. One example is the sodium/potassium pump. A receptor molecule binds with sodium ion and changes its form to enable it to pass through the phospholipid membrane. Once on the inner surface of the membrane the combined ion/receptor reverses this process to release the sodium ion into the cell. It is these chemical reactions that use the energy.

Diffusion

Diffusion (Box 1.1) occurs in areas of the body where there are gaseous concentration gradients, e.g. alveoli in the lungs and blood capillaries. In the lungs, when an animal breathes in there will be high concentrations of

DEFINITIONS

Diffusion

Movement of molecules from an area of high concentration to an area of low concentration such that eventually the molecules are evenly distributed, i.e. both molecules are in equilibrium

Osmosis

Movement of solvent molecules from an area of high concentration to an area of low concentration through a selectively (or semi-) permeable membrane until evenly distributed

oxygen molecules in the alveoli whilst in the blood capillaries surrounding them there will a low concentration of oxygen. The oxygen molecules will attempt to achieve 50% quantity in the alveoli and 50% quantity in the capillaries, therefore there will be movement of oxygen molecules from the lungs to the blood capillaries.

Diffusion is an example of a passive transport method as no energy is expended by the cells to facilitate movement of the gases.

Osmosis

- A solvent is the liquid component of a solution
- A solute is the solid component of a solution
- Osmosis is the movement of water molecules through a semipermeable membrane to an area of low concentration from an area of higher concentration (Box 1.1)
- Osmotic potential is a measure of the pressure required to stem the flow of water across the membrane and which can be measured.

Osmotic potential within the body is described relative to plasma. A high osmotic potential will result in quick movement of the molecules and conversely a low osmotic potential will have a slower transfer rate.

Isotonic solutions

An isotonic solution is a solution which is in equilibrium with plasma, i.e. the concentration of solutes in the cell is equal to the concentration of solutes outside the cell.

Hypertonic solution

A hypertonic solution has a higher concentration of solute than plasma, i.e. there is a higher concentration

DEFINITIONS

Allele

Differing form of the same gene, e.g. gene for hair colour: allele for black hair and allele for red hair

Chromosome

Structures in the cell nucleus containing long molecules of DNA (genetic material)

Chromosome number

The number of chromosomes within the nucleus. It is unique to each species

Deoxyribonucleic acid (DNA)

Genetic material, blueprint of characteristics

Diploid number

Normal chromosome number of a somatic cell

Gene

Unit of hereditary material, located on the chromosomes

Haploid number

Half the number of chromosomes of a somatic (diploid) cell

Locus (plural: loci)

Area or point upon the chromosome where the gene/allele is located

Zygote

Fertilised ovum

of solutes outside the cell and a lower concentration of solutes within the cell. Therefore water molecules would be drawn out of the cell.

Hypotonic solution

A hypotonic solution has a lower concentration of solutes than plasma. The concentration of solutes inside the cell is higher than in its environment, therefore water is drawn into the cell.

Exocytosis

This is a process by which the cell ejects waste products or secretions. A vesicle or vacuole fuses with the plasma membrane and opens on the external surface of the membrane, releasing its contents into the external environment.

Endocytosis

This is a process by which materials are taken into the cell. There are several types of endocytosis.

Phagocytosis

- The cell engulfs or ingests material
- The cell membrane forms pseudopodia or false feet which extend around a pathogen or antigen
- These eventually encompass the foreign material and fuse with each other. The inner membrane surrounding the object becomes a vesicle or vacuole containing the material
- A lysosome will fuse with this vesicle and digest the membrane to allow the digestive enzymes access to the antigen or pathogen, which they will destroy
- Macrophages and neutrophils are examples of phagocytic cells.

Pinocytosis

- This is a similar process to phagocytosis but involves the intake of liquid, not solid, materials and can be known as cell drinking
- Tiny droplets of fluid are tapped within folds of the plasma membrane, pinched into a vacuole in the cytoplasm and slowly transferred into the cell.

Receptor-mediated endocytosis

- This is another method of protein intake into the cytoplasm
- It depends on the interaction of that molecule with a specific binding protein in the cell membrane, called a receptor.

CELL DIVISION

Cells replicate in two ways – mitosis and meiosis. It is important in mitotic cell replication that the genetic material is copied exactly, otherwise the new cell would not have the same characteristics. In meiosis the genetic information is not copied exactly, which gives rise to genetic variation (allowing evolution to occur).

Mitosis

- Process of cell replication in the body, except for in the sex cells or gametes
- There are five stages but only four stages show activity in the cell.

The stages are:

1. Interphase (resting)
2. Prophase
3. Metaphase
4. Anaphase
5. Telophase.

Helpful hint!

To remember the stages of mitosis remember:
    I P M A T
    Figure 1.1 shows an overview of stage duration during mitosis and Figure 1.2 shows the stages of mitosis.

Interphase

- Interphase is the resting phase
- No chromosomes are visible as chromatin is dispersed throughout the nucleus
- Near the end in interphase the chromatin organises and begins to become visible under the light microscope.

Prophase

- Prophase is the beginning of division – it is the longest of the active stages
- Nuclear membrane breaks down and the nucleolus disappears
- Chromatin contracts so chromosomes appear separate and they become visible as long threads

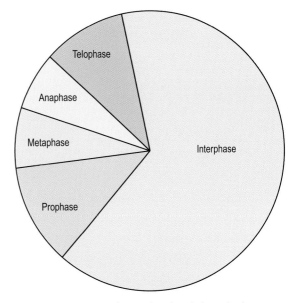

Figure 1.1 Overview of stage duration during mitosis.

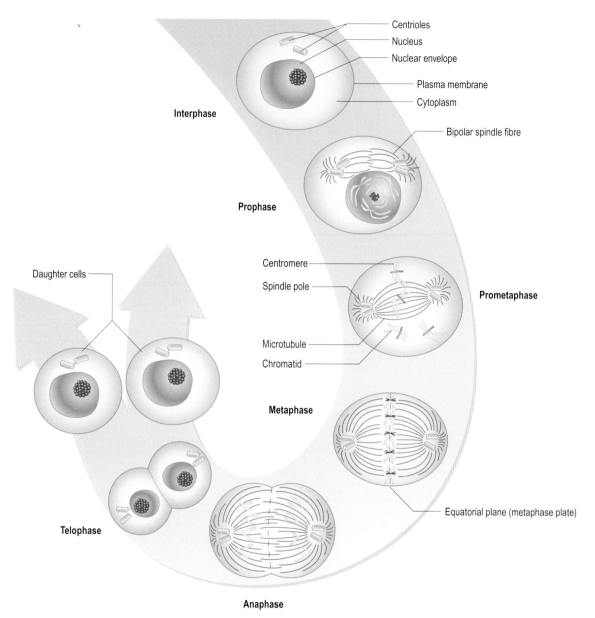

Figure 1.2 Mitosis. (Reproduced from Aspinall V 2006 *The Complete Textbook of Veterinary Nursing*. Butterworth Heinemann, London, with permission.)

- Chromosomes then start to coil and become shorter and thicker
- Centrioles divide and move to the opposite poles (ends) of the cell
- Protein microtubules develop from each centriole, to become spindle fibres
- Chromosomes are copied
- Copied chromosomes are joined to originals at the centromere and called chromotids.

Metaphase

- This is the shortest of the active phases
- The chromatids line up in the middle of the cell along the equator
- Chromatids repel each other and attach to spindle fibres via the centromere
- You should be able to see the chromatids under the light microscope.

Anaphase

- Chromatids are attached to the cell spindle fibres and the centromeres divide
- Free chromatids move to the poles, centromere first
- The spindle apparatus contracts, pulling the chromatids apart and towards the different poles (ends) of the cell.

Telophase

- This is the reverse of the prophase
- Chromatids at the poles are now regarded as chromosomes
- New nuclear membranes start to form around the chromosomes at each pole of the cell
- Nucleolus reappears and the chromosomes uncoil to diffuse chromatin, i.e. the chromatin disorganises (becomes invisible again)
- The cytoplasm divides, in a process called cytokinesis
- This results in two identical daughter cells
- Daughter cells have the same number of chromosomes as the original 'normal' cell, therefore the daughter cells are *diploid* cells.

Areas of the body where mitosis occurs

- All dividing cells, except for the gametes
- Particularly in the intestine, lungs and areas of wear and tear to replace damaged cells.

Meiosis

Meiosis is the process of cell division that occurs within the gametes (Figure 1.3). Meiosis involves two divisions of the cell, in contrast to the singular division during mitosis. Meiosis is a longer and more complicated process than mitosis, and results in four daughter cells which have a haploid chromosome number, i.e. they contain one-half the normal chromosome number of somatic cells. This is because during fertilisation the two gametes (sperm and ovum) will fuse, giving the resulting zygote a diploid or normal chromosome number.

Stages

1. Interphase I
2. Prophase I
3. Metaphase I
4. Anaphase I
5. Telophase I
6. Interphase II (often not noted as very brief)
7. Prophase II
8. Metaphase II
9. Anaphase II
10. Telophase II.

Interphase I

- Interphase I is the resting phase prior to division
- Chromatin organises near to the end.

Prophase I

- Prophase I is the longest active stage
- Nuclear membrane and nucleolus disappear
- Chromosomes contract down by coiling
- Homologous (the same) chromosomes lie side by side
- In each pair of homologous chromosomes, one is bivalent
- In bivalent chromosomes there are four strands, which would be two chromosomes, or eight strands, which would be four chromosomes
- As the chromosomes pair up they become intertwined, shortening and twisting around each other
- As this happens portions of themselves can become exchanged, i.e. genetic material is swapped
- This process is known as crossing over (twisting and turning) and the sites where information is exchanged are called chiasmata
- Crossing over mixes up the genetic material, giving rise to new characteristics
- The homologous chromosomes then pull apart.

Metaphase I

- Homologous chromosomes line up down the centre of the cell at the equator
- Then they attach to the spindle fibres.

Anaphase I

- The spindle fibres contract and begin to separate the homologous chromosomes
- When the homologous chromosomes separate, it is the chromosomes in each bivalent that separate, *not* the chromatids
- The separated chromosomes then move to opposite poles of the cell
- Therefore each pole receives only one of each homologous pair of chromosomes, i.e. a haploid number of chromosomes.

Telophase I

- The cytoplasm begins to divide and the nuclear membrane reforms around each group of haploid chromosomes

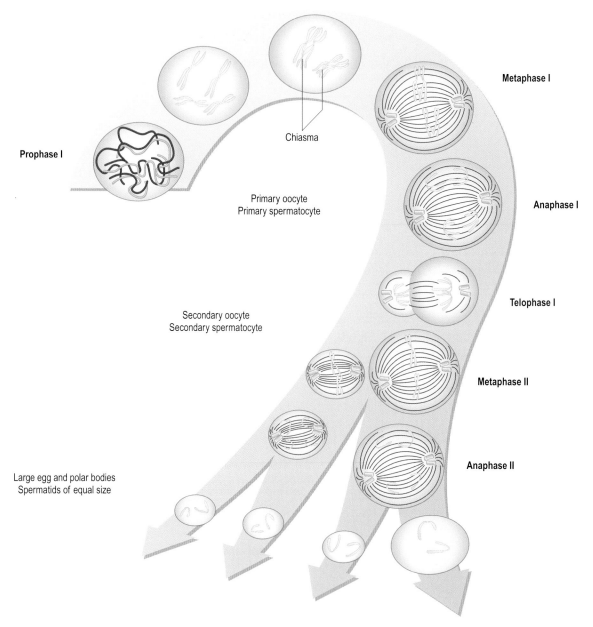

Prophase I

Chiasma

Primary oocyte
Primary spermatocyte

Metaphase I

Anaphase I

Telophase I

Secondary oocyte
Secondary spermatocyte

Metaphase II

Anaphase II

Large egg and polar bodies
Spermatids of equal size

Figure 1.3 Meiosis. (Reproduced from Aspinall V 2006 *The Complete Textbook of Veterinary Nursing*. Butterworth Heinemann, London, with permission.)

- Cytokinesis can occur, resulting in two haploid cells, or the cell can remain fused in a dumbbell shape
- The cell or cells now undergo the second division immediately.

Second meiotic division

Interphase II

- This phase is virtually non-existent as the second active stage of division occurs immediately.

Prophase II

- The chromosomes are already contracted
- Chromosomes are replicated
- New spindle fibres form at 90° to the old spindle apparatus.

Metaphase II

- The chromosomes line up in the middle of the cell
- Chromosomes attach to the new spindle apparatus by the centromere
- Chromatids repel each other and start to pull apart.

Anaphase II

- The centromeres divide and the spindle fibres contract
- Chromatids pull apart fully and move to the opposite poles of the cell.

Telophase II

- At the poles, chromatids lengthen and become indistinct
- The spindle fibres disappear
- The nuclear membrane reforms
- Cytokinesis occurs
- The result is four daughter cells which have a haploid number of chromosomes. Each will have a different genetic make-up.

Meiosis

The first meiotic division results in two haploid cells. The second meiotic division results in two haploid cells divided by mitosis, resulting in four haploid cells. Genetic variation occurs because of:

- Random segregation of homologous chromosomes as they line up (chance). If you consider two pairs, one pair of red and one pair of blue chromosomes, you could get:

R	B
R	B
R	B
B	R

- Therefore from two pairs you get 2^2 chances, i.e. four options. If an animal has 23 pairs of chromosomes (as do humans), you get $2^{23} = 8\,000\,000$ options!
- Crossing over – cutting and pasting of genetic material give rise to new combinations and increase variation.

Meiosis occurs in the:

- Ovary of the female – ovum
- Spermatogenic cells of the testes on the male – spermatozoa.

BODY TISSUES

Figure 1.4 shows the structure of the body.

Tissues have many different structures, which are held together by extracellular matrices. There are four main tissue groups:

1. Epithelial (epithelium)
2. Connective
3. Muscular.
4. Nervous

Epithelia (epithelium)

- Diverse tissue types form this group
- Each type of epithelium is embedded on to a basement membrane
- Epithelium is lining tissue for both internal and external body surfaces
- It lines body cavities, tubes and surfaces
- It can act as a biological interface for reactions
- It allows absorption, e.g. diffusion, osmosis (in simple epithelial tissue)
- It acts as protection in areas of wear and tear (in multilayered epithelial tissue).

Types of epithelia

Epithelia can be classified by the amount of cell layers:

- Simple: one cell thick
- Stratified (compound): two or more layers thick.

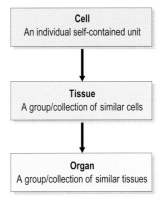

Figure 1.4 Structure of the body.

It is also classified by cell shape when it is taken in section perpendicularly, as different types have different shapes. Where the epithelium is present in many layers, i.e. stratified, the top layer is examined to provide the classification according to shape.

Epithelial tissue can also be classified according to specialisation, as some epithelial tissues are specialised for a particular function (Figure 1.5).

Therefore an overall description would be:

- Number of cell layers + description of cell shape + any specialisation.

Simple epithelium

- Surface epithelium is only a single cell or layer thick
- Its function is absorption or secretion
- It is found lining tracts, organs and tubes
- It provides little protection
- It may have surface specialisation present.

Simple squamous epithelium

- One cell layer thick
- It looks like flattened cells, giving a 'pavement' effect
- It is very thin, making it ideal for absorption to occur via diffusion
- It is found lining blood vessels, alveoli and body cavities.

Simple cuboidal epithelium

- One cell layer thick
- Cuboid in shape
- It possesses ideal properties to facilitate secretion and absorption functions
- The increased width of the tissue offers slightly more protection than simple squamous epithelium
- It is found lining the renal tubule.

Simple columnar

- One cell layer thick
- Column-like or elongated in shape
- Its shape provides protection for the areas it lines and it often has a secretion function
- It is found lining the gastrointestinal tract and the respiratory tract.

Ciliated columnar epithelium

- It is found in the respiratory tract
- Air current produced by cilia moves dust from the lungs
- It is interspersed with specialised unicellular glands called goblet cells which produce mucus.

Stratified squamous

- More than one layer thick, and provides protection
- It is found in areas subject to friction and wear and tear

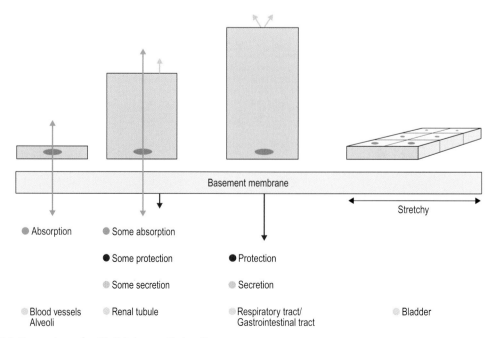

Figure 1.5 Comparison of epithelial shape with function.

- The top layers lose their cellular outline: these layers will be sacrificed to give protection
- It may be keratinised to provide extra toughness, e.g. in the epidermis
- It is found in the epidermis, lining the vagina and the rectum
- Stratified epithelium function is protection and it is usually squamous in shape at the top layer but cuboidal in shape above the basement membrane
- It can be moderately permeable to water and small molecules.

Transitional epithelium

- This is elastic and therefore very stretchy
- It returns to its original shape after stretching
- It provides protection by allowing stretching
- It is found lining the bladder and in the uterus.

Glands

These are specialised epithelial structures. Glands can be unicellular or multicellular.

Unicellular glands

- These are found in epithelial linings, e.g. goblet cells, in digestive tract
- Unicellular glands are modified epithelial cells.

Multicellular glands

- These are also of epithelial origin
- They lie within layers of epithelial tissue
- They have ducts connecting them to the epithelial surface
- Multicellular glands are classified according to their shape:
  ○ Tubular
  ○ Alveolar or saccular
  ○ Coiled
- And on how many shapes are present:
  ○ Simple: only one
  ○ Compound: more than one.

Glands are also split into two groups according to where their secretions are released (see Chapter 7, Figure 7.3).

Connective tissue

The connective tissue provides structural and metabolic support for tissues and organs. Connective tissue is made of cells embedded in a matrix or around a substance which holds them in place.

Types

- Loose connective tissue or areolar tissue
- Fibrous or dense connective tissue

- Cartilage – hyaline/elastic/fibrous
- Blood – erythrocytes/leukocytes/thrombocytes/plasma
- Bone – compact/spongy or cancellous.

Loose connective or areolar tissue

- This forms a layer between the skin and the tissues beneath
- It supports the viscera
- It consists of a loose network of collagen fibres (tough and not stretchy) and elastic fibres
- It contains fibroblasts, cells which produce collagen fibres, and fat cells
- The tissue has its own blood and nerve supply
- An example of loose connective tissue is the omentum found in the abdominal cavity
- Another example is adipose tissue. Adipose tissue is a specialised form of loose connective tissue where gaps in the matrix are filled up with an excess of fat cells
- Adipose tissue can be white or brown:
  ○ White adipose tissue is stored fat, and therefore provides an energy source plus protection plus insulation
  ○ Brown adipose tissue plays a role in the thermoregulation of neonates.

Fibrous or dense connective tissue

- As the name suggests, this is a dense material packed full of collagen fibres and forming a dense matrix
- It comprises collagen fibre bundles with fibroblasts in between
- It is strong and non-elastic
- The fibres can be arranged in parallel to increase strength
- It is found in tendons and joins muscle to bone
- It is found in ligaments and joins bone to bone
- It is found in muscle fascia, making up the outer layer or jacket of the muscle.

Figure 1.6 illustrates loose connective tissue and dense connective tissue.

Cartilage

- This is a tough substance which is a blue-white colour
- It is produced by cells called chondrocytes
- It has no blood supply, therefore is covered in a fibrous lining, the perichondrium, which is vascular
- There are three types of cartilage:
  1. Hyaline cartilage
  2. Elastic cartilage
  3. Fibrous or fibrocartilage

Loose connective tissue

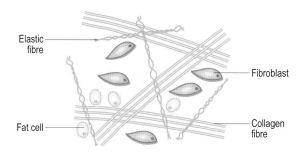

- Between skin/tissues
- Support viscera

Dense connective tissue

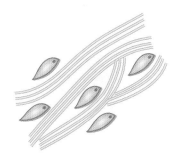

- Dense collagen fibres ➡ non-elastic and strong
- Fibre bundles in parallel ⬆strength
- Found: tendons
  ligaments
  muscle fascia

(B)

Adipose tissue

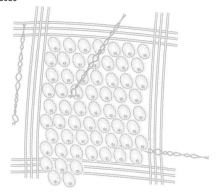

- Specialised loose connective tissue

White ➡ storage/energy/insulation/protection

Brown ➡ thermoregulation in neonates

(A)

Figure 1.6 (a) Loose connective tissue. (b) Dense connective tissue.

Hyaline cartilage

- This is the most common form of cartilage
- It is found in joints, covering the articular surfaces of bones
- It is a very smooth substance which aids in the reduction of frictional forces
- It is also found in the nasal septum, the larynx, the tracheal rings and the sternal ends of the ribs.

Elastic cartilage

- Elastic fibres are added to the hyaline matrix to form elastic cartilage
- This gives elastic cartilage the ability to bend and return to its original shape
- These fibres give flexibility but reduce the strength of the material
- It is found in the pinna, epiglottis, laryngeal cartilage and walls of the eustachian tube.

Fibrous cartilage

- Lots of collagen fibres are added to hyaline matrix to form fibrous cartilage
- These fibres give added strength but with no or little flexibility
- It is found in the intervertebral discs, pubis symphysis, joint capsules and connecting ligaments/tendons.

Blood

Blood consists of erythrocytes, leukocytes, thrombocytes and plasma. It has a normal pH of 7.35, making it slightly alkaline, and an animal's blood volume comprises approximately 7% of an animal's total body weight. The functions of blood are varied and include:

- Transportation of oxygen and carbon dioxide
- Transportation of nutrients
- Transportation of water
- Transportation of waste
- Homeostasis: thermoregulation + pH acid–base balance
- Clotting
- Transportation of hormones/enzymes
- Protection via the immune system.

Erythrocytes

- Red blood cells
- Biconcave discs that have no nucleus in mammals (nuclei are present in the erythrocytes of birds, reptiles and fish)
- They contain haemoglobin for oxygen transportation
- Average lifespan 120 days
- Produced in erythropoietic tissue – in the spleen and liver before birth then in the bone marrow afterwards
- Destroyed by the spleen.

Leukocytes

- White blood cells
- Two types: granular and agranular
- Granular: granulocytes have granules present in cytoplasm:
  - Neutrophils – phagocytic action
  - Basophils – increased numbers seen in allergies
  - Eosinophils – increased numbers seen with parasitic burdens
- Agranular: no granules in cytoplasm:
  - Lymphocytes: T and B lymphocytes have a role in immunity
  - Monocytes: phagocytic, mature into large cells called macrophages which can move between tissues 'eating' bacteria and debris.

Thrombocytes

- Commonly known as platelets
- Role in haemostasis (blood clotting).

Plasma

- Liquid component of blood
- Straw-coloured
- If clotting factors are removed, plasma is classified as serum
- Plasma consists of:
  - Water
  - Minerals
  - Plasma proteins
  - Nutrients
  - Gases in solution
  - Urea and creatinine
  - Hormones, enzymes
  - Antibodies and antitoxins.

Bone

There are two types of bone – spongy or cancellous bone and compact bone. Bone is made of:

- Minerals: calcium and phosphorus
- Collagen fibres
- A matrix of mucopolysaccharide polymer
- Osteocytes, bone contained within lacunae
- It is covered by a fibrous membrane – the periosteum.

Compact bone

- Compact bone is a hard white substance
- It contains a series of canals running the length of the bone – these are the Haversian canals
- These are surrounded by layers of bone tissue
- Haversian canals contain the blood supply, nerves and lymph
- They are made of calcium phosphate, collagen fibres, mucopolysaccharide polymer (base material) and osteocytes in the spaces or lacunae
- Osteocytes are bone-producing cells
- Compact bone is found in the outer layer of all bones.

Spongy or cancellous bone

- Haversian canals are spread further apart
- Spaces in between are filled with red bone marrow
- Red bone marrow comprises fat cells and cells that produce blood cells
- It is found in the ends of long bones and the core of short and flat bones

All bones are covered by a tough fibrous membrane called periosteum.

15

Muscular tissue

There are three types of muscle tissue:

1. Skeletal or striated or voluntary muscle (movement is under voluntary control)
2. Smooth or involuntary muscle (movement is *not* under voluntary control, i.e. unconscious)
3. Cardiac muscle.

   Muscular tissue function is to allow movement of the body in conjunction with the skeletal system.
   This is facilitated by the contraction of muscle tissue.
   Muscle tissue is made up of myofibrils.

Skeletal muscle

- This makes up the large muscle masses attached to the bones
- It is under the control of the animal, i.e. under voluntary control
- Skeletal muscle cells have many nuclei and lie parallel in bundles, held together by a fibrous tissue sheath
- The tissue has striations (which give a stripy appearance under the microscope).

Smooth muscle

- This tissue is found all over the body, comprising part of body organs and systems
- It is not under voluntary control, e.g. digestive tract, uterus, blood vessels
- Smooth-muscle cells are spindle-shaped and have less connective tissue than striated muscle.

Cardiac muscle

- This is only found in the walls of the heart
- It is not under voluntary control
- Its cells are short and cylindrical and the tissue does have some striations present.

Nervous tissue

- Nervous tissue is composed of neurons or nerve cells
- Neurons are specialised cells for conducting electrical nerve impulses
- Connective tissue or neuroglia run between them
- Neurons exist in a variety of shapes and sizes
- Synapses are junctions between the neurons which electrical impulses have to cross with the help of neurotransmitters (chemicals)
- Nerve consists of many neurons bound together in a connective tissue sheath
- Nerves can be unipolar, bipolar or multipolar depending upon the number of dendrites and their position in the body.

Bibliography

Aspinall V 2006 The complete textbook of veterinary nursing. Butterworth Heinemann, London

Aspinall V, O'Reilly M 2004 Introduction to veterinary anatomy and physiology. Butterworth Heinemann, Oxford

Campbell N, Reece J, Mitchell L 1999 Biology, 5th edn. Benjamin Cummings, San Francisco

Colville T, Bassett J M 2002 Clinical anatomy and physiology for veterinary technicians. Mosby, St Louis

Dyke K M, Sack W O, Wensing C J G 1996 Text book of veterinary anatomy, 2nd edn. W B Saunders, Philadelphia

Green N P O, Stout G W, Taylor D J 1991 Biological science. Cambridge University Press, Cambridge

Lane D R, Cooper B, Turner L 2007 BSAVA Textbook of Veterinary Nursing. BSAVA, Oxford

Moore M 2000 Manual of veterinary nursing. BSAVA, Oxford

Pratt P W 1998 Principles and practice of veterinary technology. Mosby, Philadelphia

Roberts M B V 1986 Biology: a functional approach. Nelson, Surrey, UK

Simpson G 1994 Practical veterinary nursing, 3rd edn. BSAVA, Oxford

Chapter | 2 |

Jane Williams

Locomotor system

This chapter discusses the development of bone and identifies the bones that comprise the skeleton with discussion of species variation. It also considers the structure of muscles and how these interact with the skeleton to produce movement.

COMPOSITION OF BONE

There are two types of bone tissue – spongy (cancellous) bone and compact bone. The basic structure of both types is similar and they contain the same components:

- A chondrin matrix laid down by chondroblasts
- Organic material
- A mixture of calcium phosphate and calcium carbonate salts (these serve to harden the matrix) embedded within a mucopolysaccharide polymer.

Both types have Haversian systems, which are concentric circles of the bone lamellae layered cylindrically around a Haversian canal. The lamellae are interspersed with osteoblasts in characteristic 'holes' or lacunae. The canal in the centre contains the vascular and nervous supply of the tissue as compact bone is avascular.

Compact bone has tightly packed longitudinal Haversian canals to give strength to the outer cortex as the majority of stress in the long bones where it is found will be placed upon the shaft. Spongy bone is less compacted and softer than compact bone; the Haversian systems are effectively spaced out, giving rise to interconnecting channels known as trabeculae with bone marrow filling the spaces. Bone marrow consists of fat cells and blood cells (erythropoietic tissue). A tough fibrous membrane surrounds the bone cortex to allow attachment of connective tissue, e.g. tendons, ligaments. Compact bone is found in the cortex of long bones and spongy bone is found in the epiphyses of long bones and in flat bones.

DEVELOPMENT OF BONE

There are two methods of bone formation:

1. Endochondral ossification
2. Intramembranous ossification.

In endochondral ossification a cartilage model of the bone forms first and then calcifies partially within the embryo.

In intramembranous ossification, membrane bones are formed between two membrane layers of the periosteum which then calcifies, e.g. skull.

Bones in the embryo consist of a fibrous membrane and hyaline cartilage, which are bone-shaped but are not strong.

Endochondral ossification in the long bone

Stage 1

- Stage 1 takes approximately 4 weeks (in embryo)
- In the fetus the bone consists of a cartilaginous shaft
- The primary ossification centre occurs in the diaphysis
- When a complete ring has formed around the diaphysis, periosteum forms
- Internal to the periosteum the cartilage cells begin to disintegrate.

Stage 2

- Osteoblasts migrate from the periosteum into the cartilaginous shaft and convert cartilage tissue to bone by laying down calcium salts
- The result is a long, hard, narrow tube
- The original space will eventually become the medullary cavity and fill with bone marrow cells due to the activity of osteoclasts (bone-destroying cells).

Stage 3

- Secondary sites of ossification occur in either one or both of the epiphyses
- The layer of tissue that remains between the diaphyseal and epiphyseal ossification sites will remain as cartilage and is termed the growth plate or metaphysis or epiphyseal plate
- The metaphysis will eventually fuse when the animal reaches skeletal maturity.

Stage 4

- Chondrocytes in the epiphyseal plate enlarge and mature
- As they enlarge the epiphysis is pushed away from the plate
- When chondrocyte growth stops the growth plate is replaced by bone and the epiphysis and diaphysis fuse.

CLASSIFICATION OF BONE

There are seven classifications of individual bones:

1. Long bones
2. Short bones
3. Flat bones
4. Irregular bones
5. Sesamoid bones
6. Pneumatic bones
7. Splanchnic bones.

Long bones

- Examples include the femur, radius, ulna and tibia
- Long bones consist of diaphysis and epiphyses
- The shaft contains a medullary cavity which contains bone marrow.

Short bones

- Examples include carpals and tarsals
- Short bones consist of compact bone enclosing a spongy bone core with no medullary cavity
- They aid with absorption of concussion and movement.

Flat bones

- Examples include scapula, skull, pelvic bones and ribs
- Flat bones consist of outer layers of compact bone which enclose a layer of spongy bone; they have no medullary cavity.

Irregular bones

- Examples include vertebrae and ear ossicles
- Irregular bones consist of two layers of compact bone with spongy bone between them.

Sesamoid bones

- Examples include the patella and fabella
- Sesamoid bones consist of very smooth small bones, which are 'free-floating' and often found embedded in muscle
- They assist with the smooth passage of tendon working.

Pneumatic bones

- Pneumatic bones are specialised bones that contain air spaces to lighten them and reduce the weight
- They are found in the skull, e.g. maxillary and frontal bone.

Splanchnic bones

- These are bones that develop in soft tissue and remain unattached to the skeleton
- An example is the os penis in the dog.

The skeleton

See Tables 2.1 and 2.2 for terminology relating to the skeleton. Figure 2.1 illustrates the skeleton of the dog and Figure 2.2 the skeleton of the horse.

Functions

- Support
- Protection
- Locomotion
- Production of erythrocytes and granular leukocytes
- Storage facility for calcium and phosphorus.

Parts of the skeleton

The skeleton can be divided into three parts:

1. The axial skeleton, consisting of the skull, vertebral column, ribs and sternum
2. The appendicular skeleton, consisting of the limbs

Table 2.1 Skeletal terminology	
Condyle	Rounded projection of a bone which often articulates with another bone
Epicondyle	Lateral articular surface located above the condyle
Foramen	Hole or opening or passage through a bone
Fossa	An indent or hollow on a bone
Ligament	Connects bone to bone
Tendon	Connects bone to muscle
Trochlea	Structure on the bone over which or through which tendons pass
Trochanter Tubercle Tuberosity	'Lumps or bumps' on bones where muscles attach to them

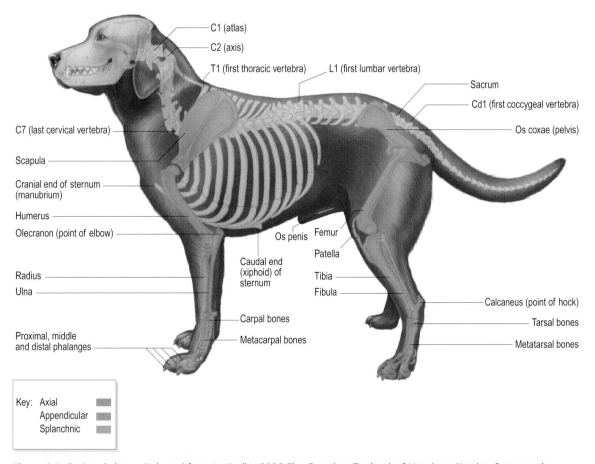

Figure 2.1 Canine skeleton. (Adapted from Aspinall V 2006 *The Complete Textbook of Veterinary Nursing*. Butterworth Heinemann, London, with permission.)

Table 2.2 Bones of the appendicular skeleton in the dog/cat

Shoulder region

Scapula
- Shoulder blade
- Large flat bone that has a spine running down the middle of the lateral surface; on either side of the spine there are hollows – the supraspinous (above) and infraspinous (below) – which provide muscular attachment
- The narrow end of the scapula forms the glenoid cavity which forms the shoulder joint

Clavicle
- Can be vestigal in some species, e.g. the dog
- Does not articulate with other bones

Foreleg

Humerus
- Long bone of the proximal foreleg
- Articulates proximally with the scapula and distally with radius and ulna at the elbow

Radius
- Long bone of the distal foreleg
- Lies parallel to the ulna but slightly shorter

Ulna
- Long bone of the distal foreleg
- Lies parallel to the radius
- At the proximal end of the ulna is a projection – the olecranon

Olecranon
- Proximal ulna
- Forms the point of the elbow joint

Carpus
- 'Wrist'
- Made up of the carpal bones

Metacarpus
- Consists of five small long bones
- They are numbered I–V, with I being the most medial and V the most lateral

Phalanges
- Also known as digits
- They are long bones
- Each phalange comprises three bones, except for the first, which comprises two bones
- They are numbered I–V, with I being the most medial and V the most lateral
- The dew claw in dogs is the first digit
- The distal phalanx ends in the ungular process, which forms the nail

Hindleg

Femur
- Long bone found in the proximal hindleg (thigh)
- Articulates with hip joint
- Held in place by the round ligament
- Articulates with the tibia at the stifle joint

Tibia
- Forms the lower or distal hindlimb
- Larger of the two lower-limb bones
- Lies parallel to the fibula (slightly more medial)

Fibula
- Forms lower hindlimb
- Smaller of the two lower-limb bones

Patella
- Kneecap
- Situated in trochlear groove within the patellar ligament
- Sesamoid bone

Tarsus
- 'Ankle' or hock
- Seven short tarsus bones arranged in three rows
- Proximal row of talus and calcaneus articulate with tibia and fibula at hock joint
- Os calcaneus or tuber calcis: point of the hock

Metatarsus
- Five bones, although many breeds only have four

Phalanges
- Five bones, although many breeds only have four

Pelvis

Ischium
- One of three bones that form the hip
- Paired on each side of the pelvis
- Ischium forms the arches at the caudal (back) of the pelvis

Ilium
- One of three bones that form the hip
- Paired on each side of the pelvis
- Forms the wings of the pelvis at its cranial (front) aspect

Pubis
- One of three bones that form the hip
- Paired on each side of the pelvis
- Forms the base of the hip socket

Acetabular bone
- Small bone around which the ischium, ilium and pubis form the hip joint

Acetabulum
- Articular socket of the hip joint

Pubic symphysis
- Joint where two sides of the pelvis join

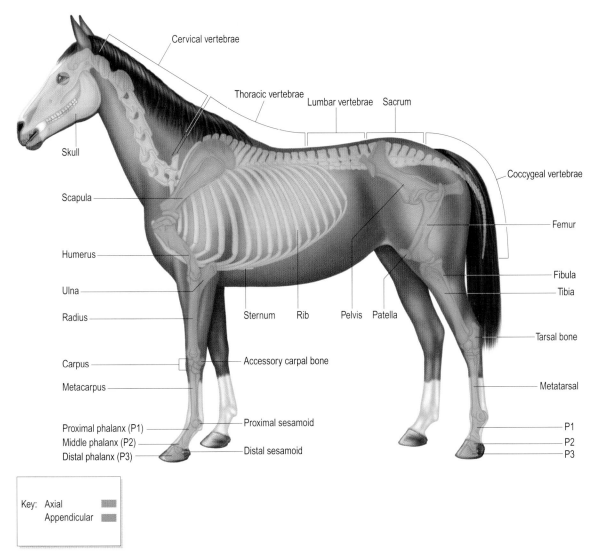

Figure 2.2 Equine skeleton. (Adapted from Aspinall V 2006 *The Complete Textbook of Veterinary Nursing*. Butterworth Heinemann, London, with permission.)

3. The splanchnic skeleton – bones that develop in tissue but are unattached to the skeleton.

The skull

The skull comprises a number of bones that serve to protect and house the brain, sensory organs and teeth (Table 2.3). It contains a number of bones that are joined by fibrous joints which allow very little movement. Skull shape varies between animal species and within breeds. In dogs three skull shapes are recognised: brachiocephalic (shortened skull with rounded cranium and squashed muzzle (Figure 2.3), e.g. Pug), mesaticephalic ('normal', e.g. Collie) and dolichocephalic (elongated skull, e.g. Greyhound). In many large animals, e.g. horse, whose head would weigh a significant amount and could become a disadvantage as prey species, the skull has developed to include numerous sinuses which are large and air-filled to reduce the weight of the head.

The vertebrae

The spine or vertebral column runs along the midline of the body from the occipital condyles which articulate with the atlas, the first vertebra, to the cauda equina. The

Table 2.3 Bones of the head

Parietal	• Comprises sides (lateral aspects) and back (dorsal aspect) of the skull
Temporal	• Found below the parietal bone • Forms tympanic bulla which houses the middle ear
Frontal	• Forehead • Contains the frontal sinus which connects to the nasal chamber
Occipital	• Found at the base of the skull • At the bottom is the foramen magnum, a large hole, through which the spinal cord passes
Sphenoid	• Forms the floor of the cranial cavity
Sagittal crest	• Bony crest at the top of the cranium
Zygomatic	• Cheekbone
Lacrimal	• At base of eye • Lacrimal fluid (tears) drain through this region
Orbit	• Eye socket • Provides bony protection for the eyes
Maxilla	• Upper jaw
Mandible	• Lower jaw • Comprises two halves which are joined in the middle by the mandibular symphysis • Divided into the body (horizontal section) and the ramus (vertical section) • Teeth are sited in the alveoli (sockets) in the lower jaw
Temporomandibular joint	• Articulation point for maxilla, mandible and associated muscles to achieve mastication
Hyoid apparatus	• Located inside the mandibular space • Moves the larynx and tongue

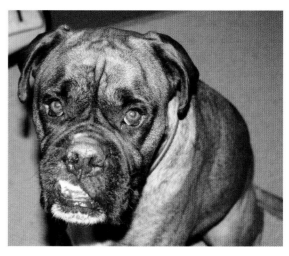

Figure 2.3 Boxer: brachiocephalic skull shape.

vertebrae provide postural support, house the spinal cord and form a protective case for its delicate structure. Spinal nerves arise from between the vertebrae along its length. The structure of the vertebrae varies according to function, especially linking to the muscular attachments within the region it is located. Every species has a distinctive number of vertebrae that can be written as a formula linking to the different types and number of vertebrae present. There are five types of vertebra:

1. Cervical vertebrae – neck region; includes atlas (first) and axis (second) which has a specialised peg known as the dens which articulates with atlas; they have short spinous processes and wide transverse processes
2. Thoracic vertebrae – thoracic region; long, pronounced spinous processes and moderate transverse processes which articulate with their equivalent rib
3. Lumbar vertebrae – abdominal region; moderate spinous processes with long transverse processes
4. Sacral vertebrae – pelvic region; these are fused together to form the sacrum
5. Caudal or coccygeal vertebrae – tail region; short spinous and transverse processes.

Each vertebra has is rounded with a ventral body: the caudal end of this body is concave and the cranial end convex to allow the vertebra to interlink. Above the vertebral body is the vertebral foramen, a hole through which the spinal cord runs. Each vertebra has transverse (side) processes and a neural spine or spinous process (dorsal/top surface) arising from the neural arch – these allow muscular attachment. The vertebrae are interspersed with intervertebral discs which reduce friction. The discs comprise a tough fibrous connective tissue case, the annulus fibrosus, which surrounds the nucleus pulposus, its gelatinous core.

Ribs and sternum

The sternum is found on the ventral surface of the thoracic cavity and comprises eight bones called the sternebrae, which are linked by intersternebrae cartilages. The first sternebra is the manubrium and the last is the xiphisternum or xiphoid process – both are useful anatomical landmarks when navigating the animal body.

The ribs form a bony cage protecting the thoracic cavity and aiding in the mechanics of respiration. They are paired and the number varies between species, e.g. there are 13 pairs in the dog and 18 in the horse. Ribs are flat bones; they have a bony dorsal component and a cartilaginous ventral portion or costal cartilage. The costal cartilages of the ribs articulate with the sternum, although not all are directly attached to it, and these are known as 'false' ribs. The false ribs attach to their adjacent rib to form a costal arch. The last pair of ribs are not attached to each other or to the sternum and are known as 'floating' ribs. The space between pairs of ribs is called the intercostal space and contains the intercostal muscles which help to move the ribcage during breathing.

Bones of the limbs

The bones of the foreleg, hindleg, the shoulder and the pelvis comprise the appendicular skeleton. The foreleg does not connect to bones in the trunk of the body but uses muscular attachments to enable movement; the hindleg does articulate with the pelvis but also utilises muscular attachments to enable movement. The individual bones are described in Table 2.4.

Joints

A joint or arthrosis can be defined as an area where two articulating bones meet. There are a number of different types of joint (Table 2.5):

- Synovial joints
- Cartilaginous joints
- Fibrous joints.

Synovial joints or diarthroses

These occur where articular (joint) surfaces of the bones involved are covered with hyaline cartilage. They are found throughout the limbs, in the temporomandibular joint (jaw) and in the first two joints of the vertebral column. The entire joint is surrounded by a joint capsule whose outer layer is a continuation of the periosteum and whose inner layer comprises a synovial membrane.

Table 2.4 Definitions of individual bones

Epiphysis	Proximal or distal end of the bone
Metaphysis	Growth plate
Diaphysis	Shaft
Periosteum	Dense white fibrous covering around surface of bone: inner layer contains osteoblasts; outer layer contains blood vessels. Lymph vessels and nerves
Cortex	Compact bone 'outer'
Medullary cavity	Bone cavity containing bone marrow. Two types: • Yellow – mostly fat • Red – blood-forming cells
Articular cartilage	Smooth hyaline cartilage covering area prone to frictional damage
Nutrient foramen	Small channels between compact bone and bone marrow through which blood vessels pass

Table 2.5 Joint movement and types

Flexion	Decreases the angle between two bones
Extension	Increases the angle between two bones
Abduction	Moves the limb away from the body
Adduction	Moves the limb into/towards the body
Rotation	Can be inward or outward; one end of the bone swivels around the joint, allowing the opposite end to circle around
Gliding or sliding	One articular surface moves over another
Hinge joints	Allow movement in one direction only, e.g. elbow
Condylar joints	Allow flexion, extension to straight line and overextension, e.g. carpal joint
Pivot joints	Allow rotation, e.g. radiohumeral joint
Ball-and-socket joints	Allow most movement: flexion, extension, rotation, adduction and abduction, e.g. hip joint
Plane joints	Allow restricted amount of gliding of one bone over another, e.g. small bones in carpus

The synovial membrane lines the joint cavity and secretes synovial fluid which acts as lubrication and a nutrient source for the articular cartilage. The consistency of the fluid varies; it should be thick and viscous but can become thin and sparse in animals as they age or if they are unathletic. Synovial joints often have stabilising ligaments associated with them; these can be on the inside or the outside of the joint. Collateral ligaments are most common: they lie on either side of nearly all hinge joints. Fibrocartilage menisci may also be present; these increase the range of movement and reduce wear and tear on the articular surfaces, e.g. in the stifle and the jaw.

Cartilaginous joints

These comprise bones connected by cartilage and may or may not have movement associated with the joint. Synarthroses allow little or no movement, e.g. the pubic symphysis, whereas amphiarthroses allow a reasonable amount of movement between the bones, e.g. the intervertebral joints.

Fibrous joints

These are formed by bones joined together by dense fibrous connective tissue. They allow little or no movement, e.g. between the flat bones of the skull. Both fibrous and cartilaginous joints may become ossified or may develop pockets of synovial fluid.

Species variation – skeletal system

All animals have evolved a shape which best suits their lifestyle. The skeleton and its muscular attachments enable the animal to move and function. In birds bone structure has adapted to reduce weight to enable flight; the bones are reduced in number, they are less dense and therefore lighter and many are hollow and filled with air sacs. In reptiles bony prominences have evolved to form protection, e.g. shells, and in large animals the lower limb is significantly different from that of the dog (considered previously).

Lower-limb skeletal structure in the horse

The horse's limb consists of the same bones as in the dog but their design is different. Figure 2.4 shows the equine distal forelimb. The lower limb has elongated from the knee, with the distal third comprising the carpals and digits. The cannon bone and splint bone, carpal bones, are located from the knee to the fetlock with the phalanges. The fetlock joint connects the cannon bone with the first of the three pastern bones. The first pastern bone fits

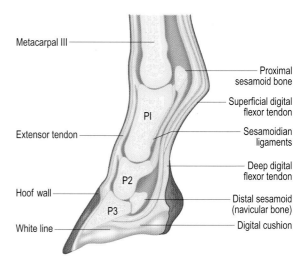

Figure 2.4 Equine distal forelimb. P1, first pastern bone; P2, second pastern bone; P3, third pastern bone. (Reproduced from Aspinall V 2006 *The Complete Textbook of Veterinary Nursing*. Butterworth Heinemann, London, with permission.)

into the second pastern bone via the pastern joint and the third pastern bone, the coffin bone, interconnects with the second via the coffin joint. The leg has a complicated pulley system, the stay apparatus, which consists of muscles, flexor tendons and the proximal sesamoid bones which allow the horse to stand and sleep upright using minimal effort. The distal sesamoid bone or navicular bone is located within the hoof at the junction of the short pastern and coffin bone, and provides another pulley for the deep digital flexor tendon.

The hoof

The hoof is a modification of the integument; its functions include protection of the underlying soft tissues, digging, scratching, use as a protective weapon and as a means to reduce concussion from locomotion. Hoofed animals are known as ungulates.

The junction between the hoof and the skin is called the coronary band or coronet. The wall of the hoof comprises the epidermis and it grows downwards from the coronet. The inner layer of the wall of the hoof, the corium, is modified dermal tissue and attaches to the distal phalanx (coffin bone) underneath. The corium is connected to the hoof wall by laminae, which are also essential in the attachment of coffin bone to the hoof. The dermal laminae are sensitive structures and inflammation leads to the condition laminitis.

The hoof can be divided into three sections: the toe, quarters and heels. The dorsal section is the toe; at the back of the hoof the hoof wall creates bars and forms the heel. There is a central v-shaped frog which is in contact with the floor. The frog is divided by the central sulcus and has a thick pad of fat and fibrous tissue, the digital cushion, underneath it. The sole is concave and fills the gaps between the frog, bars and hoof wall. The white line is where the sole meets the hoof wall.

MUSCULAR SYSTEM

There are three types of muscle: skeletal muscle (Figures 2.5 and 2.6), smooth muscle and cardiac muscle, which are considered in Chapter 1.

All muscle is stimulated to contract by nervous impulses. These stimulate the thin actin fibre and thicker myosin fibres which form a sacromere (unit of contraction) in the myofibril to slide over each other. As the two types of fibres move, the actin fibres pull past the thicker myosin, and this has the effect of shortening the sacromere and thus the muscle. The process requires energy and calcium ions are essential for the process to occur.

Muscle tone describes the state of tension in the skeletal muscles responsible for body posture as if these relaxed the animal would fall over. Not all of the mus-

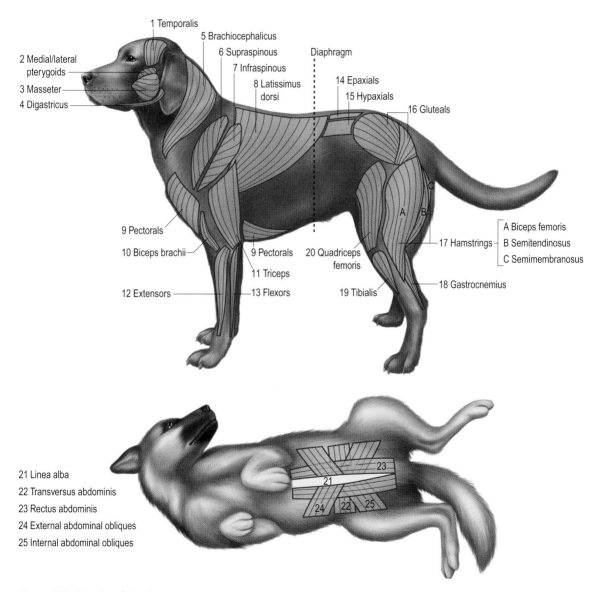

1 Temporalis
2 Medial/lateral pterygoids
3 Masseter
4 Digastricus
5 Brachiocephalicus
6 Supraspinous
7 Infraspinous
8 Latissimus dorsi
Diaphragm
14 Epaxials
15 Hypaxials
16 Gluteals
9 Pectorals
10 Biceps brachii
9 Pectorals
11 Triceps
12 Extensors
13 Flexors
20 Quadriceps femoris
19 Tibialis
17 Hamstrings
A Biceps femoris
B Semitendinosus
C Semimembranosus
18 Gastrocnemius

21 Linea alba
22 Transversus abdominis
23 Rectus abdominis
24 External abdominal obliques
25 Internal abdominal obliques

Figure 2.5 Muscles of the dog.

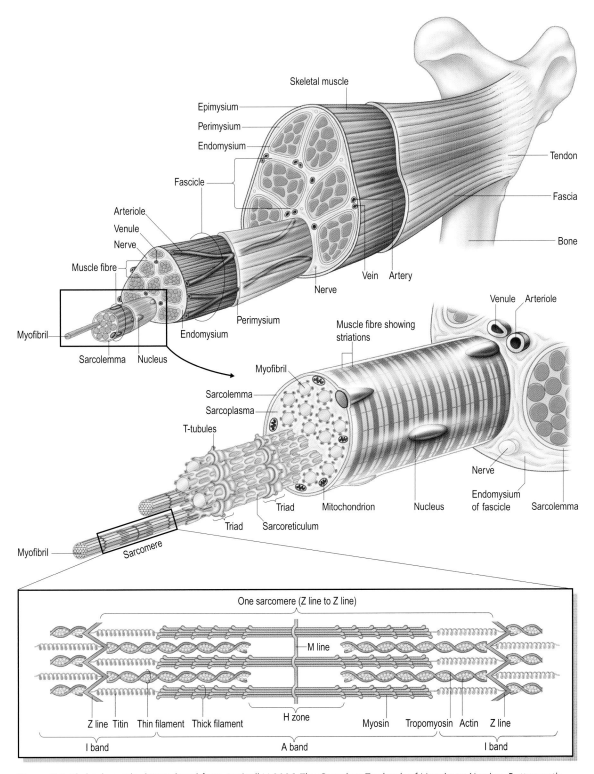

Figure 2.6 Skeletal muscle. (Reproduced from Aspinall V 2006 *The Complete Textbook of Veterinary Nursing*. Butterworth Heinemann, London, with permission.)

Table 2.6 Muscles of importance

Mastication	• Chewing
	• Muscles involved are digastricus, masseter, temporalis and medial/lateral pterygoids
	• Masseter – closes jaw
	• Temporalis – largest and most powerful muscle in the head
	• Medial/lateral pterygoids – sideways movement
		Forelimb	• Extrinsic muscles of the forelimb
			  – Trapezius: draws foreleg forward and protracts the limb
			  – Pectorals: adduct limb and hold forelimb into body
			  – Latissimus dorsi: retracts the forelimb
			  – Brachiocephalicus: with limb on the ground, flexes neck and bends it laterally; with limb up it draws forelimb forward or protracts the leg
			• Intrinsic muscles of the forelimb
			  – Supraspinatus: extends the shoulder and stabilises the shoulder joint
			  – Infraspinatus: stabilises shoulder joint and flexes shoulder joint
			• Lower-limb movement
			  – Triceps brachii: extends the elbow
			  – Biceps brachii: flexes elbow joint
			  – Brachialis: flexes elbow joint
			• Carpus and digits
			  – Carpal extensors
			  – Digital extensors
			  – Carpal flexors
			  – Digital flexors

Movement of the eyes	• Extrinsic muscles move the eye in its socket • Extrinsic muscles are dorsal rectus, ventral rectus, medial rectus and lateral rectus • Rotation of the eye – dorsal oblique and ventral oblique • Pull the eye back into its socket – retractor bulbi • Ciliary muscles – change shape of lens		

Vertebral column	• Epaxial muscles – dorsal to transverse processes of the vertebrae; support the spine and allow sideways movement and extension
	• Hypaxial muscles – ventral to transverse processes of the vertebrae; flex the neck and tail and help flex the spine
		Hindlimb	• Upper hindlimb
			  – Gluteals: superficial, middle and deep gluteals: extensors of hip joint
			  – Hamstrings: biceps femoris, semitendinous and semimembranous
			  – Biceps femoris: extends hip, flexes stifle and extends hock
			  – Semitendinous: extends hip, flexes stifle and extends hock
			  – Semimembranous: extends hip and flexes stifle
			  – Quadriceps femoris: extends stifle
			• Lower hindlimb
			  – Gastrocnemius: extends hock and flexes stifle
			  – Achilles tendon: string tendon runs down the back of the hindleg
			• Hock and digits
			  – Anterior tibialis: flexes hock and rotates the paw medially
			  – Digital extensors
			  – Digital flexors

Thorax	• External intercostals – raise thorax up and out during inspiration • Internal intercostals – move thorax in and down during expiration; largely passive movement		
Diaphragm	• Sheet of muscle with tendinous centre • Separates thorax and abdomen • Main muscle of inspiration		
Abdomen	• Four large, broad muscles which support internal structures • Situated in such a way that they maximise the support • All terminate on linea alba (white line) central tendon • External abdominal oblique – most superficial • Internal adominal oblique – under the external and at opposite oblique angle • Transversus abdominis – deepest • Rectus abdominis – forms the floor of abdomen		

cle's fibres are contracted during rest: only sufficient are used to maintain the animal's posture. This demonstrates that there are two types of muscle activation within the animal body. The first is defined as isometric contraction and can be described as a muscle which has tension or muscle tone but does not shorten. The second is isotonic contraction, which is where the muscle shortens to produce a movement. Muscle size will increase with use or exercise and this is known as hypertrophy. Conversely muscle mass will decrease through lack of use: this is called atrophy.

Muscles are attached to bones by tendons which join to the muscle heads at the points of origin and insertion. The origin is the end which moves the least during contraction and the insertion is the end which moves the most. Muscles can have multiple bellies and heads which insert at the same point; for example, the biceps brachii has two heads.

Muscles can also be described as intrinsic or extrinsic (Table 2.6). Intrinsic muscles are found completely within the region of the body where they have both their origin and insertion, and produce movement within that region only. Extrinsic muscles are not limited to one region and produce movement that is not limited to one region. It should also be considered that muscles may be circular in structure, known as sphincters; these normally control the passage of substances in and out of organs, e.g. pyloric sphincter of the stomach. Muscles can also be flat, such as those associated with the diaphragm; the tendon attachment needs to be the same structure and in this case the diaphragm is a flat tendon or aponeurosis. Bursae are not muscles but are associated with them; they are sacks of connective tissue filled with synovial fluid to form a cushion or cushioning sheath, as in some tendons, to reduce friction.

Bibliography

Aspinall V 2006 The complete textbook of veterinary nursing. Butterworth Heinemann, London

Aspinall V, O'Reilly M 2004 Introduction to veterinary anatomy and physiology. Butterworth Heinemann, Oxford

Campbell N, Reece J, Mitchell L 1999 Biology, 5th edn. Benjamin Cummings, San Francisco

Colville T, Bassett J M 2002 Clinical anatomy and physiology for veterinary technicians. Mosby, St Louis

Dyke K M, Sack W O, Wensing C J G 1996 Text book of veterinary anatomy, 2nd edn. W B Saunders, Philadelphia

Green N P O, Stout G W, Taylor D J 1991 Biological science. Cambridge University Press, Cambridge

Lane D R, Cooper B, Turner L 2007 BSAVA Textbook of Veterinary Nursing. BSAVA, Oxford

Moore M 2000 Manual of veterinary nursing. BSAVA, Oxford

Pratt P W 1998 Principles and practice of veterinary technology. Mosby, Philadelphia

Roberts M B V 1986 Biology: a functional approach. Nelson, Surrey, UK

Simpson G 1994 Practical veterinary nursing, 3rd edn. BSAVA, Oxford

Cardiovascular and respiratory systems

This chapter discusses the anatomy of the heart and blood vessels and the components of the respiratory system. The physiological processes that occur to enable oxygen to be provided at cellular level and waste carbon dioxide to be excreted are explained.

BLOOD AND THE CIRCULATORY SYSTEM

The circulatory system comprises blood, blood vessels and the heart (Table 3.1).

Blood (Figure 3.1)

- Blood is a red fluid
- Arterial blood is a brighter red colour than venous blood because it is transporting more oxygen

- Total circulating blood volume is equivalent to 7% of an animal's body weight – this is about how much oil the average car would have in its engine!

Blood comprises:

- Blood cells
- Plasma.

Plasma

- This is the liquid component of blood
- It is normally a straw-coloured fluid
- It contains numerous chemical compounds in solution and in veterinary practice it is often used for biochemistry assays to ascertain their circulating levels as an indicator of health
- It can be separated from the blood cells by centrifugation
- In the body it is constantly mixed with the blood cells as it circulates in the blood vessels
- It is in dynamic equilibrium with the interstitial fluid (the fluid that bathes the cells) and intracellular fluid (the fluid within the cells) to allow the passage of substances throughout the body.

Composition of plasma

- Water (approximately 92%)
- Plasma proteins
- Mineral salts
- Foodstuffs
- Gases
- Waste products
- Hormones and enzymes
- Antibodies and antitoxins.

Table 3.1 Blood vessels that comprise the systemic circulation

Artery/vein	Area blood is supplied to and taken away from
Coronary artery/vein	Heart
Carotid artery	Brain
Subclavian artery/vein	Forelimbs
Mesenteric artery/vein	Intestines
Renal artery/vein	Kidneys
Hepatic artery/vein	Liver
Iliac artery/vein	Hindlegs
Inguinal artery/vein	Groin
Vena cava	Heart
Hepatic portal vein	Intestine to the liver

Plasma proteins

Plasma contains several kinds of proteins, including:

- Albumins and globulins, which help regulate fluid balance
- Fibrinogen and prothrombin, which have roles in blood clotting.

Plasma proteins are large molecules which cannot pass through the walls of blood vessels. They exert an osmotic pressure and are important in maintaining blood volume. (In the body, if there is little circulating fluid but lots of proteins, the osmotic potential created will act to draw fluid from the interstitial fluid into the blood volume.) The liver produces most of the plasma proteins with immunoglobulins (part of the immune system) being produced by plasma cells.

Mineral salts

- Sodium (Na^+): main extracellular cation (positive ion)
- Chloride (Cl^-): main extracellular anion (negative ion).

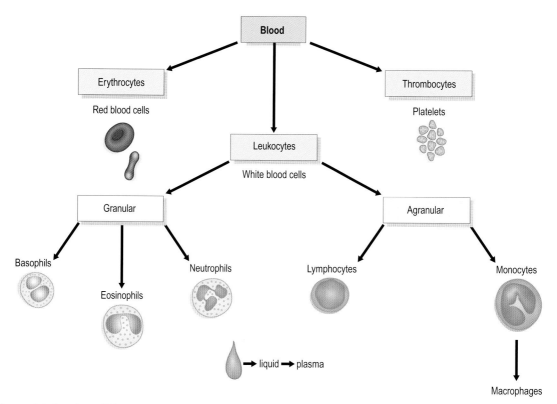

Figure. 3.1 Overview of blood cells.

Potassium (K^+), calcium (Ca^{2+}), phosphate and carbonate are also found as ions in plasma. Mineral salts act as acid–base buffers maintaining the correct pH of body fluids. The normal pH of blood is approximately 7.35.

Foodstuffs

The end products of food breakdown – amino acids, fatty acids and glucose – are transported via the plasma around the body.

Gases

Carbon dioxide is carried in plasma bound as bicarbonate molecules.

Waste products

Urea and creatinine from cells and tissues are taken to the kidneys for excretion.

Hormones and enyzmes

Hormones and enzymes utilise plasma as a transport mode to travel to their target cells/organs.

Antibodies and antitoxins

Antibodies and antitoxins also use plasma as a transportation method around the body.

Serum

Serum is the fluid which separates from blood when the process of clotting takes place or plasma minus the clotting proteins/agents.

Blood cells

Blood contains many different types of cell. These can be divided into three categories:

1. Red blood cells or erythrocytes
2. White blood cells or leukocytes (also spelled leucocytes)
3. Thrombocytes or platelets.

Red blood cells or erythrocytes

- Erythrocytes are highly specialised cells whose function is oxygen transportation
- In mammals they have no nuclei but in birds, fish and reptiles they do normally have nuclei
- They are biconcave discs
- They are small in size – approximately 7 μm or 0.007 cm
- It is the *haemoglobin*, which is an iron-containing protein that gives the cells their red colour, contained in red blood cells, that binds with oxygen molecules to allow it to be transported around the body
- The average red blood cell has a lifespan of approximately 21 days.

Erythrocyte production

In animals before birth erythrocytes are produced in the spleen and liver whilst after birth they are only produced in the bone marrow (Figure 3.2).

- Cells called erythroblasts containing nuclei take up haemoglobin: their nuclei shrink and they become normoblasts
- The nuclei then disappear completely, leaving behind a network of fine strands of nuclei material in the cytoplasm. The cell is now a reticulocyte
- The network gradually vanishes and the cell is now a mature erythrocyte and is released into the blood stream.

Note Reticulocytes are numerous in the blood when an animal is anaemic, indicating that the body is trying to restore the red blood cell count to normal levels.

- *Erythropoiesis* is the process of red blood cell production
- *Haemopoiesis* relates to the production of red blood cells.

Erythrocytes are broken down in the spleen or lymph nodes at a rate of approximately 2.4 million cells a second. Erythrocyte production is regulated by oxygen levels in the body tissues and is stimulated by a hormone called erythropoietin. Bone marrow is haemopoietic tissue, i.e. it produces erythrocytes or red blood cells. Myeloid tissue is tissue that makes blood cells and contains cells similar to those found in bone marrow, e.g. the spleen and liver produce erythrocytes prior to birth.

White blood cells or leukocytes

These can be divided into two groups:

1. Granulocytes
2. Agranulocytes.

Granular leukocytes

- These comprise approximately 70% of white blood cells
- They have an average lifespan of 21 days
- They are also known as polymorphonuclear leukocytes
- They possess large distinctive granules in their cytoplasm
- They are manufactured in the red bone marrow

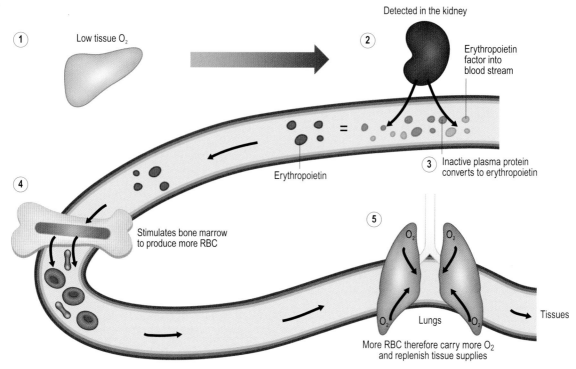

Figure 3.2 Hormonal control of red blood cell (RBC) production.

- There are three types: neutrophils, eosinophils and basophils.

Neutrophils

- These have a lobulated nucleus and cytoplasm remains clear after staining
- They are phagocytic cells which ingest bacteria and dead cells, e.g. during infection or injury.

Eosinophils

- These are present in allergic reactions and parasitic infections
- The granules in their cytoplasm stain red, making them identifiable via microscopy.

Basophils

- The granules in their cytoplasm stain blue, making them identifiable via microscopy
- They play a role in allergic reactions as they contain large amounts of histamine which they release in response to allergy
- They also contain heparin (anticoagulant) and it is believed they play a role in preventing blood clotting inappropriately in blood vessels.

Agranular leukocytes

- These have clear cytoplasm and a rounded or kidney-shaped nucleus
- There are two types: monocytes and lymphocytes.

Monocytes

- These are the largest white blood cells and are produced in the bone marrow
- They mature into macrophages
- Their role is to engulf bacteria and dead cells.

Lymphocytes

- These comprise 80% of agranular leukocytes
- There are two types: T lymphocytes and B lymphocytes
- They are produced in the fetus but mature in the thymus (T lymphocytes) and in the spleen (B lymphocytes)
- They play an important role in antibody production and therefore in the body's defence mechanism.

The white blood cell count is a measure of the circulating volume of white blood cells. This can be a useful clinical tool when compared with average leukocyte count for an individual species. Increases may suggest infection or inflammation whereas decreases could suggest neoplasia or autoimmune problems.

Thrombocytes or platelets

- These are cell fragments that are essential for blood clotting
- They are produced in the bone marrow (together with other blood cells) from cells called megakaryocytes
- They are small oval bits of cytoplasm that lack a nucleus and are enclosed by a membrane.

The clotting process

- When a blood vessel is damaged, platelets stick to damaged walls of blood vessel. Simultaneously broken platelets release a substance called thromboplastin
- Prothrombin (a circulating plasma protein) converts to thrombin in the presence of thromboplastin and calcium (which is also circulating in the blood)
- Thrombin is an active enzyme that acts on the plasma protein fibrinogen, producing insoluble strands of fibrin
- Fibrin strands form a net-like mesh over the damaged area, trapping platelets and blood cells, forming a clot
- The clot shrinks and serum is released.

Vitamin K is an essential requirement for the manufacture of prothrombin. Clotting time is influenced by:

- Speed of platelet arrival
- Nature of damage to vessel
- Presence of clotting factors
- Presence of vitamin K.

Remember that clotting occurs within the body to repair minor damage to vessels, e.g. in the lungs.

Functions of blood

- Gas transport – oxygen to tissues from lungs and carbon dioxide from tissues to lungs
- Food transport – the blood transports the end products of food breakdown around the body
- Removal of waste material – urea and creatinine are removed from the tissues to the kidneys for excretion
- Transportation of hormones, enzymes, antibodies and antitoxins around the body.

Blood vessels

Blood is transported around the body via a network of vessels. These are the:

- Arteries
- Arterioles
- Capillaries.
- Venules
- Veins.

Arteries

- These carry oxygenated blood away from the heart
- The only exception is the pulmonary artery, which carries deoxygenated blood from the heart to the lungs
- Arteries have thick muscular walls, containing much elastic tissue
- They have a small lumen relative to their diameter
- They are capable of constriction but are not permeable, i.e. substances cannot pass in and out of them
- They do not contain valves, with the exception of the aorta and pulmonary artery, which do
- Blood in arteries is under high pressure, moves in pulses and flows rapidly.

Arterioles

- The distributing artery branches within an organ or tissue form very small arteries or arterioles
- They determine the amount of blood distributed to a tissue
- The smooth muscle in the tunica media can contract or relax, changing the diameter of the lumen and therefore controlling the volume of blood passing through it
- Arteriolar contraction produces vasoconstriction – the diameter of the lumen is decreased, i.e. the arteriole decreases in size
- Arteriolar relaxation produces vasodilation – the diameter of the lumen is increased, i.e. the arteriole increases in size
- This helps to maintain blood pressure throughout the body.

Capillaries

- Arterioles deliver blood into microscopic vessels called capillaries
- These consist of thin walls of single-cell epithelium which permits the exchange of nutrients, gases and waste products between blood and the tissues – therefore they are permeable
- They contain no muscle and no elastic tissue
- They have a large lumen and contain no valves
- Capillaries are sites of exchange: blood changes from oxygenated to deoxygenated across the capillary bed

- The blood pressure reduces due to the reduction in size of the vessel and blood within them is also slow-flowing – ideal conditions for diffusion to occur
- They also have no pulse as the blood is under low pressure, not moving in waves.

Venules

- Capillaries link directly into venules or small veins
- These have precapillary sphincters – smooth-muscle cells which can open or close to regulate the passage of blood into them.

Veins

- Venules link to veins
- At any one time approximately 50% of blood volume will be present in the veins
- They have thinner, less elastic walls than arteries and blood within them is under low pressure
- Muscular activity aids venous blood flow by compressing veins but they cannot constrict themselves
- They are equipped with valves to prevent backflow of blood
- Their function is to transport blood to the heart and they contain deoxygenated blood
- The only exception is the pulmonary vein which carries oxygenated blood from the lungs to the heart
- They have no pulses and blood is flowing slowly.

THE HEART

The function of the heart is to pump blood around the body under pressure. Figure 3.3 shows the structure of the heart.

Structure of the heart

The mammalian heart is a hollow, muscular, four-chambered organ located in the mediastinum between the lungs. It is conical in shape with the apex pointing downwards and lies to the left at the level of rib 7. It is enclosed by a tough connective tissue sac – the pericardium. The inner surface of the pericardium is covered by a smooth layer of epithelial cells or epicardium or serous pericardium. The epithelial inner lining of the heart is the endocardium. Between the endocardium and the epicardium is the pericardial cavity. This is filled with fluid that acts to reduce friction as the heart beats. The muscle of the heart is the myocardium. The heart has a right and left side, both of which are divided into two chambers. The top chambers or atria have thinner walls than the thick-walled bottom chambers or ventricles. The right atrium and ventricle are separated from the left atrium and ventricle by a wall or septum.

Blood flow in the heart (Figure 3.4)

- Deoxygenated blood enters the right atrium via the anterior and posterior vena cava
- It passes through the right atrioventricular (AV) valve (or tricuspid valve) into the right ventricle
- Then it passes through the semilunar valves or pulmonary valve into the pulmonary arteries and is taken to the lungs
- At the lungs carbon dioxide is excreted and oxygen diffuses into the blood, which is now oxygenated and travels back to the heart via the pulmonary vein
- The pulmonary vein enters the left atrium and blood goes through the left AV valve (or bicuspid valve) into the left ventricle
- The left ventricle has a thick muscular wall to enable it to pump blood all around the body. The ventricle

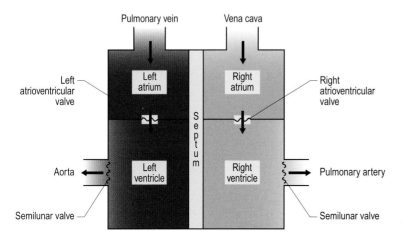

Figure 3.3 Structure of the heart.

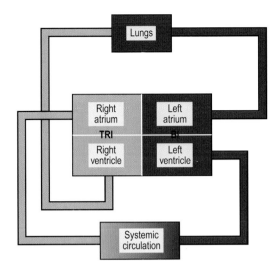

Figure 3.4 Cardiac and pulmonary circulation.

contracts and blood goes through the semilunar valves or aortic valve and onward to the systemic circulation via the aorta.

How does blood not flow back into the heart?

- The AV valves are held in place by chordae tendinae, which are attached to the ventricle walls by papillary muscles
- When blood fills the atrium the increase in blood pressure forces the AV valves open, therefore filling the ventricles
- As the ventricles contract, blood is forced back on the AV valves, pushing them closed. The papillary muscles contract and hold the chordae tendinae taut, preventing the AV valves from opening back into the atria
- When blood passes out of the ventricles, the semilunar valves are pushed aside and offer no resistance to blood flow
- When the ventricles are relaxing and filling with blood from the atria, the blood pressure is higher in the atria than it is in the ventricles
- Blood fills pouches in the semilunar valves, stretching them across the artery so that blood cannot flow back into the heart
- Heart murmurs can result from backflow of blood into the ventricles due to damage to the semilunar valves.

How the heart beats

Cardiac muscle can contract rhythmically without a constant nerve supply. (Note: the autonomic nerves to the heart only control heart rate.) To ensure the heart beats in a regular and effective rhythm, there is a specialised conduction system.

1. Each beat is initialised by the pacemaker – sinoatrial (SA) node – a small mass of specialised cardiac muscle in the posterior wall of the right atrium near the opening of the superior vena cava. The SA node fibres fuse with atrial muscle fibres and produce atrial contraction
2. The impulse activates the AV node located in the right atrium along the lower part of the septum. The transmission is briefly delayed to allow the atria to contract
3. The impulse from the AV node spreads into specialised muscle fibres called Purkinje fibres. These large fibres make up the bundle of His or AV bundle
4. The bundle of His divides, sending branches into each ventricle at the end of the Purkinje fibres. The impulse spreads into the cardiac muscle fibres of the ventricles, causing them to contract.

The whole process is known as the cardiac cycle.

Heart sounds

If you listen to your heart with a stethoscope, you will hear two main heart sounds – 'lub' and 'dub', which repeat rhythmically.

- Lub: low-pitched, fairly long sound. This corresponds to the closing of the AV valves and the beginning of ventricular systole
- Dub: higher-pitched, shorter sound. This is the closing of the semilunar valves and the beginning of ventricular diastole.

Arterial pulse

Each time the left ventricle pumps blood into the aorta, the elastic wall of the aorta expands and this expansion moves down the arteries as a wave. The artery snaps back into place as the wave passes, producing the pulse.

Blood pressure

Refer to Box 3.1 for useful definitions.

- Blood pressure is determined by blood flow and resistance to that flow
- Blood flow depends on the pumping action of the heart
- Therefore, when cardiac output increases, blood flow increases and blood pressure increases

DEFINITIONS

Blood pressure

Force exerted by the blood against the inner walls of the blood vessels

Diastole

Portion of the cycle when relaxation takes place

Heart rate

Number of pulsations/heart beats in an artery in a minute

Pulse

The alternate expansion and recoil of an artery

Systole

Portion of the cycle in which contraction takes place

- Or, if circulating blood volume drops (there is less resistance to blood flow), the blood pressure will drop
- Or, if the volume of blood increases (overinfusion with intravenous fluids), this will lead to increased blood pressure
- Changes in blood pressure are sensed by baroreceptors present in the arterial walls.

PULMONARY CIRCULATION

Deoxygenated blood is pumped from the right ventricle into the pulmonary circulation. It emerges via the pulmonary arteries at one of the lungs. In the lungs, blood is pumped through the pulmonary arteries to the pulmonary arterioles and then to the pulmonary capillaries in the alveoli (air sacs). Carbon dioxide diffuses out of blood into the air in the alveoli and oxygen diffuses into blood from the air in the alveoli.

Oxygenated blood is carried back to the heart from the pulmonary veins. To summarise:

right atrium → right ventricle → pulmonary artery → pulmonary capillaries in lung → diffusion/gaseous exchange → pulmonary veins → left atrium → left ventricle → rest of body.

SYSTEMIC CIRCULATION

Blood enters the systemic circulation from the *aorta*. Arteries branch off the aorta to carry blood to all regions of the body. Blood returning from the capillary networks to the heart travels via the main veins in the body: the jugular vein returns blood from the brain and the subclavian veins returns blood from the arms. These veins merge with other upper-body veins to form the *superior vena cava* which empties into the right atrium. The renal vein, iliac vein, hepatic vein and other lower veins merge to form the *inferior vena cava*, which delivers blood into the right atrium.

The azygos vein runs along the right side of the aorta and collects blood from the intercostal spaces. It empties either directly into the right atrium or into the vena cava.

CORONARY CIRCULATION

Heart muscle is supplied with oxygen and nutrients by the coronary arteries. These arise directly from the aorta at the point it leaves the heart. The deoxygenated blood is returned via the coronary veins which join to form the coronary sinus, which empties directly into the right atrium.

Hepatic portal system

The function of the hepatic portal system is to enable the end products of digestion to be absorbed by the gut and thus transported directly to the liver for storage and/or use.

1. Blood flows from the heart to the capillaries in the stomach and intestine
2. It enters the hepatic portal vein, which transports it to the liver into another capillary bed where nutrients are exchanged
3. Blood from the liver drains into the hepatic vein then into the posterior vena cava.

FETAL CIRCULATION

In the fetus the lungs are not yet in use; there is a hole in the septum between the atria and an additional vessel, the ductus arteriosus, which interconnects the inferior aorta and the pulmonary artery (Figure 3.5). Oxygenated blood arrives via the umbilicus from the placenta into the caudal vena cava then flows through the right atrium to left atrium and then into the left ventricle. Here it is pumped to the head and body. Deoxygenated blood from the fetus travels along the cranial vena cava into the right ventricle but as the lungs are not working it

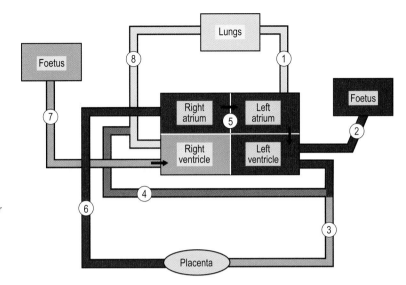

Figure 3.5 Fetal circulation. 1, Pulmonary vein (not active); 2, superior aorta (oxygenated to foetus head); 3, inferior branches of the aorta; 4, ductus arteriosus; 5, foramen ovale; 6, caudal vena cava; 7, cranial vena cava; 8, pulmonary artery.

needs to be taken back to the placenta to be removed. The extra vessel, the ductus arteriosus, acts as a short cut from the pulmonary artery to the inferior aorta and connects back to the placenta. After birth the ductus arteriosus closes and the normal systemic circulation begins. At the same time the foramen ovale seals, separating the two atria. Occasionally a small hole may remain, leading to cardiac problems, and the ductus arteriosus can remain patent or partially patent.

Species variation – heart and circulatory system

Reptilian hearts comprise two atria and only one ventricle. The ventricle effectively consists of three chambers receiving blood from both atria. Blood from the hindlimbs and tail can drain straight into the kidneys.

RESPIRATORY SYSTEM

Box 3.2 contains a list of respiration definitions.

All cells have an essential requirement for oxygen to react with nutrients to produce energy. To provide the oxygen, gases must be exchanged continuously between the organism and its environment. Oxygen is taken from the environment and transported to the cells whilst carbon dioxide, the byproduct of respiration, must be excreted into the environment. The supply of oxygen and elimination of carbon dioxide are facilitated by the respiratory system and cardiovascular system working together.

Box 3.2

RESPIRATION DEFINITIONS

Anatomical dead space

Structures containing volumes of air drawn in at each respiration that never undergo gaseous exchange: nasal cavity, nasopharynx, laryngopharynx, larynx, trachea, bronchi, bronchioles and terminal bronchioles

Apnoea

Cessation of breathing

Bradypnoea

Decreased respiratory rate compared to normal

Dyspnoea

Difficulty breathing

Orthopnoea

Open-mouthed breathing

Respiratory rate

Number of complete breaths (inspiration + expiration) in 1 minute

Tachypnoea

Increased respiratory rate compared to normal

Functions of the respiratory system

Acid–base balance

- Carbon dioxide dissolves in the blood to form carbonic acid (H_2CO_3), thus lowering the pH. Respiration helps balance the body pH by adjusting the extent and rate of carbon dioxide removal from the body.

Body temperature regulation

- Panting cools the body; inhaling warmed air heats the body.

Olfaction (sense of smell)

- Olfaction receptors are located in the upper respiratory tract. As air containing chemical 'smells' passes over them during inspiration these receptors sense the 'smell'.

Voice production (phonation)

Immunity

- This has a role in body defence via the alar fold and turbinates where the specialised epithelium traps dust, dirt and pathogens in mucus and wafts them out of the respiratory system.

Gaseous exchange facility

Respiration is the exchange of gases between an organism and its environment.

- External (organismic) respiration is the process of getting oxygen into the body and to the cells and removing from the body carbon dioxide from the cells
- Internal (cellular) respiration is a complex series of chemical reactions by which the cell breaks down fuel molecules, releasing carbon dioxide and energy which require oxygen (Figure 3.6).

Respiratory pigments

- These combine reversibly with oxygen
- They increase the capacity of blood to transport oxygen
- Haemoglobin is the respiratory pigment utilised in vertebrate species.

Physiological control of respiration

Figure 3.7 illustrates control of respiration.

Nervous control of respiration

The respiratory control centres are located in the pons and medulla oblongata and are thought to overlap in their control of respiratory function. Respiration is involuntary, although voluntary control can be initiated. The inspiratory centre is constantly being activated unless stimuli cause it to be inhibited. It is the inspiratory centre that initiates the neural impulse that travels to the respiratory muscles (intercostals, diaphragm) and causes these to contract.

As the lungs are stretched, stretch receptors in the elastic tissue are stimulated and this triggers an impulse to be sent along the vagus nerve to the expiratory centre of the brain. The expiratory centre in turn releases an impulse to the inspiratory centre, inhibiting its function. When the inhibitory effect is strong enough inspiration is interrupted, i.e. stopping the animal breathing in. This is known as the *Hering–Breuer reflex*. This establishes a cyclic pattern of respiration.

Chemical control of respiration

Chemical control centres upon partial pressure of gaseous agents found in the cardiovascular system – specifically carbon dioxide and oxygen. Partial pressure is the pressure exerted by a specific gas in a mixture of gases. The

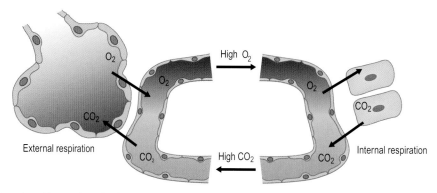

Figure 3.6 External and internal respiration.

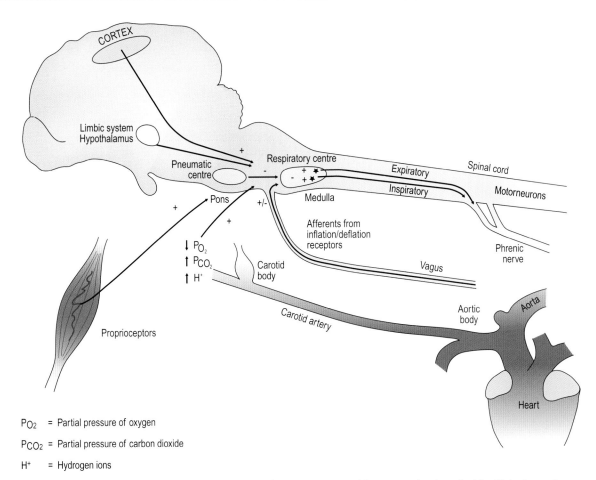

PO₂ = Partial pressure of oxygen

PCO₂ = Partial pressure of carbon dioxide

H⁺ = Hydrogen ions

Figure 3.7 Control of respiration. P_{O_2}, partial pressure of oxygen; P_{CO_2}, partial pressure of carbon dioxide; H⁺, hydrogen ions.

concentration of the gas dissolved in a liquid is proportional to the pressure of that gas in the fluid; therefore concentrations of gases in fluids are also expressed as partial pressures. The respiratory centres of the brain also respond to partial pressure of carbon dioxide and oxygen and directly influence respiration. There are peripheral chemoreceptors located in the carotid arteries and aortic arch, the *aortic* and *carotid bodies*, which monitor and respond to:

- Decreased partial pressure of oxygen (low blood concentration)
- Decreased perfusion rates (reduced flow of blood through vessels and to organs)
- Increased partial pressures of carbon dioxide (high concentrations in blood)
- Increased concentrations of hydrogen ions (acidaemia/acidosis).

In response the aortic and carotid bodies send impulses to the brain and initiate reactions within the respiratory centres. There are central chemoreceptors which lie in the brainstem and are more specifically sensitive to the pH of the cerebrospinal fluid and respond to increasing levels of carbon dioxide by increasing the respiration rate. The major contributory factor for altering respiratory rates and patterns is fluctuating levels of carbon dioxide. Oxygen levels only really affect the system when they reach critically low values.

Structure of mammalian respiratory systems

The respiratory tract is divided into the upper and lower portions.

The upper respiratory tract contains:

- External nares
- Nasal cavity with paranasal sinuses
- Pharynx, particularly nasopharynx and laryngopharynx

- Larynx
- Trachea.

The lower respiratory tract contains:

- Lungs – everything distal to the two main stem bronchi
- Bronchi
- Bronchioles
- Alveolar ducts
- Alveolar sacs
- Alveoli.

Respiratory tract anatomy

External nares

- These form openings for air to enter the respiratory system
- There are two comma-shaped alar folds of skin that cover the alar cartilages – the nostrils
- These protect the entrance to the nasal cavity from foreign bodies
- They open into the nasal cavity.

Nasal cavities

- These are also known as the internal nares
- These are paired into a right and left cavity. They are separated by a wall of cartilage, the nasal septum, which becomes bony as it progresses caudally
- Conchae (projections) extend from the lateral wall of each cavity, increasing the surface area air that travels over
- Surface area is important as the olfactory epithelium is located in the roof of the nasal cavity and contributes to the sense of smell.

Turbinates

- These are highly convoluted (twisted), very fragile bones which almost fill the nasal cavity
- Cavities have a mucous lining whose role is to trap dirt particles that have been inhaled
- The cilia move the mucus along to the back of the throat where it is swallowed with saliva
- Their function is to warm, filter and moisten air as it enters the respiratory tract.

Function of the nasal cavities

- Transfer of air to respiratory tract
- Warm and humidify inhaled air
- To trap particles from inhaled air, e.g. dust, pollen
- To transfer trapped particles via cilia currents and mucus to the pharynx to be swallowed.

Paranasal sinuses

- The nasal cavities connect to the nasal sinuses – small cavities in the bones of the skull filled with air
- They are lined with ciliated, mucous epithelium
- The frontal sinus is located above the eyes on either side of the midline, within the frontal bone
- The maxillary sinus is located within the maxilla on either side of the true nasal cavity
- Mucus from the sinuses drains into the nose (in allergies and colds)
- The function of the sinuses is unclear but they do:
  ○ Protect the orbit, nasal and cranial cavities
  ○ Reduce the weight of the head
  ○ Affect the resonance of the voice.

Pharynx

- Air continues from the internal nares across the pharynx
- This is the area at the back of the mouth utilised by both the respiratory and digestive tracts
- The nasal chamber, the mouth, the eustachian tubes, the oesophagus and the larynx open into the pharynx
- The pharynx enables air to be mouth-breathed to gain access to the respiratory tract
- It consists of three regions which interconnect with each other:
  1. Nasopharynx – where the pharynx connects to the nasal cavity: it begins at the caudal choana and the eustachian tube opens into the lateral wall (protected by flaps of mucosa-covered cartilage)
  2. Oropharynx – portion of the pharynx which connects to the oral cavity; it contains tonsils and the bony hard palate extends caudally as the soft palate to separate the oropharynx from the nasopharynx
  3. Laryngopharynx – portion which lies over, under and around the larynx; it communicates with the larynx at the glottis cranially and with the oesophageal opening caudally
- Functions of the pharynx:
  ○ Nasopharynx conveys air to larynx
  ○ Oropharynx conveys food/liquid to laryngopharynx (over the epiglottis) when swallowing
  ○ Laryngopharynx conveys food/water if swallowing or air if breathing
  ○ Auditory tube (eustachian tube) adjusts pressure on both sides of the tympanic membrane (eardrum)
  ○ Tonsils – lymphoid tissue.

Larynx

- The larynx is a rigid, hollow structure constructed from cartilage
- It is the opening to the lower respiratory tract
- It comprises the single epiglottis cartilage, paired arytenoid cartilages, single thyroid cartilage and single cricoid cartilage plus muscles and mucous membrane
- It is attached to the skull by the hyoid apparatus which allows it to move forward and backward in a swinging motion
- It contains the vocal cords. These are folds of epithelium that vibrate and produce sound as air passes over them. They are found in the lumen of the larynx. Pitch can be determined by the attached muscles varying the tension of the vocal cords
- The epiglottis is the first of the laryngeal cartilages. It is a piece of elastic cartilage that covers the entrance of the respiratory tract during swallowing
- The glottis is the opening into the larynx
- Swallowing causes the larynx to swing forward, pulling the epiglottis over the glottis. As the larynx moves back the epiglottis falls forward and the glottis is open again, allowing passage of air
- The epiglottis is triangular and lies above the soft palate when in the resting position (it is often seen during intubation)
- Foreign material contained in inspired air will initiate the cough reflex when it touches the larynx.

Trachea

- Air leaves the larynx and enters the trachea
- This is a permanently open tube which begins at the laryngeal cartilage and runs through the thoracic inlet where it divides at the bifurcation into left and right bronchi
- It is kept from collapsing by incomplete rings of hyaline cartilage (on the dorsal aspect) separated by fibrous connective tissue and smooth-muscle fibres
- It is lined with ciliated mucous epithelium
- It needs to be supported open as air contained within it will be at a lower pressure than atmospheric air during inspiration
- The trachea lies in the ventral neck along the midline with the oesophagus on its left
- It divides into two cartilaginous bronchi at the level of rib 1.

Bronchus (bronchi)

- This is a large airway formed by the bifurcation of the trachea
- One bronchus goes to each lung

- They are similar in structure to the trachea, comprising cartilage and smooth muscle
- They are lined by ciliated mucous epithelium
- When the bronchus enters the lobes of the lung it divides into smaller bronchi and eventually gives rise to tiny bronchioles.

Bronchioles

- The bronchioles are narrower than bronchi and contain only smooth muscle in the wall and no cartilage
- Bronchioles branch repeatedly into smaller passageways throughout the lung tissue
- Eventually they give rise to clusters of alveoli
- Cilia lining the respiratory tract move foreign particles back up the tract to the pharynx to be swallowed
- Terminal bronchiole is a very thin smooth-muscle wall
- Respiratory bronchiole is an intermittent smooth-muscle wall broken up by communication with alveolar ducts.

Alveolar ducts

- The alveolar ducts are a long dilated tube which opens off the respiratory bronchiole and on to many alveolar sacs
- Some smooth muscle may be found in the walls.

Alveolar sacs

- The alveolar sacs are chambers/sacs on to which several pulmonary alveoli open.

Pulmonary alveolus (alveoli)

- This is where gases are exchanged
- They are only one cell thick to facilitate diffusion of gases and are lined with pulmonary membrane
- They are coated with a surfactant of phospholipid that lowers the surface tension within them, allowing easier dilation
- Each alveolus is encapsulated within a capillary network
- Only two membranes separate air from alveolus – the epithelium of alveolar wall and endothelium of capillary wall (both are only one cell thick and ideal for diffusion to occur)
- They are perfect for diffusion as they have a high surface area
- Alveolar macrophages remove dust and potential pathogens
- Certain drugs and hormones are metabolised and excreted by the alveoli (Figure 3.8).

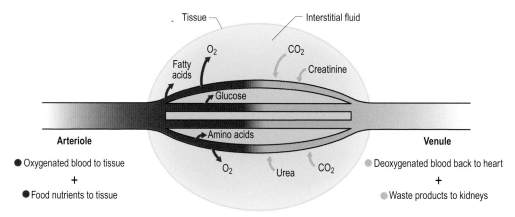

Figure 3.8 Oxygen and carbon dioxide transfer in the capillary bed.

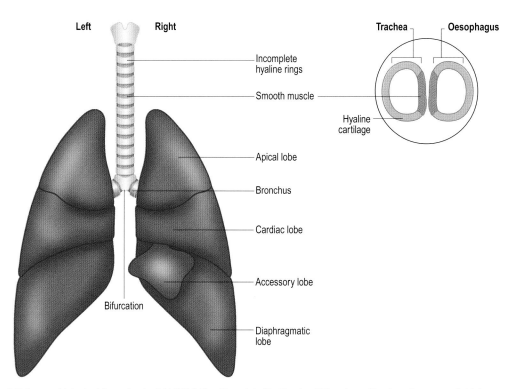

Figure 3.9 Lungs. (Adapted from Aspinall V 2006 *The Complete Textbook of Veterinary Nursing*. Butterworth Heinemann, London, with permission.)

Lungs (Figure 3.9)

- These large, paired organs occupy the thoracic cavity, one lying on either side of the mediastinum
- Each lung is divided into several lobes:
  - Right lung – cranial, caudal, middle and accessory
  - Left lung – cranial and caudal

- They are covered by a layer of smooth epithelium – the visceral pleura
- The space between the pleura lining the thorax and the pleura lining the lung is known as the pleural cavity
- It is covered by a film of fluid to reduce friction during breathing

- Pleurisy is inflammation of the pleura
- All structures are supported by connective tissue rich in elastic fibres
- They have a vast surface area for gas exchange (in humans, the equivalent of one tennis court)
- Branches of the pulmonary artery and vein follow the bronchi in and out of the lung lobes to provide support for gaseous exchange; the lung's blood supply is provided by the broncho-oesophageal artery.

Mechanism of respiration

Breathing is the mechanical process of taking air into the lungs (*inspiration*) and letting it out again (*expiration*). Oxygen needs to be continuously available.

Mammals have the ability to control movement of the ribs, chest muscles and diaphragm and hence can control the volume of the chest cavity. The main muscles are the intercostal muscles between the ribs and the diaphragm – a flat sheet of muscle that separates the thoracic cavity from the abdominal cavity.

Lung tissue contains no muscle tissue itself, but is very elastic and will spring back to its collapsed state when not filled with air. The intrathoracic pressure inside a normal thoracic cavity is always more negative (less) than atmospheric pressure, giving a partial vacuum within the thorax. Negative intrathoracic pressure is needed for breathing as it pulls the lungs tightly out against the thoracic wall and keeps them inflated.

Inspiration

- Breathe in
- Thoracic cavity volume increases
- The diaphragm contracts and flattens caudally
- The ribs move outwards (cranially and slightly dorsally) as external intercostal muscles contract, increasing the diameter of the thorax
- As the thorax expands the pleura pulls the lung tissue out along with the chest walls, increasing the volume of each lung
- In the lungs air molecules have more space to move about and air pressure decreases to make intrathoracic pressure more negative (even lower than atmospheric air)
- Air from outside rushes in to equalise the pressure within the lungs
- In the resting animal there is a 75% change in volume due to diaphragmatic movement; during exercise the role of the ribs/intercostals increases intrathoracic capacity
- Also during inspiration abductor muscles in the larynx open the glottis to allow air into the trachea whilst the alar cartilages move to dilate the nostrils

- Increase in potential space in the thorax allows expansion of lungs, aided by elastic fibres, production of surfactant to reduce surface tension and the serous membrane (pleura) of the thoracic cavity and covering lungs allow friction-free movement
- Compliance is the 'stretchability' of the lungs.

Expiration

- Diaphragm relaxes
- The internal intercostal muscles relax, returning ribs to their normal position
- The chest cavity volume decreases, simultaneously increasing air pressure in the lungs (intrathoracic pressure becomes less negative)
- Distended alveoli return to their normal size, expelling air that was inhaled and returning air pressure to equilibrium
- Glottis and nostrils both close.

Exchange of gases

- Oxygen diffuses into capillaries; carbon dioxide diffuses into air in the alveoli
- Oxygen binds with haemoglobin molecules in blood and is transported to cells for use as oxyhaemoglobin (which is bright scarlet in colour).

Factors that affect respiration

A number of factors can affect an animal's respiratory rate (Table 3.2) and should be considered when measuring respiration as a clinical tool or during the management of animal collections. Exercise will result in an increased respiratory effort in the short term but as an animal's fitness increases then the difference from the resting respiratory rate with exercise will reduce. Other factors which can increase rate and depth of respiration include stress, disease and environmental conditions. External temperature and humidity can influence breathing, e.g. on a hot and humid day the respiratory rate would be increased. Young animals tend to have faster respiratory rates than their adult counterparts.

Table 3.2 Normal respiratory rates	
Dog	15–30 breaths/minute
Cat	20–30 breaths/minute
Rabbit	38–65 breaths/minute
Horse	8–15 breaths/minute

Species variation – respiratory system

In birds air enters via the nostrils on the beak into the nasal chambers through a cleft called the choana into the oral cavity. The trachea enlarges just above the sternum into the syrinx, then splits into two bronchi which enter the lungs. There are numerous air sacs which do not allow gaseous exchange but can act as an air reservoir. The bronchi eventually subdivide into parabronchi then terminal air capillaries where oxygen and carbon dioxide are exchanged. Reptiles have lungs but no diaphragm present and snakes have one functional right lung and a vestigial left lung. The anterior of the right lung is where gas exchange occurs and the remainder can act as an air store.

Bibliography

Aspinall V 2006 The complete textbook of veterinary nursing. Butterworth Heinemann, London

Aspinall V, O'Reilly M 2004 Introduction to veterinary anatomy and physiology. Butterworth Heinemann, Oxford

Campbell N, Reece J, Mitchell L 1999 Biology, 5th edn. Benjamin Cummings, San Francisco

Colville T, Bassett J M 2002 Clinical anatomy and physiology for veterinary technicians. Mosby, St Louis

Dyke K M, Sack W O, Wensing C J G 1996 Text book of veterinary anatomy, 2nd edn. W B Saunders, Philadelphia

Green N P O, Stout G W, Taylor D J 1991 Biological science. Cambridge University Press, Cambridge

Lane D R, Cooper B, Turner L 2007 BSAVA Textbook of Veterinary Nursing. BSAVA, Oxford

Moore M 2000 Manual of veterinary nursing. BSAVA, Oxford

Pratt P W 1998 Principles and practice of veterinary technology. Mosby, Philadelphia

Roberts M B V 1986 Biology: a functional approach. Nelson, Surrey, UK

Simpson G 1994 Practical veterinary nursing, 3rd edn. BSAVA, Oxford

Chapter | 4 | Jane Williams

Digestive and lymphatic systems

This chapter outlines the major components of the mammalian digestive system with consideration of ruminant variation. The response of the animal body to pathogenic attack is considered with respect to the immune system and the role the lymphatic system plays in the maintenance of health.

DIGESTIVE SYSTEM

The digestive system varies between animal species depending upon their nutritional habits. The function of the digestive system is to provide the body with useable energy that it has obtained from the breakdown of food-stuffs ingested and the end products of digestion for the reparation and growth of body tissue.

The digestive system comprises the following parts:

- Mouth, teeth, tongue and lips
- Pharynx
- Oesophagus
- Stomach
- In ruminants: rumen, omasum, abomasum and reticulum
- Small intestine – duodenum, jejunum and ileum
- Large intestine – caecum, colon, rectum and anus.

Functions of the digestive system

- Ingestion: take food/liquid into the body by swallowing
- Digestion: the physiological act of breaking down food into a form that can be absorbed and used or excreted
- Absorption: the physiological passage of materials through the lining of the intestine into the blood
- Metabolism: the series of chemical reactions that provide energy and nutrients that living organisms require to stay alive
- Excretion: act or process of discharging waste matter from tissues/organs.

The digestive system requires the following organs or glands to function effectively:

- Salivary glands (salivary amylase for carbohydrate digestion)
- Pancreas (produces enzymes that aid digestion)
- Liver
- Gallbladder.

Non-ruminant digestive system
Mouth, teeth, tongue and lips

All teeth have a similar structure. They have a sensitive centre, the pulp cavity, which contains the blood and nervous supply for the tooth. This is surrounded by the dentine and then the enamel which is the shiny white covering most visible in the mouth. Each tooth is firmly rooted into a depression, or alveolus, in the maxilla or mandible by a sticky substance called cementum and further held in place by the periodontal ligament. Only the enamel outer covering of the tooth is visible above

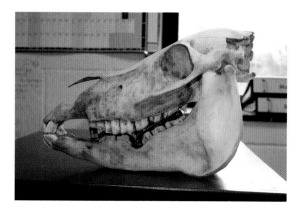

Figure 4.1 Equine skull showing dentition.

the gingival membrane. Figure 4.1 shows equine dentition.

Tooth shape and function

There are three types of tooth:

1. Incisors
2. Canines
3. Molars, including:
   - Premolars
   - Carnassials
   - Molars.

Incisors

- These are found at the front of the jaw
- They are usually small and pointed with a single root
- They are used for fine nibbling and grazing
- In rodent and lagomorph species they are 'open-rooted', i.e. they grow continuously.

Canines

- These are curved teeth with a single root
- There is one on each side of the upper and the lower jaw in carnivore species
- They are used for holding prey firmly in the mouth and to administer puncture wounds during hunting.

Premolars

- These have a flatter surface
- They have several cusps
- They normally have two or three roots
- The shape varies between carnivorous and herbivorous species; they are used for tearing flesh in carnivores and for grinding in herbivores.

Carnassial

- This is the largest tooth in the jaw
- It is the first lower molar and last upper premolar
- It is primarily used for cutting and shearing.

Molars

- These have a similar structure to premolars but are larger with three roots
- They are used for shearing or grinding depending upon species.

Teeth

Dogs, cats and horses have two sets of teeth during their lives:

- Milk or 'baby' teeth: deciduous teeth
- Permanent teeth: these replace the deciduous teeth.

Looking at teeth can provide an approximation of age in animals.

Dental formulae for dog
Upper/lower per side

Permanent I3/3 C1/1 PM 4/4 M2/3
Total = above × 2 = 42 teeth
Deciduous I3/3 C1/1 PM 3/3
Total = above × 2 = 28 teeth

Dental formulae for cat

Permanent I 3/3 C 1/1 PM 3/2 M 1/1
Total = above × 2 = 30 teeth
Deciduous I 3/3 C 1/1 PM 3/2
Total = above × 2 = 26 teeth

The oral cavity

Functions include:

- Picking up food
- Breaking food into small boluses to facilitate swallowing
- Lubricating the food bolus to enable ease of swallowing.

The tongue

- The tongue is a muscular organ that is situated on the floor of the oral cavity. It comprises striated muscle and is attached to the hyoid apparatus by the root and is incredibly dexterous
- It is covered by a layer of mucous membrane. It has a dense dorsal surface comprising papillae which provide a rough surface to aid grooming and the formulation of the food bolus

- The sublingual artery and vein are located on the ventral surface of the tongue. They can be utilised during anaesthesia to administer drugs, in venepuncture or for monitoring the pulse
- The tongue aids ingestion of food
- It contains tastebuds, which are specialised cells that 'sense' different sensations: sweet, salt, bitter, sour. This allows taste or gustation to occur. This is an important aspect of digestion as in some species if the food is not appetising it can lead to inappetance
- It aids in the formation of the food bolus by muscular action
- It is used for self-/allogrooming in some species
- It plays a role in thermoregulation. For example, panting helps reduce body temperature
- It helps produce vocalisation in conjunction with vocal cords and larynx.

Salivary glands

Table 4.1 lists the names and locations of the salivary glands.

- These consist of paired glands, one on each side of the head: the zygomatic, sublingual and mandibular salivary glands
- Their function is to secrete saliva
- Saliva comprises 99% water and 1% mucus
- Saliva contains salivary amylase in omnivores and herbivores. This is an enzyme which begins to digest starch (carbohydrate) and aids in the lubrication of the food bolus, but this is not the case in the dog and cat.

The pharynx

- The pharynx links the oral cavity and the oesophagus
- It has a shared function with both the gastrointestinal tract and the respiratory tract
- It plays an important role in the mechanics of swallowing

Table 4.1 Location of the salivary glands	
Zygomatic	Near the eye, beneath the orbit
Sublingual	Medial to the mandible, under the mucous membrane of the ventral tongue surface
Mandibular	Caudal to the point of the mandible
Parotid	Cranial to the mandibular salivary glands but underneath the ear

- It prevents food entering the trachea and air entering the oesophagus
- The soft palate, situated on the dorsal surface of the oral cavity, divides the pharynx into the oropharynx (communication with the oral cavity) and nasopharynx (communication with the nasal cavity)
- The pharynx contains lymphoid tissue known as the tonsils which play a role in an animal's defence mechanisms against pathogens
- The epiglottis, an elastic cartilage flap, is stimulated to close when the food bolus is passed to the back of the oropharynx, thus preventing food entering the larynx and the respiratory system
- Once the bolus has been swallowed the epiglottis flips back, exposing the larynx and trachea
- The bolus is swallowed or deglutinated and a wave of muscular contraction or peristalsis continues the food's passage into the oesophagus.

The oesophagus

- This is located caudal to the trachea and follows approximately the same path
- It enters the stomach via the cardiac sphincter
- It comprises a smooth-muscle tube which has the capacity to expand when a food bolus is present. It sits behind the trachea in the section where the hyaline rings are incomplete, which also allows for it to expand without compromising respiratory function
- The lining is stratified squamous epithelium as it is subject to damage as the boluses pass along it
- There are mucous glands present on the lining to aid lubrication
- The food bolus is moved along its length via peristalsis
- It passes through the diaphragm via the oesophageal hiatus.

Stomach

Figure 4.2 illustrates the canine digestive system.

- The stomach is a sac-like organ
- In the dog and cat it is simple and monogastric, i.e. it is made up of one compartment
- The function of the stomach is to act as a food store, to break up food, to introduce digestive enzymes and to begin protein digestion
- It is located on the left-hand side of the cranial abdomen and consists of four parts:
  1. Cardia, which controls the entry of food (cardiac sphincter)
  2. Fundus, which secretes gastric juices and mucus

47

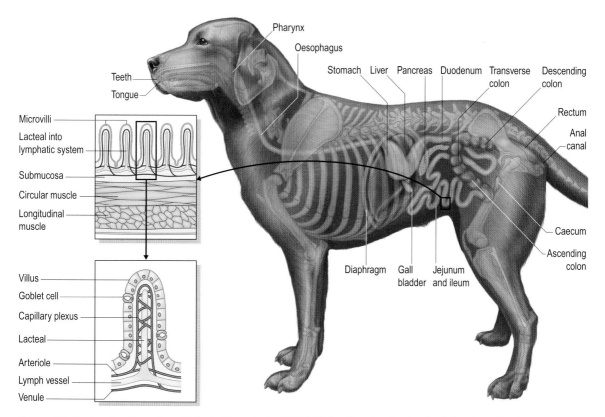

Figure 4.2 Canine digestive system. (Adapted from Aspinall V 2006 *The Complete Textbook of Veterinary Nursing.* Butterworth Heinemann, London, with permission.)

3. Corpus (body), the continuation of the fundus
4. Pylorus, where mucus and gastrin are secreted; this joins the duodenum

- The stomach is coated in a visceral peritoneum or mesentery; the layer on the inner curve of the fundus is called the lesser omentum and that on the outer curve is the greater omentum
- Within the folds of the greater omentum the spleen can be found
- The pyloric sphincter controls the passage of chyme (partially digested food) out of the stomach
- The function of the stomach is to begin digestion by mixing food and gastric juices to produce chyme.

Stomach contents are produced within gastric pits in the stomach mucosa:

- Hydrochloric acid is secreted from parietal cells in the fundus; it protects from harmful bacteria, denatures protein before digestion and provides an acidic pH which is essential for pepsin to work effectively
- Mucus is secreted from goblet cells; it lubricates food and protects against self-digestion

- Pepsinogen is secreted from chief cells in the fundus; this enzyme starts to digest proteins
- The result is chyme, which is a mixture of partially digested food plus digestive juices and is acidic
- Food can return from the stomach to the mouth via regurgitation, reflux and vomiting.

Small intestine

- The small intestine comprises three parts: the duodenum, the jejunum and the ileum
- Its main function is digestion and absorption of nutrients, and it is here that the majority of enzymatic digestion occurs.

Duodenum

- Located on the right-hand side of the abdomen, the duodenum is a u-shaped tube
- It incorporates the pancreas, which lies inside the 'u'
- The presence of chyme (and the sight, smell and taste of food) stimulates production of pancreatic juices

and bile which are added to the partially digested food via the bile duct and pancreatic duct

- Bile and pancreatic juices are alkaline, therefore they neutralise the acidity of the chyme and provide a suitable environment for the multitude of digestive enzymes, secreted from Brunner glands, to begin to work.

Jejunum/ileum

- It is difficult to establish morphologically the two distinct sections
- They make up a long mobile tube which loops around the abdominal cavity filling the peritoneum
- The walls contain crypts of Lieberkühn which secrete digestive enzymes
- The ileum ends at the ileosacral junction where it joins the caecum
- The tube is invaginated to increase surface area and is lined with villi which incorporate lacteals
- The products of fat, protein and carbohydrate digestion are absorbed into the blood stream via the lacteals
- Chyme continues to move along via peristalsis towards the colon.

Remember that nutrients break down to their basic components:

- Fats break down into fatty acids and glycerol
- Carbohydrates/sugars break down into simple sugars
- Proteins break down to amino acids.

Absorption

- Absorption occurs in the walls of the villi: amino acids and simple sugars are absorbed into the blood capillaries and then transported to the liver via the hepatic portal vein
- The lacteals absorb the products of lipid digestion – glycerol and fatty acids
- These go into the lymphatic system as a milky substance called chyle (note: don't confuse chyle with chyme!) and are returned to the systemic circulation via a lymphatic duct.

Role of the gallbladder and the pancreas

- The exocrine section of the pancreas secretes digestive enzymes and bicarbonate (which aids in the production of an alkaline environment) into the duodenum through the pancreatic duct
- The gallbladder is located in the folds of the liver; bile produced in the liver drains into the gallbladder, which acts as a bile reservoir

- Bile is a green colour due to the presence of bilirubin, a byproduct of erythrocyte destruction in the liver
- Bile contains bile salts which are needed for fat digestion
- It is secreted into the duodenum along the common bile duct.

Pancreatic juice consists of:

- Bicarbonate, which neutralises acid and creates a beneficial alkaline environment
- Trypsinogen, which acts with enterokinase to form trypsin, used in protein digestion
- Lipases, which are activated by bile salts, used in fat digestion
- Amylases, which act on carbohydrate, used in carbohydrate digestion
- Maltase, sucrase and lactase convert sugars to glucose
- Aminopeptidase breaks down peptides to amino acids.

Large intestine

- The remaining contents pass along the caecum and into the colon then the rectum
- At this stage only indigestible material and fluid remain
- Water is reabsorbed into the body in the colon
- The caecum has no role in carnivore digestion but in herbivores it is a site of fermentation by microbes to break down grass.

Colon

- The colon consists of three parts (which describe the location in the abdomen of each part):
  1. Ascending colon
  2. Transverse colon
  3. Descending colon
- The function of the colon is to absorb water and electrolytes, then push the remaining waste into the rectum by peristalsis
- The lining is folded and contains goblet cells to produce mucus for lubrication
- There is a commensal bacterial population to help degrade the remaining undigested food.

Rectum

- There is a short conclusion to the rectum; it is located in the pelvis
- Its function is to store semisolid faeces before defecation
- It terminates in the anal canal

- This has two anal sphincters: an internal and external sphincter
- The internal sphincter is smooth muscle which is under involuntary control where the external sphincter is striated muscle which is under voluntary control, allowing some control of toilet habits
- There are also anal glands which produce a sticky substance containing pheromones that coat the faeces and are thought to play a role in communication.

The process concludes when the animal defecates, passing the faeces, the indigestible remnants of digestion.

The liver

The liver is the largest organ in the body. It is located in the cranial abdomen in close proximity to the stomach, duodenum and right kidney. It is divided into several lobes or folds surrounding the falciform ligament (the remnants of the fetal umbilical blood supply). The gallbladder is situated in the lobes near the centre of the liver. The hepatic portal vein concludes in the liver, bringing the end products of carbohydrate digestion glucose to the liver. The hepatocytes or liver cells receive the glucose molecules and use them for metabolism.

Functions of the liver

- Carbohydrate metabolism – conversion of excess glucose to glycogen and vice versa when required
- Protein metabolism – producing plasma proteins, combining amino acids to make new proteins for growth and repair
- Deamination – removal of surplus amino acids by changing them to ammonia then to urea which is excreted in the urine
- Fat metabolism – conversion of fatty acids and glycerol into phospholipids to be used or for storage as excess fat
- The liver creates bile and stores it in the gallbladder
- It destroys old erythrocytes
- It creates new erythrocytes
- It acts as a vitamin store for fat-soluble vitamins A, D, E and K
- Storage of iron
- It plays a role in thermoregulation
- Detoxification of substances, e.g. steroid hormones and drugs.

PROCESS OF DIGESTION

Figure 4.3 illustrates the digestion process.

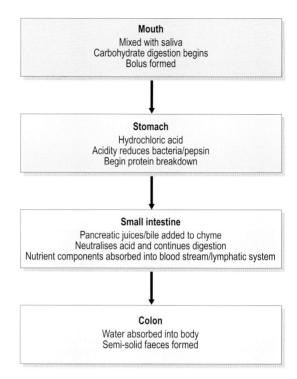

Figure 4.3 Process of digestion.

Digestive enzymes

- Trypsin: converts protein into amino acids
- Amylase, maltase, sucrase and fructose: convert carbohydrates and complex sugars into simple sugars and glucose
- Bile salts and lipase: convert fats into glycerol and fatty acids
- The gastrointestinal tract comprises:
  - Oral cavity
  - Pharynx
  - Oesophagus
  - Stomach
  - Small intestine
  - Large intestine
- Digestion requires each component to function effectively and enzymatic action to be successfully achieved.

Ruminant digestion

In ruminants, e.g. cattle, food passes through three forestomachs before arriving at the true stomach (Figure 4.4). The forestomachs comprise the rumen, the reticulum and the omasum, with the true stomach being called the abomasum. The oesophagus communicates

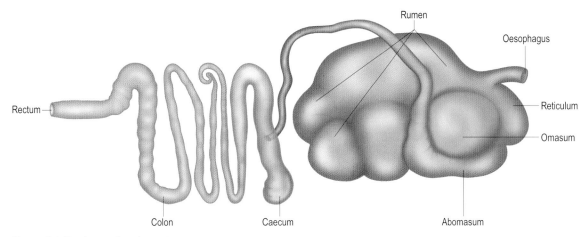

Figure 4.4 Ruminant digestive system.

directly with the largest forestomach, the rumen; the rumen is the site of microbial fermentation to break down the complex cellulose that forage contains. From here the food enters the reticulum, which is the smallest chamber and is lined with honeycomb-like folds that trap foreign materials and also further ferment the foodstuffs. Food can move freely between the rumen and the reticulum. The omasum is the final chamber: this is lined by muscular folds which grind the food further and is also a site of water absorption. The food finally enters the true stomach or abomasum, which is the equivalent of the stomach in a monogastric animal and has the same functions.

Ruminant animals exhibit different mastication patterns to monogastric animals; when they graze the food is chopped and lightly chewed. It enters the rumen and is regurgitated and chewed thoroughly approximately 40–50 times and then reswallowed. This process is called rumination or chewing the cud. In cattle up to 8 hours per day can be spent ruminating; a side-effect of this process is the production of gases (methane and carbon dioxide). Eructation or belching must take place to remove these gases or a life-threatening condition called bloat can occur.

Species variation – digestive system

Some herbivore species such as the rabbit are monogastric hindgut fermenters. The basic anatomy of the digestive tract is the same as that of the dog but the caecum is enlarged. The caecum has a large surface area and is responsible for microbial fermentation to digest or break down the tougher plant material ingested. In rabbits hard faeces will be passed within 4 hours of ingestion

but softer, more fluid faeces will remain in the digestive tract and be passed back through the caecum where enzymatic microbial digestion occurs again. The soft faeces or caecotrophs are excreted and ingested by the rabbit (coprophagy or caecotrophy); the caecotroph is protected by a layer of mucus so is not affected by the digestive processes in the stomach, thus allowing the dense fibrous material they contain to be digested twice and maintain healthy digestive tract function.

The horse's diet comprises mainly forage materials such as grass, hay or haylage. Unlike ruminant species it is incapable of rumination but must still break down the complex cellulose fibres present in its diet. The horse must effectively chew the food before swallowing and produces copious amounts of saliva to aid this process. The colon and caecum are enlarged and act as areas of microbial digestion. Horses cannot vomit or regurgitate so any gas which is produced must escape via the digestive tract as they cannot belch; horses will only digest the equivalent of 85% of forage when compared to a similar amount in a ruminant (Figure 4.5).

Birds' digestive tracts have an additional diverticulum off the oesophagus – the crop; the crop can be used for food storage. Birds' stomachs are divided into two parts: the proventriculus and the gizzard. The proventriculus begins protein digestion and the gizzard grinds up food and may contain grit to aid this process. The digestive system ends at the cloaca which is shared with the urinary and reproductive systems. The coprodeum (anterior) receives faeces, the urodeum (middle) collects urogenital discharges and the proctodeum (posterior) collects and stores substances from al three systems prior to defecation through the anus. Reptiles' and snakes' digestive tracts also end in the cloaca.

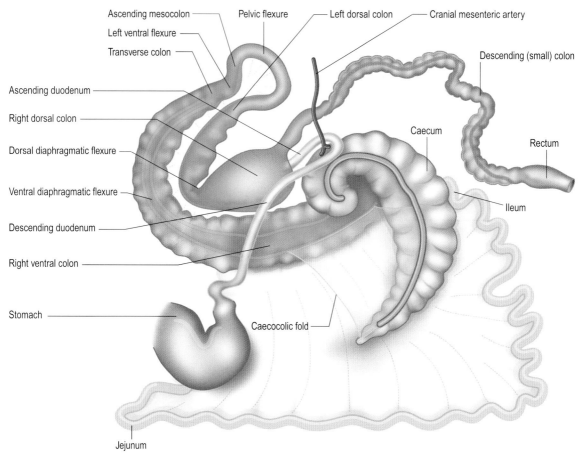

Figure 4.5 Equine digestive tract. (Reproduced from Aspinall V 2006 *The Complete Textbook of Veterinary Nursing.* Butterworth Heinemann, London, with permission.)

LYMPHATIC SYSTEM

Tissue fluid is the fluid that has leaked from the capillary bed into the surrounding tissue.

Some tissue fluid is returned to capillaries by osmosis but it still leaves a deficit that needs to be removed from the tissues and returned to the circulation (or blood volume would decrease). The lymphatic system is a system of vessels that return tissue fluid to the circulation. Lymph is the fluid within the lymphatic vessels (Figure 4.6).

Functions of the lymphatic system

- To return excess tissue fluid to circulation
- To filter bacteria and foreign antigens out of fluid in the lymph nodes
- To produce lymphocytes
- To transport digested food (particularly fat).

The lymphatic system consists of:

- Lymphatic capillaries
- Lymphatic vessels
- Lymphatic tissues (spleen and lymph nodes)
- Lymphatic ducts.

Lymphatic capillaries

These are a series of fine channels that collect tissue fluid; they join together to form lymph vessels. Lymphatic capillaries are also found in the villi of the ileum where they are known as lacteals. The lacteals absorb fatty acids and glycerol from digested fat in the intestine and transport it to the cisterna chyli as minute fat droplets, then to the thoracic duct and back to the blood stream.

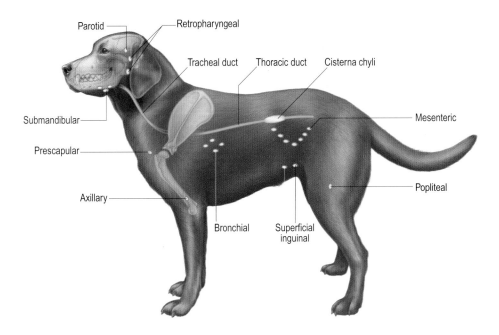

Figure 4.6 Location of lymphatic glands, lymphatic ducts and lymphoid tissue.

Lymphatic vessels

Lymphatic vessels have a similar structure to veins: they have thin walls with valves distributed throughout their length. The walls contain no smooth muscle and the passage of the lymphatic fluid requires the 'milking' or contraction of surrounding tissues to push the fluid along the vessel past the non-return valves. Lymph vessels are numerous in the body tissues.

Lymphatic nodes

The lymphatic vessels return the lymph to the circulation via the lymph nodes. Lymph nodes are collections of lymphocytes joined together by connective tissue. Afferent vessels always enter lymph nodes, regardless of the side of entry; there is one efferent vessel that leaves the lymph node from the same location, the hilus. Lymph nodes serve to filter bacteria and antigens from the lymphatic fluid and also produce lymphocytes. Each node is surrounded by a connective tissue capsule – the trabecula. The node consists of cortical and medullary regions which have different functions. The cortex produces lymphocytes from lymph nodules whilst the medulla contains a network of sinuses packed full of phagocytic cells to filter pathogens.

Lymph nodes are located at various sites throughout body (Table 4.2), mainly at the proximal end of the limbs and body portals, usually where the inside meets the outside, e.g. the groin. Some lymph nodes are pal-

Table 4.2 Location of lymph nodes	
Submandibular nodes	Group of 2–5 nodes below the jaw bone
Parotid node	Caudal to temporomandibular joint of the jaw
Superficial cervical nodes or prescapular nodes	One is located on the cranial aspect of the scapula
Superficial inguinal nodes	Two nodes situated on each side of the groin
Popliteal node	Caudal to stifle joint

(Reproduced from Aspinall V 2006 *The Complete Textbook of Veterinary Nursing*. Butterworth Heinemann, London, with permission.)

pable in normal animals but they are normally easier to palpate when infection or disease is present.

Lymph nodes in the animal body

- Submandibular lymph node
- Prescapular lymph node
- Axillary lymph node
- Bronchial lymph node
- Mesenteric lymph nodes

- Popliteal lymph nodes
- Superficial inguinal lymph nodes
- Retropharyngeal lymph nodes
- Parotid lymph nodes.

Lymphatic ducts

The lymphatic fluid enters one of two lymphatic ducts after it travels through the lymph nodes. The smaller right lymphatic duct drains the right forelimb and right-hand side of the head and neck, whilst the larger left lymphatic duct drains the whole of the rest of the body. The left lymphatic duct is known as the cisterna chyli whilst it is in the abdomen, collecting all lymph; then it becomes the thoracic duct after it crosses the diaphragm via the aortic hiatus where it drains the left-hand side of the upper body. Both right and left lymphatic ducts empty into either the right jugular vein or the right vena cava. There are also two smaller tracheal ducts that aid in drainage of lymph from the head and neck.

Lymphatic tissue

Lymphatic tissue is also found in the spleen, tonsils and thymus.

Spleen

The spleen is located in the abdomen next to the greater curvature of the stomach. It is not essential to life and can be surgically removed (splenectomy). Its functions are storage of erythrocytes, destruction of erythrocytes, production of lymphocytes and phagocytosis of bacteria and foreign antigens.

Tonsils

The tonsils are located in the pharynx, near the root of the tongue in the tonsillar fossae. They are easily seen when enlarged and act as the primary defence in the oral cavity against pathogens.

Thymus

The thymus is located in the anterior part of the thoracic cavity. Its function is to produce T lymphocytes in the first few months of life. After this it shrinks and the lymphoid tissue is replaced by fat. T lymphocytes play an important role in cell-mediated immunity.

IMMUNITY

A pathogen is a disease-causing organism and an antigen is a foreign protein. The body's defence system will react to the presence of either of these and will trigger a range of defence mechanisms to counteract the invaders.

The body has two types of self-defence mechanism:

1. Non-specific: activates against a multitude of foreign organisms
2. Specific: activates against a particular entity or pathogen.

Non-specific defence mechanisms include phagocytosis and inflammatory responses. Specific defence mechanisms are grouped together as immune responses. Immune derives from the Latin word meaning safe and immune responses are tailor-made by the body to target specific pathogens and are therefore highly effective and keep the body safe.

Immunology is the study of specific defence mechanisms.

Requirements of an immune system

An immune system must have the ability to distinguish between itself and non-self, i.e. the body's own cells and pathogens. Every organism is biochemically unique and there are macromolecules embedded into the cell membranes which enable cells from the same organism to recognise each other. There are two types of immunity: innate immunity and acquired immunity. Innate immunity is inherited from the parents and will vary according to genetic factors and is characterised by physical barriers and the inflammatory response. Acquired immunity or specific immunity is the process which occurs whenever an animal encounters a pathogen throughout its life.

Invertebrates

These animals tend to react to invasion by non-specific immune responses such as phagocytosis and an inflammatory response. Some have haemolymph, which contains non-specific substances that kill bacteria, e.g. coelomocytes (amoeba-type organism).

Particles too large for phagocytosis can be encapsulated and contained in this manner.

Vertebrates

These tend to be more complex organisms and they produce specific and non-specific immune responses in response to pathogens. They have more sophisticated defence mechanisms, enabled by the presence of a specialised lymphatic system.

Non-specific defence mechanisms

These are the first line of defence and can be as simple as the outer covering of the organism, e.g. skin. Commensal bacteria inhabit the skin, inhibiting 'bad' bacteria from colonising the skin, but these can gain an upper hand in times of stress or illness, leading to skin infections. The skin also acts as a barrier to pathogens. The mucous lining of the respiratory tract also serves to remove foreign pathogens; acidity within the gastrointestinal tract can destroy pathogens by acidity and enzymes. If a pathogen makes it into the tissues, further mechanisms are then activated. Interferons are a special type of protein that stimulate other cells to produce antiviral proteins and become natural killer cells, which kill cells that have been altered by a virus or bacterium.

Barriers to invasion

- Skin
- Mucous membranes
- Hairs
- Secretions.

Phagocytosis

- Phagocytic cells, e.g. neutrophils, will speed to the infected area
- Pseudopodia extend from the cell and engulf the pathogen/antigen
- The cell completely surrounds the antigen; the membrane breaks off and leaves the antigen/pathogen within a vacuole
- The vacuole containing the pathogen is called a phagosome
- Lysosomes adhere to the vacuole; these digest the membrane and the bacterium
- Neutrophils can phagocytise >20 bacteria before being inactivated
- Macrophages can phagocytise > 100 bacteria before being inactivated
- The phagocytic cells are eventually inactivated by the lysosome enzymes spilling into the cytoplasm of the cell and self-digesting it.

Inflammation

- A pathogen invading tissue stimulates an inflammatory response
- The blood vessels in the local area dilate, thereby increasing blood flow, which is why skin often looks red or feels warm when infection is present
- Capillaries become more permeable in the area, which allows more fluid into the tissues from the circulation
- This leads to oedema (fluid swelling) as the volume of interstitial fluid increases
- The oedema causes pain characteristic of inflammation as the swelling presses on pain receptors in the localised area, stimulating the nervous system pain response
- The increased blood flow brings lots of phagocytic cells (neutrophils then monocytes) to begin to fight the infection.

Specific defence mechanisms

Non-specific mechanisms can be thought to 'hold the fort' for the animal whilst the specific defence mechanisms are mobilised. Immune responses require several days to activate. There are two main types:

1. Cell-mediated immunity: lymphocytes attack pathogen directly
2. Antibody-mediated immunity: lymphocytes produce antibodies to attack pathogen.

Several types of cell play a direct role in immunity, as follows.

Monocytes

- These are large mononuclear cells
- They are 10–18 μm in diameter
- They have a kidney-shaped nucleus
- They develop into macrophages and are phagocytic.

Lymphocytes

- These are small mononuclear cells
- They are approximately 6–10 μm in diameter
- There are two types: T and B lymphocytes
- T lymphocytes are produced in the thymus during the first few months of life
- B lymphocytes are produced in the bone marrow
- T cells are responsible for cellular immunity and there are hundreds of different types
- They have antigen-binding molecules on their surfaces, called T-cell receptors
- There are three main types of T-cell receptors:
  1. Cytotoxic T cells: these recognise cells with antigens on the surface and destroy them
  2. Helper T cells: these assist T and B lymphocytes in their response to antigens
  3. Suppressor T cells: these inhibit the immune response
- B cells are responsible for cell-mediated immunity
- B cells effectively clone antigens
- These B-cell clones then develop into plasma cells
- The cloned plasma cells have highly developed endoplasmic reticulum within them to synthesise proteins, which will manufacture the antibodies
- Macrophages help in immunity by stimulating antigen-sensitive leukocytes and secreting substances that help regulate the immune response.

Antibody-mediated immunity (humoral-mediated immunity)

- B cells are also responsible for this process
- Antibody-mediated immunity interacts with cell-mediated immunity
- Cell-mediated immunity fights against foreign cells and viruses whereas antibody-mediated immunity produces antibodies in the fight against disease
- Macrophages and T cells are needed to produce antibodies
- The antibodies modulate the function of the macrophages and T cells.

How does it work?

- Bacteria enter the body
- Macrophages engulf some of them
- When a macrophage destroys a bacterial cell some of the bacterial antigen goes to the surface of the macrophage
- The macrophage now has its own surface proteins and bacterial antigens
- The protein produced in response to the pathogen is the antibody
- The antibodies on the surface of the B cell serve as receptors
- Each antibody is specific to an individual antigen
- The macrophage displaying antigen and a helper T cell results in the secretion of interleukins
- Interleukins activate helper T cells to detect B cells that are bound with antigen on the surface of the macrophage
- Helper T cell binds with B cells, releasing lymphokines (these can also be secreted by lymphocytes)
- These activate competent B cells
- B cells increase in size and divide by mitosis
- Some mature into plasma cells, producing antibodies for the original antigen
- Others become memory cells – these continue to produce small amounts of antibody after the infection has passed (allowing the body to retain immunity to specific infections)
- Antibodies are immunoglobulins
- Vaccinations work in this manner.

Cell-mediated immunity

- This is performed by T cells and phagocytic cells, e.g. monocytes, macrophages
- It is very effective against viruses, fungal infections and bacteria that live within host cells.

How does it work?

- Invading pathogens alter the host cell's macromolecules
- The host cell then becomes a foreign cell and the T cells destroy it
- Helper T cells are again involved
- In this case the destruction stimulates the T cells to divide and clone, thereby producing memory T cells
- These are sent to the infected area, accompanied by lymphocytes and macrophages stimulated by inflammatory response
- Suppressor T cells are stimulated by the presence of an antigen
- They regulate B and T cells
- They multiply more slowly than other types
- It generally takes approximately 1 week before they are present in sufficient numbers to suppress an immune response.

Types of immunity

Remember that there are two types of immunity: innate and acquired immunity. Innate immunity is characterised by genetic factors and physical barriers, e.g. skin and the inflammatory response. Acquired immunity can be subdivided into four categories:

1. Natural active immunity
2. Artificial active immunity
3. Artificial passive immunity
4. Natural passive immunity.

Natural active immunity

- This is immunity developed following exposure to specific antigens
- For example, if a dog is exposed to leptospirosis, then it will produce antibodies in response and if it survives the infection it will retain a memory of the antibodies that code for this disease.

Artificial active immunity

- Again, this is immunity that has developed from exposure to specific antigens
- In this case, a version of the pathogen that has reduced virulence is introduced into the animal and will not cause clinical symptoms but will stimulate the production of antibodies
- This is how vaccination works, as the vaccine is the inactive form of the disease
- Vaccinations may be attenuated (modified live pathogen), usually requiring one dose and not advised in pregnant animals, or inactivated (dead pathogen), which require two doses and which are usually considered safe in pregnant animals.

Artificial passive immunity

- The body is given antibodies actively produced by another organism
- It can be thought of as 'borrowed immunity'
- It only provides short-acting immunity as the body will break down the introduced antibodies as these are foreign to it, e.g. tetanus antitoxoid.

Natural passive immunity

- Antibodies are passed from mother to fetus via placental blood supply, inferring some immunity
- Antibodies are also provided by colostrum (first milk). The neonate has an optimum period during the first few hours of life when its digestive system has increased permeability to allow the large immunoglobulin molecules, of which antibodies are made, to pass through into the offspring's blood stream
- Passive immunity has a duration of 8–12 weeks, allowing the neonate the opportunity to produce its own antibodies in response to newly encountered pathogens.

Vaccinations

The incubation period is the time lapse between acquiring an infection and the presence of symptoms. It will depend upon the disease, i.e. the virus/bacterial multiplication rate. An animal is immune after the infection has occurred when the body produces antibodies specific to that infection.

A vaccine consists of modified bacterial/viral culture that stimulates immunity but the agent included is incapable of producing the disease, i.e. it is avirulent.

Dead vaccines are produced from organisms in culture that have been killed by heat or chemicals. Live vaccines are produced by laboratory-cultured virus grown then transferred repeatedly to new tissue until their virulence is reduced so that they will induce an immune response but have lost the ability to produce clinical symptoms, i.e. attenuated. Adjuvant is an additional chemical that is added to live/dead vaccines to increase their efficacy. It acts to delay the disappearance of antigen from the body, allowing a longer period of time for antibody production.

Autogenous vaccine is prepared from bacteria/virus from an individual animal for injection back into the same animal, and is commonly used in animals with chronic skin infections. Heterotypic vaccine is prepared from one animal to use in another, e.g. the use of human measles vaccine for dogs to provide rapid immunity against distemper, for instance, in an exposed puppy which has not been vaccinated (only short-term protection is afforded). The vaccine manufacturer's instructions should always be read and the administrator should consult with the manufacturer before deviating from the norm.

Vaccination of puppies/kittens

The aim is to provide active vaccine-derived immunity as soon as possible.

The problem is that maternal-derived antibodies may block the vaccination response. As the levels of maternal-derived antibodies decrease, young animals enter a susceptible period or 'immunity gap'. Historically this is when we choose to vaccinate, between 8 and 12 weeks, but new research has indicated that vaccination from as early as 6 weeks can provide an adequate immune response and has several other benefits.

Extra doses of the vaccine can be given if an animal is a member of a susceptible group, e.g. parvovirus in Dobermans, or if the risk to an animal of a specific pathogen is increased, i.e. there has been a recent outbreak. Most vaccinations require annual or biannual boosters to maintain immunity. Animals may exhibit a vaccination reaction which is often categorised by a transient pyrexia and lethargy and vaccination failure may also occur.

Bibliography

Aspinall V 2006 The complete textbook of veterinary nursing. Butterworth Heinemann, London

Aspinall V, O'Reilly M 2004 Introduction to veterinary anatomy and physiology. Butterworth Heinemann, Oxford

Campbell N, Reece J, Mitchell L 1999 Biology, 5th edn. Benjamin Cummings, San Francisco

Colville T, Bassett J M 2002 Clinical anatomy and physiology for veterinary technicians. Mosby, St Louis

Dyke K M, Sack W O, Wensing C J G 1996 Text book of veterinary anatomy, 2nd edn. W B Saunders, Philadelphia

Green N P O, Stout G W, Taylor D J 1991 Biological science. Cambridge University Press, Cambridge

Lane D R, Cooper B, Turner L 2007 BSAVA Textbook of Veterinary Nursing. BSAVA, Oxford

Moore M 2000 Manual of veterinary nursing. BSAVA, Oxford

Pratt P W 1998 Principles and practice of veterinary technology. Mosby, Philadelphia

Roberts M B V 1986 Biology: a functional approach. Nelson, Surrey, UK

Simpson G 1994 Practical veterinary nursing, 3rd edn. BSAVA, Oxford

Chapter | **5** | *Jane Williams*

Urogenital system

This chapter considers the anatomical features and the physiological control of the urinary system with particular reference to water balance and sodium retention. The anatomy of the male and female reproductive systems is discussed and the mutual components of the urogenital system are identified.

The urinary and reproductive systems are often collectively known as the urogenital system as there are a number of shared components between the two.

THE URINARY SYSTEM

The urinary system consists of:

- Kidneys (a pair)
- Ureters (a pair)
- Bladder
- Urethra.

Kidneys

The kidneys filter blood. They lie against the dorsal wall of the abdomen attached by a fibrous covering called the capsule. The right kidney is situated about half its own length in front of the left kidney. The hilus is an indentation through which the renal artery, vein, nerves and ureters enter and leave the kidney. Each kidney has a pad of fat located next to it for protection and as an energy store.

The internal structure of the kidney comprises three distinct areas (Figure 5.1):

1. Cortex (outer)
2. Medulla (middle)
3. Renal pelvis (inner).

The kidney is surrounded by a dense fibrous connective tissue covering the capsule. The cortex contains the renal corpuscles and convoluted tubules of the nephron. The medulla contains the collecting ducts and pyramids located between them and the loops of Henle of the nephrons. The renal pelvis is a whitish colour and made of dense connective tissue. It is effectively a funnel through which urine collects and drains from the kidney into the ureter.

Functions of the kidneys

- Formation (excretion) of urine
- Production of renin
- Conversion of vitamin D to its active form
- Production of erythropoietin
- It plays a role in homeostasis (balancing the pH of the body).

The kidneys produce urine from water, salts and wastes that they filter from the blood. By adjusting the amount of water and salts they excrete, the kidneys perform a vital homeostatic service in maintaining the internal chemical balance of the body (Table 5.1). Urine is excreted in a continuous trickle, collecting in the renal pelvis.

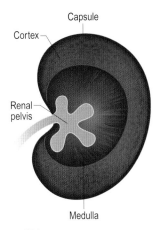

Capsule
Cortex
Renal pelvis
Medulla

Figure 5.1 Gross kidney anatomy.

Ureters

From the renal pelvis peristaltic contractions move the urine along the ureters. The ureters connect the kidneys to the urinary bladder; the length of ureters varies depending on the species. The ureters have thick walls of smooth muscle and are lined with mucous membrane and transitional epithelium to allow them to expand as the urine passes. They enter the bladder close to its neck on the dorsal aspect where there is a simple flap valve to prevent backflow of urine.

Bladder

The bladder is located in the lower, anterior portion of the pelvic cavity. It is made up of a double layer of smooth muscle and transitional epithelium (that allows stretch) that continues into the urethra. It is covered with peritoneum and its lining is invaginated (folded upon itself) which allows for great expansion. The trigone is the area between the ureteral openings and the neck of the bladder. As the volume of urine held increases, distension of the muscle wall stimulates nerve endings which in turn send impulses to the brain, producing a feeling of fullness. Impulses may then be sent back to stimulate urination. Urination is also known as *micturition*. Micturition is defined as the expulsion of urine from the bladder.

Urethra

The urethra leads from the bladder to outside the body in males and to the urethral orifice in females (which opens into the genital tract at the junction of the vagina and the vestibule).

The urethra has two sphincters close to where it leaves the bladder:

1. The internal sphincter, which is under involuntary control
2. The external sphincter, which is under voluntary control.

The urethra is shorter in females than in males. In females it only transports urine but in males it transports semen (sperm plus seminal fluid) and urine. The length of urethra in the male discourages bacterial infection due to its length whereas the female urethra is shorter, leading to a higher incidence of infection. Conversely the length and smaller diameter of the male urethra encourage blockages along its length and particularly at areas where the urethra curves, e.g. the ischial arch. Bladder control depends upon an animal's learned ability to facilitate or inhibit the reflex action that causes micturition. In dogs and cats this ability is not inherent and requires time to learn.

Table 5.1 Urine analysis	
pH	Cat/dog 5–7 Slightly acidic due to carnivorous diet Horse 7.42–7.45 Slightly alkaline due to diet
Specific gravity	A measure of density or concentration of urine Cat 1.020–1.040 Dog 1.016–1.060 Horse 1.020–1.060
Protein	Should not appear in a healthy animal Can be present if the urinary tract is damaged, or if there is increased permeability of glomerulus, chronic renal disease and cystitis
Blood	Not normal It can be due to physical damage, contaminant (prostate) or because an animal is in season (bitch)
Bile	Can be due to liver disease or blockage of bile duct
Glucose	Present if the renal threshold is exceeded, e.g. in diabetes mellitus
Ketones	Produced when fats are oxidised (used for energy) Can appear in diabetes mellitus and in malnutrition cases where fat is used by the body as a food source
Deposits	Calculi, cells, casts of renal tubules may all be present

Nephron

Each kidney contains millions of nephrons that regulate the composition of the blood and excrete waste. A nephron comprises a renal corpuscle and a renal tubule.

Renal corpuscle

- The renal corpuscle is made up of a Bowman's capsule and a glomerulus
- The Bowman's capsule is a double-walled, hollow cup of cells
- The glomerulus is a spherical tuft of capillaries fed by an afferent arteriole and drained by an efferent arteriole
- The glomerulus projects into the kidney capsule.

Renal tubule

This consists of three main regions:

1. The proximal convoluted tubule
2. The loop of Henle (which goes from the cortex into the medulla and loops back into the cortex)
3. The distal convoluted tubule.

The proximal convoluted tubule is lined with simple cuboidal or columnar epithelium which has microvilli to increase the surface area for absorption. The loop of Henle is lined with simple squamous epithelium and the distal convoluted tubule is lined with cuboidal epithelium but contains no microvilli. Each distal convoluting tubule empties into a collecting duct, lined with columnar epithelium, with lots of distal tubules which empty into each collecting duct. The collecting ducts drain into the renal pelvis at the apices of the pyramids of the medulla. The calyces are defined as the indentations between the pyramids of the medulla.

Renal filtration and absorption

Figure 5.2 shows absorption in the renal nephron.

- An afferent arteriole delivers blood to the glomerulus. It then drains from the glomerulus into a much narrower efferent arteriole, producing a high hydrostatic pressure within the glomerulus. The hormone renin can also be employed by the body to constrict the glomerulus further and increase the pressure
- Blood is under high pressure in the glomerulus and under low pressure in the Bowman's capsule
- The result is the passage of fluid or ultrafiltration; the fluid produced is known as the glomerular filtrate or primitive urine and drains into the Bowman's capsule

- The glomerular filtrate consists mainly of plasma minus the larger plasma proteins and blood cells. It contains 99% water and 1% chemicals in solution
- The amount of glomerular filtrate produced vastly exceeds how much urine is produced. Therefore the reabsorption system must be highly effective to prevent excessive water loss from the body.

Note: the renal blood supply is via the renal artery and vein which travel past the glomerulus to the kidney.

Reabsorption

Reabsorption is the passage of substances from the lumen of renal tubules into the renal capillaries to return them to the systemic circulation.

- Reabsorption occurs in the renal tubule
- Substances are reabsorbed by active transport or by passive diffusion
- Water is reabsorbed in the proximal convoluted tubule: some reabsorption occurs in the distal convoluted tubule by active transport under the control of antidiuretic hormone (ADH)
- Sodium ions are reabsorbed in the proximal convoluted tubule by active transport and the ascending limb of the loop of Henle. A small amount is reabsorbed in the distal convoluted tubule. Potassium ions are secreted into the filtrate in the distal convoluted tubule to replace the reabsorbed sodium ions
- Chloride ions are reabsorbed in the proximal convoluted tubules by diffusion as a secondary result of sodium absorption due to ionic attraction
- Glucose is reabsorbed in the proximal convoluted tubule when it exceeds the renal threshold. The renal threshold is the 'normal' concentration of a certain chemical or substance that should be in the body; once this is exceeded it is excreted. In diabetes mellitus, due to the failure in insulin production, excessive glucose is circulating in the blood and is not converted to glycogen but will be filtered within the glomerular filtrate, thus exceeding the renal threshold, and it is excreted in the urine
- Amino acids are reabsorbed in both proximal and distal convoluted tubules and should be completely absorbed back into the body
- Any protein that is filtered, which is a small amount, is reabsorbed in the proximal convoluted tubule
- A small amount of urea is reabsorbed in the proximal convoluted tubule then secreted into the loop of Henle
- Acids and bases are selectively absorbed and secreted, e.g. hydrogen, bicarbonate and ammonia ions to aid the body acid–base balance

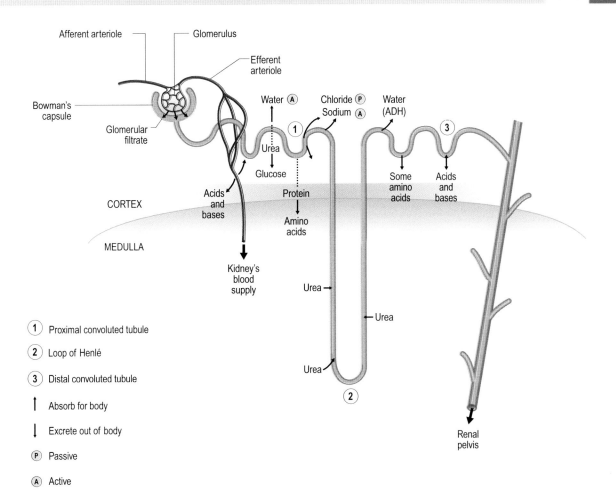

Figure 5.2 Absorption in the renal nephron. A, active; P, passive; 1, proximal convoluted tubule; 2, loop of Henle; 3, distal convoluted tubule.

- Drugs and toxins are actively secreted *into* the filtrate to remove them from the body.

Remember – substances that are reabsorbed in the nephron are taken *back* into the body, usually via the blood, to be utilised; they are normally substances which are useful.

Water reabsorption

- The loop of Henle regulates the volume and concentration of urine that will be produced in response to the body's status
- Water is reabsorbed by passive and active transport: passive (osmosis) in the proximal convoluted tubule and active in the distal convoluted tubule
- Water is reabsorbed by osmosis in the descending loop of Henle, resulting in very concentrated filtrate

in the loop; in the ascending limb the walls are impermeable to water molecules but actively reabsorb sodium ions. As a result of this process water molecules are drawn back into the filtrate. On balance the concentration of the filtrate will be constant at the beginning and end of the loop of Henle but the volume of urine will be reduced. This aids certain species, e.g. gerbils, which have long loops of Henle which help to preserve body water

- Water reabsorption in the distal convoluted tubule is under the control of ADH
- ADH is secreted from the posterior pituitary gland in response to water balance in the body
- The tubules of the distal convoluted tubule are lined with simple epithelial cells and microvilli to increase their surface area
- There are also lots of mitochondria to provide the energy required for active transport

- When the body needs to conserve water, ADH is secreted and it acts upon the distal convoluted tubule, increasing its permeability to water and resulting in very concentrated urine
- If the body needs to get rid of excess water, ADH production will be reduced, therefore less water will be reabsorbed by the distal convoluted tubule
- For example, in diabetes insipidus, the body cannot make sufficient ADH and is therefore unable to concentrate urine regardless of the intake volume.

The distal convoluted tubule can be thought of like a tube containing holes that can change their diameter. Under normal circumstances the holes are small and water molecules cannot fit through them back into the blood. However when times are hard and water is scarce, ADH increases the diameter of the holes and they are now big enough for the water molecules to fit through, increasing the amount of water in the blood stream.

Sodium reabsorption

- This is under the control of aldosterone and has a secondary effect on water reabsorption
- Aldosterone is produced in the adrenal cortex
- When plasma sodium levels fall the kidney produces a substance called renin (note the spelling difference between this renin and rennin, which is produced in the digestive system)
- Renin acts on substances in the plasma (angiotensin) that stimulate the renal cortex to increase the secretion of aldosterone
- Aldosterone acts on the distal convoluted tubule and increases the rate of absorption of sodium and chloride ions
- Angiotensin also increases blood pressure, thereby increasing the glomerular filtration rate and pressure.

Osmoregulation is an important aspect of homeostasis and the control of water and sodium reabsorption in the body plays an important role in the regulation and balance of body water.

Species variation – urinary tract

The urinary system of the bird has a pair of kidneys, a pair of ureters but no bladder; they excrete nitrogenous waste in the form of uric acid and urates suspended in urinary water. The semisolid fluid leaves the ureters and enters the urodeum of the cloaca, then returns to the colon for more water reabsorption to occur before excretion. Reptile kidneys do not possess loops of Henle and therefore produce very dilute urine; snakes also do not have a bladder.

THE REPRODUCTIVE SYSTEM

Many generalisations can be made for sexually reproducing animals even though the details of the reproductive process vary with species.

The basic components of the male reproductive system are:

- Male gonads or testes which produce spermatozoa
- Transport of sperm to exterior of body via the sperm duct
- A specialised area of the sperm duct which produces nourishment – the seminal vessels
- A copulatory organ into which the sperm duct empties – the penis.

The basic components of the female reproductive system are:

- The female gonads or ovaries which produce ova
- A tube for transporting ova, called the oviduct
- An area for storage of the ova and development of the fertilised egg – the uterus
- The terminal portion of the oviduct which opens to the exterior of body – the vagina.

Not all male and female animals possess all the modifications. Some simple animals have complex reproductive systems whereas some complex animals have simple reproductive systems. The reproductive systems of the male and female will be considered individually, taking the dog as an example of a mammal.

Male reproductive system

Figure 5.3 shows the male reproductive tract.

Functions of the male reproductive system include:

- Production, storage and nourishment of the spermatozoa (male gamete)
- Transport of spermatozoa to the female genital tract for fertilisation to occur.

It comprises the:

- Testes
- Epididymides
- Vasa deferentia/deferent ducts
- Prostate gland
- (In some species, e.g. the cat, there is an additional gland – the bulbourethral gland)
- Urethra
- Penis
- Prepuce.

Note: the urethra and penis are common to both the urinary and reproductive tracts.

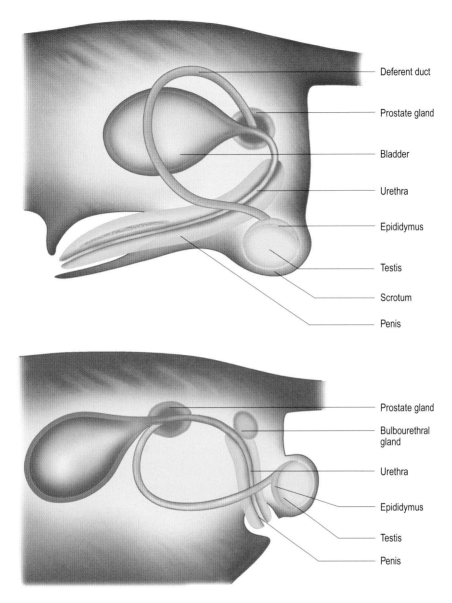

Figure 5.3 Male reproductive tract. (Reproduced from Aspinall V 2006 *The Complete Textbook of Veterinary Nursing*. Butterworth Heinemann, London, with permission.)

Testes

These descend from the abdomen through the inguinal ring which then closes as the animal develops. They are developed from undifferentiated gonad tissue in the fetus. When the testes move through the inguinal ring the perineum lining that is pulled through with them develops into the scrotum.

The scrotum has two layers, an inner and an outer layer:

1. Internal tunica vaginalis – the inner layer
2. External tunica vaginalis – the external layer.

At the same time the blood vessels, nerves and ducts of the glands also descend through the inguinal ring and collectively form the spermatic cord. The testes may remain in the abdomen for various reasons:

* A cryptorchid animal has no testes descended
* A monorchid animal has only one testis descended

- A rig is an animal (usually a horse) that has some testicular tissue still present in the abdomen and exhibits sexual characteristics postcastration.

Testes normally begin their descent around 8–10 weeks of age and should be palpable within the groin if not actually present in the scrotum. The testes remain relatively small until puberty (but this is dependent on breed and species). Running concurrent with the spermatic cord is a thin strip of muscle originating from the external oblique, called the cremaster muscle. The cremaster muscle retains the ability to move the testes closer to or away from the body to help control the temperature at which the spermatozoa are stored.

In small mammals the inguinal ring remains open and the cremaster muscle can withdraw the testes into the abdomen.

Temperature control of the testes is important as spermatozoa production and storage can be affected by fluctuations. Ideally the temperature of the testes should be lower than body temperature. The blood supply to the testes originates from the abdominal aorta along the spermatic cord to the associated epididymus where it becomes involuted and forms the pampiniform plexus. The pampiniform plexus allows the blood to cool and pulsations to smooth out before entering the gonad, preserving the lower temperature required for optimum sperm production and storage.

Surgical removal of testes is commonly known as castration or orchidectomy. Early castration can prevent the development of the secondary sexual characteristics:

- Thickening of muscle mass
- Development of erectile tissue in the penis (dog)
- Distinctive urine smell and voice of tomcat.

The scrotum comprises the testis and epididymus within the tunica vaginalis.

Internal structure of the testis

The testis is made up of hundreds of convoluted tubules called seminiferous tubules. These are supported by connective tissue and cells. There are two types of cell that line the seminiferous tubules:

1. Spermatogenic cells: these divide by meiosis to produce the male gametes or spermatozoa
2. Sertoli cells: these produce oestrogens and part of the spermatic fluid (nourish spermatozoa).

The cells located within the connective tissue matrix are called the cells of Leydig. Cells of Leydig are interstitial cells which produce testosterone. Testosterone is thought of as male hormone and is responsible for regulating spermatogenesis and for the development and maintenance of the secondary sexual characteristics. Testosterone has an inhibitory effect on the hypothalamus and subsequently the anterior pituitary gland from producing interstitial cell-stimulating hormone (ICSH) and luteinising hormone (LH) until puberty.

ICSH and LH are responsible for the development of the seminiferous tubules, where the sperm are produced, i.e. no sperm are produced until after puberty.

When puberty is achieved, testosterone no longer inhibits the hypothalamus and the production of ICSH and LH results in the development of the seminiferous tubules and increased testosterone production by the cells of Leydig, i.e. sperm are produced and male characteristics are formed.

Testosterone

- Testosterone is a male hormone
- It is responsible for spermatogenesis
- It produces the secondary sexual characteristics
- Testosterone controls the descent of the testes
- It inhibits the hypothalamus from stimulating the anterior pituitary to produce ICSH and LH until puberty.

Epididymus

One epididymus is located upon each of the testis. It may be palpable during examination of the testis. It consists of many coiled tubules where the spermatozoa are stored. Spermatozoa are transported to the epididymus via the vas efferentia (efferent ducts).

Vas deferens (deferent duct)

The vas deferens lie within the spermatic cord. They transport the sperm from the epididymus through the inguinal ring to the urethra. They empty into the urethra through the tissue of the prostate gland.

Structure of spermatozoa

Sperm comprise a head (acrosome and nucleus), a mid-piece(mitochondria) and a tail (flagella for movement).

Spermatogenesis is the process of sperm production. It is a complicated process with many stages. The age of the animal affects the number of spermatozoa produced, with fertility levels declining as animals age. The size of an animal may also play a role: large dogs produce more sperm than small dogs. High or low temperatures, radiation, drugs, toxins, vitamin A deficiency and limited diets can affect spermatozoa production. Abstinence reduces fertility due to blockage of tubules by old spermatozoa and it is normal practice for two coverings to occur to negate this issue.

Prostate gland

The prostate gland produces a large proportion of the seminal fluid – the fluid that nourishes the sperm and provides it with a transport medium. The ejaculate comprises spermatozoa and seminal fluid. The prostate is a bilobed structure that surrounds the urethra at the level of the pelvis brim. It can often be palpated and may cause problems in older uncastrated animals as it may develop neoplasia which results in an increase in size and excretory problems, as enlargement can cause obstruction to faeces.

Bulbourethral glands

These are only found in certain species, e.g. cat. Their function is to contribute a proportion of the seminal fluid and they are located further down the urethra than the prostate, near to the perineum.

Penis

The penis runs from the ischial arch through the perineum to its conclusion between the hind legs. It differs greatly in structure between species. The distal portion is protected by the prepuce. The prepuce is a sheath or covering constructed from abdominal skin tissue suspended from the ventral abdominal wall. It is lined with mucous epithelium for lubrication and its function is to protect the distal penis or glans penis. It is pushed back to expose the glans penis during coitus. Problems can occur if the prepuce is too small for the erect penis and surgical intervention may be necessary.

Structure of the penis

The penis comprises the following structures:

* Urethra
* Os penis
* Corpus cavernosum penis
* Corpus spongiosum penis
* Retractor penile muscle.

Two strips of erectile tissue or crura run along the penis from the root to almost the tip. This tissue is known as the corpus cavernosum and houses the urethra in the middle of the two layers. The corpus spongiosum runs beneath the corpus cavernosum and urethra and expands proximally to form the bulb (important to achieve the tie) and the tip or glans penis. At the glans penis the corpus spongiosum completely engulfs the urethra. The os penis is a small bone found within penile tissue in some species, e.g. the dog. It is v-shaped with the urethra running along a groove upon it.

Retractor penis muscle

The retractor penis muscle originates from the first coccygeal vertebrae and its role is to pull the penis back into the protective prepuce.

Female reproductive system

The female reproductive system (Figure 5.4) comprises the following:

* Ovaries (female gonads)
* Oviducts or fallopian tubes
* Uterus (horns and body and cervix)
* Vagina
* Vestibule
* Clitoris
* Vulva.

Functions of the female reproductive system

* Production of ova (female gametes)
* To provide a location for fertilisation (fallopian tubes)
* To prepare the genital tract for implantation
* To provide a location for implantation and subsequently pregnancy to develop.

Ovaries

The ovaries are located in the abdomen, one behind each kidney. They are held in place by the ovarian ligament which attaches the ovary to the kidney capsule. Their blood supply is provided by the ovarian artery developed from the aorta; it is very convoluted and runs alongside the ovarian ligament to the ovary itself. The ovaries lie within a fold of the mesentery called the mesovarium, which has an opening within it to allow the mature ova to depart. This opening is known as the ovarian bursa. When an animal is born it has a definitive number of undeveloped ova within each ovary. Depending upon species ova may be released individually or in a multitude.

A primary ovarian follicle develops into a mature or ripe ovarian follicle or graafian follicle under hormonal influence. The almost ripe follicle bulges out of the surface of the ovary until it is ready to pop and release the ovum (female gamete). The follicle consists of the ovum and a large quantity of fluid. The rupture of the follicle and release of the ovum occur at ovulation. The ovum is ejected and usually caught by the hair-like projections or fimbriae of the infundibulum at the head of the oviduct. The ruptured follicle then develops into the yellow body or corpus luteum (which has a role in pregnancy by producing progesterone).

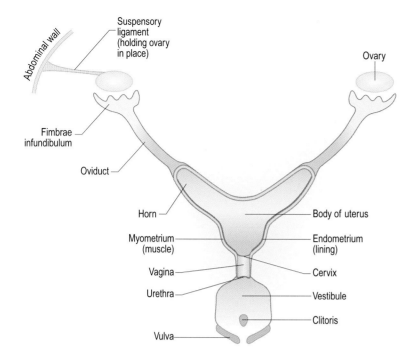

Figure 5.4 Overview of female reproductive tract.

Oviduct or fallopian tube

The oviduct is a narrow tube that transports the ovum from the ovary to the horn of the uterus. It consists of the infundibulum that encloses the ovary and the tube portion that runs to the uterus.

Uterus (womb)

Most animals are multiparous, i.e. they give birth to many young, including the cat and the dog. These animals have a uterus comprising two uterine horns. The uterine horns lead to the body of the uterus which in turn leads to the cervix or entrance of the uterus. The uterus is located within the broad ligament or mesometrium of the uterus and is dorsal to the abdomen. The exception to this location is when the uterus is enlarged during pregnancy, when the weight of the uterus brings it into a more ventral position.

The uterus consists of layers of smooth muscle, the myometrium and a mucous epithelial lining or endometrium. The cervix is located at the base of the uterus and is a muscular sphincter that closes the uterus except during mating or parturition. The round ligament runs from the ovary through the inguinal ring where it terminates in a pad of fat known as the vaginal process. The round ligament is the female equivalent of the cremaster muscle.

Vagina

The vagina extends from the cervix to the external urethral orifice. It is completely contained within the pelvis. At the end of the vagina the genital tract deviates sharply downwards and passes into the vestibule. The vestibule is utilised by both the urinary and reproductive systems. The muscles in the wall of the vestibule are very strong and help maintain the tie during mating in the dog.

Vulva

The vulva forms the boundary between the genital tract and the outside world. It takes the form of protective folds of skin or vulval lips. Contained within the vulval lips is the female equivalent to the penis, the clitoris. The clitoris is a piece of erectile tissue and lies in the clitoral fossa, a small cavity just inside the base of the vulva. The vulval lips are normally soft but during oestrus become enlarged and turgid.

Reproductive variations
Birds

* Sexing is difficult and a number of methods are employed:
  ○ Visual inspection of cloacal anatomy

- Examination of chromosomal karyotype and/or comparison of hormone levels from blood sampling
- Surgical sexing under anaesthetic by laparoscopy
- DNA techniques (feathers) are used in most parrot species
- Stress and aggression are often seen when mixing birds:
  - Birds may be incompatible
  - One may dominate the other, which may be species-dependent
  - Stress can lead to infertility
- Birds can form permanent pair bonds which take time to establish (1–2 years, e.g. swans)
- Reproductive cycles depend on daylight, quality, quantity, temperature and an increase in food supply
- Generally larger birds lay one egg
- Another generalisation is the higher the latitude, i.e. the longer days, then the more eggs are produced
- Some birds will lay more if eggs are removed from their nest, e.g. chickens
- Most lay one clutch of eggs a year and some on alternate years, e.g. penguins
- The interval between laying eggs is approximately 24 hours but all will hatch at the same time (chicks can communicate with each other while still in their shells and synchronise their watches!)
- Size, colour and shape of eggs vary
- Male birds can either have or not have a phallus
- In the intromittent form (those with protruding phallus), e.g. ducks, geese, swans:
  - The phallus lies on the floor of the cloaca and is erected by engorgement of lymphatic fluid
- In the non-intromittent form, e.g. domestic fowl and Passeriformes:
  - Two lateral folds become momentarily engorged at ejaculation and protrude to meet the protruding oviduct of the female and internal fertilisation occurs.

Reptiles

- Copulatory organs of male snakes and lizards are paired and found at the sides of the base of the tail just behind the tail vent
- At rest they are retracted and it is possible to palpate a pocket-like sac which can be used to determine sexing (females won't have one if you probe, except for pythons where it is half-depth in females compared with the males)
- In chelonians and crocodiles the hemipenes are situated in the ventral wall of the cloaca; these can be extruded into the female's cloaca to facilitate passage of sperm
- Internal fertilisation occurs

- The nesting place is important to all reptiles – they usually dig holes
- They often have problems whereby they become egg-bound because captive animals keep hold of eggs looking for an ideal nesting place, or due to stress, infections of the oviduct or mineral imbalances (calcium)
- Ova are fertilised in the salpinx (located anterior to the cloaca)
- Reproductive cycles are closely related to environmental conditions:
  - Mature, good condition and healthy
  - Space and habitat
  - Daylight length and quality
  - Temperature
  - Moisture
  - Food
- Eggs can be laid or develop in a female who subsequently will give birth to live young.

Fish

- External/internal fertilisation occurs
- Hit-and-miss process
- Gonads produce normal hormones which can also play a role in colour changes
- Most species have a male and female but hermaphroditism, bisexuality, parthenogenesis and gynogenesis occur
- Sex reversal in adults is not uncommon
- The number of eggs produced is usually determined by the amount of parental care given, e.g. cod release millions of eggs into open water but sticklebacks that build nests and protect them only produce a few tens of eggs
- Some fish will brood their young in their mouths
- Fertilisation methods vary:
  - Eggs and sperm are released into water
  - Copulation: fertilised eggs are released
  - Copulation: internal incubation – live young are released, e.g. guppy
- Testes are found adjacent to the swim bladder and can weigh up to 12% of total body weight
- Sperm are carried from the testes by the vas deferens to the external environment by a genital opening at the urinary papilla
- In some primitive species these ducts are absent and sperm are released into the body cavity before leaving through the genital opening
- Ovaries vary in complexity but are usually paired and can account for up to 70% of adult weight
- In advanced species a small oviduct conducts eggs to the genital opening whilst in others ova are released into the peritoneal cavity, then find their way through to the genital opening.

67

Bibliography

Aspinall V 2006 The complete textbook of veterinary nursing. Butterworth Heinemann, London

Aspinall V, O'Reilly M 2004 Introduction to veterinary anatomy and physiology. Butterworth Heinemann, Oxford

Campbell N, Reece J, Mitchell L 1999 Biology, 5th edn. Benjamin Cummings, San Francisco

Colville T, Bassett J M 2002 Clinical anatomy and physiology for veterinary technicians. Mosby, St Louis

Dyke K M, Sack W O, Wensing C J G 1996 Text book of veterinary anatomy, 2nd edn. W B Saunders, Philadelphia

Green N P O, Stout G W, Taylor D J 1991 Biological science. Cambridge University Press, Cambridge

Lane D R, Cooper B, Turner L 2007 BSAVA Textbook of Veterinary Nursing. BSAVA, Oxford

Moore M 2000 Manual of veterinary nursing. BSAVA, Oxford

Pratt P W 1998 Principles and practice of veterinary technology. Mosby, Philadelphia

Roberts M B V 1986 Biology: a functional approach. Nelson, Surrey, UK

Simpson G 1994 Practical veterinary nursing, 3rd edn. BSAVA, Oxford

Chapter | 6 |

Jane Williams

Nervous system

This chapter considers the anatomy of the nervous system and how it is structured and assesses the effect of each aspect upon the normal function of an animal. The individual sensory systems of sight, sound, smell, touch and taste are described and their respective anatomy is detailed.

OVERVIEW

The function of a nervous system is to enable an animal to function in its external environment and to maintain equilibrium in its internal environment.

A simple nervous system would:

- receive information about the external environment
- receive information about the tissues and organs of the animal's own body
- interpret the information received
- send impulses throughout the body via the nervous system to stimulate activity of some kind.

The nervous system can be divided into a number of parts:

- Neurons: cells that transmit nerve impulses
- Receptors: these collect information from the internal/external environment, e.g. pain receptors in fingers.

The sensory nervous system comprises receptors and neurons. The information that the sensory information gathers is sent to the central nervous system (CNS) where it is processed. The CNS can initiate responses to the information it has received. This is done by the motor nervous system along effectors.

The motor system is divided into two parts:

1. Autonomic nervous system: activates involuntary (not under your control) responses
2. Somatic nervous system: activates voluntary responses.

Consider what would happen if you pricked your finger with a drawing pin. In the sensory nervous system a receptor will receive a stimulus of pain. This information will be sent via a sensory neuron as a nervous impulse to the CNS where the impulse will be interpreted and what action to take will be formulated. The CNS will instruct the motor nervous system via the somatic system along a motor neuron to your hand and you will withdraw your hand from the pin.

- Afferent neurons carry information to the CNS and will always be sensory neurons
- Efferent neurons carry information away from the CNS and will always be motor neurons.

$$Sensory \rightarrow CNS \rightarrow motor$$

Nervous tissue

A neuron is a nerve cell (Figure 6.1). Nerve cells contain all the normal organelles which would be found in a eukaryotic cell but also have specialised parts which aid in the transmission of nervous impulse, which is their function. Neurons may be unipolar, bipolar or multipolar depending on where they are located in the body and the number of dendrites they possess.

Dendrites

These are several short processes where nerve impulses enter the neuron.

Axon

An axon is a long process along which the nerve impulse travels. Axons can be myelinated, surrounded by a fatty sheath made of myelin, or unmyelinated. Nervous impulses travel faster in myelinated axons.

Myelin is produced by specialised cells called Schwann cells. Axons vary in length from less than 1 mm to many centimetres. The entire axon is surrounded by a sheath of connective tissue known as the neurilemma. There are gaps in the myelin sheath, called nodes of Ranvier, where the axon is in direct contact with the neurilemma. The nodes of Ranvier allow oxygen and nutrients to enter the axon, which uses a lot of energy transporting the nervous impulse. The ends of the axon branch into nerve endings ready to pass the impulse on to the dendrites of the next neuron.

A nerve consists of lots of neurons bound together in a connective tissue sheath. The gaps between neurons are known as synapses. Nervous impulses are carried across synapses by chemical messengers or neurotransmitters.

Nervous impulses

Stimuli from the internal and external environment are carried around the nervous system as impulses of electric

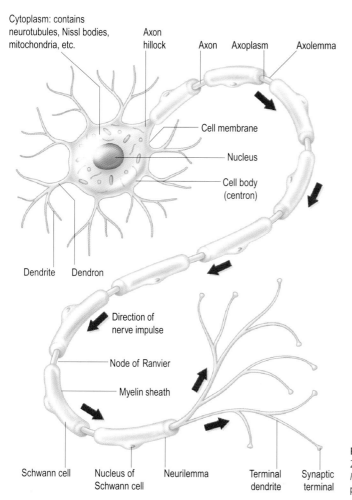

Figure 6.1 Neuron. (Reproduced from Aspinall V 2006 *The Complete Textbook of Veterinary Nursing*. Butterworth Heinemann, London, with permission.)

charge. They pass along the neuron due to changes in electrical charge along it. When the impulse is generated the sodium and potassium ions in the axon become excited, generating electrical potential; once this has exceeded the resting threshold there is sufficient energy for the impulse to travel onwards. This process occurs all the way along the axon. When it arrives at a synapse the impulse needs a 'piggyback' across the gap: this is the role of the neurotransmitter (Figure 6.2). The impulse combines with the chemical to enable it to bridge the synaptic cleft and at the other side the reaction reverses to enable the impulse to continue on its journey. This is a simplified description: in reality a number of complex

reactions occur and the presence of calcium ions is required. The most common neurotransmitter is acetylcholine; others include adrenaline (epinephrine), serotonin and dopamine.

ORGANISATION OF THE NERVOUS SYSTEM

- The CNS consists of brain and spinal cord
- The peripheral nervous system consists of paired nerves which arise either directly from the cranium (cranial nerves: Table 6.1) or from the spinal cord (spinal nerves)

Neurons can be

- Unipolar
- Bipolar
- Multipolar

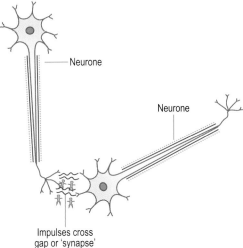

Figure 6.2 Impulse conduction across synapse.

Table 6.1 Cranial nerves	
I Olfactory	Runs from the olfactory tissue to the brain. Smell and taste
II Optic	Eyes to the brain via optic chiasma. Sight
III Oculomotor	Extrinsic muscles of eye. Enables eye to focus as appropriate
IV Trochlear	Extrinsic muscles of eye
V Trigeminal	Sensory from face and skin around the eyes. Motor to the temporal and masseter muscles involved with mastication
VI Abducens	Extrinsic muscles of eye
VII Facial	Motor action on the muscles which give facial expressions
VIII Vestibulocochlear (auditory)	Senses balance and hearing from semicircular canals and cochlea respectively
IX Glossopharyngeal	Senses taste from the tastebuds. Motor action on the muscles in the pharynx
X Vagus	Sensory from pharynx and larynx. Motor to the larynx. Parasympathetic role with heart beat
XI Accessory	Motor action on the muscles of the neck and shoulder
XII Hypoglossal	Motor action on the muscles of the tongue

- The efferent nervous system is divided into the somatic and the autonomic nervous systems
- The autonomic nervous system can be further divided into the parasympathetic nervous system and the sympathetic nervous system
- Sympathetic and parasympathetic nervous systems act antagonistically, i.e. if one slows the heart rate, the other speeds it up.

CENTRAL NERVOUS SYSTEM

The CNS comprises the brain and the spinal cord.

Brain

The brain is made up of three parts: the forebrain, the midbrain and the hindbrain. The forebrain consists of the right and left cerebral hemispheres, or cerebrum, and the hypothalamus; the midbrain joins the fore and hindbrains and is located deep between the two structures and the hindbrain consists of the cerebellum, pons and medulla oblongata (Figure 6.3).

The brain and spinal cord are surrounded by three layers of protective membranes known as the meninges. These are the outer layer (the dura mater), the middle layer (the arachnoid layer) and the inner layer (the pia mater). The dura mater is a tough fibrous membrane which contours closely with the periosteum of the cranium. The epidural space is a hollow filled with fat and blood vessels between the dura mater and the vertebrae and is sometimes used for drug administration. The arachnoid layer is made of a layer of collagen fibres and blood vessels that is closely attached to the pia mater; beneath it is a space, the subarachnoid space, filled with cerebrospinal fluid. It supplies the surrounding areas with nutrients. The final layer is the pia mater, a delicate and very vascular membrane which is closely attached to the brain itself.

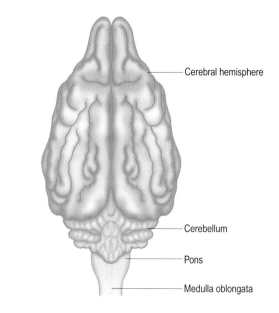

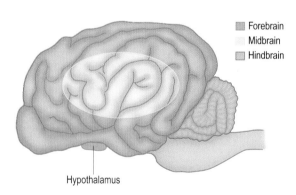

Figure 6.3 Mammalian brain.

Cerebral hemispheres

- The paired cerebral hemispheres together make up the cerebrum
- This is the largest part of brain
- It senses heat, touch, sight, hearing, taste and smell
- It also initiates control of skeletal muscles, i.e. voluntary movement
- It contains centres concerned with mental activities such as speech, consciousness, emotions and memory.

Hypothalamus

- The hypothalamus synthesises numerous hormones
- It plays an important role in osmoregulation and homeostasis and is closely linked to the endocrine system.

Midbrain

- This section of the brain conducts impulses between the fore and hindbrains
- It has centres associated with vision and auditory reflexes.

Cerebellum

- The cerebellum acts with the cerebrum to produce movement of the skeletal muscles
- It helps to coordinate balance and posture of the body.

Pons

- This consists mainly of nerve fibres between the two main parts of the cerebellum
- It contains centres which help to control respiration.

Medulla oblongata

- This is the continuation of the pons and comprises nerve fibres that pass to the spinal cord
- It has reflex centres that control depth of breathing and heart rate
- It is associated with reflex actions such as sneezing and coughing.

Ventricles and cerebrospinal fluid

The brain is an essential structure for the body to survive and it needs to be well protected. Within the brain there is a ventricular system of four large fluid-filled spaces or ventricles. The ventricles are continuous with the central canal of the spinal cord and both are filled with cerebrospinal fluid which is secreted by choroid plexuses located in the roof of the ventricles.

Function of cerebrospinal fluid

- The fluid provides protection by acting as a supporting cushion to brain and spinal cord
- The fluid also supplies nutrients and oxygen to the nervous tissue
- The brain monitors levels of chemicals within CSF and can make changes accordingly.

Spinal cord

The spinal cord is found within the vertebral canal of the spine, running through the foramen magnum. It consists of a central area of grey matter and an external area of white matter. In the centre there is a canal containing cerebrospinal fluid. Grey matter consists of the cell bodies of motor nerve cells which contain no myelin, giving the grey coloration. The white matter consists of columns of sensory nerve fibres which are myelinated and which provide the white coloration.

There are 31 pairs of spinal nerves arising from the spinal cord which leave the spinal cord through gaps in the vertebral column. These nerves separate into two close to the spinal cord. The top root into the spinal cord is called the dorsal root and the bottom one is called the ventral root. The dorsal root always carries sensory or afferent neurons and the ventral root always carries motor or efferent neurons. Dorsal root ganglion contains the cell bodies of the sensory neurons that occur within the dorsal root, forming a swelling. The spinal cord terminates in the cauda equina, which is a collection of terminal spinal nerves, so called as they resemble the hairs in the tail of a horse.

Reflex arcs

Reflexes are nervous responses that occur a lot within the normal functioning of the body and because of this a pathway has been firmly established for the neurons involved and the whole process occurs without conscious thought very quickly. Reflexes can be learnt or innate (not learnt). Examples of learnt reflexes could be withdrawing your hand from a pin or ducking your head to go under a low door in your house. Examples of innate reflexes include the palpebral reflex and coughing reflex. A reflex arc is the name given to the 'right of way' established for a reflex action. A reflex arc could be defined as a fixed, involuntary response to certain stimuli.

Simple reflex arc

- Stimulus
- Receptor receives stimulus and converts it to an electrical impulse
- Impulse to spinal cord is sent via a sensory neuron
- It travels into the spinal cord via a dorsal root ganglion
- The impulse to the brain initiates a response
- The impulse leaves the spinal cord via a ventral root
- The impulse travels to the effector via a motor neuron
- The effector removes the stimulus: this is the response.

SENSES

Sense organs link organisms with the outside world and enable them to receive all kinds of information about their environment.

What is a sense organ?

A sense organ is a specialised structure that consists of one or more receptor cells and often accessory cells. It detects changes in the environment and transmits this information to the nervous system. For example, rods and cones in the retina are receptor cells and the cornea and lens act as accessory structures to enhance their versatility as a sense organ.

How are sense organs classified?

Sensory organs can be classified according to the location of the stimuli affecting them.

Exteroreceptors receive stimuli from the outside environment and assist in the following functions:

* Explore world
* Search for food
* Find a mate
* Recognise friends/enemies
* Learn.

Proprioceptors are located in sense organs within muscles, tendons and joints:

* They enable the animal to perceive the position of body parts, individually and as a whole
* They enable animals to eat in the dark.

Interoreceptors are located in sense organs within body organs. They help in the following:

* Detect changes in pH
* Regulating body temperature
* Maintaining osmotic pressure
* Composition of blood
* Controlled by CNS (under unconscious control to maintain homeostasis).

Sense organs can also be classified according to the type of energy they respond to, as shown in Table 6.2.

How do sense organs work?

Receptor cells absorb various types of energy and convert the energy into an electrical receptor potential. Energy or receptor potential stimulates the nervous system, which converts it into a response to the stimulus.

Mammalian sense organs

The integument

The integument is the covering of the body. It includes:

* Skin
* Hair (Table 6.3)
* Feathers
* Claws and nails.

Skin

Skin forms an external covering layer over the body, merging with the mucous membranes at the body openings, e.g. mouth. Figure 6.4 shows the structure of the skin.

Skin has several functions:

* It protects the surface of the body
* It protects against invasion by microorganisms
* It has a role in controlling body temperature (homeostasis)
* It prevents excessive water loss
* It manufactures vitamin D
* The hair and pigment in the skin (melatonin) protect the body against ultraviolet radiation
* It contains specialised receptors which are sensory cells that detect changes in the environment, e.g. pressure, temperature, pain

Table 6.2 Classification of sense organs according to energy		
Type of receptor	**Examples**	**Effective stimulus**
Mechanoreceptors	Tactile receptors Semicircular canals Proprioreceptors in muscle spindles	Mechanical energy – touch, pressure, gravity, stretching, movement
Chemoreceptors	Tastebuds Olfactory epithelium	Chemical stimuli – a multitude
Thermoreceptors	Pit organs in vipers(tongue) Nerve endings in skin	Heat/cold
Electroreceptors	Organs in fish	Electrical energy
Photoreceptors	Retina of vertebrates	Light energy

Table 6.3 Types of hair

Guard hairs	Long hairs of topcoat One from each follicle	Hackles raised Bottlebrush tail of cat
Wool hairs/undercoat	Insulating layer Shorter, softer hairs Trap air between them, creating warmth Can be lots from one follicle	Puppy coat In adult more in winter than summer
Vibrissae	Tactile hairs Thickest hairs Project beyond rest of coat Grow from specialised follicles Nerve endings at base Sensory organs	Should never be cut Mostly on head Upper lip Above eyes

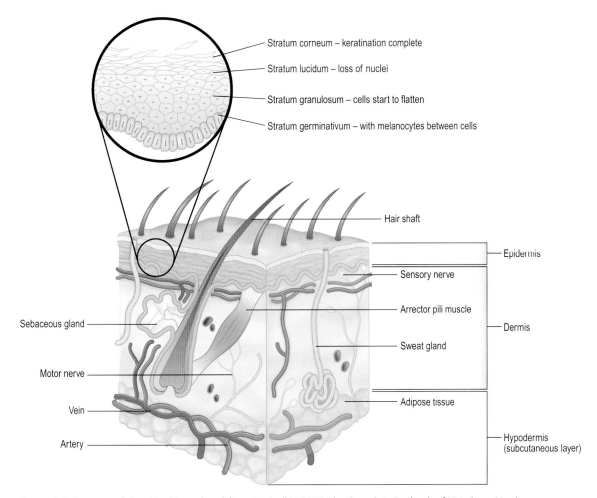

Figure 6.4 Structure of the skin. (Reproduced from Aspinall V 2006 *The Complete Textbook of Veterinary Nursing.* Butterworth Heinemann, London, with permission.)

- It contains glands (sebaceous and sweat glands) which give it a secretory function
  - These glands produce sebum (sebaceous glands)
  - They produce pheromones.

Skin consists of three layers:

1. Epidermis
2. Dermis
3. Hypodermis.

The epidermis

- This is the outer layer of the skin
- It contains no blood vessels and consists of stratified squamous epithelium
- The thickest areas are the pads of the feet and the nose.

The dermis

- This is the layer underneath the epidermis which is firmly attached to it
- It is composed of fibrous dense connective tissue with some elastic tissue for shock absorption and some fat cells for insulation
- It also contains blood vessels, nerves, muscles, hair follicles, glands and pigment cells.

The hypodermis

- This is not a true layer of skin
- It is the layer underneath the dermis
- It consists of layers of loose connective tissue, often with fat cells between the layers.

Temperature control Skin plays an important part in temperature control. Heat is maintained by fur acting as an insulator and fat acting as an insulator. Heat is lost by evaporation of sweat but this process requires heat; latent heat from the body is used and the body cools down effectively. The body must have mechanisms to cope with overheating and overcooling to enable it to maintain a constant body temperature.

There are two types of glands present within the skin: sebaceous and sweat glands. They are both examples of exocrine glands.

Sebaceous glands

- These are located alongside hair follicles
- They produce sebum
- For the hair to stand erect a papillary muscle contracts within the hair follicle and simultaneously squeezes sebum out and along the hair shaft
- Other sebaceous glands are found in the tail and the anal glands (both of which can become blocked due to overproduction of sebum)
- Sebum aids in thermostatic control.

Functions of sebum

- It keeps the skin and hair soft
- It helps protect the integument against drying out
- It can produce a smell, playing a role in territory marking
- It waterproofs the coat
- It contains pheromones.

Sweat glands or sudoriferous glands There are two types – eccrine and apocrine glands.

Eccrine glands

- These empty directly on to the skin and are not connected to the hair follicle
- They are found in hairless areas, e.g. footpads and nose.

Apocrine glands

- These empty into the hair follicle
- They are found in haired skin and in specialist areas
- They help to provide a protective film over the body.

The ear

The functions of the ear are to enable hearing and control balance in the animal. All mammals have a pair of ears located on the dorsal aspect of the head; other species have a rudimentary ear consisting of only the middle and inner ear, such as reptiles. The ear can be divided into three chambers:

1. Air-filled outer ear
2. Air-filled middle ear
3. Fluid-filled inner ear.

The outer or external ear

Pinna The internal ear is protected by the ear flap or pinna. This is a flap of skin that is given shape by elastic cartilage which also allows it to be flexible as it plays a role in body language. It is mobile and can be adapted to enhance the collection of sound waves. The inner surface has fine hairs and outer longer hairs which provide protection against pathogens and foreign bodies (Figure 6.5).

External auditory meatus At the base of the pinna there is a ring of cartilage called the annular cartilage which leads to the external auditory meatus. This consists of a vertical canal which starts at the base of the pinna connected to a horizontal canal which communicates with the tympanic membrane (eardrum). It is filled with air and if it becomes infected this would be classified as otitis externa. The skin inside contains ceruminous glands which are modified sebaceous glands that secrete wax which acts to protect the ear canal.

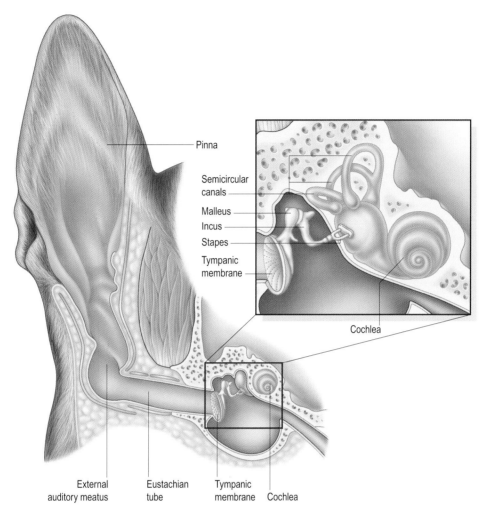

Pinna

Semicircular canals

Malleus

Incus

Stapes

Tympanic membrane

Cochlea

External auditory meatus   Eustachian tube   Tympanic membrane   Cochlea

Figure 6.5 Cross-section through the dog ear. (Reproduced from Aspinall V 2006 *The Complete Textbook of Veterinary Nursing*. Butterworth Heinemann, London, with permission.)

Tympanic membrane

- This is also known as the eardrum
- It comprises a stretched sheet of tissue that forms a barrier between the middle ear and the outer ear
- The eardrum vibrates when sound waves hit it and it effectively transfers the sound into the middle ear via the ear ossicles
- The eardrum can be ruptured.

Middle ear

The middle ear is located within the temporal bone of the skull. It contains air, the auditory ossicles or bones (malleus, incus, stapes) in the tympanic cavity and the opening of the eustachian tube. The auditory ossicles are three small bones which have synovial joints between

them: the malleus or hammer, the incus or anvil and the stapes or stirrup. The ossicles transmit the sound waves they have collected from the eardrum to the oval window of the inner ear.

Eustachian tube

- This is also known as the auditory tube
- It connects the middle ear to the pharynx
- It allows regulation of pressure which is achieved via swallowing
- It keeps ear pressure at atmospheric pressure, i.e. in equilibrium on either side of the eardrum.

Inner ear

The inner ear is situated within the temporal bone and it contains the hearing apparatus. It is a fluid-filled sealed chamber comprising a membranous labyrinth which is inside a bony labyrinth. The bony labyrinth is made up of the vestibule, containing the semicircular canals, the cochlea and the round window. The membranous labyrinth contains a fluid called endolymph and the space between the membranous and bony labyrinth is filled with a fluid called perilymph. Sound waves are transferred into the inner ear from the oval window. It is in the inner ear where the sound waves are interpreted for pitch and balance is maintained.

Balance

The inner ear consists of two sac-like chambers – the saccule and the utricle – three semicircular canals and the snail-like cochlea. The vestibular apparatus comprises the saccule and the utricle and the semicircular canals. The saccule and utricle contain gravity detectors called otoliths. Otoliths are small calcium carbonate stones.

The pull of gravity causes the otoliths to move and press on different sensory hair cells sited upon a gelatinous cupula, stimulating them to send nervous impulses to the brain. When the head is tilted the pressure of the otoliths on the hairs enables the animal to perceive the direction of gravity.

The direction the head is turning in is sensed by the semicircular canals. Each canal is linked to the utricle. The three lie at right angles to each other. Each canal is filled with a fluid called endolymph. At the opening to the utricle there is a specialised bulb called the ampulla, which contains sensory hairs similar to those in the utricle and saccule but without the otoliths. These sensory hairs are called crista and connect to receptor cells that are stimulated by movement within the endolymph. When the head turns, the endolymph within the semicircular canals will be slightly delayed in its movement. As the fluid flows the cristae are stimulated, giving the feeling of rotation and causing the eyes to move. Because there are three semicircular canals, whenever the head is moved one of the canals will detect movement within the endolymph. It is the movement of endolymph that causes motion sickness and the dizzy feeling associated with alcohol.

Hearing

Birds and mammals have highly developed senses of hearing. Sounds are detected within the inner ear in a structure called the cochlea. The cochlea is a spiral tube within the inner labyrinth of the inner ear. It looks like a snail's shell and contains specialised mechanoreceptor hair cells that detect pressure waves. If the cochlea was uncoiled, it would consist of three canals separated by thin membranes which come to almost a point at the apex.

The outer canal and inner canal, the vestibular canal and tympanic canal, are connected to one another at the apex and are filled with perilymph. The middle canal, the cochlear duct, is filled with endolymph and contains the actual organ of hearing – the organ of Corti.

Each organ of Corti contains 24 000 hairs arranged in rows running the entire length of the coiled cochlea. The hairs rest upon the basilar membrane, which separates the cochlea from the tympanic canal. Overhanging the hair cells is another membrane, the tectorial membrane – this is attached to the hair cells on one side and unattached on the other. The hair cells initiate impulses in the fibres of the cochlear (auditory) nerve.

How do we hear?

* Sound waves are detected in the specialised pinna and directed down the external auditory meatus (outer-ear canal) and progress to the eardrum
* The eardrum (tympanic membrane) vibrates
* The vibrations are transmitted across the middle ear by the malleus, incus and stapes. The malleus is in contact with the tympanic membrane and the stapes with the fenestra ovalis (oval window)
* The vibrations or sound waves pass the oval window into the fluid filling the vestibular canal. Since fluids cannot be compressed there must be an escape valve for the pressure that builds up. This is provided by the round window at the end of the tympanic canal
* The pressure wave presses upon the round window causing it to bulge
* The pressure wave causes movements in the endolymph within the organ of Corti and stimulates the cells upon the basilar membrane, which in turn stimulate the cochlear nerve, and as a result we hear!

Sounds vary in pitch, loudness and tone quality. Animals can detect a much wider range of pitch than human beings. Pitch is determined by frequency of sound waves; the higher the frequency, the higher the pitch and vice versa. Loudness produces amplitude waves of a greater intensity that cause a different pattern of hair stimulation, helping the body to recognise the level of noise produced.

Deafness This is caused by damage to the hearing apparatus. This could include:

* Very loud noise which can injure the organ of Corti
* Infection in the middle or the inner ear
* A blockage of wax in the outer ear
* Genetic defects: cats with a white coat and blue eyes are usually deaf
* Old age
* Some drugs/toxins.

Species variation

Birds have a very similar hearing system to mammals, although the external ear and pinna are not present. They do have a three-compartment ear and have highly specialised hearing as they communicate a lot via sound, e.g. bird song. Reptiles do not have an external ear and the internal ear comprises only the middle and inner sections; hearing is probably their poorest sense and it is thought that they only detect vibrations rather than pitch.

Taste and smell

The sensitivity of chemoreceptors varies greatly between species. Chemoreceptors are responsible for the senses of taste and smell.

Taste

In higher vertebrates, taste is detected by specialised cells known as the tastebuds. They are found predominantly in the mouth on the tongue in tiny elevations or papillae. They are replaced approximately every 10–30 hours.

A tastebud consists of an epithelial capsule containing several taste receptors. It has microvilli at its free surface and a hair-like projection that extends to the tongue surface. Each taste receptor is connected to a sensory neuron with a complicated interlocking system so that more than one neuron can be stimulated by a certain taste. Certain tastes are detected in certain areas of the tongue. Flavour is a combination of taste, smell and thermoreception.

Smell

Smell or olfaction occurs in the olfactory epithelium located on the upper surface of the nasal cavity (internal nares). Nasal epithelium contains approximately 20 million specialised olfactory cells connected to the axons of the olfactory nerve. On the end of each olfactory cell are a number of hairs that are thought to react to specific odours (chemicals) in the respired air. Certain animals have more specialised senses of smell than others.

Species variation – organ of Jacobson

This is a specialised organ in the roof of the mouth of some species, e.g. reptiles and horses. It enables further evaluation of the inspired air as it is packed full of specialised sensory receptors. In reptiles the organ of Jacobson is used to taste and smell their environment; the animal uses its tongue to push air back into the cavity below the organ of Jacobson and it is here the sensory cells interpret the information it contains. This advanced sense can enable prey to be detected, mates to be detected and the animal's environment to be fully explored. In horses the organ of Jacobson is also used to evaluate smells further; the horse raises its top lip and snorts in extra air which it transfers to the cavity containing the organ of Jacobson. Flehmen is often exhibited during reproduction or when a new object is encountered.

Some reptiles, e.g. vipers, have sensory pits in their head which can detect their prey's body heat, enabling them to hunt very effectively.

Vision

There are many different types of vision apparatus within the animal kingdom depending on the species under consideration; in this section the mammalian eye will be examined (Figure 6.6).

The eyeball is located within the orbit of the skull and is embedded in a pad of fat, leaving it very well protected with only its anterior exposed. It is supplied by the second cranial nerve. The eye consists of three layers:

1. An outer fibrous coat – the sclera and the cornea
2. A middle vascular layer – the choroids, tapetum lucidum, the ciliary body and the iris
3. An inner nervous layer – the retina.

Sclera This is the outer coating of the eye; it is made of tough connective tissue. It is an opaque white colour. The sclera helps to maintain the rigidity of the eyeball. The extrinsic and intrinsic eye muscles are attached to the sclera; the extrinsic muscles move the eyeball and the intrinsic muscles change the shape of the lens. The epithelium of the sclera is continuous with the inner layer of the eyelids and anteriorly it is continuous with the cornea.

Cornea This is a continuation of the sclera and covers the front or anterior of the eye. It is thinner than the sclera and transparent to allow light to enter. It has no blood supply but does contain a large number of nerves to protect against dust and dirt. The cornea receives nourishment and lubrication from the lacrimal glands (which produce tears) and the aqueous humour. It has a very thin layer of conjunctiva covering it. The junction between sclera and cornea is called the limbus.

Choroid This is a thin pigmented layer, which lines the inner surface of the sclera. It is extremely vascular and has a brown coloration due to the presence of dark pigment cells that absorb light that passes through the retina, preventing internal infections. It supplies the retina with nutrients.

Ciliary body The ciliary body is located behind the limbus. It is a projection of the choroid and is circular in structure. It comprises lots of involuntary muscle

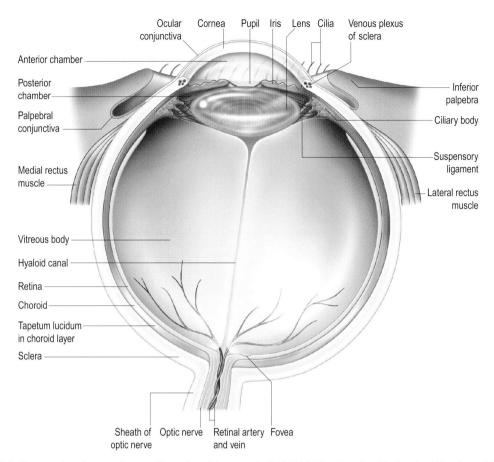

Figure 6.6 Cross-section through the eye. (Reproduced from Aspinall V 2006 *The Complete Textbook of Veterinary Nursing*. Butterworth Heinemann, London, with permission.)

fibres and has suspensory ligaments that attach to its inner surface. The intrinsic muscles of the eye alter the shape of the lens by pulling the suspensory ligaments to focus light entering the eye on the retina.

Iris This is part of the intrinsic muscle group of the eye. It is a thin pigmented disc which is attached to the anterior margin of the ciliary body. It contains the pupil in its central aperture. It has two groups of involuntary muscles, the radial and circular muscles, which alter the size and shape of the pupil to control the amount of light entering the eye.

Retina This is the innermost coating of the eye. It lines the choroid and is a delicate membrane. It consists of nerve fibres and specialised cells known as rods and cones which detect light. It also contains sensory nerve endings that pass the electrical impulses that translate to vision to the brain via the optic nerve.

Cones These are colour-sensing cells. Every cone connects to the optic nerve. They are densely packed together

around the fovea or yellow spot where colour vision is most acute. They aid animals who have colour vision to perceive their environment as accurately as possible.

Rods These are the most common light receptor cell. They lie outside the fovea and their function is to perceive as much light as possible. They detect black and white, enable some degree of night vision and act to provide retinal convergence – a process by which all their signals are added together to give a cumulative effect.

Nerve cells Ganglion and bipolar cells conduct impulses from rods and cones to the brain via the optic nerve.

Fovea This is the area of ultimate vision. It is located in a depression in the centre of the posterior part of the retina and comprises only cones.

Optic disc The optic disc is the area where all the nerve fibres join together to leave the eye and form the optic nerve. It is also known as the blind spot as it contains neither rods nor cones and cannot detect vision. The ophthalmic artery and vein also leave the eye through the optic disc.

Aqueous humour The aqueous humour is the fluid that fills the anterior chamber of the eyeball. It is clear and watery in consistency and is found between the cornea and the lens. It is secreted in the posterior chamber behind capillaries in the ciliary body. It is constantly flowing and provides nourishment for the cornea. It exerts a constant pressure on the front of the eye and drains into the canal of Schlemm.

Vitreous humour Vitreous humour is the fluid that fills the posterior chamber of the eye. Its consistency is different to that of aqueous humour, being thick and viscous or jelly-like. It is transparent to allow light through the eye to the retina. By filling the larger posterior chamber of the eye it helps maintain the shape of the eye. It also supports the delicate retina against the choroid.

Lens The lens has a biconvex shape; it is transparent and enclosed in a protective capsule. It is suspended by the suspensory ligaments from the ciliary body. Both the capsule and lens are elastic, allowing the shape to be altered depending on what the animal is focusing upon.

Tapetum lucidum This is a layer of specialised cells present in the choroid layer; the cells are iridescent, i.e. they give the eye the ability to glow in the dark. The tapetum covers approximately one-third of the choroid's layer. The function is to reflect light in the eye at night or in darkness to utilise the light present to its optimum capacity, thereby helping to improve night vision. It develops after birth and in dogs gives the eye at night a green/yellow/pinkish colour and in cats a brighter more metallic colour, often yellow.

Eyelids The eyelids provide protection for the delicate eyeball. They reduce secretions and distribute them over the eye surface. They are mobile folds of skin that protect the front of the eye. They play a role in the corneal reflex which innately shuts the eye when an object approaches it. The upper and lower lids meet at the medial (nearest to the nose) and the lateral (corner) canthus. The lids are lined with mucous membranes continuous with the conjunctiva. The formix is the junction between the conjunctiva and the eyelid which contains sebaceous glands (tarsal and meibomian glands) that produce a waxy substance that prevent lacrimal fluid running down the animal's face.

Nictitating membrane This is also known as the third eyelid and is present in many species. It projects from the medial canthus and consists of a plate of hyaline cartilage covered by a conjunctival layer. It is held in place by a pad of fat. It is often seen during illness or

disease when fat is displaced, causing it to cover the animal's eye partially.

Lacrimal glands These are found on the dorsolateral surface of the eyelid and produce lacrimal fluid (tears). Lacrimal fluid is spread over the eye by blinking.

The lacrimal canaliculi are small ducts in the medial canthus where tears pass into the lacrimal sacs and the nasolacrimal duct is a duct that drains tears from the lacrimal sac into the nasal passages. Lacrimal ducts can become blocked or have poor conformation, leading to insufficient drainage and resulting in euphoria.

Muscles of the eye

- Intrinsic: ciliary body, which controls the shape of the lens
- Extrinsic: six opposing pairs, which hold the eyeball in the socket (the strongest is the retractor bulbi)
- Palpebral: voluntary and involuntary muscles, used in blinking.

How do we see?

When humans or animals look at an object they perceive an upright vision of that object instantaneously. Light rays travel in straight lines and are refracted (bent) by the object being viewed and a certain number of them will enter the eye through the pupil. The light rays are then refracted again by the lens, which can alter shape to increase the clarity of the image to be projected on the retina. The light rays then hit the retina, stimulating the rods and cones. Impulses from the rods and cones are sent to the brain, resulting in an inverted image of the original image. The brain organises the stimuli and reinverts the image so the object is perceived the correct way up.

The position of the eyes on the head directly influences the range of vision an animal detects. Predators such as dogs whose eyes are situated at the front of the head have good three-dimensional vision, enabling perception of distance, which is favourable for hunting, but poor peripheral vision. Conversely, herbivore species often have eyes located on the sides of the head; this provides a narrower field of three-dimensional vision to the front of the head, blind spots directly underneath the head but enhanced fields of peripheral vision which would allow detection of predators whilst grazing.

Species variation

Reptile vision varies between species but in those that hunt binocular vision is often provided by eyes located at the front of the head; some species such as chameleons can move each eye independently. Some species have a single transparent scale or 'spectacle' which takes the role of an eyelid protecting the eye whereas others have none.

Bibliography

Aspinall V 2006 The complete textbook of veterinary nursing. Butterworth Heinemann, London

Aspinall V, O'Reilly M 2004 Introduction to veterinary anatomy and physiology. Butterworth Heinemann, Oxford

Campbell N, Reece J, Mitchell L 1999 Biology, 5th edn. Benjamin Cummings, San Francisco

Colville T, Bassett J M 2002 Clinical anatomy and physiology for veterinary technicians. Mosby, St Louis

Dyke K M, Sack W O, Wensing C J G 1996 Text book of veterinary anatomy, 2nd edn. W B Saunders, Philadelphia

Green N P O, Stout G W, Taylor D J 1991 Biological science. Cambridge University Press, Cambridge

Lane D R, Cooper B, Turner L 2007 BSAVA Textbook of Veterinary Nursing. BSAVA, Oxford

Moore M 2000 Manual of veterinary nursing. BSAVA, Oxford

Pratt P W 1998 Principles and practice of veterinary technology. Mosby, Philadelphia

Roberts M B V 1986 Biology: a functional approach. Nelson, Surrey, UK

Simpson G 1994 Practical veterinary nursing, 3rd edn. BSAVA, Oxford

Chapter | **7** | *Jane Williams*

Endocrine and exocrine systems

This chapter considers how the animal body maintains physiological equilibrium and operates at normal values via the process of homeostasis. The role that both the endocrine and exocrine systems play within homeostatic control is examined as well as specific examples of common hormonal mechanisms in operation.

HOMEOSTASIS

Homeostasis is the name given to the collective processes which occur within the animal body to maintain its equilibrium and functioning correctly. The body needs to regulate temperature, water, acid–base balance and the circulating levels of glucose in the blood, amongst other things.

Fluid balance and disposal of metabolic wastes

Water is essential for life and determines what type of life is present and its distribution on earth. It is the medium where metabolic reactions take place.

The simplest life is found in the sea, utilising sea water for oxygen and food requirements. Such animals release excretory products directly into the sea and use passive transport methods such as diffusion and osmosis to facilitate these processes.

Complex life has also colonised the land; it could be said it has its own 'internal sea' provided by the blood and extracellular fluid. These organisms still require processes to take in oxygen and nutrients and to remove excretory products. Terrestrial animals obtain water from drinking and from the diet and it is created as a byproduct of metabolic reactions (the transformation of adenosine diphosphate to adenosine triphosphate creates metabolic water).

Osmoregulation is defined as control of the water content of the body and control of the concentration and distribution of ions within the body.

Different animals utilise different systems. For example, freshwater protozoa have contractile vacuoles to pump out excess water. Other species have specialised structures designed to rid the body of excess water and ions are usually adapted to rid the body of metabolic wastes. Organs that get rid of waste products are part of the animal's excretory system. If waste metabolites from cells were not excreted they would rise to toxic levels and therefore threaten homeostasis (balance) so it is important that they are continuously excreted from the body.

Excretion is the process of removing metabolic wastes from the body (Figure 7.1). Elimination is the removal of undigested or unabsorbed food materials from the body in the faeces; these have merely passed through the digestive system and did not undergo any metabolic reactions, e.g. fibre.

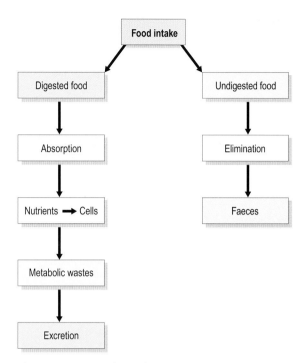

Figure 7.1 Process of excretion.

Functions of an excretory system

The main function of an excretory system is to contribute to the maintenance of homeostasis. This is achieved by:

- Excreting metabolic wastes
- Performing osmoregulation (fluids and salts)
- Regulation of the concentration of most body fluids (constituents).

The specific excretory organ collects fluid, e.g. blood in the kidney, interstitial fluid in the lymphatic system and then adjusts its composition by reabsorbing substances, e.g. glucose in the renal tubule. The adjusted excretory product is expelled from the body, e.g. as urine from the renal tubule.

Waste products

The principal waste products created in the body are water, carbon dioxide and nitrogenous waste. Water is excreted via the kidney and through involuntary losses, e.g. respiratory losses. Carbon dioxide is excreted by diffusion during respiration. Nitrogenous waste includes ammonia, urea and uric acid; it requires deamination before it is excreted via the kidney.

Process of deamination

Figure 7.2 shows the process of deamination.

Uric acid

Uric acid presents as a paste that can be excreted in conjunction with faeces, e.g. birds have no urinary bladder and frequently excrete uric acid and faeces to decrease their weight to facilitate flight. It is also non-toxic and therefore it is a good evolutionary adaptation for egg-laying species as, when their developing young are enclosed in the egg, they will have increasing levels of uric acid; therefore any substance that is excreted needs to be non-toxic as it will increase in concentration.

Vertebrates

Metabolic waste disposal and fluid balance are controlled by an excretory or urinary system in conjunction with the skin, the respiratory system and the digestive system. Some vertebrates also have special salt glands that excrete salt. All these organs help maintain homeostasis.

Excretory organs

The function of the mammalian kidney is to excrete nitrogenous waste and excrete and absorb water, salts and other substances such as glucose, amino acids and ketones which influence homeostasis. The functional units of the kidney are the nephrons, which filter and facilitate reabsorption and secretion of substances from the blood. Blood is filtered in the glomerulus to form the glomerular filtrate. The filtrate passes through coiled tubules in the nephron, where reabsorption back into the circulation and secretion into filtrate occur. Waste products are excreted as urine.

Fish

Fish have a constant problem with osmoregulation. Marine bony fish have blood and body fluids which are hypotonic to sea water and therefore lose water osmotically, leading to dehydration. They compensate for this process by continually drinking sea water; they retain water and excrete salt through special cells located in the gills. Their kidneys are usually very small and only a small volume of urine is produced.

Marine chondrocytes such as sharks and rays experience the same osmotic problem with an accumulation of urea in the blood and the interstitial fluid. They therefore become hypotonic to sea water and water enters their body by osmosis via the gills. Their tissues have evolved to function at levels of urea which would prove toxic for other species; they excrete copious amounts of hypotonic urine and excess salts are excreted by the kidney and a specialised rectal gland.

Freshwater fish are hypertonic to water, therefore water enters their body by osmosis. They have an impervious covering of mucus to stop water entering through

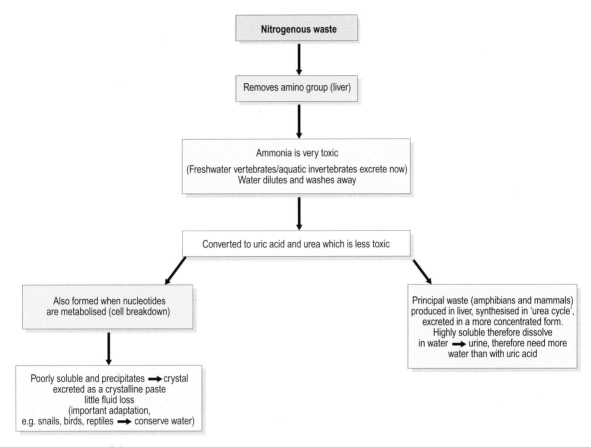

Figure 7.2 Process of deamination.

the body but it will still enter through the gills. Their kidneys reabsorb salts but not water and therefore they produce copious, dilute urine. They also lose salt into the water but have specialised cells in their gills which counteract this by obtaining salt via active transport from the water.

Amphibians

Amphibians are usually semiaquatic; they have a similar osmoregulation mechanism to freshwater fish, producing large quantities of copious urine.

Reptiles and marine birds

These species often have salt glands in the head in response to osmotic stress. Because they drink sea water or eat salty food, they actively secrete salt.

Whales, dolphins and marine mammals

These species ingest sea water with their food. Their kidneys produce very concentrated urine which is hypertonic to sea water (i.e. it is saltier).

This is an important physiological adaptation, especially for marine carnivores which have a high-protein diet of meat and produce large quantities of urea (by deamination). This needs to be excreted via the urine as it is toxic.

THERMOREGULATION

Thermoregulation is the process of maintaining body heat. There are two categories of animals: exothermic and endothermic. Exothermic or cold-blooded species take on the temperature of their environment and examples of animals in this group are reptiles. They require external heat sources, e.g. sun or warm rocks, to allow them to absorb sufficient heat to enable their body to have enough energy to function. Endothermic or warm-blooded animals maintain a constant internal temperature; to enable this a number of mechanisms are in place to increase or decrease temperature.

The hypothalamus plays an important role in thermo-regulation. When the body is too hot or too cold the hypothalamus innervates a response in the skin. If it is too hot, the papillary muscles in the skin relax, laying the hair flat so it does not trap air, glands secrete sweat on to the skin surface, facilitating heat loss through evap-oration and the blood vessels in the skin dilate, giving them a larger surface area through which heat from the blood can dissipate into the air. If it is too cold the opposite effects occur: hairs are stood on end to trap an insulating layer of air, sweat production ceases and the peripheral blood vessels vasoconstrict to conserve heat. The hypothalamus will also stimulate muscles to shiver if cold, thereby generating heat to warm the body up.

ENDOCRINE SYSTEM

See Box 7.1 for definitions relating to the endocrine system.

There are three types of hormones:

1. Hormones secreted by endocrine glands, e.g. thyroxine
2. Hormones secreted by neurons, e.g. antidiuretic hormone
3. Chemical messengers secreted by individual cells, e.g. testosterone.

Trophic hormones act on nerves to get reactions in tissues and trophin hormones act on glands themselves.

Role of hormones

Hormones have an important role in maintaining equi-librium within body systems. They are effective at very low concentrations. Chemically they are composed of proteins or lipids:

- Proteins: amines, peptides, proteins
- Lipids: derived from fatty acids or steroids.

Note: pheromones are chemicals produced by exocrine glands and do not regulate any metabolic activities and are therefore not classified as hormones.

How do hormones work?

At any one time in the body there will be approximately 30 different hormones circulating within the blood. Some hormones are free-travelling whereas others bind to the larger plasma protein molecules to be transported around the circulatory system. When the hormone arrives at its location, the hormone molecules diffuse out of the blood into the interstitial fluid around the target organ and then act upon the target organ cells. The target organs recognise their own hormones using specialised receptor cells embedded along the surface of the cell membrane of the organ cells. These recognise the hormone and bind to it. The hormone will only have an effect if it is bound correctly and allowed access into the organ.

This process can be compared to a lock-and-key mechanism, with the receptor protein being the lock and hormones being different keys. Only the specific hormone or key that fits the lock will allow the meta-bolic activity door to open.

How does an endocrine gland know how much of a hormone to secrete?

Hormone secretion is monitored by negative-feedback mechanisms. This works by special receptor cells in the body feeding back information about the level of hormone currently circulating to the endocrine gland from which it came. This is known as negative feedback because the effects are opposite to the stimulus. The gland then responds homeostatically, i.e. if low levels are present then more is produced; if high levels are present then production will be stopped.

Example: circulating calcium levels

Circulatory calcium levels are regulated by the parathy-roid gland production of parathyroid hormone. Parathy-roid hormone stimulates the release of calcium from the bones and also increases the rate of reabsorption of calcium from the kidneys. These two actions will increase the calcium concentration in the blood.

When the calcium levels drop, even if only slightly, the parathyroid gland will increase the rate of parathy-

---

Box 7.1

DEFINITIONS

Endocrine gland

A ductless gland that secretes one or more hormones that are transported by the blood

Endocrinology

Study of endocrine activity – including endocrine glands and neurons that produce hormones

Hormone

A chemical messenger transported by the blood to a target organ or a chemical messenger produced by one type of cell that has a specific regulatory effect on the activity of another type of cell

roid hormone secretion. Alternatively if the calcium levels exceed normal levels, the parathyroid glands are inhibited and slow the rate of production of parathyroid hormone.

Roles of hormones

- Hormones regulate metabolic/body activities, e.g. growth, metabolic rate, utilisation of nutrients by cells and reproduction
- Their main role is to regulate fluid balance and to maintain homeostasis
- They also help the body to cope with stress.

Principal endocrine glands

The location of the main endocrine glands is shown in Figure 7.3. The main endocrine glands are:

- Pituitary gland
- Thymus
- Thyroid
- Parathyroid
- Pancreas
- Adrenals
- Ovary
- Testes
- Pineal gland.

Before considering the individual endocrine glands, the role of the hypothalamus should be discussed.

Hypothalamus

The hypothalamus links the hormone and nervous system and is not actually an endocrine gland. It does produce hormones but does not release them. It produces antidiuretic hormone (vasopressin) which increases absorption of water in the renal tubules. It also produces oxytocin, which causes contraction of smooth muscle. These substances are then stored in the posterior pituitary gland.

Pituitary gland

The pituitary gland is approximately the size of a pea and is located in front of the hypothalamus. It has two parts: the anterior pituitary or adenohypophysis and the posterior pituitary or neurohypophysis. It secretes at least nine hormones. The posterior lobe releases:

- Antidiuretic hormone and oxytocin.

The anterior lobe produces and releases:

- Growth hormone somatotrophin, which controls rate of growth and acts on epiphysis of bones
- Prolactin, which controls milk letdown
- Gonadotrophin – one of the sex hormones

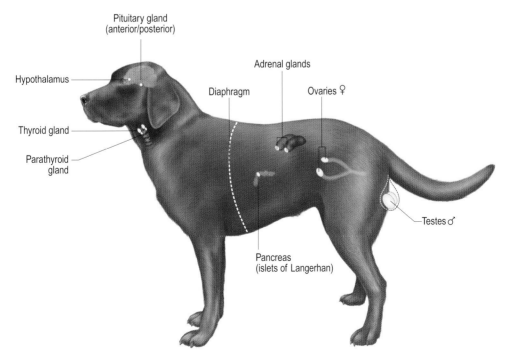

Figure 7.3 Location of major endocrine glands.

- Thyroid-stimulating hormone (TSH)
- Adrenocorticotrophic hormone, which regulates the adrenocortex hormones
- Luteinising hormone, which causes secretion of testosterone in the male and in the female is responsible for the development of the corpus luteum
- Follicle-stimulating hormone
- Interstitial cell-stimulated hormone.

Thyroid glands

These are located in the neck, either side of the midline, on the ventral aspect of the first tracheal rings and just below the larynx. They are essential for normal growth and development to occur in the animal as they stimulate the rate of metabolism within the body. They are also necessary for cellular differentiation and they promote protein synthesis and enhance growth hormone. They produce the hormones thyroxine and triiodothyronine which act together to regulate metabolism; they also produce thyrocalcitonin which decreases the level of plasma calcium by slowing its reabsorption from bone.

Regulation

The thyroid hormones are regulated by a feedback system between the anterior pituitary and the thyroid gland. The pituitary secretes TSH which promotes the synthesis and secretion of thyroid hormones and increases the size of the thyroid gland. When the concentration of thyroid hormones in the blood rises above normal, cells in the anterior pituitary are inhibited and TSH release is decreased. Too much thyroid hormone in blood affects the hypothalamus, inhibiting the secretion of TSH-releasing hormone. Hypothyroidism results in a low metabolic rate and retarded mental and physical development. Hyperthyroidism results in a high metabolic rate – a skinny but ravenous animal which often has a goitre.

Parathyroids

These lie on either side of and very close to the thyroid glands. They produce parathormone which regulates the metabolism and distribution of calcium in the body. Secretion increases as plasma calcium levels decrease; this increases the absorption of calcium from the digestive tract, bone and the kidney tubules.

Pancreas

This gland is located in the mesentery of the duodenum and has both exocrine (digestive enzymes) and endocrine functions. The endocrine section is called the islets of Langerhans. The islets of Langerhans secrete insulin, glucagons and somatostatin.

Insulin produced by beta cells controls the uptake of blood glucose (storage of glucose to glycogen). Glucagons produced by alpha cells increase blood glucose levels by stimulating glycogen stores to become glucose. Somatostatin is produced by delta cells and inhibits the production of both insulin and glucagon, thus preventing large swings in blood sugar levels which could be detrimental to health.

Insulin

Insulin facilitates the uptake of glucose into skeletal muscle and fat cells. It stimulates cells to take up glucose from the blood whilst insulin lowers the blood glucose level. It also stimulates protein synthesis and promotes fat storage.

Glucagon

Glucagon acts antagonistically to insulin. It increases the concentration of glucose in blood and stimulates glycogenolysis (conversion of glycogen to glucose) in the liver. Glucagon also mobilises fatty acids and amino acids.

Regulation

The production of insulin and glucagon is controlled by the concentration of blood sugar. After a meal, blood glucose level increases and beta cells are stimulated, increasing insulin secretion. As the cells remove glucose from blood, the glucose concentration drops and insulin secretion decreases.

If an animal hasn't eaten for a long time, blood glucose is low and the alpha cells secrete glucagons. Glucose is mobilised from the liver stores and blood sugar levels return to normal. Hyperglycaemia is characterised by an abnormally high blood glucose level and hypoglycaemia is an abnormally low blood glucose level. Hypoglycaemia can be the result of excess insulin and can be fatal.

Somatostatin

Somatostain is secreted by delta cells. It inhibits the secretion of insulin and glucagons and eliminates large swings in blood glucose. It also decreases motility of gut and secretion of digestive juices to prevent further sugar entering the circulation which could enhance the problem.

Adrenal cortex

The adrenal glands are located at the top of each kidney; they have an inner region, the medulla, and an outer region, the cortex. They act independently of each other. The cortex produces three hormones, all of which are steroids:

- Glucocorticoids – cortisol (hydrocortisone) and corticosteroid
- Mineralocorticoids – aldosterone
- Adrenal sex steroids.

The medulla produces adrenaline (epinephrine) and noradrenaline (norepinephrine) which are responsible for the fight-or-flight response in animals.

Glucocorticoids

- These are always present in the blood stream
- They are increased by stress
- They increase glucose levels in the blood
- But they decrease glucose in the cells by stimulating gluconeogenesis (amino acids are transformed to glucose)
- They mobilise fatty acids from the adipose tissue
- They can depress the inflammatory healing response when present in huge amounts.

Mineralocorticoids

- Aldosterone regulates electrolyte levels, especially the levels of sodium and potassium ions in the body
- It stimulates the reabsorption of sodium ions in the kidney tubule and increases excretion of potassium ions
- Chloride ions accompany sodium ions due to ionic attraction and movement of water molecules is also affected.

Adrenal sex steroids

- These make up the male and female sex hormones
- They are produced by both sexes
- Generally they are of no importance but the exception can be in the neutered animal.

Ovary

The female gonad produces hormones after puberty:

- Progesterone from the corpus luteum
- Oestradiol (oestrogens)
- Relaxin.

Progesterone

Progesterone is essential for maintenance of pregnancy; it is produced by the corpus luteum and acts on the lining of the uterus and mammary tissue.

Oestradiol/oestrogens

These hormones prepare the genital tract for coitus and the reception of the fertilised egg; they are produced by cells in the wall of the developing ovarian follicle.

Relaxin

This is produced by the corpus luteum in late pregnancy; it relaxes the sacrosciatic and other ligaments around the birth canal, allowing the pelvis to dilate to allow the fetus out.

Testis

The male gonad produces hormones after puberty:

- Testosterone (interstitial cells)
- Oestrogens (Sertoli cells).

Testosterone

Testosterone is produced by interstitial cells in the testis, called the cells of Leydig. It stimulates the development and maintenance of the male secondary sexual characteristics, e.g. thickening of muscle and bulk, and enlargement of the testes.

Oestrogens

Oestrogens are produced by Sertoli cells in the testes. Sertoli cell tumours can cause increased oestrogen production which can lead to a male animal exhibiting female characteristics, including increased nipple size and coat changes.

Endocrine disorders

Endocrine disorders affect the rate of hormone secretion. Hyposecretion is a reduced output and occurs if target cells are deprived of needed stimulation. Hypersecretion is an abnormal increase in output and occurs if target cells are overstimulated. A normal amount of hormone could be secreted but the target cells may lack receptors or have faulty receptors and therefore cannot take up the hormone. Any abnormality will lead to predictable metabolic malfunctions and clinical symptoms.

Endocrine problems tend to be due to an overproduction of hormones or hypersecretion or an underproduction of hormones or hyposecretion. Alternatively there can be a breakdown in the mechanics of the process. For example, the target cells may lack the necessary receptors to bind to the hormones to facilitate the action required.

EXOCRINE GLANDS

These are specialised epithelial structures. The glands can be unicellular or multicellular.

Table 7.1 Location of exocrine glands	
Simple tubular	Wall of stomach and ileum
Simple alveolar	Sebaceous glands
Simple coiled	Sweat glands
Compound alveolar	Salivary glands
Compound tubular	Duodenal glands

Unicellular glands

- Found in epithelial linings, e.g. goblet cells, in digestive tract
- Unicellular glands are modified epithelial cells.

Multicellular glands

- These are of epithelial origin
- They lie within layers of epithelial tissue
- They have ducts connecting them to the epithelial surface
- They are classified according to shape:
  - ○ Tubular
  - ○ Alveolar/saccular
  - ○ Coiled
- They are also classified by how many shapes are present (see Table 7.1):
  - ○ Simple – only one shape
  - ○ Compound – more than one shape.

Bibliography

Aspinall V 2006 The complete textbook of veterinary nursing. Butterworth Heinemann, London

Aspinall V, O'Reilly M 2004 Introduction to veterinary anatomy and physiology. Butterworth Heinemann, Oxford

Campbell N, Reece J, Mitchell L 1999 Biology, 5th edn. Benjamin Cummings, San Francisco

Colville T, Bassett J M 2002 Clinical anatomy and physiology for veterinary technicians. Mosby, St Louis

Dyke K M, Sack W O, Wensing C J G 1996 Text book of veterinary anatomy, 2nd edn. W B Saunders, Philadelphia

Green N P O, Stout G W, Taylor D J 1991 Biological science. Cambridge University Press, Cambridge

Lane D R, Cooper B, Turner L 2007 BSAVA Textbook of Veterinary Nursing. BSAVA, Oxford

Moore M 2000 Manual of veterinary nursing. BSAVA, Oxford

Pratt P W 1998 Principles and practice of veterinary technology. Mosby, Philadelphia

Roberts M B V 1986 Biology: a functional approach. Nelson, Surrey, UK

Simpson G 1994 Practical veterinary nursing, 3rd edn. BSAVA, Oxford

Chapter | **8** | *Donna de Haan and Lucy Dumbell*

The animal and equine industry

This chapter defines what an industry is and then moves on to evaluate the modern animal and equine industries.

DEFINING AN INDUSTRY

The word 'industry' is a generic term used to describe a distinct group of economic activities. Industries can be described and classified by their primary activity or product, for example the equine industry or the animal industry. Industries tend to be broad in definition, covering lots of different types of businesses or activities, which can be grouped together to form sectors or further industry groupings. For example the Royal Society for the Prevention of Cruelty to Animals (RSPCA) is a registered charity whose vision is to 'work for a world in which all humans respect and live in harmony with all other members of the animal kingdom'. We could say the RSPCA's primary product is 'animals' and the primary activity is 'charity'; the organisation could therefore fall under discussion in both the animal industry and the charity industry. Defining an industry is therefore very subjective and although there are some international similarities, industries may be defined differently in different countries.

THE EQUINE INDUSTRY

Obviously equids are animals and we could choose to group these two industries (the animal industry and the equine industry) together. Indeed there will always be an overlap between the two, but because there is so much business activity linked to just equids, it tends to be referred to as a separate industry. In the UK, for example, it is estimated that:

- 43% of the British population have an interest in some aspect of equestrianism
- 7% of the population are riders (4.3 million people)
- 2.8 million households contain at least one rider
- The horse population is around 1.35 million
- Horses are owned or cared for by 720 000 people, or 1.2% of the UK population
- The industry's gross output is £3.4 billion per annum.

When describing an industry it sometimes helps to define the structure of the industry diagrammatically. In 2003 the Henley Centre was appointed to undertake research to provide information that would feed into the development of a long-term strategy for the horse industry in the UK. The commissioned report begins by defining the equine industry as 'encompassing all activity that has the horse as its focus and activity that, in some reasonable capacity, caters for such an industry'. In relation to this definition the equine industry can further be described through core and peripheral functions. Core functions are defined as all activities based on the use, possession or ownership of horses, ranging from professional through to leisure. Peripheral activities include the suppliers of horse-related goods and services for those core activities.

We could also describe and define the equine industry according to structure: which organisation is in charge, which organisations have power over others, which organisations work independently and which work together. This is similar to an organisational chart, which may show the chief executive at the top, then middle managers or department heads, followed by shop floor workers. Figure 8.1 shows what the UK equine industry might look like if we took this approach to define it.

According to a report published by the British Horse Industry Confederation in 2005, the UK equine industry directly employs approximately 50 000 people and indirectly employs in the region of 150 000–250 000 people. Within these employment figures will be a range of job opportunities, from office-based roles, such as being the chief executive officer of a governing body or working as a racing secretary, to very practical positions, such as

being a farrier, equine dental technician or riding instructor (Box 8.1).

THE ANIMAL INDUSTRY

Throughout this next section we will look at different aspects of the animal industry. In order to provide structure we have created a flow diagram based on the function and use of the animal (Figure 8.2).

Number of animals

The word 'animal' comes from the Latin word *animal*, of which *animalia* is the plural, and is derived from *anima*, meaning vital breath or soul. In everyday colloquial usage, and for the purpose of this chapter, the word 'animal' will refer to non-human animals. Around 1.5 million species of animals have been named, over a million of which are insects. However, we do not know exactly how many species of animals there are in the world.

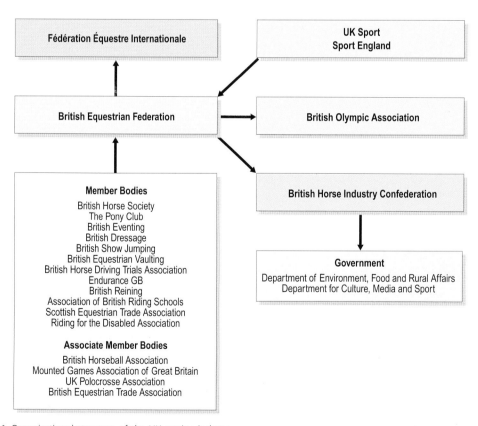

Figure 8.1 Organisational structure of the UK equine industry.

JOB IN FOCUS – RIDING INSTRUCTOR

The British Horse Society (BHS) examination scheme is one of the UK's most recognised riding instructor qualification systems. Through a series of vocational examinations designed for, and aimed at, persons wishing to pursue teaching as a career or who simply wish to explore the extent of their equestrian knowledge, candidates are tested on their skills and competencies in relation to working as a riding instructor and/or groom and/or stable manager. In relation to a career as a riding instructor, the BHS currently offers qualification levels of assistant instructor (BHSAI), intermediate instructor (BHSII), instructor (BHSI) and fellow (FBHS).

The International Group for Equestrian Qualifications (IGEQ) is an independent organisation of national equestrian federations worldwide. It currently has 32 members. The BHS qualifications sit within the qualifications matrix and consequently are recognised as valid and fit for purpose within the member countries. An equestrian passport is available for instructors of riding, driving, vaulting and therapeutic, with eligible certification which confirms and recognises the holder's qualifications, ensuring recognition and acceptance in all IGEQ member countries.

In relation to defining animal-related industries, we could group animals in a classification system along a spectrum of increasing domestication:

- Wild populations experience their full life cycle without deliberate human intervention
- Populations raised in captivity are nurtured and sometimes bred under human control, but remain as a group which is essentially indistinguishable in appearance or behaviour from their wild counterparts
- Domesticated populations are bred and raised under human control for many generations and are subsequently altered as a group in appearance or behaviour.

Each of these groups of animals could be defined as an industry. In relation to this chapter we will look more closely at domesticated animals.

Domestic animals

The term 'domestic animal' applies to animals that live in physical proximity to humans, such as companion animals, pets and guard animals, working animals, animals used in sport or even food species kept very close to humans. Again the category of domestic animals can be subdivided into three sections: socioeconomic uses, sport and leisure and intrinsically non-profit uses.

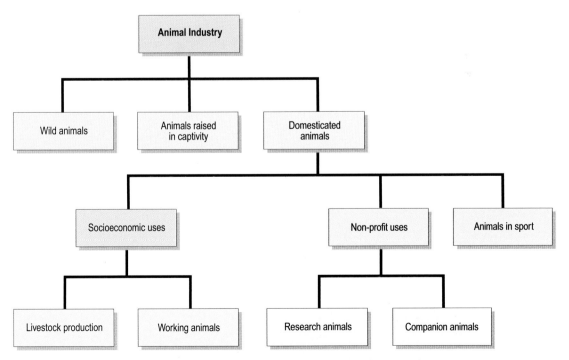

Figure 8.2 Flow diagram of the animal industry based on the function and use of the animal.

Socioeconomic uses

The body and natural produce, as well as the labour and senses, of various animals have been found to be useful for a wide variety of human activities. In this section we have defined an industry that uses animals predominantly for their economic value. This section of the animal industry includes livestock production and working animals.

Livestock is the term used to refer (singularly or plurally) to a domesticated animal intentionally reared in an agricultural setting. Raising animals (animal husbandry) is an important component of modern agriculture and is practised in many societies. Livestock are defined in part by their end purpose in relation to the production of a food source (meat, dairy) or a commodity (fibre, wool, mohair, leather, bones, horns, fertiliser) (Table 8.1).

In agriculture, agribusiness is a generic term that refers to the various businesses involved in food production, including farming, farm machinery, wholesale, marketing and retail. Agribusiness is widely used to refer to a range of activities and disciplines encompassed by modern food production.

Working animals are kept by humans and trained to perform tasks. Around the world millions of animals

work in a relationship with their owners. Domesticated animals are often specifically bred to be suitable for different uses; Golden Retrievers and Labradors for example are often the breed of choice for guide dog training. Some semidomesticated animals can also be classed as working animals, such as logging elephants.

Working animals may be selected and used for their physical strength; these are often referred to as draught or draft animals. This type of working animal is used to provide transport and haulage, such as pulling carts or sleds and ploughing fields, and is sometimes known as a beast of burden.

A pack animal is a beast of burden used by humans as a means of transporting materials. A packhorse refers generally to an equid such as a horse, mule, donkey or pony, used for carrying goods on its back, in sidebags or panniers. Typically packhorses were used to cross difficult terrain.

Packhorses were heavily used in the UK in the 18th century to transport goods. In North America packhorses, mules or donkeys were seen as a critical tool in the development of the Americas. Packhorses were used by Native American people when travelling from place to place, and were also used by traders to carry goods to both Indian and white settlements. Today in North America and Australia the packhorse still plays a major

Table 8.1 Estimated date of domestication and current commercial use of livestock

Animal	Estimated date of first captivity/domestication	Area of first captivity/domestication	Current commercial uses
Bison	Late 19th century	North America	Meat, leather,
Camel	Between 4000 BC and 1400 BC	Asia	Mount, pack animal, meat, dairy
Cattle	6000 BC	South-west Asia, India, North Africa	Meat (beef, veal, blood), dairy, leather
Goat	8000 BC	South-west Asia	Dairy, meat, wool, leather
Horse	4000 BC	Ukraine	Mount, pack animal, meat, dairy
Llama	3500 BC	Andes	Light mount, pack animal, meat, wool
Pig	7000 BC	Eastern Anatolia	Meat (pork) and bacon, leather
Rabbit	Between AD 400 and 900	France	Meat, fur
Reindeer	3000 BC	Russia	Meat, leather, antlers, dairy
Sheep	8000 BC	South-west Asia	Wool, dairy, meat (mutton and lamb)
Water buffalo	4000 BC	China (Tibetan plateau)	Mount, meat, dairy

role in recreational pursuits, particularly to transport goods and supplies into wilderness areas; they are even used by the US Forest Service. In the Third World, pack-horses and donkeys are still heavily used to transport produce to market and carry supplies for workers, and may even be used in modern warfare to take supplies into areas where roads are poor or fuel supply is uncertain. Arabian and Bactrian camels are also used as pack animals, as are llamas in the Andes and yaks in the Himalayas. Dogs, reindeer and goats are also used around the world to carry packs.

Working animals can also be harnessed, singly or in teams, to pull or haul sleds or wheeled vehicles. Harness animals predominantly include equids but dogs, reindeer and oxen are also used in harness. Equids, elephants, camels, oxen and yaks can all be utilised as ridden working animals.

Working animals can also be used for their senses and instincts. Working dogs are used around the world for a variety of purposes. Search dogs are trained to find missing people by following scent which is carried on the air. Dogs can work equally well in daylight or dark as they use their senses of smell and hearing. It is believed that in good search conditions, a dog is equivalent to about 20 human searchers, and can pick up a human scent from around 500 metres. Search dogs can be deployed to find missing people in a variety of situations in locations all around the world.

The National Search and Rescue Dog Association (NSARDA) is an umbrella organisation for air-scenting search dogs in the UK. Its members are the Search and Rescue Dog Associations (SARDAs) which are located throughout the UK. Each of the individual SARDAs is a voluntary organisation responsible for training and deployment of air-scenting search and rescue dogs to search for missing persons in the mountains and high moorlands of the UK as well as lowland, rural and urban areas (Box 8.2).

Another type of working dog is an assistance dog. Assistance Dogs International (ADI) is a worldwide coalition of non-profit organisations that trains and places assistance dogs. ADI categorises assistance dogs into three groups: guide dogs for the blind and visually impaired; hearing dogs for the deaf and hard of hearing; and service dogs for people with disabilities other than those related to vision or hearing. Assistance Dogs (UK) is the umbrella organisation for registered charities training assistance dogs in the UK.

The Guide Dogs for the Blind Association is a registered charity which was established in 1931. Here are some facts and figures about the charity you may not know:

- There are currently around 5000 working guide dogs in the UK today

JOB IN FOCUS – NATIONAL SEARCH AND RESCUE DOG ASSOCIATION (NSARDA) HANDLER

The entry requirements for becoming a handler vary slightly from association to association. In general, to become a trainee handler you must be proposed and supported by a mountain rescue (MR) team and have been a full-time member of that MR team for more than 12 months. This is because during training and upon qualification you will be expected to be familiar with MR techniques, and operate in potentially severe and dangerous environments. This normally means training takes 2 years in total – 12 months as a trainee, 12 months as a full member.

Ideally handlers would not get their dog for training until they start training with Search and Rescue Dog Associations (SARDAs). It is much better to start off on the right foot with your new dog, training with SARDA, than it is to set off doing one thing on your own and then try to change it later.

- The estimated lifetime cost of a guide dog is around £35 000 (including all breeding and training costs, vet and feeding bills)
- Guide Dogs for the Blind Association employs around 900 professional staff in the UK
- The charity is supported by around 10 000 volunteers
- The charity campaigns for the rights of visually impaired people in relation to mobility and access issues
- Guide Dogs for the Blind Association funds major research projects looking into the prevention and cure of eye disease
- The charity receives no government funding and is entirely dependent on voluntary donations
- Guide Dogs for the Blind Association requires over £50 million a year to provide its service
- The most common breed for guiding is a Labrador/Retriever cross, Labradoodles – a cross between a Labrador and a Poodle, which does not shed its hair – are also used, especially for people who may be allergic to traditional breeds of dogs
- The working life of a guide dog is about $6\frac{1}{2}$ years, and many owners will have several dogs during their lifetime. Retired dogs are placed with voluntary 'adopters'.

Dogs aren't the only animal used to assist the visually impaired. In 1999 the Guide Horse Foundation was established as an experimental programme to assess the abilities of miniature horses as assistance animals.

According to the Guide Horse Foundation there is a critical shortage of guide animals in the USA, and they believe miniature horses can provide the same level of assistance as dogs.

Non-profit uses

In the previous section we defined an industry that uses animals predominantly for their economic value, referred to as socioeconomic uses. In this section we look at industries which use animals in non-profit ways, including animals used in research and companion animals.

Research

The public debate on animal research sometimes becomes so heated that the facts can be forgotten. Animals have been used to help advance medical science since the 17th century. Many of the drugs and procedures we see as commonplace in modern medicine practice can trace their development back to research carried out on animals. As we have come to understand more about animal welfare, our use of animals in research has changed.

Trying to estimate the numbers of animals used in research worldwide is difficult because many countries do not provide comprehensive statistics. However, we know that the major centres for research are the USA (about 15 million procedures), the EU (about 11 million procedures) and Japan (about 5 million procedures), and that animals are also used in research in Canada (2 million), Switzerland (less than 1 million) and Australia (less than 1 million). If we make a generous estimate that other countries might carry out 10 million animal procedures every year, the total worldwide maximum is unlikely to exceed 50 million animal procedures per year.

The Research Defence Society (RDS) is the UK organisation representing medical researchers in the public debate about the use of animals in medical research and testing. They provide information about the need for animal research, the controls under which this research is carried out and the benefits to medicine which have resulted. The RDS also helps government and animal welfare groups to promote best practice in laboratory animal welfare and develop non-animal techniques.

According to the RDS, in 2006 just over 3 million scientific procedures using animals were carried out in the UK. The annual number of animal experiments has almost halved over the last 30 years. This is due to higher standards of animal welfare, scientific advances and stricter controls. There have been small rises in the last 5 years, so there now seems to be a gradual upwards trend following a few years when the numbers appeared to level off. The year 2006 marked the first time in 15 years that the number of procedures topped the 3 million mark. The recent rises in animal procedures are due to the increased production and use of animals with genetic modifications or defects; the numbers of genetically normal animals continue to fall year on year.

While nearly all species can potentially be involved in research related to their natural behaviour, there are a limited number of species that are frequently chosen, for convenience and/or as representative substitute for tests which would be unethical to perform on human test subjects. According to the RDS, the following list shows facts and figures relating to the types of animals used in medical research in the UK in 2006:

- 83% rats, mice and other rodents – all specially bred laboratory species
- 14% fish, amphibians, reptiles and birds (including many fertilised hen's eggs)
- 1.9% sheep, cows, pigs and other large mammals
- 0.7% small mammals other than rodents, mostly rabbits and ferrets
- 0.3% dogs and cats specially bred for research. No strays or unwanted pets can be used
- 0.15% monkeys, such as marmosets and macaques. Chimpanzees, orang utans and gorillas have not been used in the UK for over 20 years and their use is now banned.

The Animals (Scientific Procedures) Act 1986 protects all living vertebrate animals (plus one species of octopus) used in scientific procedures in the UK. Other invertebrate animals such as fruitflies and worms are also used in research, but are not protected under British law.

Guinea pigs, which would fall into the first RDS category above, have been used to advance medical research since the 17th century. In fact, the term 'guinea pig' has even been used as a metaphor in English for a subject of experimentation since the first half of the 20th century. Here are some facts and figures about guinea pigs and research you may not know:

- Guinea pigs have contributed to 23 Nobel prizes for medicine or physiology
- Studies on guinea pigs led to the discovery of vitamin C, the tuberculosis bacterium, and adrenaline (epinephrine)
- Guinea pigs were used in the development of vaccines for diphtheria, tuberculosis, replacement heart valves, blood transfusion, kidney dialysis, antibiotics, anticoagulants and asthma medicines
- Today guinea pigs are used mostly in research and testing to develop new medicines. The whole living animals are used as well as isolated tissues
- Guinea pigs were used in just over 27 000 scientific experiments in the UK in 2004, representing less than 1% of total animal research

- The use of guinea pigs has fallen by over three-quarters since 1988, mostly due to a reduction in their use in safety testing.

Companion animals

A companion animal or pet is an animal kept for companionship and enjoyment (Figure 8.3). Whilst in theory any animal could provide companionship, in practice only a relatively small number of mammals and other small animals can practically be kept as pets. In veterinary medicine, dogs and cats are often considered 'household' pets, whilst birds and reptiles are referred to as 'exotics'.

In the UK alone just over half of households own a pet, ranging from dogs, cats and rabbits to the more exotic snakes and spiders. Dogs and cats have traditionally been the most popular British pets. Over the past 10 years changes in lifestyle and how households are structured have affected the relative populations of dogs and cats. Urban living and modern working lifestyles favour the free-living, independent cat over the more dependent dog. As a result the cat population is gradually increasing to outnumber dogs. According to the American Veterinary Medical Association (AVMA) there are more than 72 million pet dogs in the USA and nearly 82 million pet cats. According to the Pet Food Manufacturers Association, in the UK in 2004 there were 6.1 million cat-owning households, 5.2 million dog-owning households, 4.1 million fish-owning households, 1.96 million rodent-owning households and 1.39 million bird-owning households. There is also a growing trend among pet owners towards owning unusual or exotic animals: snakes, reptiles and tropical fish are all growing in popularity.

There are several sectors of the animal industry which have specifically developed to cater for companion animals, such as pet food and pet care. Despite a general stagnation in pet numbers in the UK, the pet food and pet care market is one of the most robust sectors of the animal industry.

Today's pet owners are increasingly likely to consider their pets as part of the family and will go to greater efforts to care for them. According to AVMA nearly half of American pet owners consider their pets to be family members. With anthropomorphism (the attribution of uniquely human characteristics and qualities to non-human beings, such as animals) gathering pace, manufacturers are increasingly able to persuade pet owners to trade up to super-premium products which will drive sales of value products. Anthropomorphism is also contributing to the rise of the pet superstore as pet owners want to ensure that all their pet's requirements are met. This, however, is luring consumers away from small independent pet stores, which cannot stock wide ranges, particularly with the advent of lifestage products that pet owners are demanding. Marketeers expect to see an increasingly segmented market as manufacturers with similar high-quality products seek to drive value by diversifying their products (Box 8.3).

Therapy animals may also fall under the category of companion animals. Dogs are the most common type of therapy animal. The concept of a therapy dog is often attributed to Elaine Smith, an American who worked as a registered nurse in England. Smith noticed how well patients responded to visits by a certain chaplain and his canine companion, a Golden Retriever. Upon returning to the USA in 1976, Smith started a programme for training dogs to visit institutions. Animal Assisted Therapy (AAT) and Animal Assisted Activities (AAA) remain

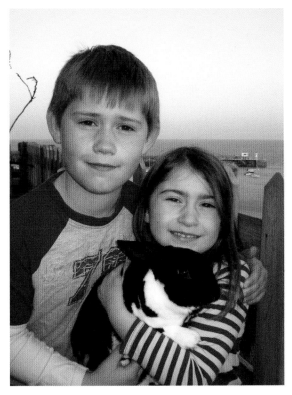

Figure 8.3 Children benefit from pets as they teach life skills and responsibility.

Box 8.3

FAST FACT

2006 saw the release of the world's most expensive television pet food advertisement – £1 million to support the Sheba cat food brand.

popular in the USA and are growing in popularity in the UK.

Animals used for sport and leisure

The final sector of the animal industry, 'animals used for sport and leisure', loosely falls under our 'domesticated' sector of our industry model. It's clearer to discuss domesticated animals in relation to leisure activities, although some animals used in sport could be classed as wild. Indeed, this section could also have fallen under 'working animals' as many of the animals, at least in more commercial sports, are highly trained and have often been selected for sport based on the same desirable characteristics which enable them to work. However, we placed working animals directly under 'socioeconomic use' and, although there may be socioeconomic gains to be made as a result of the commercialisation of sport (through sponsorship, ticket sales, prize money and merchandise), not all sport is commercialised.

Animals used in sport

According to the European Sports Charter, 'sport' means all forms of physical activity which, through casual or organised participation, aim at expressing or improving physical fitness and mental well-being, forming social relationships or obtaining results in competition at all levels. We may assume that this definition refers to human sport; it's very difficult to get a clear definition of animals and sport.

Spotlight on sport – equestrianism

There are many sports involving horses, including endurance riding, racing, reining, show jumping, dressage (Figure 8.4), eventing (Figure 8.5), horseball and polo. As with human sports, equestrian sports have governing bodies which control and manage the sports at both national and international level. The Fédération Equestre Internationale (FEI) is the international governing body of equestrian sport and is currently the only sporting governing body to represent both able-bodied and disabled athletes. The FEI currently represents 134 nations, each of which has its own national governing body (Figure 8.6).

Each country is only allowed one national governing body which reports directly to the FEI. Most sports are organised in such a way that the national governing body only represents the one sport and reports directly to the international governing body. So, for example, organisations such as the England and Wales Cricket Board and the Lawn Tennis Association only govern and oversee one sport each, cricket and tennis. Equestrian governing bodies appear to be structured differently. The US Equestrian Federation, for example, currently has 54

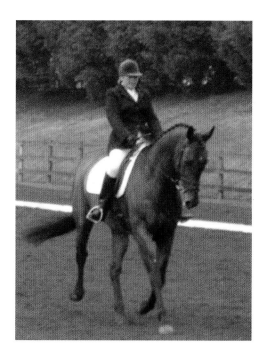

Figure 8.4 Dressage.

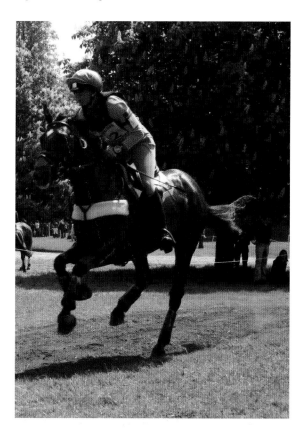

Figure 8.5 Three-day eventing.

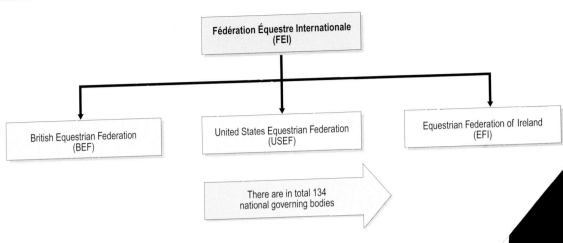

Figure 8.6 Equestrian international and national governing bodies.

FAST FACT

Equestrianism as a sport made its début at the summer Olympics in 1900 and, although it failed to appear in the next two summer Olympics, equestrian sport has been consistently present at the summer Olympics since 1912. The 1912 Olympics in Stockholm introduced the three equestrian disciplines with which we are currently familiar: dressage, show jumping and eventing (Figure 8.6). This format has been consistent apart from the 1920 Olympics in Antwerp, which also saw the introduction, and only appearance, of equestrian vaulting.

member bodies and the British Equestrian Federation has 16 member bodies, including:

- Three Olympic and Paralympic discipline organisations: British Eventing; British Dressage; British Show Jumping Association (Box 8.4)
- Seven non-Olympic discipline organisations: British Equestrian Vaulting; British Reining; Endurance GB; British Horse Driving Trials Association; UK Polocrosse Association; British Horseball Association; Mounted Games Association of GB
- Six non-discipline-specific organisations: British Horse Society; Pony Club; Association of British Riding Schools; British Trade Association; Scottish Equestrian Association; Riding for the Disabled Association (Box 8.4).

Racing is a popular sport involving animals, most commonly h_____ h____ but it may also include camels and e_

Horse racing in the UK

There is evidence that horse racing became ___ UK as early as the 12th century, when the E_ returned from the Crusades with Arab h_ show that racing took place in that period in London and at the famous Roodeye tra_ of Chester (Box 8.5).

In the UK horse racing is predomina_ racing or national hunt racing.

The late 18th century saw certain flat ___ the ultimate tests for racehorses. These 'classic' races and are still run today. The_ were for 3-year-old horses. The oldest o_ Leger, which was founded around 177_ famous and world-renowned race is _ 8.6).

Horse racing was one of only two s_ ued during both world wars. In the _ television brought horse racing into t_ rooms and it is now second only to fo_ widely televised sport. In 1961 bettin_ courses became legalised as the first b_ high street opened. Today, online hor_ tinues to draw new audiences to the _

There are now 60 racecourses i_ reported turnover on the day of the _ June, is approximately £50 million_ many in the racing calendar is the C_ Hunt Festival in March. This is raci_ fences and hurdles, and continues _ highlight being the Cheltenham G_

National hunt racing developed _ Irish pastime of foxhunting, when h_ speed of their mounts during the _ Organised steeplechase racing be_

Box 8.5

FAST FACT

Horse racing is known as the 'sport of kings'. This nickname originated from the association of King James I with the sport. The monarch had a palace built near a little-known village called Newmarket. This town was beginning to become prosperous, especially after a neighbouring village called Exning caught a plague, and all weekend markets had to be moved to another nearby town – Newmarket.

Newmarket became the home of organised horse racing in the UK, and during the reigns of Charles I and Charles II continued to grow in popularity. Under the reign of Queen Anne, spectators were finally allowed to place racing bets, and racecourses were founded in the UK. This included Ascot, which was founded by Queen Anne in 1711.

Racing's elite met at Newmarket to form the Jockey Club. They wrote a comprehensive set of rules and code of conduct for horse race meetings. In this way, the Jockey Club became the controlling body of horse racing in England and it is thought that this early formation of a regulatory body became the first regulated sport in the UK. The Jockey Club was released from its regulatory duties in 2006, and the British Horseracing Authority now governs the sport, and the Jockey Club now focuses on its other business interests.

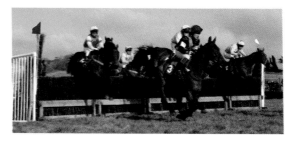

Figure 8.7 Point to point racing.

- The average number of horses in training is approximately 14 658
- The number of race horse owners is approximately 9403
- In 2005 there were 569 licensed trainers in the UK
- Of the 620 full-time jockeys, 121 have professional licences for flat racing and 99 for jump racing. The remainder have either apprentice or conditional licences
- Over 18 000 are employed on a full-time basis within the core horse-racing industry
- The total economic impact of British racing is approximately £2.8 million

After football, British horse racing attracts the highest-paid attendance of any sport, and provided four of the 10 sporting events by attendance in 2005

The UK's newest racecourse, Great Leighs, opened in Essex in 2008 and became the first course to open for 80 years, taking the number of race courses to 60.

Box 8.6

FAST FACT

The story of how the race was named after football, British horse racing Bunbury and the Earl of Derby tossed a race. The Earl of Derby won the toss, but it was Sir Charles Bunbury won the inaugural running of the Derby in 1780 when owning the winner Diomed.

The most famous steeplechase in the world is the Grand National which started in 1839 and is run at Aintree in Liverpool.

Point to point races are for amateurs and are run on over 100 courses throughout the British Isles (Figure 8.7). Originally run across the country from one point to another (hence the name), they are often found on farmland with built-in fences.

In 2006 Deloitte published a report *Economic Impact of British Racing*. Here are some facts and figures from the report which highlight the size of the horse-racing industry in the UK:

Horse racing around the world

As previously highlighted the most popular types of racing in the UK are flat and national hunt. Harness racing is also very popular in the USA, Australasia, and European countries, predominantly France, Sweden. Horse racing, in its various forms, is also popular in countries around the world, such as:

- India
- South Korea
- Japan
- Pakistan
- United Arab Emirates
- Many European countries

Horse racing in North America dates back to the establishment of a course in Long Island, New York, in 1665. In the USA, races can occur on flat surfaces of dirt, polytrack or grass. Unlike the UK there is no jump racing and the most popular type of racing is thoroughbred racing on the flat, although there is also quarter horse racing and harness racing. Racing with other breeds, such as Arabian horse racing, is found on a limited basis.

Ireland has a rich history of horse racing; point to pointing originated there and even today, jump racing (national hunt racing) is marginally more popular than racing on the flat. As a result, every year Irish horse-racing fans travel in huge numbers to the highlight event of the national hunt calendar, the Cheltenham Festival, and in recent years Irish-owned or bred horses have dominated the event. Ireland has a thriving thoroughbred breeding industry, stimulated by favourable tax treatment. The world's largest thoroughbred stud, Coolmore Stud, is there.

Blood sports

In most countries the act of two or more animals fighting each other, such as cockfighting, is seen as cruel and is therefore illegal. On 18 February 2005, the Hunting Act was passed to make illegal the hunting of fox, deer, hare and mink in England and Wales. Fox hunting is often viewed as a typically traditional British activity, but hunting with hounds takes place in many countries, including the USA, Canada and India, France, Italy and Ireland. In many regions of France, deer, hares and wild boar are also hunted with hounds.

There are several other blood sports in history that were intended as entertainment, many of which involved baiting by dogs. Many different types of animal were placed into a pit, sometimes tied to a post, and set upon by dogs. This ranged from rat-baiting and badger-baiting to bear-baiting and lion-baiting.

Some legal animal fights take place around the world; cow fighting, for example, is legal in Switzerland (Box 8.7).

There are also some legal forms of sport where humans fight animals, such as bull fighting, which has a long history in Spanish and Portuguese tradition. Not all animals are large, however, with cricket fighting being a popular (though illegal) sport in Macau and Hong Kong.

CONCLUSION

As we outlined at the start of this chapter there is no clear definitive definition of either the 'animal' or 'equine'

Box 8.7

FAST FACT

Cow fighting is a traditional Swiss event which determines the leader of the herd. Unlike bull fighting, in which humans fight bulls, cow fighting pits cow against cow. With their horns blunted, the fights often become nothing more than a pushing contest. Any cow that backs down from a fight is eliminated until one cow is left standing in the ring. Each year, the Swiss state of Valais hosts a series of cow fights known as les combats de reines (combat of queens), which began in the 1920s and have drawn as many as 50 000 spectators in a year. The winner is called la reine des reines (the queen of queens) and increases dramatically in worth. At the end of the year, a grand final is held in Aproz, where the six best from seven districts do battle in six weight categories.

---

industries. However this chapter has given us an insight into a functional-based view of the animal industry. It has also helped demonstrate the wide variety of roles animals play in our modern society, whilst highlighting interesting differences between countries and cultures.

Bibliography

American Veterinary Medical Association. Available online at: www.avma.org

Assistance Dogs International. Available online at: www.adionline.org

British Horse Industry Confederation strategy for the horse industry in England and Wales 2005. Available online at: www.defra.gov.uk/rural/horses

British Horse Society. Available online at: www.bhs.org.uk

Economic impact of British racing 2006 Available online at: www.kempton.co.uk/downloads/economic-impact-june-2006.pdf

Fédération Equestre Internationale. Available online at: www.fei.org

Guide Dogs for the Blind Association. Available online at: www.gdba.org.uk

Henley Centre 2004 A report of research on the horse industry in Great Britain. Available online at: www.defra.gov.uk/rural/horses

National Search and Rescue Dog Association (NSARDA). Available online at: www.nsarda.org.uk

Research Defense Society. Available online at: www.rds-online.org.uk

Chapter | 9 |

Jane Williams

Companion animal health and welfare

This chapter introduces the general principles of animal health and welfare, and then continues to apply these to dogs and cats specifically. The impacts of the five needs for the average pet owner are considered to promote responsible pet ownership. Routine prophylactic measures that should be employed in companion animal species are described and the pathogens they often serve to prevent are discussed.

BUYING AND CHOOSING A PET

For many people buying a pet happens as a result of a 'spur of the moment' decision. Pets can become ideal companions or your worst nightmare. Pet owners have a legal responsibility to their pet to keep it in good health and in suitable conditions; in the UK this is governed by the Animal Welfare Act 2006.

The Animal Welfare Act 2006 states that all animal owners have a legal 'duty of care' to ensure the welfare of their pet. It identifies the five freedoms or key needs of every animal:

1. The need for a proper diet (including water)
2. The need for somewhere suitable to live
3. The need to be housed with, or apart from, other animals (as appropriate)
4. The need to express their normal behaviour
5. The need to be protected from pain, suffering, injury and disease.

While many pet owners already provide for these needs, anyone who fails to do so could be liable for a fine or even a prison sentence. The duty of care can be applied to the owner of the animal, any person in charge of the animal in lieu of the owner, e.g. veterinary surgeon or boarding kennels, and a parent or guardian if the owner is under 16 years of age and legally not an adult.

The five key needs provide legal definitions which quantify animal health and welfare not just for companion animal species but for all farm animals and wild animals kept in captivity. The achievement of some of the key needs, for example the need for a proper diet, can appear relatively clear to the pet owner whilst others require a more thorough understanding of the animal species, for example the need to express normal behaviour. The definition of the key needs has provided a forum for animal welfare organisations to police pet owners and animal keepers to enable animals to be seized and prosecution to occur if intent or neglect is intended without the need for suffering to have actually taken place. Tables 9.1 and 9.2 identify some of the factors prospective pet owners should consider when choosing a suitable pet.

SPREAD OF INFECTION

Disease in animal species is the result of the infiltration of pathogens into the body systems. Pathogens are disease-causing microorganisms; the most common

Table 9.1 Factors to consider when choosing a pet

Who is the pet for?	Young family Elderly person Working owner
Does the owner work?	Full-time Part-time Can the pet go to the workplace? Would there be a pet sitter?
Is the owner disabled?	How severely? Does the owner have any assistance?
Will there be contact with children? What are their ages?	Own children Neighbours Friends or family
Who is going to be responsible for the pet?	Adult Children (legally, pet owners must be over 16 years of age)
How much time will be dedicated to looking after the pet?	Cleaning Walking Training Companionship
How often do the owners go on holiday? Will the pet go with them?	Pet travel scheme Cost of kennels/cattery Who will look after the pet?
Where do the owners live? What type of house?	Garden Back yard Flat Communal Neighbours
What type of pet would be considered?	Species Breed Short or long hair Age Specialist knowledge/equipment required Rehoming

Table 9.2 Factors to consider when assessing suitability of animals as family pets

Family	Children: will they treat the animal as a toy? Could they be bitten? Lack of free time Possible behavioural/hierarchy problems Teach responsibility
Working owners	How much spare time will they have? Housing animal whilst at work Provision of exercise
Financial implications	Vet bills: provision of basic annual cost and emergencies throughout the pet's life Feeding costs Housing/bedding costs Lighting costs Insurance – legal cover in case the pet causes an accident Other pets – lots of potential problems
Dogs	Age Neutered or intact Breed suitability Long/short-haired Amount of exercise required Insurance costs Vet bills – microchip, vaccinations, neuter, worm, flea How much food will the dog need? Hereditary problems
Cats	Age Neutered or intact Breed suitability Long/short-haired Does the cat require company? Vet bills Insurance Food
Rabbits	Food Housing Indoor or outdoor pet? Vet bills Management, e.g. stop breeding, keep in same-sex groups or individually
Exotic species	Housing – special tanks and environmental considerations, e.g. light, humidity More expensive and specialised veterinary care Special diet Disease implications (zoonoses)/handling, e.g. *Escherichia coli*, *Salmonella* Growth – too small for tank Moral ground

encountered in companion animal species are bacteria, viruses, fungi and protozoa. The animal body is adapted to fight infection from pathogens via a range of strategic defences (Box 9.1).

Carrier status

Animals may occasionally come into contact with a microorganism and not exhibit any clinical signs of the disease – these animals are termed carriers.

DEFINITIONS

Infectious disease

Disease caused by microorganisms/microbes, e.g. *Salmonella*

Non-infectious disease

Disease not caused by microorganisms, e.g. diabetes mellitus

Contagious disease

Disease that is capable of being transmitted by direct contact or indirect contact from one animal to another

Incubation period

The interval of time between the animal coming into contact with a microorganism and the development of the clinical signs of the disease

---

Carriers are important in veterinary medicine because even though they show no clinical signs they may still shed/excrete the microorganism and infect other animals. There are two types of carrier: healthy carriers and convalescent carriers. A healthy carrier is an animal that has been exposed to an infectious disease but has never shown any clinical signs. Healthy carriers will carry the microorganism and shed it into the environment, posing a potential health risk, e.g. *Haemobartonella felis* and *Campylobactor*. Convalescent carriers are animals that have recovered from a clinical disease; these animals may shed large quantities of microorganism for variable time periods after recovery, e.g. leptospirosis.

Routes of transmission

Animals do not magically become infected by microorganisms. The microorganism has to find a way into the animal's body and a multitude of methods are utilised. When considering how a microorganism has passed to an animal you have to establish:

- The routes by which an organism may have left an animal
- The routes of transmission from one animal to another
- The routes of entry into the new host.

Routes by which a microorganism may leave an animal include the following:

- Oral, nasal and ocular discharges, e.g. distemper
- In urine, e.g. leptospirosis

- In faeces, e.g. parvovirus
- In vomitus, e.g. parvovirus
- In blood, e.g. *Haemobartonella felis*
- Via the skin, e.g. ringworm
- In milk (from dam to pup), e.g. *Toxocara*, feline leukaemia virus (FeLv)
- Venereal contact (semen/parturition), e.g. *Brucella*
- From dead animals, e.g. *Echinococcus granulosus*.

Routes of transmission from one animal to another include:

- Direct contact
- Indirect contact
- Aerosol transmission
- Contamination of food and water
- Carriers.

Direct contact involves actual physical contact from an infected animal with an uninfected one, usually via body secretions or parasites. Indirect contact involves spread from one animal to another one via other objects, known as fomites, e.g. food bowls and bedding, or spread from one animal to another through other animals, known as vectors, e.g. mice, fleas and sheep.

Routes of entry into a new host include:

- Ingestion
- Inhalation
- Through the skin
- Via mucous membranes
- Congenital route.

Ingestion

The infectious microorganism is taken into the body. The level of clinical disease depends on the quantity of microorganism ingested and the health status of the animal.

Inhalation

The number of air changes in animal accommodation can also affect the numbers of pathogens present in the environment.

Through the skin

The skin is one of the body's defence mechanisms to prevent pathogenic infections penetrating the skin.

Congenital

Congenital transfer of pathogenic organism occurs from dam to fetus during pregnancy via the placenta.

At this point it worth remembering that the incubation period for any disease will depend upon:

- The dose of microorganisms
- Immune status of the animal
- General health of the animal
- Age of the animal
- Route of entry.

Methods used to control infection

The study of animal diseases has provided clues on how to prevent them spreading. These include:

- Avoiding direct contact between animals, i.e. isolation/quarantine
- Very high hygiene levels for animals and fomites
- Housing – reducing numbers in an area and ensuring good air movement
- Early and effective treatment
- Routine vaccination/control
- Strict import controls into a country
- Routine health checks.

Routine hygiene

The use of safe but effective disinfectant products combined with strict hygiene controls is essential to reduce the risk of infection. Schedules of work for any animal establishment should detail what is to be cleaned, the order of cleaning (cleanest to dirtiest to prevent contamination) and a record of cleaning. The disinfection of housing, bedding, feeding utensils and equipment, use of disinfectants at the correct dilution for the appropriate contact times, good practice between animals by staff washing their hands or using alcohol gels to reduce spread of infections and isolation protocols can reduce risk.

Isolation/quarantine

The availability of an isolation facility can aid in the control of infectious disease outbreaks and provides a relatively safe environment for the assessment of animals whose previous infection status is not known. Quarantine enables the isolation of potential disease-harbouring animals, thus reducing the risk of introducing a disease into a population. Strict controls are required to manage the facility, including:

- Limiting the people who can enter
- Strict controls between animals
- No direct contact
- No indirect contact
- Barrier nursing
- High standards of hygiene
- Simultaneous treatment with drugs.

What happens when an animal is exposed to a disease?

The animal body has a range of non-specific defence mechanisms that aim to prevent infection or combat the initial invasion. These include:

- Phagocytosis – neutrophils/monocytes
- Natural barriers – skin, mucous membranes
- Skin secretions, which prevent the multiplication of pathogens
- Blood clotting
- Mucus secretion in the respiratory system
- Ocular secretions
- Wax in ear
- Stomach acids
- Macrophages in tissues
- Inflammatory response.

These are complemented by specific defence mechanisms; these are mechanisms that are activated within the body in response to the entry of a pathogen. They are collectively known as the immune system and involve the lymphatic and circulatory systems. There are different types of immune response and these vary depending on:

- The age of the animal – young and old are less effective
- The health status of the animal.

An antigen is a foreign protein that initiates an immune response. Antibodies are complex proteins produced by B lymphocytes. Specific antibodies are produced for specific diseases and their role is to destroy or inactivate specific antigens.

T lymphocytes play an active role in immunity and have the ability to destroy virus-infected cells and tumours without antibodies. The immune system begins to act the instant a foreign pathogen invades the body but it takes time for the levels of T and B lymphocytes to build up to sufficient numbers to be effective. During this time the animal will feel unwell and demonstrate the clinical signs of the disease.

The body has special memory cells that remember which diseases the body has encountered in the past and if that disease invades again the antibody response is triggered by these memory cells. Memory cells can remember some diseases for a lifetime, e.g. smallpox, but others need to be regularly updated by booster vaccination.

Vaccination

Vaccination introduces specially treated non-infective versions of diseases to initiate an immune response to achieve antibodies and give memory cells an encounter with the disease. Vaccination does not begin in very young animals because there are two types of immunity. Active immunity occurs due to stimulation of T and B lymphocytes whereas passive immunity is a short-lived immunity which can be transferred from dam to off-spring or by an injection of antibodies. There are many different brands of vaccine available and each has a specific protocol that should be adhered to.

Zoonotic infection

A zoonosis is an infectious disease that can be passed from animals to humans. If an animal has a zoonotic disease then strict protocols should be adhered to when handling, cleaning and generally doing anything with that animal. Examples of zoonotic diseases include:

- Leptospirosis or Weil's disease
- *Cheyletiella* spp.
- *Sarcoptes scabeii*
- Dermatophytosis (ringworm)
- *Toxocara canis*
- Toxoplasmosis
- Salmonellosis
- *Feline chlamydophilia*.

PROMOTION OF HEALTH

A number of generic factors can be considered by the informed observer regardless of the animal species; refer to Tables 9.3 and 9.4. The evaluation of the specific

Table 9.3 Types of immunity

Type	Description
Active	Active response by immune system
Naturally acquired	Active response due to natural exposure, e.g. infection
Artificially acquired	Active response due to artificial exposure, e.g. vaccination
Passive artificial	Ready-made antibodies, e.g. tetanus antitoxin injected
Passive natural	Antibodies cross the placenta or are present in milk and transmitted from dam to offspring
Innate	Certain species are immune to certain diseases

animal and the observer's responses can provide essential clues to animal health, particularly in wild species housed in captivity where comprehensive health checks are prohibitive for safety reasons. The physical and clinical parameters for individual animals can be considered to provide a picture of the animal's health status, but the environment the animal has had access to may directly influence health. Good husbandry is essential to health and knowledge of species and breed requirements is required by handlers and keepers. The five key needs must be met by the animal accommodation but their implementation will vary depending on the ultimate destination of the animal; for example, an intensively farmed pig would experience a very different environment than a free-range pig.

All handlers and keepers should be trained in systems to ensure consistency of practice; this can be achieved by utilising schedules of work for common tasks, staff training, mentor schemes and monitoring the environment. Careful consideration of construction materials, the order of work, products used for disinfection, equipment employed, sharing of utensils and food bowls can improve or reduce the probability of cross-contamination. Establishing strict hygiene controls in association with a quarantine or isolation protocol if disease is suspected and for new arrivals should reduce the risk of infection spreading. Prophylactic measures should be employed via vaccination, routine parasite control and regular health checks to promote health.

Disinfection

Disinfection can be defined as the destruction or reduction of microorganisms that are pathogenic, not including bacterial spores. Transient bacteria numbers will be affected. Disinfectants are classified into different compound groups, each of which is developed for a specific use:

- Phenolics offer a wide range of bactericidal action but have a variable action against viruses and are a poor response to reducing bacterial spores. They are relatively inexpensive but are absorbed by rubber and some plastics, therefore equipment choice needs to be considered. They have a distinctive strong smell and can be toxic to some species, e.g. cats
- Halogens: this group includes iodines and iodophors. These are solutions that have a wide range of activity, often stain and are utilised for skin disinfection e.g. Pevidine
- Hypochlorites: this group includes bleach. They show good action against pathogens and are inactivated by organic material. They are often used for environmental cleaning

Table 9.4 Factors that indicate health status

Factor	Good health	Poor health
Appetite	Normal	Increased Decreased Dysphagia Mastication problems Vomiting Regurgitation Pica
Skin/coat condition	Groomed Shiny Complete	Alopecia Greasy Scurf/flaky Matts Dull Pustules Parasite in faeces Pruritus
Mobility	Normal gait	Lameness Reluctance to move Abnormal gait
Activity levels	Normal	Reduced Increased Abnormal patterns
Urinary output	Normal	Oliguria Anuria Polyuria Haematuria
Faecal output	Normal	Tenesmus Diarrhoea Constipation Presence of endoparasites Presence of blood
Behaviour	Normal interactions observed	Abnormal reactions Stereotypies Lethargy Hyperactive Unreactive to stimuli Hyperreactive to stimuli
Injury	No signs	Wounds Haemorrhage Fractures
Temperature	Normal range considering animal's activity, e.g. if temperature is slightly increased after exercise, this would be considered normal	Outside normal range
Pulse rate	Normal range	Outside normal range Abnormal rhythm Disparity to heart rate

Continued

Table 9.4 *Continued*

Factor	Good health	Poor health
Heart rate	Normal range and heart sounds	Abnormal range, rhythm or heart sounds
Respiratory rate	Normal range	Abnormal range, pattern or noise
Inflammation/localised heat	None	Presence suggests injury or infection
Sleep patterns	Normal for activity level, environment	Abnormal – prolonged or shortened
Social interaction	Normal for species	Inappropriate behaviour Solitude Negative response to social stimuli Reduction in social position within hierarchy
Discharges	None observed	Presence of discharges, e.g. ocular, aural
Environment	Clean Recommended density Safe materials Hygiene practice implemented Shelter and warmth Quarantine/isolation employed for illness/new arrivals	Dirty Presence of pathogens Infected/ill animals Overstocked Inadequate shelter/warmth
Vocalisation	Normal	Excessive vocalisation No vocalisation Whimpering, crying
Capillary refill time	1–2 seconds	3+ seconds
Mucous membrane colour	Salmon pink	Brick red – poisoning, cyanotic (blue), grey, white – all may be due to reduced oxygen Petechia – pinpoint haemorrhage

- Quaternary ammonium compounds: these are used in the environment and on the skin, with a wide range of action e.g. Trigene. Their cost is relatively low and they are inactivated by hard water, organic material and soap
- Peroxides are oxidising agents with a wide range of bactericidal, fungicidal and virucidal activity, but this is reduced if organic matter is present
- Alcohols are very effective except for bacterial spores and some viruses but organic material must be removed as it inactivates them. They are often employed in hand rubs and solutions for personal hygiene between patients. Care should be taken as they are flammable
- Aldehydes are another group which have a wide range of bactericidal action, including spores and virucidal activity. However they are relatively slow-acting and require longer contact times than other products. Organic matter does not greatly reduce efficiency but they do have high toxicity and may irritate skin, mucosa and eyes. They are not often used as a

general disinfectant but may be used as a method of cold sterilisation.

Using a disinfectant can still be ineffectual if you do not follow the core steps listed below or ignore the manufacturer's instructions.

Prior to disinfection

1. First clean with soap or detergent to remove any organic material
2. Rinse thoroughly with plain water
3. Make up the disinfectant solution accordingly to the manufacturer's instructions
4. Check Control of Substances Hazardous to Health regulations and adhere to them
5. Use disinfectant for appropriate contact time.

Inactivation of disinfectants

Disinfectant compounds vary in the extent their efficiency can be compromised by external factors. The presence of organic material, mixing products, the addition of detergent, hard water, dilution rate, contact time, temperature and presence of bacteria can all inactivate specific products and it is essential that the manufacturer's instructions and datasheet should be meticulously followed to ensure the product used is effective.

How can you categorise the risk?

Any indidivual who is responsible for cleaning and reducing the risks of cross-contamination and infection within the animal environment should be able to identify and categorise risk areas within the business and select suitable products and suitable cleaning regimes.

Low-risk areas

- Areas of general traffic
- No specific points of multiple contact
- Product used usually has detergent action and some bactericidal action.

Medium-risk areas

- Areas of concentrated traffic
- Areas of possible multiple contact
- Areas where there is no continuous risk of body fluids/material present
- Instruments used on intact skin surfaces
- Product usually has detergent action, some bactericidal action, some virucidal action.

High-risk areas

- Areas of concentrated traffic
- Areas of repeat multiple contact
- Confined spaces of known infection
- Areas of continuous risk of contact with mucosal membranes, body fluids or material
- All areas known to have been in contact with an infected animal or material
- Equipment, instruments or hands likely to enter the body cavity
- Product usually has detergent, bactericidal, virucidal and fungicidal action (sterilisation maybe!).

How often should you clean?

Cleaning regimes, including frequency, should be considered on an individual basis but a general guideline would be:

- Weekly: areas of low use or low risk
- Daily: areas of concentrated traffic and low/medium risk

- Twice daily: areas of concentrated traffic and medium/high risk
- Between clients/animals: areas of multiple contact and high risk.

INFECTIOUS DISEASES OF COMPANION ANIMAL SPECIES

An infectious disease is defined as a disease that is capable of being passed from one animal (it may be restricted to one species) to another and that can be described as contagious (Box 9.2).

Feline infectious diseases

There are numerous feline infectious diseases that should be considered, including:

- Feline infectious respiratory disease
- *Feline chlamydophilia*
- Feline panleukopenia
- Feline coronavirus (FeCoV)
- FeLv
- Feline immunodeficiency virus (FIV)
- Toxoplasmosis
- Feline infectious anaemia
- Feline infectious peritonitis.

Feline infectious respiratory disease

This is a viral respiratory disease, of which there are two types: feline calicivirus and feline rhinotracheitis virus or

---

Box 9.2

DEFINITIONS

Aetiology
Investigation of the cause or orgin of a disease

Epidemiology
Study of disease origin and spread, including the pattern of disease development

Pathogenesis
The cause, development and effects of a disease

Lability
Liable to change: a measure of how long a pathogen can survive away from its ideal environment

Virulence
A measure of strength or infectiveness of a pathogen

feline herpesvirus (FHV). The condition can also be known as feline upper respiratory tract disease, feline influenza or cat flu.

Feline rhinotracheitis

Aetiology

- Alpha-herpesvirus: double-stranded DNA and glyco-protein lipid envelope
- Only one serotype but different strains are identified
- Labile for up to 24 hours depending on temperature and humidity
- Envelope is affected by common disinfectants, including hypochlorites and quarternary ammonium compounds
- It only affects the cat family.

Pathogenesis and pathology

- Infection is via intranasal, oral or conjunctival contact
- The virus replicates in the nasal passages, then travels to mandibular lymph nodes and the trachea
- Mucupurulent exudates are produced from nasal passages and the nasal turbinates
- It results in inflammation in the trachea and conjunctiva.

Clinical signs

- Severe upper respiratory disease, particularly in young animals
- Incubation period is 2–6 days, but can be up to 12 days
- Depression, sneezing, inappetence, pyrexia
- Ocular and nasal discharges
- Leukocytosis with left shift
- Mortality rate is not high
- Resolution is usually within 2–3 weeks: the animal may present with a chronic rhinitis/sinusitis and recurrence is a possibility.

Treatment

- Broad-spectrum antibiotics
- Vitamin supplementation
- Fluid therapy, as often the cat will be dehydrated
- Tender loving care (TLC)
- Strong-smelling food to tempt the animal to eat, as nasal discharge reduces olfaction
- Nebulisers/steam/decongestants.

Prevention

- Annual vaccination
- Isolation of infected individuals.

Feline oral calicivirus

Aetiology

- Small undeveloped, single-stranded RNA virus
- One main serotype but there is antigenic variation
- Can survive up to 1 week in the environment
- Susceptible to low pH but not all disinfectants
- Only affects cats
- Incubation period: 2–12 days.

Pathogenesis/pathology

- Intranasal, oral or conjunctival infection
- Virus multiplies in the oral cavity and upper respiratory tract and conjunctiva
- Ulcers are a common symptom.

Clinical signs

- Feline calicivirus can be mild or severe in presentation
- It presents as a general malaise
- Transient pyrexia, mild sneezing, conjunctivitis
- Less ocular and nasal discharge
- Mouth ulceration present.

Treatment

- As per FHV.

Carriers

- Carriers shed virus continuously
- Some are lifelong carriers whilst some spontaneously recover.

Prevention

- Vaccination as per FHV.

Feline chlamydophilia

Aetiology

- Highly specialised obligate intracytoplasmic bacteria
- Similar to Gram-negative bacteria
- Has the potential to be zoonotic in felines but is not common (the avian strand is zoonotic).

Epidemiology

- Problem in colonies of cats
- Transmitted by direct and fomites contact from ocular discharges
- Natural immunity is ineffective.

Pathogenesis

- Bacteria multiply in the conjunctiva and oral cavity
- Incubation period: 3–10 days
- Persistent conjunctivitis
- Secondary infections
- Acute – serous ocular discharge, blepharospasm

- Can be unilateral or bilateral discharges
- Can display mild nasal discharge, sneezing, pyrexia, coughing
- Takes 3–4 weeks to recover and the animal often suffers episodic recurrences.

Treatment

- Systemic and topical antibiotics
- All cats in a household must be treated simultaneously for at least 3–4 weeks or until 2 weeks after the clinical signs have disappeared.

Prevention

- Annual vaccination
- Colony testing
- Colony control – isolation of infected individuals and treating all cats.

Feline panleukopenia

This is also known as feline infectious enteritis and also affects cats, mink, ferrets and racoons. It is characterised by a decrease in white blood cells or a panleukopenia and the destruction of intestinal mucosa or enteritis.

Aetiology

- Parvovirus, 20 nm (small), undeveloped, single DNA
- Only one serotype
- Closely related to canine parvovirus
- Very stable in the environment; can last for up to a year
- Requires active mitotic cells to multiply
- Hypochlorite, gluteraldehydes and formaldehydes are effective.

Pathogenesis

- Mitotic cells required primarily in intestine, lymph and bone marrow.

Pathology

- Changes are slight
- Dehydration
- Vomiting and fetid diarrhoea
- Intestines have petechial haemorrhage
- Mesenteric lymph nodes are enlarged.

Clinical signs

- More severe in young animals
- Incubation period: 2–10 days
- Lethargy, fever, anorexia, thirsty but refusal to drink
- Vomiting
- Enlarged abdomen (due to gas/fluid)

- After 2–3 days diarrhoea may develop, which may lead to dehydration
- Subnormal temperature
- Very poor prognosis with a mortality rate of 25–75%.

Treatment

- Supportive
- Control of secondary infections
- Fluids/antiemetics to combat dehydration
- Correction of electrolyte imbalance
- Vitamin therapy
- TLC.

Epidemiology

- Direct contact in the environment or with immune carriers.

Vaccination

- Very successful
- Natural and vaccine-induced immunity is high and long-lived.

Feline coronavirus

This virus predominantly affects young cats. It has intra-uterine transmittal and has a variable incubation period. There are two types:

- Feline infectious peritonitis virus (FIPV)
- Feline enteric coronavirus (FECV).

Pathogenesis

- Dependent upon age, immune status, strain, dose of virus
- Cell-mediated immunity (CMI) response plays an important role
- Infection is transplacentally or via oronasal direct contact
- The virus replicates in lymph nodes in the gastrointestinal tract, then the endothelium, throughout the body, kidneys, eyes and blood vessels
- If there is a moderate CMI response, the condition is dry FIP
- If there is a poor CMI, the condition is wet FIP
- Dry FIP can easily progress to wet FIP
- Individuals can become persistently shedding carriers and pose a significant disease risk to other animals.

Clinical signs
Dry FIP

- Granulomatous lesions on viscera, e.g. liver and kidneys
- Central nervous system infection produces neurological signs, e.g. ataxia, paresis, fits.

Wet FIP

- The cat may develop ascites and lose weight, and have depression and anaemia, leading to death
- Pleural/pericardial effusion, causing dyspnoea
- Uveitis
- Jaundice.

With wet FIP a peritoneal tap is often performed aseptically to obtain a fluid sample:

- Fluid is generally cloudy and straw- or yellow-tinged
- It foams when shaken due to increased protein
- It clots on exposure to air.

Treatment

- Non-specific, symptomatic treatment – the condition has a poor prognosis.

Vaccination

- A temperature-sensitive vaccine is available in the USA and some EU countries; effectiveness is debatable
- It gives good mucosal immunity although poor systemic immunity, but still appears to be effective.

Feline leukaemia

This disease is often seen in the younger members of multicat households and in cats that have direct contact with other felines as it is spread by direct contact.

Aetiology

- Retrovirus
- Three subtypes: A, B, C – only FeLv A is transmissible in felines.

Pathogenesis

- Route may be direct infection, transplacental or transmammary
- Virus is shed in saliva, urine, faeces, milk, by licking and via close contact
- Virus multiplies in the oropharynx and lymphoid tissue, particularly the bone marrow
- A transient viraemia is observed between 2 days and 8 weeks
- Others will present with a persistent infection then clinical disease and will be a main infective source for other cats
- Kittens are more susceptible; once over 16 weeks of age only 1 in 5 cats get persistent infection
- Dose is dependent on environmental and colony conditions
- FeLv is the most common cause of death in young cats.

Clinical signs

- Often die within 4 years
- Infection occurs in the haemopoietic system
- Neoplasia (lymphosarcoma) is often present
- Anaemia and leukopenia resulting in reduced weight, anorexia, pyrexia
- Immunosuppression leading to secondary infection, which is often the cause of death
- Associated reproductive failure.

Treatment

- Non-specific, supportive therapy
- Poor prognosis.

Diagnosis

- Enzyme-linked immunosorbent assay (ELISA)/serum assays
- Should retest after 12 weeks to determine if viraemia is transient or persistent.

Control

- Test all cats
- Separate positive from negative cats
- Retest after 12 weeks
- Remove all positive cats
- Retest all cats every 6–12 months
- Test and isolate new members then retest after 12 weeks before introducing to others.

Vaccination

- Recommended from 9 weeks of age
- Pre-blood test advised
- Vaccines are not live, therefore do not give lifelong protection.

Feline immunodeficiency virus

This disease is most common in entire cats aged between 5 and 9 years which are allowed to roam.

Aetiology

- Retrovirus
- Related to human immunodeficiency virus (HIV) but is not zoonotic.

Epidemiology

- Domestic and wild felines are affected
- More common in male, unneutered cats over 5 years as free-roaming and sexually active
- Main route of transmission is via inoculation of the virus, i.e. bites/sexual transmission
- Incubation periods vary from a few weeks to a few months.

Clinical signs

- Lymphadenopathy
- Mild pyrexia, depression, leukopenia after 4 weeks
- Less severe in older cats
- Can be healthy for years
- Usually die from secondary infections
- Clinical signs seen in middle-aged plus cats
- Common ones:
  - Chronic stomatitis and gingivitis
  - Chronic upper respiratory tract disease
  - Muscle wasting
  - Pyrexia
  - Lymphadenopathy
  - Anaemia
  - Chronic skin disorders/diarrhoea
  - Neurological signs
  - May increase risk of neoplasia.

Diagnosis

- ELISA kits are available
- Assays are sent to external labs.

Pathogenesis

- Not fully understood
- Initial lymphadenopathy between 4 and 6 weeks which resolves after 2–3 months
- The cat can be healthy for several years before exhibiting clinical signs and only presenting with secondary infections.

Treatment

- Systemic and supportive therapy
- Surgery to remove neoplasms
- Corticosteroids may have a short-term beneficial effect
- Nothing will cure the disease.

Prevention/control

- No vaccine available
- Avoid cat-to-cat transmission
- Prevent infective cats roaming
- Same-cat household should be OK (if they get on and no fighting occurs!).

Toxoplasmosis

Aetiology

- Caused by a protozoan – *Toxoplasma gondii*.

Pathogenesis

- Transmission is by ingestion of infected cat faeces to other species
- Transmission is by eating raw meat from an infected animal in felines

- Incubation period of 2–5 weeks
- The cat is the end host where the protozoan remains in the small intestine.

Clinical signs

- Asymptomatic but diarrhoea, lethargy and jaundice may occur.

Treatment/control

- Diagnosis by blood test
- Treat with antibiotics and ensure cooked-meat diet to prevent
- Regular cleaning of litter trays removes the faeces before the oocysts reach their infective stage
- Pregnant women should avoid cleaning litter trays for this reason.

Canine infectious diseases

There are a number of canine infectious diseases that should be considered, including:

- Canine parvovirus
- Canine distemper
- Canine leptospirosis
- Infectious canine hepatitis
- Canine infectious tracheobronchitis (kennel cough)
- Borreliosis (Lyme's disease)
- Leishmaniasis
- *Giardia*

Canine parvovirus

Aetiology

- Canine parvovirus type 2 (CPV-2).

Pathogenesis

- Virus is related to feline panleukopenia and was first seen in the 1970s with a high mortality rate
- Virus is shed in the faeces during the incubation period and can survive in the environment for up to 6 months
- It is very virulent and correct disinfectant protocols and barrier nursing of patients are essential to control spread of infection
- Transmission is via direct or indirect contact with faeces
- The incubation period is 4–7 days
- The virus requires mitotic cells to replicate and concentrates in the lymph nodes, bone marrow and linings of the lungs, liver and intestines
- It has an increased incidence in puppies and there appears to be a breed prevalence to greater susceptibility in Rottweilers, German Shepherds and Dobermans.

113

Clinical signs

- Depression, vomiting, anorexia
- The disease is characterised by profuse, violent haemorrhagic diarrhoea
- Animals become severely dehydrated and it is this which most often is the cause of death
- Diagnosis is via history and ELISA test.

Treatment

- Isolation
- Barrier nursing
- Antibiotics for secondary infections and fluid therapy.

Prevention

- Vaccination of breeding females and puppies.

Canine distemper

Aetiology

- Morbillovirus (related to measles).

Pathogenesis

- The virus is labile and is quickly destroyed by sunlight, heat and desiccation
- It can remain in a chronic form in infected animals for many years
- Transmission is via aerosol droplets and ingestion
- The virus replicates in lymphoid tissue (tonsils and lymph nodes) causing a viraemia
- If an animal has a compromised immune status then the virus continues to replicate in respiratory and gastrointestinal epithelial cells and causes keratinisation of the nose and pads; hence the lay term 'hard pad'
- If an animal has a good immune status mild signs are often seen
- The nervous system is affected by the virus in all animals.

Clinical signs

- Pyrexia, nasal discharge, coughing, vomiting, diarrhoea, chorea (twitching) and hyperkeratosis of pads
- Chronic signs include encephalitis and rheumatoid arthritis
- Diagnosis is by blood test, which will exhibit a lymphopenia and cells will have inclusions present.

Treatment

- Supportive therapy – antibiotics, fluids, antiemetics, antitussives and anticonvulsants
- Euthanasia.

Prevention

- Vaccination.

Canine leptospirosis

Aetiology

- Bacterial infection with multiple serotypes, of which there are two types most common in the UK:
  - *Leptospira canicola* – affects the kidneys
  - *L. icterohaemorrhagiae* – affects the liver
- The disease is zoonotic and the bacterium is a spirochaete and can penetrate intact skin (it works its way through like a corkscrew).

Pathogenesis

- Transmission is by direct or indirect contact with contaminated urine or water
- It is also known as Weil's disease and can be spread via rat urine and lamppost disease (as dogs tend to urinate on and sniff lampposts)
- It can also be transmitted via transplacental and transmammary routes
- The bacteria can be shed for months or years after recovery
- Bacteria penetrate the skin or mucous membranes and replicate in the liver and kidney, depending on which species is implicated
- This causes acute kidney failure, hepatitis and intravascular coagulation.

Clinical signs

- Pyrexia, vomiting, shock, interstitial nephritis and hepatitis
- Diagnosis via blood test to evaluate liver and kidney enzyme levels.

Treatment

- Fluid therapy, including plasma or blood (to correct intravascular coagulation)
- Antibiotics, antiemetics and prescription diets.

Prevention

- Vaccination
- Good hygiene.

Infectious canine hepatitis

Aetiology

- Canine adenovirus (CAV-1).

Pathogenesis

- Transmission is by direct or indirect contact with faeces, urine, saliva and fomites
- Incubation period: 5–9 days

- Virus enters via the oral cavity and replicates in lymphoid tissue (nodes and tonsils) causing viraemia
- It then travels to the vascular epithelium and replicates, causing pericardial effusions, hepatitis and vasculitis.

Clinical signs

- Anorexia, pyrexia, vomiting and diarrhoea, hepatomegaly, conjunctivitis, photophobia, petechia and jaundice
- Death can be imminent
- Diagnosis via blood evaluation of liver enzymes and clinical signs.

Treatment

- Supportive therapeutic care
- Fluids, antibiotics, antiemetics.

Prevention

- Vaccination
- The live CAV-2 strain used in vaccination may cause 'blue eye' in certain breeds, e.g. Collies.

Canine infectious tracheobronchitis (kennel cough)

Aetiology

- A range of pathogens, including *Bordetella bronchioseptica*, canine herpesvirus, CAV-2 and bacterial agents.

Pathogenesis

- Transmission by aerosol droplets via direct or indirect routes
- Common in boarding kennels and multidog environments
- Incubation period is 5–7 days
- The pathogens replicate in the upper respiratory tract, resulting in secondary infections in damaged tissue.

Clinical signs

- Dry cough, often with associated retching, especially after exercise, excitement or on palpation of the trachea/larynx
- Mucopurulent nasal and ocular discharge
- May develop into pneumonia
- Diagnosis is by clinical signs and history.

Treatment

- Antibiotics, antitussives, restrict exercise and rest.

Prevention

- Vaccination – parenteral and intranasal vaccines are available.

Borreliosis (Lyme's disease)

Aetiology

- *Borrelia burgdorferi* (bacterium).

Pathogenesis

- Transmitted by *Ixodes* spp. (ticks) during feeding on the host
- No specific incubation period.

Clinical signs

- Lameness, pyrexia, lethargy, lymphoadenopathy and cardiac arrhythmias
- Diagnosis by blood tests.

Treatment

- Remove ticks
- Antibiotics and supportive therapy.

Prevention

- Prophylaxis with reputable veterinary ectoparasiticide. Vaccine available in the USA.

Leishmaniasis

Aetiology

- Protozoal parasite *Leishmania infantum*, which is transmitted by sandfly bites
- Zoonotic.

Pathogenesis

- Transmitted by sandfly bites which inhabit Mediterranean and tropical countries
- Increased movement of dogs to these countries is thought to be responsible for cases seen in the UK and USA
- Sandfly injects protozoa during feeding on the host, usually the ear or muzzle, leaving a small lesion or chancre; it then replicates in the internal organs and compromises the immune system.

Clinical signs

- Weakness
- Weight loss
- Depression
- Inappetance
- Gastrointestinal signs – vomiting and diarrhoea
- Skin disease
- Swollen legs and joints
- Respiratory signs – pneumonia, cough
- Jaundice
- Fever
- Death.

115

Treatment

- Supportive therapy
- Diagnosis – blood test.

Prevention

- Ectoparasiticide deltamethrin, available in collars, will kill sandflies.

Giardia

Aetiology

- Common in young dogs under 6 months of age and immunosuppressed animals in the USA
- Notifiable disease in the UK
- Protozoa.

Pathogenesis

- Transmission via direct contact with faeces, indirect contact with contaminated water or cysts in the environment
- Infective form: the *Giardia* trophozoite attached to the intestine of infected animals replicates and releases into the gastrointestinal tract and is passed in the faeces
- The parasite can also form infective cysts which survive longer in the environment.

Clinical signs

- Light-coloured, greasy soft faeces as population increases and interferes with absorption
- Profuse diarrhoea as it progresses
- Mild anaemia, increased eosinophil count.

Treatment

- Supportive therapy – antibiotics and fluids
- Endoparasiticide (although no product is specifically licensed for *Giardia*).

Prevention

- Vaccine is available in the USA. Its effectiveness is debatable.

Equine infectious diseases

Equine herpesvirus (EHV)

Aetiology

- There are four causal agents which are endemic worldwide:
  1. EHV-1: respiratory disease (neurological rhino-pneumonitis) and abortion, stillbirth and high mortality in neonates
  2. EHV-2: not apparently pathogenic
  3. EHV-3: genital problems

  4. EHV-4: respiratory disease (upper respiratory tract disease in young animals)
- Breeders can be heavily affected financially by the agents and they are also a major cause of lack of performance in horses
- Also known as equine rhinopneumonitis.

Pathogenesis

- Transmission is via direct contact with respiratory discharges or fetal tissue and membranes
- Virus replicates in the respiratory tract, then migrates transplacentally in pregnant mares to infect offspring.

Clinical signs

- Pyrexia, inappetance, nasal discharge, pharyngitis, depression and limb oedema
- Diagnosis is by antibody assays or histopathological examination/virus isolation of fetal tissue and membranes.

Treatment

- Symptoms are treated and antibiotic therapy indicated for secondary infections.

Prevention

- Vaccination: routine and pregnant mares should be vaccinated during the 5th, 7th and 9th month of gestation with inactivated EHV-1 vaccine but even this does not afford full protection from abortion
- Mares and stallions are usually swabbed for EHV prior to breeding.

Equine influenza

Aetiology

- Orthomyxoviruses
- Numerous versions which are constantly changing (antigenic drift)
- Outbreaks often occur in young horses (1–3 years) when mixing with others at the racecourse or shows
- Older horses can be infected but often show milder clinical signs.

Pathogenesis

- Transmission is via droplet and aerosol contact
- Incubation period: 1–5 days
- Infected animals present with a persistent cough which can result in rapid infection within populations
- Virus replicates in ciliated epithelium of the respiratory tract, causing them to lose the cilia, which causes oedema and reduces the respiratory tract's ability to

remove pathogens, thus increasing the possibility of secondary infections.

Clinical signs

- Pyrexia, coughing, serous nasal discharge which progresses to purulent discharge, inappetance, muscular soreness and enlarged mandibular lymph nodes
- Diagnosis is by nasopharyngeal swab and culture of virus.

Treatment

- One week of complete rest for every day of raised temperature
- Non-steroidal anti-inflammatories
- Antibiotics for secondary infections.

Prevention

- Vaccination – inactivated as attenuated live versions are subject to mutation
- In the USA equine influenza virus A/1 and A/2 are of importance and vaccines are available but duration of action is short-lived, with race horses and show animals required to be revaccinated every 2–3 months.

Equine viral arteritis (EVA)

Aetiology

- Virus similar to coronavirus
- Worldwide problem for the equine industry as it results in abortion
- Notifiable disease in the UK.

Pathogenesis

- Transmission is by direct contact with respiratory and venereal discharges or indirect contact via fomites; aborted fetuses and fetal membranes are also laden with the virus
- Virus tends to colonise the arterial walls, resulting in necrotic arteritis.

Clinical signs

- Range from subclinical to severe disease and death
- Pyrexia, depression, nasal discharge, lacrimation, coughing, limb oedema, stiffness in gait, inflammation of the conjunctiva
- Diagnosis is by serology and virus isolation.

Treatment

- Supportive therapy and rest; most horses recover.

Prevention

- Restriction of movement of horses from affected premises
- Vaccination (permission is required in the UK).

Tetanus

Aetiology

- Bacterium: *Clostridium tetani.*

Pathogenesis

- Bacteria are present in equine faeces and that of other herbivores and in the soil
- Bacteria are anaerobic and it is the toxins produced as they replicate which cause clinical signs
- Incubation varies from 1 to 3 weeks.

Clinical signs

- Inability to retract nictitating membrane, spasms in facial muscles, ears are pricked, muscular stiffness, dysphagia, convulsions
- Death usually occurs within 1 week of clinical sign onset and is as a result of respiratory arrest or convulsions
- Diagnosis is by bacterial culture.

Treatment

- Active immunity via injection of tetanus toxoid provides immediate protection for approximately 2 weeks.

Prevention

- Vaccination.

Streptococcus equi (strangles)

Strangles is the most common bacterial disease in horses; it is highly contagious and can spread through stables rapidly. Horses present depressed and dull, and stop eating. They exhibit pyrexia and the lymph nodes around the throat swell, forming abscesses. The horse can have difficulty breathing and swallowing (hence the name 'strangles'). A nasal discharge is at first clear and then becomes purulent after the abscesses have ruptured in the nasal passages; abscesses may be lanced. Abscesses that rupture shed highly infective pus into the environment, which can infect other horses. In some outbreaks and in up to 10% of cases, these abscesses spread to other parts of the body (a condition known as 'bastard strangles'), which is nearly always fatal. Diagnosis is via nasopharyngeal swab. Treatment is supportive therapy and strict isolation and hygiene controls in the yard.

In the USA and Canada a number of other equine infectious diseases are considered, including:

- Equine encephalomyelitis – a viral neurological disease, maintained by bird and animal vectors and transmitted via biting insects to horses; it is prevalent in South and Central America. Horses on the border states with the USA are commonly vaccinated as a preventive measure
- Potomac horse fever – equine monocytic ehrlichiosis: the causal agent is *Ehrlichia risticii*, and it is prevalent in eastern USA and near to waterways. It is thought that aquatic insects, ticks and snails are vectors for the disease. A vaccine is available
- Botulism – a bacterial disease which affects horses worldwide; the causal agent is *Clostridium botulinum* which can be present in fermented forage. A type B toxoid is available and in the USA the vaccine is often given to mares 30 days before they foal to prevent shaker foal syndrome in areas of high incidence.

Rabbit infectious diseases

Respiratory disease

Aetiology

- *Pasteurella multocida, Staphylococcus aureus, Enterobacter* spp. and *Pseudomonas aeruginosa.*

Pathogenesis

- Transmission via direct and indirect contact
- Once infected, many rabbits remain as asymptomatic carriers, leading to widespread infection
- Organisms replicate in the upper respiratory tract and often an ocular or nasal serous discharge is observed which progresses to become mucopurulent
- Nasolacrimal ducts and the inner ear may become infected and septicaemia may result, as can pneumonia.

Clinical signs

- Ocular/nasal discharge
- Rhinitis, sneezing, pneumonia, otitis media, conjunctivitis, abscesses, genital infections and septicaemia.

Treatment

- Antibiotics – though care should be taken as dysbiosis and enteritis can result, which can lead to death.

Prevention

- Isolation of new animals into a colony
- Detection and cull of carriers
- Isolation of infected animals.

Myxamatosis

Aetiology

- Poxvirus
- Endemic in European rabbit species – domestic and wild.

Pathogenesis

- Transmitted by vector – bites from mosquitoes, flies and fleas and by direct contact
- Virus replicates and damages the dermis, with lesions present in the mucous membranes and fibrous nodules occurring over the nose, ears and feet.

Clinical signs

- Physical appearance – conjunctivitis with a thick ocular discharge
- Lethargic, anorexia, abnormal behaviour, pyrexia, oedema of the lips, nose, eyes, ears and coat
- Mucopurulent discharge and dyspnoea
- Death occurs within 1–2 weeks.

Treatment

- Supportive therapy; euthanasia should be considered

Prevention

- Vaccination (every 6 months if endemic in local area).

Viral haemorrhagic disease (VHD)

Aetiology

- Parvovirus (thought to be related to porcine parvovirus).

Pathogenesis

- Aerosol and discharge transmission via direct/indirect contact; also vectors such as rodents are implicated
- Rapid replication occurs within 24–72 hours: animals are found dead although still appearing in good condition
- Lesions present in respiratory tract and liver with frothy congestion in the lungs and trachea
- Focal, coagulative hepatic necrosis is present.

Clinical signs

- Protracted cases – dyspnoea, congestion of eyelids, orthopnoea, abdominal breathing and tachycardia
- Just before death a violent episode similar to a fit occurs, with the animal flipping and turning rapidly.

Treatment

- None: the disease is always fatal.

Prevention

- Vaccination
- Quarantine for rabbits entering countries which do not have the disease.

All species: infectious diseases

Salmonellosis

Aetiology

- Bacterium: *Salmonella typhimurium*.

Pathogenesis

- Zoonosis
- Transmitted by eating raw, uncooked meat
- Salmonella organisms are transient bacteria which are normally present in the gastrointestinal tract. Immunosuppressed animals can be susceptible to infection due to increased populations or by direct contact with faeces from infected animals containing shed bacteria, e.g. foals
- Incubation period is variable.

Clinical signs

- Acute or chronic gastroenteritis
- Drooling saliva, pyrexia, colic, abdominal pain, icterus and breeding problems
- Diagnosis by faecal analysis.

Treatment

- Isolation and barrier nursing
- Fluid therapy, rest and supportive therapeutics
- Antibiotics are often not used as they destroy the normal gut flora.

Prevention

- Reduction in unnecessary antibiotic use
- Feed cooked meat.

Rabies

Aetiology

- Rhabdovirus (Lyssavirus)
- Zoonotic; notifiable in UK.

Pathogenesis

- Transmitted by direct contact with saliva from bite wounds

- Incubation varies between 1 and 6 months (this is why quarantine in the UK is 6 months for countries in which the Pet Travel Scheme does not apply)
- Endemic in North America
- Onset of clinical signs depends on the immune status, dose of virus and location of bite
- The virus replicates in the muscles before it enters the nervous system
- Antibodies are effective against the virus whilst it is contained in the muscle but once the nervous system has been entered the prognosis is death.

Clinical signs

There are two forms: furious and dumb rabies.

Furious rabies

- Hyperexcitability interspersed with periods of calm, pica, aggression often directed at unseen objects, ataxia, progressive facial paralysis, drooling, dysphagia, frothy saliva and convulsions, which may lead to death.

Dumb rabies

- Timid, often affectionate, generalised paresis leading to paralysis and ataxia; respiratory muscles become paralysed, which may lead to death
- Diagnosis is via histopathology of the brain (once the animal is dead) – lesions are present.

Treatment

- In the UK – all animals are euthanised and the Department for Environment, Food and Rural Affairs must be informed.

Prevention

- Vaccination – routine in North America and other countries
- In the UK only animals who enrol on the Passports for Pets scheme are vaccinated.

Parasites

A parasite is defined as a plant or an animal that lives on or in another, usually larger, host organism in a way that harms or is of no advantage to the host.

Ectoparasites are parasites that live on or in the body surface, i.e. the skin. There are two categories:

1. Surface parasites
2. Subsurface parasites.

Endoparasites are parasites that live inside the body, usually in the gastrointestinal tract, respiratory tract or heart.

119

Parasiticides are products that kill parasites; care should be taken as they will only kill if administered at the correct dose rate, and if the manufacturer's instructions are followed.

Ectoparasites

Most ectoparasites are of the phylum *Arthropoda*. They include fleas, lice, mites, ticks, chiggers and flies. There are many treatments available and control can be challenging, as the animal itself, its environment and the animals it has interacted with require consideration. It is recommended to consult a veterinary surgeon before choosing a suitable product as many commercial variations are available.

Fleas: **Ctenophalides canis, C. felis** Both dogs and cats are commonly infested with cat fleas, *Ctenophalides felis* (Figure 9.1). Fleas are not host-specific and prefer to inhabit a warm and humid environment akin to many human households. Fleas feed on blood, injecting an anticoagulant into the animal to prevent clotting occurring during feeding, and it is this substance which causes pruritus and allergic responses in animals, e.g. miliary dermatitis in cats and flea-allergic dermatitis in dogs. Signs of infestation include pruritus, loss of coat condition and flea dirt in the coat. In young and immunosuppressed animals a heavy flea burden can result in severe anaemia due to excessive blood loss. Flea dirt is flea faeces and a simple test is to use a fine-toothed comb to collect coat debris then place it on damp paper and the dirt will make the paper a red/brown colour as it comprises digested blood.

The flea lifecycle can be completed in favourable conditions in as little as 12–16 days; adult fleas lay eggs in the fur of animals; they are not sticky so fall off the coat into the environment. In houses with carpeted surfaces these provide an ideal environment for the flea eggs to hatch. The eggs hatch into larval stages which feed on adult flea dirt, skin flakes and organic debris in their environment; they undergo two moults before they pupate and then emerge as adults. Fleas act as an inter-mediate host for numerous diseases and parasites, including *Dipyldium caninum*. Affected animals should be treated with insecticide and their environment should be treated concurrently, placing special attention on moving furniture and not forgetting all areas they inhabit, e.g. the car. Flea eggs can remain dormant for up to 2 years in the environment until movement vibrations from animals or humans stimulate them to hatch.

Ticks: **Ixodes ricinus, I. hexagonas, Dermacentor reticulatus, Rhipicephalus sanguineus** There are many different species of tick and all species feed on blood from a host animal. The larval and adult ticks feed until engorged and can then drop off into the environment; females lay their eggs on the ground in a moist location before they die. A heavy infestation can result in anaemia and incorrect removal may leave the mouthparts in situ, and these mouthparts could become infected. Ticks are also important vectors for babesiosis. Treatment is insecticide and ticks themselves should be removed using a proprietary tick removal device.

Lice Lice are host-specific, possess claws to attach themselves to their host and feed on blood. Lice can be described as biting or sucking depending on whether their mouthparts have evolved to chew the skin to feed or to pierce the skin to enable them to suck. Lice eggs are known as nits and are sticky, enabling them to attach to the coat hairs and complete their lifecycle on the host.

The biting louse of the dog is *Trichodectes canis* and in the cat is *Felicola subrostratus*. Dogs also have a sucking louse, *Linognathus setosus*. In horses the sucking louse is *Haematopinus asini* and the biting louse *Damalinia equi*.

Animals with a lice infestation are described as having a pediculosis and exhibit pruritus; their coat condition is poor and nits or lice may be observed. Anaemia can result and young, old and debilitated animals are most affected. Treatment is a suitable insecticide and, as the nits are not usually killed, treatment should be repeated 10 days after the first application.

Mites: **subsurface and surface mites** Subsurface mites live in the dermis and present with short legs whilst surface mites live on the epidermis and tend to have longer legs.

Ear mites: **Otodectes cynotis** *Otodectes cynotis* are surface mites that possess suckers and hairs to grasp the walls of the ear canal (Figure 9.2). They present on examination as off-white dots on ear wax; infected animals will shake, scratch and rub their head and their ears will be excessively waxy and often smell. They are spread by direct contact and treatment by acaricidal product is required.

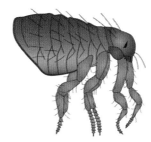

Figure 9.1 Flea. (Reproduced from Aspinall V 2006 *The Complete Textbook of Veterinary Nursing*. Butterworth Heinemann, London, with permission.)

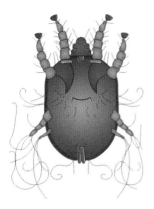

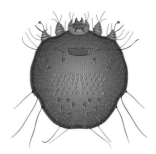

Figure 9.3 *Sarcoptes*. (Reproduced from Aspinall V 2006 *The Complete Textbook of Veterinary Nursing*. Butterworth Heinemann, London, with permission.)

Figure 9.2 *Otodectes cynotis*. (Reproduced from Aspinall V 2006 *The Complete Textbook of Veterinary Nursing*. Butterworth Heinemann, London, with permission.)

Chorioptes equi A similar surface mite to *Otodectes* which infects horses, this mite infects the skin, particularly the feathers, in heavy breeds of horse.

Psoroptes equi/P. cuniculi These are two closely related surface mites which look identical and have suckers on stalks; in the rabbit *P. cuniculi* causes ear infections and in horses *P. equi* produces a pruritic dermatitis.

Cheyletiella *spp.* These surface mites affect dogs, cats and rabbits; each has its own specific mite. They are relatively large and can just be seen with the naked eye. They cause a scurfy, flaky coat and are known as 'walking dandruff' as the mites are often found under skin debris. They are capable of surviving away from the host so both the animal and its environment should be treated.

***Harvest mites:* Neotrombiculus autumnalis** Another surface mite, this is prevalent in late summer/ early autumn and will feed then drop off infected animals. They are an orange/red colour and may result in pruritus and dermatitis.

Sarcoptes scabeii *Sarcoptes scabeii* (Figure 9.3) is a subsurface mite that is zoonotic, although it only survives for up to 3 weeks in humans. It affects dog, foxes and sometimes horses, cats and rabbits and is commonly known as mange. The mite lays its eggs in burrows it creates in the skin and it causes an erythematous, alopecic dermatitis characteristically of the pinna, hock and elbow and which expands to cover the animal. It is highly pruritic. Treatment is via application of insecticide.

Demodex *spp.* *Demodex* (Figure 9.4) is a characteristically cigar-shaped subsurface mite which is thought to be normally present with no ill effects in healthy animals. It can overpopulate at times of stress or immunosuppres-

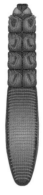

Figure 9.4 *Demodex*. (Reproduced from Aspinall V 2006 *The Complete Textbook of Veterinary Nursing*. Butterworth Heinemann, London, with permission.)

sion to produce a widespread alopecic dermatitis with secondary bacterial infections common. Treatment is by acaricide.

Endoparasites

Endoparasites can be broadly divided into four main groups:

1. Nematodes – roundworms
2. Cestodes – tapeworms
3. Trematodes – flukes or flatworms
4. Protozoa – unicellular organisms.

Nematodes Nematodes are known as roundworms as they are cylindrical in cross-section and look a little like spaghetti. Ascarids are large roundworms found in the intestines of the horse, dog and cat. Ascarids include:

- Dog: *Toxocara canis*
- Cat: *T. cati, T. leonina*
- Horse: *Parascaris equorum*.

Toxocara canis Eggs from infected animals are passed in the faeces and are ingested from the environment or

121

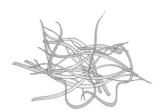

Figure 9.5 *Toxocara canis*. (Reproduced from Aspinall V 2006 *The Complete Textbook of Veterinary Nursing*. Butterworth Heinemann, London, with permission.)

via eating animals which are already infected. The larvae migrate through the liver and lungs to the gastrointestinal tract to mature to adult worms (Figure 9.5); some larvae remain in somatic cells and are stimulated during pregnancy to migrate transplacentally to the developing fetuses. They can also migrate in a transmammary route after birth, which is is why it is important to treat puppies regularly with an appropriate endoparasiticide. Heavy burdens can result in loss of condition and an enlarged abdomen or 'worm belly' and may result in intussusception or intestinal obstruction. *T. canis* are zoonotic and in humans develop in the eye and viscera, which can result in ocular and liver disease.

Toxocara cati The lifecycle is similar to that of *T. canis* but no prenatal migration occurs in cats, with infection via the transmammary route in kittens. Again there is zoonotic potential.

Toxocara leonina This may affect dogs and cats and is zoonotic; infection occurs by ingesting eggs or paratenic hosts (intermediate hosts that are not needed in the lifecycle).

Parascaris equorum These are usually only problematic for foals and younger horses. Eggs can remain viable in the soil for many years and horses usually ingest them as they graze. The eggs hatch in the gastrointestinal tract and the larvae migrate into the veins, then move to the lungs where they are coughed up, reswallowed and passed into the small intestine. Once in the small intestine the larvae develop into adult roundworms. The adults, which can grow up to about 50 cm long, lay eggs which are passed out in the faeces. Prevention by suitable anthelminthic is required as well as pasture management.

Hookworms Hookworms are named after the appearance of their mouthparts. They are parasites of the small intestine with numerous species affecting a range of animals. Eggs hatch in the environment and develop into larvae, which are ingested or may enter through the skin.

Uncinaria stenocephala This is endemic in the UK in dogs. Larvae are either ingested or can penetrate the skin: animals living in a kennel environment are most susceptible. Dogs present with diarrhoea.

Ancyclostoma caninum This is endemic in the EU and occasionally in the UK. The larvae thrive in warm environments and infection is by ingestion or skin penetration; transmammary infection can occur. Infected animals often exhibit melaena due to the presence of undigested blood in the faeces. It also occurs in foxes, coyotes, wolves and raccoons.

Ancyclostoma tubaeforme This feline hookworm affects cats in the EU and causes anaemia.

Whipworms These are so called as their anterior end is thin and whip-like. The adults inhabit the intestine.

Trichuris vulpis Canine, fox and coyote whipworm eggs are passed into the environment in faeces and require a temperate climate to develop; larvae are enclosed in a shell and may remain viable for up to a year until favourable conditions present. Heavy burdens can result in diarrhoea and metabolic disturbances.

Strongyloides *spp.* Infections are common in young animals, with *Strongyloides westeri* affecting foals through transmammary migration of larvae or ingested from the environment. Larvae mature to adult worms in the small intestine. Infection can occur by eating infective larvae or by penetration through the skin. If the larvae enter the horse's system through its skin, they move to the lungs, then up the windpipe where they are coughed up and swallowed. They mature in the small intestine, where adult females lay the eggs that are passed out in the manure.

If the larvae enter through the skin the next stop is the lungs, where they can cause bleeding and respiratory problems. Inflammation and rashes can develop where the larvae penetrated the skin. The worst damage occurs in untreated foals. Infected through their mother's milk, they can suffer diarrhoea, weakness, weight loss and failure to thrive and grow at a normal rate. Dogs may also present with diarrhoea from *Strongyloides* infestation.

Strongyles Equids can potentially be infected by a range of nematodes. Control by pasture management and regular anthelminthics is required.

Small redworms (cyathostomins) These worms are the most common horse parasites. Adults living in the large intestine lay eggs that are passed out in the faeces. The worm eggs hatch and develop through three stages, with the third being the infective stage. If a grazing horse eats the infective stage the larvae will migrate to the intestinal lining, where they can remain dormant for long periods of time. Vast numbers of larvae can potentially build up in this area, then suddenly reactivate and erupt out of the gut wall, which can cause extensive damage to the gut wall. Larvae emerge into the large intestine and develop into adults which lay eggs that are passed out in the droppings, completing the cycle.

Large redworm (Strongylus vulgari, S. equinus and S. edentatus) The large redworm differs from small redworms in size and lifecycle. Horses become infected by ingesting larvae as they are grazing. The larvae of large redworms migrate through the blood vessels to the arteries of the intestinal tract where they can cause severe damage. After about six months they return to the intestine as egg-laying adult worms. Adult worms vary in size between 1.5 and 5 cm and, in large numbers, can cause several different disease problems including clot formation in mesenteric arteries resulting in necrosis of the intestine and ulceration of intestinal tissue.

Pinworm (Oxyuris equi) Pinworms are so called as they look like carpet tacks; they are not thought to be harmful but can provoke irritation around the tail. Pinworms inhabit the large and small colon and have a relatively simple lifecycle. The females lay their eggs around the anus of the horse, using a sticky substance which is irritating to the horse. The eggs are dislodged as droppings are passed and fall on to the pasture where they are eaten by horses.

Lungworms Dictyocaulus arnfieldi The equine lungworm is long and slender; the larvae go through the walls of the intestine and into the circulatory system. They are carried in the circulatory system into the lungs, where they mature. The eggs pass through the horse's system through the manure. Female lungworms lay eggs containing larvae. The horse eats the eggs of the lungworm off damp grasses. If there are large numbers of the larvae present, the lungs may become irritated, causing the horse to have a severe cough, difficulty breathing and loss of appetite.

Infection is usually light in older horses because they develop resistance to the parasite and usually have no signs. If foals are infected, they could die from a lungworm infection because they have less immunity.

Heartworms Heartworms are nematodes that colonise the heart. There are three canine heartworms of note: *Angiostrongylus vasorum* (which can also affect foxes), *Dirofilaria immitis* and *Dipetalonema reconditum*. *D. immitis* and *D. reconditum* are not endemic in the UK but are endemic in the USA and some parts of Europe. Prevention is essential for animals inhabiting or travelling in affected areas as surgical removal and anthelminthics can be used as treatment but both pose risks.

Cestodes Cestodes are commonly known as tapeworms. They are flat in appearance and have a head or scolex and a chain of segments or proglottids. The tapeworm attaches to the intestinal wall and produces gravid segments full of eggs which move out of the animal via the anus. They resemble grains of rice and are sticky and mobile. Most have intermediate hosts and control is via an anthelminthic with cestodial action.

Anoplocephala perfoliata This is an equine tapeworm which can grow to about 8 cm long and about 1.5 cm wide. It lives in the midpart of the gut at a junction between the small and large intestine, known as the ileocaecal junction. Infected horses pass eggs on to the pasture. These eggs are eaten by tiny oribatid mites which are present in their thousands in every square metre of grass. Once inside the mite, the eggs hatch and develop into an intermediate infective stage. Grazing horses inadvertently eat mites with almost every mouthful. The adults attach in clusters to the lining of the gut at the ileocaecal junction and release eggs, thereby completing their lifecycle; recent research implicates tapeworm infestation with certain types of colic.

Dipylidium caninum This tapeworm affects both dogs and cats, with intermediate hosts being fleas and other biting lice. Infection usually occurs when an infected intermediate host is ingested and there are few signs of infestation unless present in large numbers.

Taenia *spp.* There are a number of *Taenia* spp. that affect animals:

- *T. pisiformis*: dog and fox (intermediate host – rabbit)
- *T. hydatigena*: dog and fox (intermediate hosts – cattle and sheep)
- *T. multiceps*: dog (intermediate hosts – sheep and cattle)
- *T. ovis*: dog and fox (intermediate hosts – sheep and goat)
- *T. serialis*: dog (intermediate host – rabbit)
- *T. taeniaeformis*: cat (intermediate host – rodents).

Infections occur when infected intermediate hosts are ingested.

Echinococcus granulosus This is a very small tapeworm that affects dogs and foxes and huge numbers must be present before signs of infestation are observed. It occurs worldwide and it is zoonotic; if humans ingest eggs a hydrated cyst can develop in the lungs, requiring surgery or anthelminthic treatment. Infection in dogs usually occurs by eating raw offal of infected animals (sheep is the intermediate host).

Trematodes Flukes or trematodes are found in the intestine, bile ducts, blood and lungs of domestic animals.

123

Common liver fluke: Fasciola hepatica Adult flukes in the liver lay eggs in the bile, which carries them into the intestine. They leave in the host's faeces. After hatching, the immature fluke must penetrate a snail for the lifecycle to continue. Multiplication occurs within particular species of snail. After leaving the snail the flukes encyst on grass where they are eaten by horses. The young parasites penetrate the gut and pass to the liver. The snails live in swampy, wet areas. *F. hepatica* occurs worldwide in wet areas where Lymnaea snails may exist. Animals experience anaemia and decreased growth. Liver damage results in organ condemnation at slaughter.

Protozoa These are unicellular organisms which can be parasitic.

Coccidiosis Isopora spp. are parasites of the gastrointestinal tract in dogs and cats; some animals tolerate them well whereas others will present with diarrhoea. Horses and rabbits may be infected by *Eimeria* spp., resulting in diarrhoea. *Sarcocystis neurona* produces a severe neural disease in horses – equine protozoal myeloencephalitis.

Insects Horses may be affected by parasitic infection by insects, including:

- Bots – *Gastrophilus* spp.
- *Culcoides* – midges/sweet itch
- *Habronema* spp. – fly bites.

Rabbits and sheep may be affected by:

- Myiasis – fly strike from bluebottle eggs.

Bibliography

Appleby M 1999 What should we do about animal welfare? Blackwell Science, Oxford

Appleby M C, Hughes B O 1997 Animal welfare. CABI Publishing, Oxford

Aspinall V 2006 The complete textbook of veterinary nursing. Butterworth Heinemann, London

Blood D C, Studdert V P 1998 Bailliere's comprehensive veterinary dictionary. Baillière & Tindall, London

Chandler E A, Gaskell C J, Gaskell R M 1994 Feline medicine and therapeutics, 2nd edn. Blackwell Sciences/BSAVA, Oxford

Dawkins M S 1980 Animal suffering. The science of animal welfare. Chapman & Hall. London

Garner R 1993 Animals, politics and morality. Manchester University Press, Manchester

Gaskell R M, Bennett M 1996 Feline and canine infectious disease. Blackwell Science, Oxford

Gorman N 1998 Canine medicine and therapeutics, 4th edn. Blackwell Science/BSAVA, Oxford

Lane D R, Cooper B, Turner L 2007 BSAVA Textbook of Veterinary Nursing. BSAVA, Oxford

Meredith A, Redrobe S 2002 Manual of exotic pets, 4th edn. BSAVA, Gloucester

Ramsey I, Tennant B 2001 Manual of canine and feline infectious diseases. BSAVA, Oxford

Sainsbury D 1998 Animal health, 2nd edn. Blackwell Science, Oxford

Spedding C 2000 Animal welfare. Earthscan, London

Torrance A G, Mooney C T 1998 Manual of small animal endocrinology, 2nd edn. BSAVA, Oxford

Warren D M 1995 Small animal care and management. Delmar, New York

Equine health and welfare

This chapter discusses the main principles that should be considered to promote equine health and welfare. It discusses identification of horses, provides information on basic handling and evaluates basic husbandry and management systems.

IDENTIFICATION

Identification of horses can be roughly categorised into four main areas:

1. Type
2. Breed
3. Visual appearance
4. Paper-based documentation.

Type

This refers to groups of horses such as hunters, cobs, hacks and even such a broad grouping as ponies. The type does not narrow down the individual; rather, it places them in a group with common features. This is judged more through experience than by exact measurements or features. Type is a general term applied to categorise an equine and is developed with experience of seeing many different equines (Figures 10.1–10.3).

Breed

This is a more specific and accurate grouping. If a horse is a specific breed, it is normally registered with that breed society. Most breed societies have specific criteria and regulations for acceptance and registration. There are stud registers for many breeds to allow parentage to be traced and individuals to be identified. Many breeds have grading systems that an individual must pass to qualify for status and breed recognition. This is designed to establish the most influential bloodlines for that breed. Breeds such as Dartmoor ponies have to meet certain physical criteria, such as height, to be registered and yet other breeds have to perform at a certain level and demonstrate certain levels of capability to be accepted and registered (Figure 10.4).

Visual appearance

This incorporates type, as type is a visual characteristic that would be established when visually assessing an equine. Other obvious visual signs are colour, markings, age, height and any brand or freeze markings.

Common colours are:

- Black – this is actually a rare colour for a horse as many dark bay horses may appear black but on closer inspection the hair colour is in fact dark brown. To be black the horse must have all black hair; white markings are acceptable
- Brown – this is where the main body of the horse is brown, and this can vary from lighter to dark brown. The points of the horse are also brown, as are the mane and tail, and there can be white markings. This is similar to a bay horse but without the black points

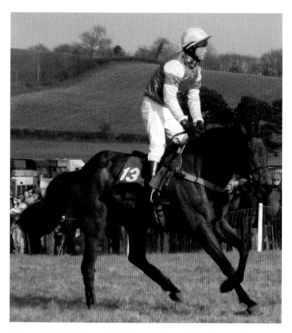

Figure 10.1 Light-weight horse: thoroughbred racehorse.

- Bay – this is a brown-coloured horse, again varying from light to dark, with black points and possibly some white markings. The mane and tail must be black for the horse to be called bay. As there is such a large variety of bays they are often described as bright bay, dark bay and light bay
- Chestnut – a yellowy, ginger or reddish colour all over the body, including the mane and the tail. White markings can be present. A darker brown colour all over is called a liver chestnut
- Grey – this covers a wide range of colours from dapple grey to iron grey and many shades in between. Grey normally indicates a coat of white, grey and black hairs mixed together to form an overall colour of 'grey'. The mane and tail are also a mixture of white and black hairs. Most grey animals are born very dark – almost black – and become a whiter shade of grey as they age; however this is not always the case. If the coat contains more black and dark grey hair the horse is known as iron grey. If the coat contains patches or circles of darker hair this is described as dapple grey and a freckled appearance is called a flea-bitten grey
- Dun – this can vary from a mousey to an almost golden, biscuit-like colour, commonly with dark, almost black points, and often a darker mane and tail. Some dun animals have a black dorsal line

- Roan – there are different types of roan such as blue roan, strawberry roan, and a range of colours in between. The predominant features of roan are that there is base colour with white hairs throughout the coat, making the colour seem almost paler. The mane and tail and points are normally the base colour but with less white dispersed amongst the hair
- Piebald – this is a black and white horse where the colours are randomly spaced and of irregular patterns
- Skewbald – this is a brown and white horse, where the colours are randomly spaced and of irregular patterns. The brown can vary from very light to very dark.

The only way to become proficient at identifying colours and markings of horses as well as recognising type and breed is to spend time viewing many different horses. This will highlight the huge individuality and range of colours and markings.

Markings

These are normally associated with either the face or limbs of the horse.

Facial markings

- Stripe: this is a narrow strip of white hair down the centre of the face
- Blaze: this is a thicker strip of white hair down the centre of the face, normally covering further down the face to the nose
- Snip: this is a small white marking in or around the nostrils. Commonly this is found in between the nostrils but it can be on either side
- Star: this is a white patch of hair on the horse's head between the eyes
- White face: this describes a very broad blaze; in most instances a white face would be the description if the blaze reached toward the eyes and/or to both nostrils.

Leg markings

- Sock – this is where there is white hair on any of the limbs extending upward from the coronet to any height below the knee or the hock
- Stocking – this is the same as for the sock above, except that it is used to describe any white features above the knee or the hock
- Ermine marks – these are black dots or marks that appear on a white marking, usually a sock. These marks commonly occur around the coronet band (Figure 10.5)

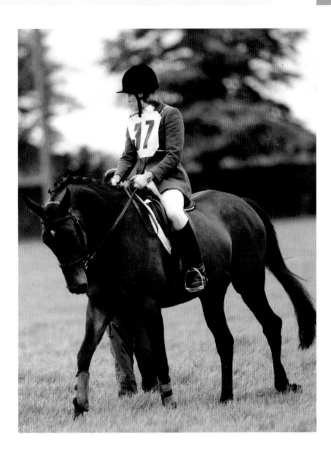

Figure 10.2 Middle-weight horse: Cleveland bay ×
thoroughbred competing at riding club showing event.

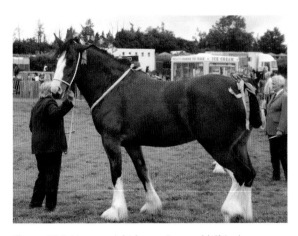

Figure 10.3 Heavy-weight horse: 2-year-old Shire horse.

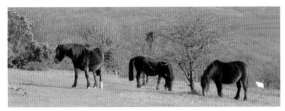

Figure 10.4 Typical Dartmoor ponies.

- White coronet – this is used to describe a white band
  around the coronet that is too small to be classed as
  a sock and is simply a 'white coronet'.

Height

This is measured in hands (hh); one hand is 4 inches
(approximately 10 cm). It is called a hand because it
originally equated to the width of a man's hand.

The measurement is taken from the highest point of
the withers of the horse: the horse should be standing

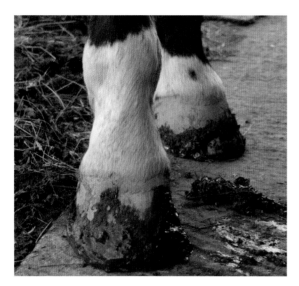

Figure 10.5 Sock and marking: note the ermine marks on the posterior hoof.

Table 10.1 Average breed heights	
Breed	**Average height**
Shetland pony	10.1 hh
Exmoor pony	12.2 hh
New Forest pony	13.1 hh
Fell pony	14.0 hh
Arab	14.2 hh
Thoroughbred	16.0 hh
Suffolk Punch	16.2 hh
Shire	17.2 hh

on a flat surface when it is being measured. The division between pony and horse is 14.2 hh. If a horse is more than an exact number of hands high, the extra inches are given after a full stop. For example, 14 hands 2 inches is written as 14.2 hh; average breed height is shown in Table 10.1.

Brands/freeze markings

These can range from small breed-associated brands or ownership brand information to a group of letters and/ or numbers associated with identification. Many horses are freeze-marked to assist in the prevention of theft and these details are then documented on their passport and can be used if the animal is stolen. It also prevents indi-

viduals being presented as one animal when in fact they are either older or younger or another animal completely. To freeze-brand a horse irons are placed in liquid nitrogen and when these are applied to the skin they destroy the pigment cells that colour the hair; this causes white hair only to grow in the treated area. There is also hot iron branding where an identifiable set of letters or numbers can be applied to the hoof wall; this grows out in time and the owner will need to repeat the process every 6 months or so.

Whorls

These are like fingerprints to humans and are areas on the horse where the hair grows in a variety of directions. Identification of whorls and their documentation on a passport can assist in ensuring the passport is actually for the horse it states. The whorls can be found anywhere on the body.

Paper-based documentation

Passports

As of 28 February 2005 all horses are required to have their own passport. The object of the introduction of passports is to ensure that any horses treated with veterinary medicines are not then slaughtered for human consumption. If the UK had not introduced passports the country would have run the risk of losing 70% of horse medicines. The idea is that the passport system will improve welfare as it may reduce the indiscriminate breeding of horses and ponies and all equines with a passport will be registered and traceable. This central database is the National Equine Database (NED). Maintaining a central database should help with the identification of disease, prevent individuals being sold with incorrect details and assist in equine breeding and development.

Breed society

This will vary depending on the society and its individual requirements.

Microchips

Many horses are now microchipped and this is an additional piece of information for their passport. A scanner is passed over the horse and the horse's identity can be determined immediately. The microchip is placed under the skin on the horse's neck and the details are added to a computer-based register. This method of identification requires that sales, slaughterhouses, vets and police use the appropriate scanners.

Note: from July 2009 it will become law that all foals born in the EU will have to be microchipped as part of the identification process.

Identification documents for most breed societies will include the following:

- Name
- Date of birth
- Colour
- Markings
- Whorls
- Height
- Owner's name and address
- Injections
- Veterinary stamp and details associated with any inoculations.

EQUINE MANAGEMENT

There are entire texts written specifically on the subject of management of the equine. Therefore, further reading is required. However, as with any animal the successful management of the equine follows a good routine. This is the basis for all equines, whether they are show jumpers, eventers or riding club horses.

Safety

Clothing and equipment

- Protective clothing such as steel toe-capped footwear, waterproofs and gloves to protect the hands, especially if lunging or leading horses, should be worn. Loose jewellery should be avoided and hair should be tied up. Footwear is of utmost importance around horses as not only is it necessary to prevent slipping but footwear must also protect feet in case a horse stands on them. Boots with steel toe caps are excellent protection for feet and should be worn when leading or handling any horse. The sole should be non-slip with a sturdy grip and if riding, jodhpur boots or long leather or rubber boots should be worn.
- Hard hats that conform to BSI standard and back protectors should be worn when riding, as should correct footwear for riding (Figure 10.6).

Yard safety

- A good routine on a yard assists in keeping order and ensures that all jobs are done in the correct manner
- Tidiness is crucial to ensure there are no hazards for the people manoeuvring around the yard or the horses
- There should be a set routine for all workers to follow that ensures areas such as the hay barn remain in order
- Maintenance of features of the yard such as water taps, gate locks and latches and electrical points is essential for the safety of both humans and equines.

The common management routines will be based around whether the horse is grass- or stable-kept. This will determine the fundamental basis of the management for the owner.

Basic handling

Correct and careful handling is essential for human safety as well as ensuring the horse is safe and correctly

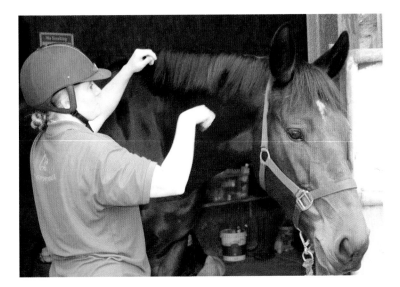

Figure 10.6 Correct protective personal equipment for working with horses.

cared for. Confident firm handling provides the horse with confidence and awareness of your location. Attempt to keep contact with the horse at all times, so that the sudden arrival of your hand doesn't startle the horse and cause it to complete its natural reaction, which is to run or to kick at the unfamiliar object that could be dangerous. Be aware of the horse and its facial and bodily expressions at all times. Most horses will provide obvious warning signs if they are not happy about a situation, allowing you the opportunity to change what is causing the problem or to ignore the situation.

Always tie the horse up when doing anything to it; this is for the safety of both the rider/handler and the horse. This should be done as part of the daily routine and not be a one-off. The head collar is placed on the horse's head with an attached lead rope. Firstly the near side shoulder/neck of the horse is approached and the horse is touched and verbally reassured. The handler should then stand beside the horse facing forward and not directly in font of the horse in case something scares the horse. The head collar is then placed over the muzzle and held up high with the left hand while the right hand flicks the head piece of the head collar behind the ears of the horse. The left hand can then catch the strap and fasten the strap to the correct fitting.

When picking out the horse's feet care must be taken to be safe. Stand facing the tail of the horse on the near side. Keep contact with the horse at all times so that the horse knows where you are and run your left hand down the back of the horse's leg. Keep your shoulder close to the horse and place a small amount of pressure under the fetlock and the horse should lift its foot for cleaning. For the hindlegs, ensure your arm is not at any time at the back of the horse's leg. For the near hindleg stand facing the back of the horse, place your left hand on the inside of the horse's leg below the hock and run it down the leg and lift as with the front leg. The main thing to remember is to be confident, approach the horse firmly and try to give clear and concise commands for the horse to follow.

Grass-kept horses

A grass-kept horse is one that lives in a more natural state, spending the majority of time out to pasture or possibly with the option of a field shelter. If horses are living out to pasture they will still require daily attention to ensure they remain healthy and uninjured.

Advantages and disadvantages of grass-kept horses

Advantages

- It is natural
- Less expense on bedding

- Less time spent mucking out
- More exercise for the horse
- Fresh air – fewer respiratory problems
- Less stereotypies

Disadvantages

- The weather means the horse is often wet and muddy
- In the dark after school or work it is difficult to inspect the horse for injuries
- Conditions such as mud fever can occur
- Rugs don't get the chance to dry out
- It is unlikely there will be adequate grass to maintain the horse for the entire winter so feeding in the field will be needed. This can lead to problems if there is more than one horse in the field or if the owners have different times for visiting the field and feeding.

The preferred system for managing horses would be to use a combination of field and stable.

The pasture

This requires careful management if it is to sustain the animals throughout the year. Approximately one acre per horse ensures enough grass, if well managed, throughout the year. The drainage of the paddock is important and can be added artificially if the field is not draining well. Although this can be disruptive at the time and may be costly, it will be worth it for the following winters if the horses are to remain living out.

Fencing

This is also important in a field. Many hedges provide good shelter; however they are often not as secure as fences. They often have brambles and thinner sections that encourage horses to investigate. The perfect fence is post and rail; however, this is costly and again needs careful care and observation to prevent the rails becoming chewed. Another option is post and wire and there are now many modern varieties of horse fence. All need careful maintenance to remain taut and safe. If other animals are to be retained in the field it is important to consider this at the time of fencing. Electric fencing can be used to divide a field for a temporary period; however it requires careful maintenance. Electric fencing should be specifically designed for horses and needs to be big and bold for the horses to see.

Water supply

This is essential for all pasture: even if the horses are stabled, at some point in the day they still require a water supply to the field. To install a trough with a water supply is initially costly but will save a great deal of effort and inconvenience in the long run. If the trough is not self-filling then all through the winter the trough will need to be washed regularly and refilled. It must be checked on cold days to ensure it has not frozen over. Ideally, for safety, the trough is incorporated into the fence and does not protrude into the field so that knocks on its sharp edges are prevented.

Paddock care

The idea is for the horse's pasture to provide a feed source for the horse for the period of time the horse is turned out. This requires careful planning and management. The grass needs to be specifically for horses and tough enough to withstand grazing and wear and tear from hooves. Another area is parasite control; this can be achieved through rotational grazing, grazing other animals with the horses and/or collecting droppings.

Grass husbandry

This usually involves dividing the land so that the horses graze some part of the pasture for a set period and then that section is left to rest and recover for a period. In the winter the paddock will become muddy; if this is a small section of the pasture then this section can be treated and allowed to recover in the following dry months. However if the horses can roam everywhere they will constantly be placing strain on all the paddock and will not allow any section the chance to recover.

Paddock treatments

Commonly paddocks should be topped if the grass has grown too long, and harrowed and rolled at a suitable time of year, in a dry period following the winter. Harrowing is basically the raking of the grass. This allows air to penetrate the soil and assists in flattening the surface. A roller flattens the pasture and again timing is essential: if it is too dry the roller will simply travel over the ridges and bumps and if it is too wet it will have the effect of causing the soil to stick to it. Many companies now offer soil analysis of your land and this can assist in deciding what, if any, treatments in the form of fertilisers are required to compensate for soil that may be lacking in certain nutrients. This analysis will also look at the acidity of the soil and advise whether lime application is needed or not. The acidity of the soil will affect the nutrient uptake of the grass. The three main components in fertiliser are nitrogen, phosphorus and potash. Nitrogen is the main nutrient related to leaf growth and potash and phosphorus are more related to general growth and root growth. The varieties of grass within the

pasture are also important. Specific seed mixtures are produced for horses and these will contain a mixture of the following:

- Perennial ryegrass
- *Fescue*
- Dog's tail
- Meadow grasses
- Cocksfoot
- Timothy
- White clover.

Herbs are advantageous for nutrients as they are deeper-rooted than grass but often are not included in the grass seed mixture. Herbs can be planted by hand at a later date.

The care of a grass-kept horse has advantages and disadvantages. Daily inspection of the horse and pasture means that the field-kept horse does not really mean spending less time than for the stable horse. The field maintenance can be costly and time-consuming, as can pasture control and care.

The stable-kept horse

Most modern ridden horses are stabled for convenience as the modern horse is groomed and often clipped, removing the natural oils and coat required to cope with cold weather. Native horses are suited to outdoor conditions but this is not the case for many 'man-made' breeds, such as the thoroughbred.

Stables are not only advantageous for protection from colder weather; the summer flies and heat are also a problem and if there is an abundance of spring grass some horses may need time away from grazing for health reasons. Stables assist in treating ill horses as there is easier access to the animal and the animal can be prevented from cavorting around the pasture. Stables also increase the security for the horse owner and the horse.

Most horse owners also have limited land to turn their horses on to and therefore need to conserve the grass and protect the land on particularly wet days or during winter months. Stables can allow horses to be fed through concentrates and forage and be turned out for a short period of time to have a roll, stretch and have some freedom and fresh air instead of turning them out to graze for nutrition.

Stables

Most stables are constructed of a brick base and wooden frame and sides. Ideally, if finances will permit, brick stables are the best but in most cases wooden ones are constructed. The advantage of solid brick or block stabling is that they can be more thoroughly steam-cleaned and disinfected than wooden stables.

As with any building, careful planning is essential. The stables need adequate drainage, access to sunlight, i.e. south-facing, be free from draughts and yet have good ventilation. Ventilation is the key to reducing respiratory disease, which is a constant problem for the majority of stabled horses.

Within the stable space needs to be considered and the majority of stables are 12 × 14 feet (approx. 3.5 × 4.25 metres) with 10 feet (approx. 3 metres) minimum height. The door should be split into a top and bottom door, with suitable latches and a kick bolt; the top of the bottom door should be covered in an antichew strip of metal. The door needs to be 4 feet (approx. 1.25 metres) wide and at least 7 feet (approx. 2.25 metres) high to allow adequate space for the horse and to prevent injury to the horse's sides. Some doors can have roll bars fitted so if the horse does collide with the stable door, the roll bars will roll to prevent damaging the horse. If stables are being built from scratch and there are plans for breeding or extra large horses to be housed, then a larger or foaling stable may be constructed. Likewise, if the stables will only hold ponies then the dimensions can be less and the traditional doors can be replaced with smaller doors to enable the ponies to stand comfortably and look out.

Other features, such as windows, lighting, position of mangers, tackroom, feedroom and tool shed, hay/straw/bedding storage, all need to be considered. Another feature worth bearing in mind is an overhang to protect from some of the weather and encourage the horses to stand looking out of the stable without being rained on.

Stabled-horse requirements

Bedding

A stabled horse will require some form of bedding in the stable. There are many different types now available: dust-free, highly absorbent and recyclable bedding. Traditionally straw and shavings were the common bedding materials and both are still used in abundance today. Storage of the new bedding, disposal of the used bedding and the system to be used in the stable need to be borne in mind.

If, for example, the owner works Monday to Friday, she may well deep litter the stable in the week and give a full muck-out at the weekend when she has more time. This will vary between individuals and personal preference; it will also need to consider the individual horse as some are cleaner in the stable than others. Cost and local availability are also considerations for the type of bedding, as shown in Table 10.2.

The stabled horse's needs

Feeding

The stabled horse will not have access to natural forage and grazing as it would in the wild or in a pasture environment and therefore this needs to be supplemented in the stable. As a horse's natural instinct is to graze for a large proportion of the day, this instinct and desire are often not met in the stable as all the nutrients can be provided in a few hard feeds that are consumed in a short time. Many racehorses that spend nearly all their time in a confined stable have been reported with stomach ulcers, believed to be related to the lack of grazing and food ingested. Therefore, providing forage in a net, maybe with small holes to increase the time taken to consume the forage, may help prevent boredom and stereotypical behaviour and allow the horse to fulfil its natural desire to graze.

Grooming

Grooming is a requirement of both stable- and grass-kept horses. However, if the horse is out at grass without a waterproof rug, grooming should be limited to help retain the natural oils in the coat and protect the horse from the weather. A stabled horse will need to be groomed regularly to help improve circulation, improve appearance, keep the horse and rugs and tack clean and to allow the horse to be checked over regularly.

There are different types of grooming depending on the desired end result. In most cases where the horse is just being exercised then quartering is adequate, where the horse is brushed off quickly and made tidy for exercise. This process is known as 'quartering' as the horse is groomed in four quarter sections. Firstly, the head and neck are groomed, then the legs, and then the feet are picked out. The rug is then undone and a quarter of the rug at a time is folded back to expose the skin and the horse is groomed in these sections. This prevents the horse becoming cold while being groomed. Quartering a horse should take around 20 minutes at the most.

Rugs

Stabled horses are often in work and therefore will probably be clipped in the winter to ease the time spent grooming and waiting for a long winter coat to dry after exercise and to reduce weight loss if the horse sweats frequently. Rugs will keep the horse warm after clipping and during the winter months and dry when in the field. Many horses will wear an exercise sheet over their quarters during exercise as well. The type and amount of rugs worn will depend on the individual and the owner's requirements. Rugs also keep the coat clean, if the rugs are cleaned regularly, and this assists in grooming and reducing sores and rubs under tack.

Table 10.2 Advantages and disadvantages of common horse bedding

Bedding	Advantages	Disadvantages
Straw	Easy to find Provides a deep soft bed Absorbent Drying for the horse's legs	Bulky to store Can be dusty Some horses may eat it Can vary in quality
Wheat straw	If it is baled correctly and not too compacted and heavy it is excellent – absorbent and soft	In most cases it is tough, coarse and heavy to handle Not easy to come by
Barley straw	Usually less dusty and of better quality than wheat straw	Can encourage horses to eat the bedding
Oat straw	Same as any other straw	Palatable to horses, becomes saturated quickly and is more expensive
Shavings	Good if the horse tends to eat the bedding Can reduce dust-associated allergies Absorbent	Can be difficult to dispose of Bulky to handle and to store, although if plastic-wrapped can be stored outside, which can save barn space
Rubber matting	Can save money on bedding No dust for the horse to breathe Removes the problem of bedding purchasing and disposal Time-saving	Not very cosy or warm Won't dry the horse's legs Horse is stood in faeces and urine while in the stable and will have to lie in mess This is very unpleasant for the horse, which, if kept in a field, would not choose to walk in fresh faeces
Paper	Dust-free and not palatable so can help with allergies Very absorbent Can be stored outside	Can be very compacted and therefore heavy and difficult to handle

There are many other modern bedding solutions and each has its own list of advantages and disadvantages. When selecting a bedding the following areas need to be assessed:

Storage facilities
Disposal facilities
Location of suppliers
Cost
Horse's individual requirements
Ease of use for owner

Disease transmission

Stabled horses are exposed to numerous respiratory pathogens, including viruses, bacteria, mould spores, dust mites and parasites. The indoor environment increases disease transmission through a lack of ventilation, fresh air and air movement. This can be assessed and prevented if the air quality is maintained through provision of vents, windows or other ventilation system. The modern stable blocks or indoor, American-style barns are now very popular for housing large numbers of horses. However, they must be designed to allow for good ventilation as their main disadvantage is the rapid spread of disease from one horse to another. The population density within the barn is also a consideration and isolation facilities are essential in a barn situation. A thorough yard routine that incorporates high standards of hygiene and cleanliness can assist in preventing the spread of diseases. General cleanliness must be an essential part of the stable horse's routine.

Management of all horses

All horses, whether in a stable or a grass field, require certain elements of care that are the same.

Health checks

Each day a horse will require a basic health check to ensure its well-being and to check for any injury (Chapter 14). You will become aware of characteristics that show that an individual is acting 'normally'.

Horses should have their feet picked out daily to ensure nothing becomes wedged between the foot and the shoe, as this could lead to lameness or bruising.

Vaccinations

Vaccinations are necessary for horses to prevent common diseases. Vaccinations are effective and cost-effective and essential if the horse is to be exposed to other horses from different areas or yards.

The most common diseases to vaccinate against are equine influenza, tetanus and equine herpesviruses 1 and 4. Some horses are also vaccinated against equine viral arteritis. The frequency and timing of the vaccinations and follow-up boosters may vary depending on the drug but generally flu vaccinations comprise three injections at the following intervals:

- First vaccination
- Second vaccination: 4–6 weeks after the first
- Third vaccination: 6 months after the second
- Booster vaccine given annually
- Some higher-level competition horses may be required to have a 6-monthly booster.

Many competitions require proof of flu vaccination. The vet should enter the details of any vaccinations on the horse's passport and sign and stamp each administration. This will provide proof of the horse's vaccination history. Foals should start their own vaccination programme from 6 months of age.

Tetanus vaccinations are as follows:

- First vaccination
- Second vaccination: 4–6 weeks later
- Third vaccination: within a year of the second
- Booster every other year – often administered with the annual flu vaccine.

Brood mares should be given a booster vaccination during pregnancy in order to provide the foal with a degree of protection from birth. This is normally administered 4–6 weeks before foaling.

Internal parasites

As well as vaccinations horses will need regular worming to control internal parasites. There are many worming programmes available and, depending on the wormer selected, the programme and advice will vary slightly. The best idea is to consult your vet for a recommended programme to suit your horses and your pasture.

Through a combination of pasture care and drug administration, worm burdens can be controlled and the horse's immune system stimulated to assist in keeping the worm burden under control (Chapter 9).

For all parasitic infestations the symptoms are similar:

- Poor doer
- Weight loss
- Colic
- Diarrhoea.

The main causes for worm burdens are:

- Poor general management
- Poor paddock management
- Density of horses
- Overgrazing pasture
- No effective worming programme.

Testing dropping samples can enable a programme to be devised but this only measures the eggs and not encysted small redworms or non-egg-producing adults, so the test should be regularly repeated.

Another method for parasite control is pasture management, which should follow these guidelines:

- Horses should *all* be well wormed
- New horses should be wormed before being turned on to the pasture
- Avoid overcrowding so horses don't need to graze dropping-contaminated grass
- Droppings should be frequently and regularly picked up. This appears to be the most effective and drug-free option
- Rotate grazing with sheep or cattle which are not affected by equine parasites, and whose parasites don't affect horses. They also graze grass not so desired by horses and are therefore good for the grass and pasture as well as assisting with reducing the worm burden. If this is not an option, resting pasture as often as possible can also assist in reducing the spread.

CONCLUSION

Good management is fundamental to ensuring the good health of horses and preventing and controlling the spread of disease. Good management results in happy and well horses which in turn should enable better performance. Careful planning should enable all horses to remain free of disease and in good health.

Bibliography

Auty I 1998 BHS complete manual of stable management. Kenilworth Press, Shrewsbury

Auty I 2008 BHS training manual stage 1. Kenilworth Press, Shrewsbury

Auty I 2006 BHS training manual stage 2. Kenilworth Press, Shrewsbury

Auty I 2006 BHS training manual stage 3. Kenilworth Press, Shrewsbury

Auty I 2006 BHS training manual stage 4. Kenilworth Press, Shrewsbury

Hastie S, Sharples J 1999 Horselopaedia. Ringpress, Singapore

Hayes M 2003 Veterinary notes for horse owners. Ebury Press, London

Jones W 1989 Equine sports medicine. Lea and Febiger, Philadelphia

Chapter | **11** | *Jane Williams and Debbie Duke*

Farm animal health and welfare

This chapter describes the methods that can be employed to handle large animal species. It discusses the differences in intensive, free-range and organic management systems and identifies breeds suitable in common species for meat, dairy and egg production. The implications and achievement of the five key needs in livestock farming are evaluated.

Modern farmers have utilised improvements in technology and advances in pharmacology and responded to economic pressures to raise productivity levels in livestock and associated produce production. Farm animal welfare is monitored and farmers must demonstrate that their management systems achieve the five key needs of animals:

1. The need for a proper diet (including water)
2. The need for somewhere suitable to live
3. The need to be housed with, or apart from, other animals (as appropriate)
4. The need to express their normal behaviour
5. The need to be protected from pain, suffering, injury and disease.

A range of farming methodologies are employed in modern agriculture, including intensive production, free-range systems and organic systems. Intensive production aims to produce the desired product as quickly and economically as possible. Free-range systems promote animal welfare and aim to produce a quality product from animals which have had the opportunity to roam and express their normal behaviour. Organic systems also promote the ideals of free-range operations but additionally meet rigorous criteria for pasture and animal production, demonstrating that no artificial chemicals or pharmaceuticals have been employed in animal management. Organic systems exclude the use of inorganic fertilisers, livestock drugs, growth regulators and feed additives. For the purposes of this chapter four livestock species will be considered: cattle, sheep (the same principles may be applied to goats), pigs and poultry species.

Common farming methods combine many of the following:

- Young animals in abundance, all with an inability to resist disease because of an undeveloped immune system
- Mixture of animals on the same site having come from many different farms
- High-density stocking (overcrowding)
- Excessive movement of animals to and from an establishment
- Poor environmental hygiene
- Insufficient bedding, ventilation, drainage and muck disposal
- Poor hygiene associated with feed and water.

HANDLING AND RESTRAINT

Cattle

Cattle are not generally approachable to halter and lead, unlike horses. They are indiscriminate about whom they trample and are quite capable of delivering a swift kick to the handler. Herds and individuals can be relatively easily driven into pens, alleyways that lead to a chute or crush. When herding, barriers should be strong enough not to be broken and ideally not made of harmful material, e.g. barbed wire. It is advisable to separate large stock from young stock before driving them into a pen to avoid injury. The chute/crush is made of strong material which comprises a metal framework with side bars, head restraint and rear restraints; the cow is locked into the frame and can be safely examined or medication administered to it. Revolving crushes are available for surgical procedures, under local or field block anaesthesia, and foot examination.

Alternatively a gated corner can be used, with the animal restrained behind the gate for examination. Cattle prods are devices which deliver an electric shock to the animal to promote movement. Cattle halters are available and are regularly used for show animals. They are similar to an equine halter, except that they are made from one single piece of rope. The halter's nose loop is placed over the muzzle and then the crown loop is flipped over the animal's head with the slack in the rope taken up as the rope comes under the jaw. Cattle should be led at arm's length to avoid stress to them and injury to the handler. Bulls must be treated with extreme caution and only handled by experienced personnel; nose rings are often in situ and can be used to lead with a rope, or a twitch can be used for restraint. Feed is a good bribe to facilitate movement.

For closer examination of the head, restraint with the halter or in the crush then grasping the tongue to one side will enable examination of the oral cavity; steel mouth gags are available for the administration of oral medication. Tail restraint can be used by pushing the tail upright in the midline, grasping the tail one-third of the way down from the tail's head and pushing into the cow. Hobbles can be used on the legs to prevent kicking and pressure on the flanks can also be a useful deterrent. Calves can be caught by flanking them and flipping them into lateral recumbency or can be restrained with an arm around the neck and holding the tail upright or with a hand under the rump.

Sheep

Sheep can also be herded successfully using people, quad bikes or trained sheepdogs. They tend to move in small groups and lambs can be quite acrobatic, which can occasionally result in trauma, and all animals in confined spaces have a tendency to climb and jump over each other or fences. Sheep can be caught in confined areas by grasping under the neck and with the other hand under the rump; avoid grabbing the fleece as it can be damaged, resulting in financial loss.

Sheep can be set on to their rump into a sitting position with their back leaning into the handler. The handler reaches under the base of the neck with the left hand and over the back to the right hindleg with the right hand; the animal is then gently lifted up towards the right whilst the right leg is simultaneously raised and the sheep is upturned. The right hand moves to the right foreleg and the left to the left foreleg and the sheep is held on its rump. This position enables shearing or examination. Lambs can be restrained, often for docking and castration, by grasping parallel hind and forelegs then bringing the hindleg forward as you hold it between hock and fetlock; the front leg is held at the elbow.

Drenching – the administration of oral medication, often anthelminthic preparations – can be achieved by straddling the sheep over its shoulders once it is backed into a corner. Restraint is achieved by applying pressure with the knees. The handler raises the head by grasping the mandible, the lower jaw, and loosely enclosing the muzzle; the syringe is inserted into the mouth and the liquid should be administered slowly, allowing the animal time to swallow. Care should be taken to keep the head parallel to the ground to prevent aspiration of the fluids.

Pigs

Piglets can be herded into confined spaces such as corners and then grasped by a hindleg. The handler then moves one hand to grasp the piglet around the body with both hands. Adult pigs can be aggressive, particularly boars and nursing sows, so care should be taken when handling. Fences and wooden panels can be used as a barrier by planting them to the ground and restraining the pig behind them as pigs will try to root out from underneath them. They will also aim for any escape routes so these should be blocked before handling is attempted. A cane can be used to drive and direct the pig by tapping it on the face or neck to steer it.

A hog snare, which has a similar construction to an equine twitch but is constructed from a metal loop, may be used to snare the upper jaw and enable the snout and thus the animal's direction to be manipulated; pigs respond very vocally to their use due to its discomfort. For castration and examination pigs can be restrained by holding their back legs off the ground with the handler standing in front of the animal with its back pushing into the handler's legs; pigs appear to struggle less when their front legs are on the ground. Pigs are very intelligent and can be easily trained to facilitate handling and this is recommended for pet animals but in intensive farming there is little room for this luxury.

Poultry

Dimming the lights in poultry sheds can aid in catching by calming birds. Spent laying birds are caught by both their legs whilst supporting their breast; broilers (meat birds) are caught by their legs and up to four birds may be carried in one hand with their feet within the fingers. Free-ranging birds may present more of a challenge and it may be prudent to attempt to catch them whilst roosting in the manner described above. Alternatively cupping the animal's thorax, thereby restraining the wings, can be used but care should be taken not to apply too much pressure and restrict breathing.

HUSBANDRY AND MANAGEMENT SYSTEMS

Farm animal management has to focus on maintaining animal welfare, ensuring increased productivity, meeting welfare standards and the requirements of welfare legislation and also ensuring the farmer achieves a profit and makes a living from the production of the animal.

Cattle

The cattle industry is divided into dairy and meat (beef) production. In the UK breed selection has engineered breeds which are fit for their specific purpose. Table 11.1 details livestock breeds and their purpose.

Dairy cattle

In the UK, modern dairy herds have declined since the introduction of milk quotas (Universities Federation for Animal Welfare 1999) and the need to supply milk at competitive prices to large supermarket monopolies. Traditionally dairy herds were milked in cowsheds and kept at pasture; this is a labour-intensive system and larger herd sizes, silage as the main forage source and economics have resulted in many adopting loose housing systems (barns), although it is recommended that access to grazing is provided for welfare.

Milk yield is an important parameter, as is breeding potential, as dairy cattle must produce offspring before they can supply milk! Puberty is attained when 40% of adult weight is achieved which with good management is on average between 10 and 12 months of age. For her

productive life an ideal diary cow would produce a calf per annum and most are culled after their fourth lactation. Female calves may be used to replace older animals but bull calves are routinely culled.

Mechanical milking systems are commonly employed within large milking parlours; hygiene is of the utmost importance. Udders must be cleaned and dried before milking to aid in reduction of bacterial counts. At her peak a dairy cow may produce 6000–12 000 litres of milk over a 10-month lactation period. Therefore dairy cows need to consume large quantities of feed to meet their physiological needs.

In the winter, forage (usually silage) is the foodstuff of choice, although hay and roots are an alternative; straights or concentrates offer supplementary nutrition. In the summer, grazed herbage or pasture is the ideal solution but poor growing conditions can have an impact on milk production. Access to water should be available at all times. Stocking density can also have an impact on production rates.

In the UK, dairy cows are normally housed inside for at least 6 months and good management is essential to reduce disease and stress and not affect production. Dairy breeds have less fat and are therefore more susceptible to cold but generate heat via digestion so they often require a thin coat, even in winter, and temperature is not a major environmental issue. Indoor housing prevents poaching of grazing and is more convenient for handlers. Loose housing systems provide animals with more space and comfort, with room to lie down during rumination (9 hours plus per day) and to exercise. Cubicle systems are also employed and care should be taken that their design does not cause injury to the cow. Ample clean, dry bedding should be provided, usually straw or shavings, to prevent injury to the hocks, and provide comfort and insulation. Each cow in loose housing should have 5 square metres plus a feeding area of 2 square metres.

Lighting should be good enough to allow inspection of the herd and buildings; increasing artificial light to 16 hours can increase production rates. Light is often provided by natural roof lighting and artificial lighting systems. Ventilation must be effective but without draught production and building design can promote this. Separate facilities for sick or calving animals are essential. Slurry needs to be removed and stored away from housing units; prevention of dampness in housing aids in the reduction of bacteria, which can contribute to mastitis.

Herd health is of significant importance both for welfare and economically. Common causes of death include hypomagnesaemia (staggers), hypoglycaemia (milk fever), mastitis, calf scour and pneumonia. Infectious disease is considered later in this chapter. Animals must be identified by ear tag and calves should be tagged

Table 11.1 Livestock breeds and their purpose

Cattle	Meat	Dairy	Dual-purpose
	Aim for a rapid growth rate, low fat and good appetite Dairy cows (Friesian/Holstein) with beef bull crosses are common Hereford Aberdeen Angus Limousin Charolais Simmental Belgian Blue	Individuals selected on conformation – breeding potential and performance: milk production and fertility Friesian Holstein Holstein Friesian cross Dairy shorthorn Ayrshire breeds Jersey Guernsey	Dairy shorthorn Friesian

Sheep	Meat	Breeding	Wool
	Hill Blackface Welsh Mountain Cheviot Swaledale **Sires of cross-bred ewes** Border Leicester Blue-faced Leicester Teeswater Wensleydale **Fat-lamb sires** Oxford Down Suffolk Texel Dorset Down Southdown **Self-contained flocks (upland/lowland)** Clun Forest Romney Marsh Devon Longhorn Dorset Horn **Cross-bred lowland flocks** Mule Greyface Welsh half-bred Scottish half-bred	Hill Blackface Welsh Mountain Cheviot Swaledale **Fat-lamb sires** Oxford Down Suffolk Texel Dorset Down Southdown **Self-contained flocks (upland/lowland)** Clun Forest Romney Marsh Devon Longhorn Dorset Horn **Cross-bred lowland flocks** Mule Greyface Welsh half-bred Scottish half-bred	Hill Blackface Welsh Mountain Cheviot Swaledale

Pigs	Meat	Breeding	
	Large White Landrace Welsh cross-breeds with Pietrain, Hampshire, Duroc, Lacombe, Meishan **Traditional breeds** British Saddleback Tamworth Gloucester Old Spot Large Black		

before leaving the farm or within 20 days, whichever is sooner. Routine disbudding (horn removal) occurs.

Beef cattle/veal calves

Conformation and fatness determine the value of a beef animal as they correlate with musculature and therefore meat quantity. Meat quality is graded according to taste, tenderness and juiciness, with age at slaughter, location and fat content important factors in determining these.

There are two types of management systems commonly employed: semi-intensive and intensive. Semi-intensive systems combine time at pasture, one or two summers, with yard housing in between, with date of birth being the main deciding factor. Cattle may be slaughtered at the end of the second summer (mid- to late-winter calves) or second winter (September to December calves) at approximately 20–24 months of age. Pasture-housed animals feed in grass alone for the first summer, for the second summer they receive silage, vitamins and mineral supplementation and when in yards they are fed forage and concentrates.

Intensive calf systems aim to produce finished calves as quickly as possibly by rearing them in confinement with highest-quality feed that is economic. Intensive beef systems confine animals indoors for the duration of their life at high stocking densities, increasing the risk of disease, especially pneumonia. Calves from beef cows (suckler cows) usually remain with their dam until late summer or winter and are then transferred to yards to complete the finishing process.

Ideally beef cattle would be housed on bedding but indiscriminate urination and defecation are economically prohibitive and promote pathogens. Housing beef animals on slatted concrete floors (over 6 months of age) is common practice. Most European veal calves are crate-reared individually and fed only a milk replacer diet deficient in iron to obtain white meat. This practice is illegal in the UK, where they are fed milk replaced in buckets but given no solid food and often housed in groups; the veal produced is often described as 'pink' veal.

INFECTIOUS DISEASE

Cattle

Cattle are routinely castrated and dehorned. They are mainly affected by disease as calves; it is essential that calves receive adequate amounts of colostrum to assist in building an efficient immune system. Calves can be susceptible to diphtheria, a bacteria that can be fatal. Bacteria can also infiltrate the navel and, if hygiene is not good, this can be infected. Ringworm is a very common

fungal condition of the skin associated with cattle and which is zoonotic. The spores can be present in housing for a long time and can cause localised irritation and become sore and infected if rubbed. Coccidiosis is a form of dysentery that normally affects young stock and is caused by a unicellular parasitic organism; it is controlled by good hygiene and husbandry. Blackquarter is similar to black leg in sheep and is a bacterial infection of the muscles in the leg. It normally begins when there has been trauma to the muscle initially, relating back to husbandry and care of the animals. Bovine virus diarrhoea is a viral condition that mainly affects younger animals, causing mouth sores and foul-smelling diarrhoea. Another viral condition is infectious bovine rhinotracheitis; this is very contagious and causes inflammation of the eyes and upper respiratory tract. Vaccines are available to protect against this condition and it is not overly common. Respiratory conditions are common amongst cattle and are normally caused through:

- Poor housing and ventilation provision
- Overstocking and therefore lack of clean air
- Lack of bedding to absorb excreta.

The spread of respiratory diseases can be prevented by:

- Isolation and early detection of the sick animals
- Reducing the interaction of the different age groups.

Metabolic disorders are another common cause of disease. Bloat is a metabolic disorder associated with grazing lush pasture. It can lead to death if not treated quickly and appears painful and distressing for the affected animal. Gas is released through stomach tubing or rumen puncture through the left flank. Bloat can be prevented by proper pasture management and monitoring of the grazing herd.

After calving cows can get milk fever, which is associated with falling calcium and phosphorus levels and rising magnesium levels. The administration of calcium-based solution normally corrects the problem. A 'downer' cow' is an animal which has collapsed, usually due to milk fever or staggers, and is reluctant or unable to stand. Due to their size, if cattle remain in lateral recumbency on one side for prolonged periods, pooling of fluid in the lungs can result in death. Ketosis can occur when an animal's food intake is inadequate for its needs and it breaks down its own fat supplies for energy. This is commonly associated with recently calved cows. Knowledgeable stockmanship and correct feeding can help eliminate this and correct the condition quickly if it develops. A common condition for dairy cows is mastitis – infection of the udder. It is associated with poor hygiene and many incidences, as opposed to an individual occurrence, are associated with a management issue. Foot and mouth disease is a viral condition that can affect all cattle and is extremely contagious, affecting cattle, pigs and sheep; although it does not directly cause death it will lower productivity and cause persistent lameness. In the UK it is a notifiable disease. It is characterised by oral lesions and blisters on the feet; any incidences are dealt with by immediate slaughter of the affected animal and susceptible animals within the 3-km protection zone. A vaccination is available but it is not used in the UK. Leptospirosis can also affect cattle and is zoonotic; as a preventive health measure cattle can be vaccinated against leptospirosis and bovine viral diarrhoea.

Tuberculosis (TB) is another common bacterial disease associated with cattle. There are three main strains: the human strain that can also affect cattle; the cattle strain that can affect humans in some cases; and the avian strain that mainly affects birds. In the UK, cattle are routinely screened for TB at 1-, 2-, 3- and 4-year intervals depending on the incidence in their region; the single intradermal comparative cervical tuberculin (SICCT) test, which is commonly known as the tuberculin skin test, is employed. A fold of skin on the neck is measured, then cattle are injected with a small amount of tuberculin (a sterile antigenic extract obtained from a culture of *Mycobacterium bovis*) and with the avian strain the sites are reexamined 72 hours postadministration. Any animals which show an increase of over 4 mm in the bovine TB site compared to the avian site are classified as reactors and subsequently slaughtered. Inconclusive cases between 1 and 4 mm are retested in 60 days. TB-free status can only be granted when all remaining cattle successfully pass two TB-free tests.

Cattle can be affected by warble flies and lice. Warble flies can cause damage to the hide and the meat and lower cattle productivity. If the condition is noticed the maggots can be treated with an appropriate insecticide. Lice infect housed cattle and are rarely seen in those living outside; a specific insecticide can eliminate an infestation. Bluetongue is an emerging disease in the UK, although it is routine in continental Europe and Africa. It is caused by a virus spread by *Culcoides* (midges) and affects ruminants, particularly sheep, but not pigs, horses or humans.

Sheep

The sheep industry is diverse, with production occurring in a variety of habitats; sheep breeds have developed to match their habitats and 70 different breeds of sheep are recognised in the UK. The main production output is meat, with some flocks kept for wool. Specific breeds suited to upland and hill areas predominate there, whereas lowland species are often cross-breeds.

Upland and hill flocks tend to have access to free-roaming grazing which is required to source the essential nutrients from often harsh climates. Lowland sheep compete for pasture with crop production and may have a diet which is supplemented by concentrates. Sheep alternate between periods of grazing (20–90 minutes) and resting (45–90 minutes) when rumination occurs; on average they will spend between 8 and 10 hours per day grazing. Sheep display strong dietary preferences and are often reluctant to eat new foods so all young stock should be trained to eat concentrates in case supplementation is required in times of hardship.

The majority of British sheep have their breeding season from late summer/early autumn until mid to late winter; this is governed by photoperiodism. Rams are usually kept away from the main flock outside the breeding season and are fed concentrates with a vitamin and mineral supplement for energy and to promote fertility and health. Breeding rams may wear a harness containing a keel marker which deposits coloured ink on to the ewe when she has been covered or tupped to enable the handler to ascertain mating has occurred. All sheep have to be routinely drenched for parasites. Lambing will occur over a set period as the breeding operation is synchronised and ewes are moved into lambing pens for parturition; hygiene is critical in these areas. Udders and teats need cleansing after birth, lamb's navels should be sprayed with antiseptic to prevent pathogen entry and multiplication and all fetal membranes must be appropriately disposed of. Lambs are routinely castrated and docked using rubber rings within 1 week of birth. Regular observation of these animals is needed to spot the early signs of disease or rejection. Rejected lambs can be fostered or hand-reared but it is essential that they receive adequate quantities of colostrum to boost their immune system. The ewes and lambs can be turned out within a week into sheltered field near the lambing sheds. Lambs are prone to hypothermia and any exhibiting a reluctance to follow their dam or which exhibit abnormal behaviour should be checked.

Most lambs are sold for slaughter at the end of the grazing season but some will remain and be sold in the autumn as hoggets. Lambs tend to be slaughtered when they attain half their adult weight before fat deposits are established.

Internally housed flocks should have access to water, food and sufficient bedding. The temperature of the housing should mirror that of the local environment and the housing should be well ventilated but not prone to draughts. Sheep are identified by temporary dyes on their fleece, ear notches or hole punches, ear tattoos or ear tags. The removal of excess wool around the tail and medial thighs (dagging) is often performed in early spring before shearing to reduce the risk of flystrike.

Pregnant and lambing ewes and young lambs are at the highest risk for infection and ewes are vaccinated in pregnancy for the most prevalent conditions such as *Escherichia coli* infection. Clostridial diseases are also common where there are sheep and tend to affect animals in the optimum condition and which are well. Many diseases are caused by this group of bacteria, such as blackleg, black disease, tetanus and lamb dysentery. All of these conditions can be vaccinated against. Some deficiency diseases associated with sheep, such as rickets, relate to an imbalance due to insufficient calcium, phosphorus and vitamin D; swayback is another deficiency condition relating to low copper levels and pine is a condition associated with a deficiency of vitamin B_{12}. Hence a suitable and nutritionally perfected diet should be provided to ensure good health.

Sheep are infested with internal parasites such as tapeworm, liver fluke and roundworms and these can be controlled with a suitable anthelminthic programme. Scrapie is a viral condition exclusive to sheep and goats and causes the sheep to be incoordinated and to itch furiously; in the UK it is a notifiable disease, as is foot and mouth in sheep. There is no known cure and all cases should be slaughtered. Lameness is a constant concern to the sheep farmer and foot rot is a condition that causes a great deal of financial loss; it is caused by bacteria in the soil and can be spread from sheep to sheep. Treatment and control can be administered but add to the cost of sheep care and husbandry. The three most important metabolic diseases of sheep are milk fever, grass staggers and pregnancy toxaemia. These conditions often relate to the production of multiple lambs, with the dam's body unable to meet its own needs and the physiological demands of the pregnancy; it is often associated with poor nutrition.

Chlamydia psittaci causes enzootic abortion. Examination of the fetal membranes (cleansing) clearly shows infection; the membranes and fluid remain infectious for up to 2 weeks and this disease poses a significant risk to pregnant women as it also causes human abortion. Toxoplasmosis is another agent which causes abortion in sheep, usually at the end month of gestation or lambs may be stillborn or debilitated. Again this disease is zoonotic and pregnant women should be careful to avoid infection. Orf, contagious pustular dermatitis, is a common viral disease in sheep and is highly contagious. It affects the lips of lambs and teats/udders of ewes. Handlers are required to don suitable personal protective equipment during treatment and orf can be vaccinated against. Ewes may also suffer from bacterial-induced mastitis, with most cases occurring within 1 month postpartum.

Pigs

Pork is the most commonly consumed meat in the world. There are four main categories of slaughter pig in the UK:

1. Pork pig: small joints and fresh meat
2. Cutter: trimmed of fat and skin; commercial joints in supermarkets
3. Bacon pig: traditionally cured
4. Heavy hog and culled adult stock: sausages, meat pies and processed meats.

Outdoor pigs and intensively reared indoor pigs require different qualities: for example, thicker skin and pigmentation to avoid sunburn, whereas breeding sows should be agile and careful mothers to avoid damaging their offspring but timid enough to be handled and trained. Large White (Boar) and Landrace, Saddleback, Hampshire and Duroc crosses are common to maximise the beneficial qualities for outdoor sows. The number of piglets a sow successfully rears per year is an important indicator of productivity.

Pigs are natural foragers and this behaviour can be satisfied in outdoor pigs but in intensive systems the lack of opportunity to forage can result in misdirected aggression, bar biting and stereotypies. Indoor pigs with limited access to food will often spend abnormal time periods drinking, so access to drinking water is an important consideration. Pigs should be habituated to the presence of the handler so it does not promote stress. Sows have a matriarchal society with boars often living separately except for breeding seasons. Management systems mirror this, with young boars often kept in straw yards together and older boars housed separately; they are introduced to gilts in their second season.

Outdoor rearing systems require electric fencing for security and pigs must be ear tagged for identification. Smaller groups of 15–20 sows are optimum for welfare. Adequate allocation of space, a skilled stockman and an appropriate breed should produce successfully reared litters. Most systems include a rounded hut for shelter and an associated foraging area. Piglets are usually weaned at 3–4 weeks then transferred to weaner accommodation which may involve selling them to intensive fattening units. Mortality in neonatal piglets is often correlated with lack of suckling so administration of colostrum via a stomach tube or putting weak specimens to other sows may improve survival rates. In the initial 24–48 hours the umbilicus is trimmed and disinfected to prevent navel ill, ears maybe notched, incisor teeth are trimmed to prevent injury to the sow's teats, iron injections are given to prevent anaemia, and tail docking and castration occur. Piglets are sensitive to cold temperatures as they are hairless and pig lamps (ultraviolet lamps) may be used to provide warmth.

Indoor systems should have adequate temperature, ventilation but not draughts and lighting. Floors should be comfortable for the pig to stand, lie down and walk upon, provide grip but not cause skin damage and any form of slatting must be suitable for the foot size to reduce the risk of injury. Straw bedding is recommended for behavioural enrichment as well as for comfort but can become contaminated with waste and slurry. Regular removal of waste, slurry and soiled bedding is essential for good hygiene and to reduce disease. Farrowing crates are common for sows in intensive systems. The sow will be able to lie and stand but cannot turn around. The crates are located in one temperature-controlled room and incorporate a creep area for the piglets to prevent them being squashed by their dam (Figure 11.1).

Most pigs are fed on cereal-based concentrates supplemented with animal protein (bone meal, milk byproducts), vegetable oil and lysine. Root crops are often provided to outdoor pigs. Vitamin and mineral supplementation is required.

As with all livestock, contamination from disease due to new arrivals and via airborne pathogens should be considered, particularly as piglets are often transported for fattening purposes. Management systems should consider the site of units and prevailing winds, isolation of new stock and good hygiene as husbandry essentials. In the UK, foot and mouth disease, Aujeszky's disease, anthrax, swine fever and swine vesicular disease are notifiable.

Farrowing fever may occur in the sow soon after farrowing. There is little milk letdown, the udder appears hard and tender and there can be infection of the uterus. Many young piglets die from transmissible gastroenteritis which causes severe diarrhoea and abdominal discomfort; very young piglets may die but as they age mortality rates reduce. *Escherichia coli* can cause numerous problems for pig farmers. In the very young piglet it can cause septicaemia, leading to death, and later in life it can cause bowel oedema. The symptoms arrive quickly and are a combination of staggering, weakness, paddling while laying on the side, coma and death. The condition is related to weaning, stress and excessive consumption of dry food. Streptococcal infections are becoming more common and are often passed from the sow to the piglets. The condition can lead to death and younger piglets are more susceptible. Pigs also suffer from respiratory conditions. Some of these conditions can be vaccinated against, such as atrophic rhinitis, but as with most respiratory conditions environmental control and management are important preventive measures. Other conditions, such as salmonellosis, ascariasis and pneumonia, often relate to environmental and management features as opposed to simply disease transmission. Pigs suffer from parasitic invasion, as do all farm animals, and again good parasite control, hygiene and management should assist in controlling any outbreaks.

Poultry

The poultry industry produces eggs and meat from chickens, turkeys and ducks; various systems are employed, ranging from small independent keepers, free-range, organic to intensive commercial operations. This section will consider chickens primarily but the principles can be applied to other species; birds which are kept for egg production are termed 'layers' and those raised for meat 'broilers'.

Laying hens kept in intensive management systems are commonly referred to as 'battery hens'; units comprise up to five layers of cages with hens inhabiting small areas, often with a density of up to 30 birds per square metre. In these systems birds produce more eggs, eat less and require less cleaning, which produces obvious economic benefits. However the hens often exhibit stereotypies and the implications for the welfare of these animals have been questioned. In this system:

- Birds are separated into small groups of 4–5 birds, providing social stability and reducing aggression, cannibalism and injury from other birds
- They are housed in cages with sloping wire mesh floors, facilitating dropping removal and allowing their eggs to roll out for collection
- They are virtually parasite-free as their droppings, which are the main cause of spread of disease, are removed very quickly
- They have no litter so there are no worries regarding dampness, which can lead to bumblefoot infections, hock burns etc.
- They have no nests and are therefore not broody
- They are housed in high densities which negates the need for heating and reduces food consumption as the birds are warm.

Barn systems allow laying hens the opportunity to express normal behaviour as they are housed within one large unit, perhaps with perches or other environmental enrichment provided. Heating, adequate ventilation and suitable lighting, as this influences laying production, need to be provided and the birds spend their life within the barn. Litter systems need to be monitored for contamination from urine and faeces as these can alter the pH, leading to problems such as hock burns and increased infections such as bumblefoot. Rations fed to

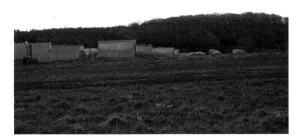

Figure 11.1 External farrowing units.

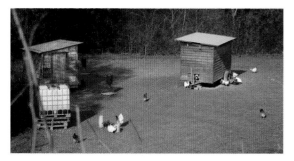

Figure 11.2 External free-range chicken production.

laying hens must provide sufficient energy for egg production but not so much that the birds increase in weight as fatness decreases egg production. They are typically fed a commercially produced cereal-based meal which is delivered to the flock by hopper and trough systems. Access to fresh water is essential and its consumption is monitored as variations can often be the first indicator of disease; water is provided by nipple or cup feeders.

Free-range birds are given access to roam, forage and perform natural behaviours, although they would still normally roost in a barn or similar at night (Figure 11.2). The external enclosure needs to be predator-proof and electric fencing is employed to prevent predation. Egg collection can be more challenging.

Laying hens

In laying hens prevention, rather than treatment, of infectious disease is essential as any disease outbreaks will often cancel out profit margins. A number of common measures are usually performed:

- Routine hygiene and disinfection of accommodation and equipment between batches of birds
- Closing the unit to wild birds, rodents and other possible vectors of disease
- Rodent and parasite control
- Prompt and hygienic disposal of dead birds; stocks are checked and dead animals are removed at least once per day
- Medicate birds: most commercial diets contain a coccidiostat as a prophylactic measure
- Vaccination of birds against all major diseases, particularly salmonellosis, Newcastle disease, Gumboro disease, infectious laryngotracheitis, avian rhinotracheitis and epidemic tremor.

Broiler chickens

Most chickens kept as broilers will be in intensive management systems whose aim is to produce birds that attain the slaughter weight as quickly as possibly. Barn systems are commonly employed, but with high-density stocking rates. The majority of birds raised are female: male day-old chicks are routinely culled. Brooding (rearing of chicks) and fattening all occur within the same unit and the same principles as discussed in the prevention of disease in laying hens apply to these birds too. The brooding broilers require an artificial heat of around 25–30°C with a measured reduction to 21°C from their fourth week onwards. The brooding period lasts for approximately 3 weeks and then the birds are allowed access to the whole housing. The environmental conditions must be monitored and a litter system at a depth of 10–15 cm on top of a damp-proof concrete floor is recommended; soft wood shavings or chopped straw are often employed. New litter is required for each batch of birds. Light requirements match productivity as chickens will continue to eat when it is light and common practice is for artificial lighting to be employed for 23 hours per day, with 1 hour of darkness to encourage weight gain. Adequate ventilation without draughts is required.

Stocking density has an impact on environmental control, disease and injury rates. Broilers are fed ad libitum from when they enter the housing unit as the aim is to gain weight as quickly as possible. Like the laying hens, a coccidiostat is included, as are growth promoters; these are antibiotics with no therapeutic purpose to the animal. Water will constitute 60–70% of the weight of the bird and therefore adequate quantities and monitoring are required, as with laying birds.

Broilers

Again, prevention of disease rather than treatment is employed as a disease outbreak can prove catastrophic financially. A number of measures are routinely employed:

- Clearing the site of all living animals at the end of the production period followed by rigorous disinfection and fumigation of all facilities and equipment
- Rearing birds of the same or close age ranges so that their immunological status is similar – this aids in the success of vaccination protocols
- Vaccination occurs in broilers but not for as many diseases as for laying hens; most day-old chicks will receive infectious bronchitis vaccine (in aerosol spray) and may subsequently be vaccinated for Gumboro disease and/or avian rhinotracheitis.

Avian flu

Avian flu or fowl plague is a zoonotic viral disease which poses a significant worldwide disease risk as it is spread via wild bird populations. There are two types of avian influenza virus: low pathogenic (LPAI) and highly pathogenic (HPAI). Within the LPAI types there is evidence that certain H5 and H7 viruses may mutate and become highly pathogenic. Typically HPAI presents suddenly, with affected birds showing oedema (swelling) of the head, cyanosis (blue discoloration) of the comb and wattles (neck and throat area), dullness, a loss of appetite, respiratory distress, diarrhoea and a drop in egg production. Birds can be infected with LPAI without showing any signs of disease.

Transmission can be via wild birds, direct contact with secretions from infected birds, e.g. faeces, or contact with contaminated vehicles, equipment, personnel, water or feed. In the UK avian flu is a notifiable disease and infected birds are slaughtered.

TREATMENT OF FARM ANIMALS

An important note worth considering during livestock production is the role of veterinary medication. Farmers and handlers often use preventive health protocols, including vaccination and parasiticides, to reduce the incidence of disease but if an animal requires veterinary treatment this can affect its productivity. Milk and meat withdrawal periods are commonly listed on large animal pharmaceuticals and these must be adhered to before the animal or its products can enter the food chain. Antibiotic resistance in livestock is another potential problem as routine prophylactic administration of antibiotics has led to a decrease in efficacy of some products.

Bibliography

Bernard E 2003 Farm animal welfare. Wiley/Blackwell/ Iowa State University Press, Iowa

Colville T, Bassett J M 2002 Clinical anatomy and physiology for veterinary technicians. Mosby, St Louis

Fraser A, Broom D 1996 Farm animal behaviour and welfare, 3rd edn. CABI Publishing, Oxford

Pratt P W 1998 Principles and practice of veterinary technology. Mosby, Philadelphia

Universities Federation for Animal Welfare 1999 Management and welfare of farm animals. Blackwell, Oxford

Chapter | **12** | *Jane Williams*

Genetics and reproductive science

This chapter explains the basic principles of inheritance of genetic characteristics and traits. Hereditary disease and the influence of genes are considered. The physiological control and fundamental principles of reproduction from mating to birth are outlined for a range of animal species.

GENETICS

Box 12.1 lists some useful definitions.

Genes comprise deoxyribonucleic acid (DNA) sequences. DNA is built up of nucleotides or building blocks of DNA and ribonucleic acid (RNA). Genes are found on the chromosomes in the cell. The genetic material can only be seen under a light microscope during cell division; when the cells are not dividing the uncoiled chromosomal material or chromatin can be viewed using an electron microscope.

Most eukaryotic cells have a specific number of chromosomes and there is a diploid number in each body cell. Chromosomes occur in pairs for identical characteristics and are known as homologous chromosomes. Genetic material is stored in eukaryotic cells as DNA arranged as a double-stranded molecule or double helix.

A chromosome has gene and non-genic areas. The specific point on the chromosome where a specific gene is located is called its locus (plural: loci). The number of different types of chromosomes is the haploid number. DNA stores genetic information using four chemical nucleotides; nucleotides are portions of DNA and RNA linked to a phosphate group. The sequences of nucleotides will make up a gene code for amino acids which will form a protein.

RNA plays an important role in protein synthesis in the cell via memory and transfer RNA.

What is genetics?

Genetics is the science of heredity or the study of how characteristics are passed on from parents to their offspring.

DEFINITIONS

Character

Heritable feature that varies among individuals, e.g. flower colour

Genes

Basic unit of heredity or a functional unit of heredity

Genetics

Study of heredity

Genome

The complete blueprint of genetic information that is inherited from the parents. These have been identified for some species, i.e. all the possible chromosome and genes are thought to be known

Heredity

Passing on of genetic factors

Hybridisation

Crossing of two varieties. Results for offspring will vary

Trait

A variant for a character, e.g. white or purple flowers

True-bred

When bred, all the offspring are of the same variety, e.g. two purple flowering plants when crossed will always produce purple flowering offspring

Where did it all begin?

The science of genetics was discovered in the 18th century by an Austrian abbott, Gregor Mendel. Gregor Mendel was a monk with an agricultural background who went to train as a teacher. During his training he encountered two scientists, Doppler (a physicist) and Unger (a biologist), who aroused his interest in the breeding of plants. Mendel experimented with breeding pea plants and observed how the offspring plants looked; he chose these plants to study inheritance, because they may have many different varieties.

Mendel engineered crosses between true-breed pea plants and observed the plants' characteristics and traits:

- If only one character's inheritance is tracked, it is termed a monohybrid cross
- If two characteristics are tracked, it is termed a dihybrid cross

- The true breeding parents are called the parental or P generation
- The first offspring produced are called the first filial generation or F1 generation
- If two of the F1 generation are crossed, their offspring are called the F2 or second filial generation.

Experiment 1

Mendel looked at pea plants which produce both white and purple flowers.

Why does this happen?

One possible reason is that the white flowers must be 'hiding' in the F1 generation. Mendel called this a recessive trait. He surmised that the purple flowers mask or overshadow most of the white flowers. Mendel called this a dominant trait. The occurrence of white flowers in the F2 generation was evidence that the heritable factor causing the recessive trait had not been diluted in any way. In further experiments, this proved the same for the following characteristics:

- Flower colour
- Seed colour
- Pod shape
- Stem length
- Flower position
- Seed shape
- Pod colour.

Remember that a *gene* is a unit of hereditary information. Therefore, each flower colour exists in two versions, i.e. there must be two different versions of the gene for flower colour. Alternative versions of genes are called alleles.

The DNA of each gene can vary in the nucleotide sequence which alters the informational content. For each character, an organism inherits two alleles, one from each parent. A diploid organism has homologous pairs of chromosomes, one from each pair inherited from each parent. Therefore the genetic locus is represented twice in a diploid cell.

- In true breeding plants, the alleles are identical: these are homozygous plants
- In F1 hybrids, the alleles are different: these are heterozygous plants
- Homozygous plants have identical alleles
- Heterozygous plants have different alleles.

If the alleles differ, i.e. in the heterozygous plant, one is said to be dominant and the other one is recessive:

- The dominant allele is expressed, i.e. its trait will be seen

147

- The recessive allele has no effect unless it is homozygous.

If the alleles are the same:

- The dominant allele will always be expressed
- The recessive allele will only be expressed in a homozygous recessive plant.

Spermatozoa and ova get only one allele of each somatic cell – this is achieved during meiosis.

Mendel's first law of genetics

This is also known as the law of segregation. It states that:

 Alleles separate to different gametes of genes and both factors are not required for the gene to be expressed.

Crosses to display inheritance can be represented schematically using Punnett square diagrams.

A character is expressed by assigning a letter to the character overall, e.g. let height of pea plants be represented by t.

- Dominant traits are always represented by the letter chosen, written as a capital letter
- Recessive traits are denoted by the same letter chosen, but represented as a lower-case letter.

The physical characteristic displayed, i.e. tallness, is known as the phenotype. The phenotype for all of the F1 generation will be tall.

The genetic make-up is known as the genotype. The genotype for the F1 generation will be Tt (heterozygous).

Remember:

- The phenotype is the physical trait: think P for photograph, i.e. what it looks like
- The genotype is the genetic make-up: think G for genes.

If the two plants from the F1 generation are crossed, for the F2 generation the following will be true:

Phenotype

- ¾ or 75% tall plants
- ¼ or 25% small plants
- This gives a phenotypic ratio for tall:small of 3:1.

Genotype

- ¼ or 25% TT: homozygous (identical) dominant (capital letters)
- ½ or 50% Tt: heterozygous (different)
- ¼ or 25% tt: homozygous (identical) recessive (lower-case letter)
- Genotypic ratio for TT:Tt:tt is 1:2:1.

Problem: what do you do if you have a purple flowering plant? How do you tell what its genotype is?

Answer: Back-cross to the recessive.

The unknown plant is crossed with a white flowering plant. The white plant must be a homozygous recessive to have white flowers since white flowers are a recessive trait.

What could the plants with purple as a phenotype have for their genotypes?

- PP: homozygous dominant
- Pp: heterozygous.

Therefore the unknown purple plant could be PP or Pp. Using a Punnett square the F1 generation can be predicted. For heterozygous purple, let P = purple flowers and p = white flowers.

- F1 offspring: 50% Pp which are purple and 50% pp which are white.

For homozygous purple, let P = purple flowers and p = white flowers.

- F1 generation 100% PP and all purple.

Therefore a back-cross to the recessive will result in:

- All dominant trait offspring, i.e. the genotype of the unknown plant is homozygous dominant
- A ratio of 1:1 dominant to recessive, i.e. the genotype of the unknown plant is heterozygous.

This can be used for more complex traits to remove inherited factors that could be detrimental to a breed or species.

Mendel's second law of genetics – law of independent assortment

This states that:

 Characteristics are inherited independently from each other

or:

 During gamete formation the segregation of the alleles of one allelic pair is independent of the segregation of the alleles of another allelic pair.

Mendel continued his studies by evaluating how traits for two related characteristics were affected during crosses. He looked at seed colour and seed shape as it would be logical to assume the two characters' inheritability could be linked in some way.

Experiment 2

This time Mendel crossed green and wrinkled seeds with yellow and round seeds (remember that these were true-bred plants). His experiment resulted in all the F1 generation being yellow, round seeds. The F1 cross resulted in nine yellow, round seeds; three yellow, wrinkled seeds; three green, round seeds and one green, wrinkled seed.

This can be considered using the same principles discussed above by using a Punnett square but with two characters considered:

Let seed colour be represented by Y for yellow, the dominant trait, and y for green seeds, the recessive trait. But also let seed shape be represented by R for round, the dominant trait, and r for wrinkled, the recessive shape.

Parental generation genotypes would be:

- Green and wrinkled: yyrr
- Yellow and round: YYRR

For the Punnett square you need to establish the possible gametes. This is done by considering all the possible combinations of the genotype if it is a haploid gamete (in simple terms, consider it as putting two different alleles together).

Parental-generation gametes would be:

- Green and wrinkled: yyrr = yr and yr
- Yellow and round: YYRR = YR and YR.

The F1 generation genotype is YyRr; phenotype would be round and yellow.

The F1 generation gametes would be: YR, yR, Yr and yr. Remember that these will be the same for both the male and female plants so *all* of them need to be represented on the Punnett square, which now needs to be twice as big (Figure 12.1).

The results of these experiments proved to Mendel that genes segregate independently of other genes even if the characteristics appear related, giving rise to his second law.

This process can also be checked using a back-cross to the recessive (Figure 12.2).

F1 cross	YR	yR	Yr	yr
YR	YYRR ◯ Yellow and round	YyRR ◯ Yellow and round	YYRr ◯ Yellow and round	YyRr ◯ Yellow and round
yR	YyRR ◯ Yellow and round	yyRR ⬤ Green and round	YyRr ◯ Yellow and round	yyRr ⬤ Green and round
Yr	YYRr ◯ Yellow and round	YyRr ◯ Yellow and round	YYrr Yellow and wrinkled	Yyrr Yellow and wrinkled
yr	YyRr ◯ Yellow and round	yyRr ⬤ Green and round	Yyrr Yellow and wrinkled	yyrr Green and wrinkled

Figure 12.1 F1 cross Punnett square.

Backcross to recessive	YR	yR	Yr	yr
yr	YyRr ◯ Yellow and round	yyRr ⬤ Green and round	Yyrr Yellow and wrinkled	yyrr Green and wrinkled

Figure 12.2 Back-cross to the recessive.

The phenotypic ratio of the back-cross would be 25% of each variation.

Mendel's third law

As a result of his experiments Mendel formulated his third law. This states that:

Each inherited characteristic is determined by two heredity factors or genes, one from each parent, which determine whether a gene will be dominant or recessive.

Genetic variation

Variation in genetic information can occur through combinations of genotypes combining, via crossing over during meiosis (Chapter 1) and via genetic mutations. Genetic drift and genetic flow also occur within populations. Gene flow refers to the passage of traits or genes between populations; this prevents high occurrences of mutation, and genetic drift. Genetic drift is random variation that occurs because the genetic population is small, leading to the proliferation of specific traits within a population which will give rise to common characteristics. For example, if the majority of a population have a long coat and they breed within their population the incidence of long coat length would increase. To prevent genetic drift, genetic material must be shared between differing populations but genetic variation can still occur. In nature, individuals within a population tend to leave at sexual maturity and mate outside their family group, which strengthens the genetic variation in the gene pool.

Gene flow should transfer 'good' genes or advantageous characteristics as the animals carrying them have survived to mate and the sharing of these genes should lead to adaptation and link to Darwin's theory of natural selection.

EVOLUTION AND NATURAL SELECTION

The theory of evolution is the single most important conceptual framework for developing hypotheses about the ultimate forces that shape the traits of organisms. It is believed that behavioural traits can evolve just like anatomical and physiological traits.

Natural selection could be defined as the change in the frequencies of different alleles in a population or species over the course of generations.

Evolution can lead to:

- Minor modifications in a population
- Speciation: larger changes which result in a new species.

Darwin had no concept of genes but realised that traits were inherited by the offspring from their parents via observational and knowledge evidence. He had travelled the world for 5 years on HMS Beagle as a naturalist and during this time he formulated his hypothesis or theory of natural selection. These original ideas have been integrated into the science of genetics. Darwin's observations were phenotypes because he wrote about what he saw, and not genotypes.

The basic principle of natural selection is that certain members of a population or species possess specific phenotypic traits or adaptations which may, or may not, equip them to be better able to survive. They possess a phenotypic adaptation. Over the passage of time if this adaptation gives the animal an advantage the genes that code for it will become more plentiful and the genotype for the adaptation will increase in frequency. These animals now possess a genotypic adaptation.

Different parameters are utilised to measure a population's or species' ability to survive. These include the following.

Reproductive success

The organism's production of offspring:

- Number of offspring born
- Number of offspring that survive to weaning
- Number of offspring that survive to mating.

'Selection' is perhaps a misleading word to quantify the process, as it implies that animals choose the path to evolve. In reality animals displaying phenotypic traits that lead to an increased survival rate will be able to mate and thus pass on that trait.

Fitness

- The probability that an organism with a particular genotype and phenotypic make-up will reproduce
- Fitness can be measured in the short term or the long term.

Short-term fitness

- The potential for each genotype to be reproduced in the next generation.

Long-term fitness

- The potential of genotypes to be reproduced in the gene pool in subsequent generations.

Remember that the relative fitness of genes will vary depending upon existing environmental factors. Fitness can be measured in a wide range of adaptations.

Competition

This is when there are limited resources that are necessary for the survival and reproduction of animals in an area. These may be required by animals of different species – interspecific competition – or by animals of the same species – intraspecific competition. Remember that competition does not necessarily indicate direct conflict between individuals. Cooperation behaviours and altruistic behaviours are often adaptive and exhibited by mated pairs or related individuals.

Causes of evolution

Natural selection

- Genetic mutations give rise to new phenotypic traits that confer advantages to individuals or increased fitness to their genetic make-up.

Mutation pressure

- This is dependent on the ratio of one allelic form to another and the resulting frequencies of these alleles within the population
- For example: A:a frequencies = 0.45:0.55 (always measured out of 1, with males and females often considered separately)
- If one individual changed, ratio = 0.5:0.5, and so on over many generations
- Eventually over thousands of generations there may be an overall phenotypic effect on the species.

Gene flow

- Animals moving from one population to another results in new alleles entering the gene pool
- This can cause a shift in allele frequencies
- It is not thought to be a major contributory factor in evolutionary change.

Genetic drift

- Variation in allele frequencies through random fluctuations
- Happens in all populations to a small degree
- Has a big effect in small population sizes
- Can occur due to chance matings.

DOMESTICATION AND SELECTIVE BREEDING

During the development of human civilisations numerous species have become domesticated. Domestication can be thought of as a specialised version of genetic drift. In this case humans have actively selected individual animals with desirable characteristics to mate to produce offspring which display these characters. Consider the horse: the Shire horse and the Thoroughbred will have a shared ancestry but have been selectively bred for working the land and racing respectively. Selective breeding is an active breeding practice employed in modern breeding. For example, dog breeders often use line breeding to mate related individuals to promote a desirable characteristic for work or showing purposes or may use an outcross to an unrelated animal to introduce wider variation to the gene pool.

Genetic determination of sex

Sex chromosomes are homologous chromosomes, i.e. they both express the same characteristic – gender. However they are not all alike in shape and size. Females have two identical sex chromosomes, XX, whereas males have a single X chromosome and a smaller Y chromosome: XY. In simple terms, maleness is determined by the presence or absence of the Y chromosome.

In exothermic animals, i.e. cold-blooded animals, such as reptiles and in birds the external temperature can also determine the sex of their offspring.

Epistasis

Sometimes a genotype at one locus may influence the effect of a second genotype at a separate locus, preventing the second genotype being expressed in the animal due to mutation and resulting in the masking of its phenotypic presentation. This is termed epistasis. It is similar to dominance but involves different genes, not different alleles of the same gene: in this case the mutation of one gene masks the effect of another unrelated one. The gene whose effects are seen is said to be epistatic whilst the one which is masked is hypostatic. Examples include inheritability of coat colour in dogs and albinism. If albinism is considered as the character it can be easily envisaged how the albino epistatic gene masks the hypostatic gene for coat colour.

Lethality

Combinations of alleles may be lethal, causing either intrauterine death or early neonatal death. For example, in the Manx cat, a heterozygous genotype for tail length translates to no tail, a homozygous recessive translates to a full tail but the homozygous dominant individuals die before birth.

Autosomal-recessive disorders

These traits require both copies of the mutated allele to express the recessive characteristic, i.e. a double recessive. Traits can skip generations but offspring will be carriers. Males and females are equally affected. Metabolic and eye genetic disorders are often inherited in this way.

X-linked recessive disorders

These traits are inherited on the X chromosome. Males are more affected than females as they only have one X chromosome and will always get the condition if their X chromosome contains the affected allele. Haemophiliac disorders are an example of X-linked recessive disorders.

GENETICS APPLIED TO THE ANIMAL INDUSTRY

The field of genetics has great potential for the animal industry as techniques become more and more advanced.

Potentially animals can be genetically engineered to remove disease, increase muscle mass for food animals, cloned from past superstars or extinct species may be reproduced.

Transgenesis is the process of introducing an exogenous gene or transgene into a living animal; the new gene codes for a desirable characteristic that the genetic engineer wishes the animal to display and if it is linked to the gametes it will be subsequently be passed into that species' gene pool. Transgenesis could prove useful, for example, in dairy farming where genetically modified cows could produce milk with added proteins that could fulfil a function for humans, or in organ donation when animals could grow organs for human implantation.

Cloning is the process of duplicating identically a known individual from a genetic sample. Other genetic technology could be used to predetermine sex of offspring or to add or remove genes that code for disease. The possibilities are endless, but the ethical side of genetic manipulation must be considered and there is much debate in both camps as to the way forward.

Reproduction science

There are two types of reproduction: asexual and sexual reproduction.

Asexual reproduction

This occurs when a single parent splits, buds or fragments to give two or more offspring. The offspring is identical to the parent; once developed it can then split from the parent to have an independent existence or remain attached but be an individual within a colony. Examples include sponges, cnidarians and hydra which reproduce by budding. Some organisms such as flatworms can regenerate new flatworms from portions of their body lost via a process called fragmentation.

Sexual reproduction

This generally involves two parents but can be a male and female section of the same organism interacting. For sexual reproduction there must be two gametes, sex cells that fuse to form a fertilised egg or zygote (Box 12.2). The female gamete is called the ovum and is a non-motile, relatively large cell which contains a nutrient base and has a haploid chromosome number (Table 12.1). The male gamete or sperm is a motile and relatively small cell which contains few nutrients but also has a haploid chromosome number.

Sexual reproduction promotes genetic variety and sexually reproducing animals should be able to adapt to environmental changes relatively quickly in evolutionary terms.

Table 12.1 Chromosome number of common species								
Dog	78 39 pairs		Horse	64		Pig	38	
Cat	38 19 pairs		Cattle	60		Rabbit	44	
Human	46 23 pairs		Sheep	54		Goat	60	

DEFINITIONS

Abortion

Expulsion of fetus and membranes before term

Embryo

Characteristics of offspring are not discernible

Fetus

Characteristics of offspring are discernible

Neonate

Animal during the first 7–10 days of life

Resorption

Resorption of entire conceptus during embryonic stages

Stillbirth

Expulsion of fetus and membranes after term

Zygote

Fertilised ovum

Fertilisation can occur inside the body (internal fertilisation) or outside the body (external fertilisation). External fertilisation has its disdvantages as the gametes are released into the environment, leaving them vulnerable to predation. To overcome this risk huge numbers of gametes are released by organisms utilising this method to ensure success. Aquatic animals often use this method. Internal fertilisation is left less to chance as the male gamete is delivered directly into the female body. This is the system used by most terrestrial animals.

REPRODUCTIVE SYSTEMS

Many generalisations can be made for sexually reproducing animals, even though the details of the reproductive process vary with species.

Basic components of the male reproductive system include:

- Male gonad – the testes, which produce spermatozoa
- The sperm duct, which transports sperm to the exterior of the body
- Specialised area of sperm duct which produces nourishment – the seminal vessels
- Copulatory organ, which sperm duct empties into penis.

Basic components of the female reproductive system include:

- Female gonad – the ovary, which produces ova
- Tube for transporting ova – the oviduct
- Area for storage of ova and development of fertilised egg – uterus
- Terminal portion of oviduct which opens to the exterior of the body – vagina.

Not all male and female animals possess all the modifications; some simple animals have complex reproductive systems whereas some complex ones have simple reproductive systems. Refer to Chapter 5 for reproductive anatomy.

Endocrinology of reproduction

Endocrinology of the male

The male drive to reproduce and the production of spermatozoa are driven by hormonal control. The anterior pituitary gland secretes luteinising hormone (LH) and follicle-stimulating hormone (FSH). Their secretion is controlled by gonadotrophin-releasing hormone (GnRH) from the hypothalamus. GnRH is present in small quantities in the young animal but an increase in production occurs at the onset of puberty. GnRH is under the negative control of testosterone. LH from the anterior pituitary acts on the cells of Leydig to stimulate steroidogenesis and testosterone production. FSH, also from the anterior pituitary, acts on the Sertoli cells to activate spermatogenesis. The GnRH from the hypothalamus acts on the anterior pituitary to initiate the release of LH and FSH. Testosterone from the cells of Leydig acts on the Sertoli cells, stimulating spermatogenesis and producing negative feedback on the anterior pituitary gland which controls GnRH production. Another hormone, prolactin, is produced by the cells of Leydig and this hormone regulates testosterone production (Figure 12.3).

Sex steroids

Androgens

- These develop the male secondary sexual characteristics, e.g. increased muscle bulk
- They play a role in spermatogenesis
- They maintain sexual libido
- The main androgen is testosterone.

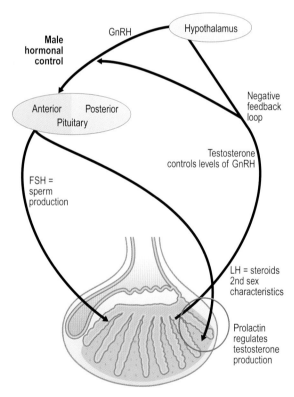

GnRH = Gonadotrophin releasing hormone

Male hormonal control

GnRH

Hypothalamus

Anterior   Posterior
Pituitary

Negative feedback loop

Testosterone controls levels of GnRH

FSH = sperm production

LH = steroids 2nd sex characteristics

Prolactin regulates testosterone production

Sertoli cells

Cells of Leydig

Figure 12.3 Hormonal control of male secondary sexual characteristics. GnRH, gonadotrophin-releasing hormone; FSH, follicle-stimulating hormone; LH, luteinising hormone.

Progesterones

- These inhibit the release of gonadotrophins
- They can be administered to control contraception in conjunction with testosterone.

Oestrogens

- These affect male physiology
- They can be used to help control behavioural problems and can also help with the treatment of prostate enlargement.

Endocrinology of the female

The oestrus cycle is a coordinated sequence of ovarian, uterus, vaginal and behavioural changes that occur to ensure the production and fertilisation of female gametes and the subsequent development of the pregnancy.

The oestrus cycle comprises a number of stages:

1. Pro-oestrus
2. Oestrus
3. Metoestrus
4. Di-oestrus
5. Anoestrus.

The oestrus cycle is controlled by a series of hormonal interactions between:

- The hypothalamus and pituitary gland
- The ovary (progesterone and oestrogen)
- The reproductive tract, accessory sex glands and brain behavioural centres.

Animals can be monoestrus, i.e. have only one oestrus cycle in each breeding season, or polyoestrus, meaning that they have more than one cycle during each breeding period.

The bitch (monoestrus, spontaneous ovulator)

Pro-oestrus

Clinical signs

- Characterised by distinct vulval reddening and enlargement of the vulval lips
- Subsequently there will be a serosanguineous vulval discharge (straw-coloured or blood-tinged discharge)
- The onset of this discharge is classified as the first day of pro-oestrus
- Behavioural changes will include restlessness, urine marking to disseminate pheromones to attract males and a wanderlust.

Reasons

- FSH is secreted by the anterior pituitary, stimulating the development of the graafian follicle
- Oestradiol is secreted from the developing follicle
- Rising oestradiol levels in blood cause the external and behavioural changes
- Within the reproductive tract the glandular epithelium grows, promoting mucosal vascularity and oedema (capillaries become fragile, leading to the discharge)
- Dramatic epithelial cell proliferation (multiplication) occurs within the vaginal mucosa; collecting and staining a vaginal smear can be a useful indicator to determine the stage of the oestrus cycle for mating
- The bitch is an example of a spontaneous ovulator; she will demonstrate peak plasma levels of oestradiol followed by peak levels of LH, after which ovulation will automatically occur. Other animals are induced ovulators: the queen is an example of this; she will ovulate after mating induces ovulation
- FSH levels are inhibited after ovulation but some FSH is still required to allow maturation of an empty follicle to develop into the corpus luteum.

Oestrus

Clinical signs

- This is the transition from attractive but unreceptive behaviour to posturally inviting and receptive, i.e. willing to stand and be mated rather than standing but running away at the last minute
- Pheromones are secreted under the influence of oestradiol in the urine and vulval discharge to attract a male
- Pheromones can also stimulate other females to come into season, so in multi-animal households females may cycle simultaneously or sequentially.

Reasons

- Pheromones are released under oestradiol control
- The brain behavioural centres are primed by the rising oestradiol levels but for full expression of oestrus the level of oestrogen must drop due to the presence of progesterone
- Once ovulation has occurred, declining oestrogen levels (no follicle) will be seen; the empty follicle develops into the corpus luteum and begins to secrete progesterone, causing levels of progesterone to rise
- The ovum has been released and is awaiting fertilisation
- There is a slight increase in progesterone levels just before ovulation

- This can be a useful detector aid and is used in some commercial mating tests to determine which stage of a cycle an animal is at
- The animal is then either pregnant or has not mated successfully.

Figures 12.4 and 12.5 summarise canine oestrus.

Fertilisation

The endometrium has thickened due to the rising levels of oestrogens, preparing for the conceptus. Simultaneously oestradiol has also increased mucosal secretions which will aid the passage and survival of the gametes. Fertilisation occurs within the oviducts. As the corpus luteum develops progesterone levels increase, altering the mucosal secretions and muscle excitability to slow the passage of the embryo (fertilised ovum) to the uterine horns until conditions are more suitable. Progesterone facilitates gamete survival and aids gamete transport and gamete fertilisation.

Metoestrus

- Phase when the female refuses to stand to be mated
- Usually 6–8 days after onset of oestrus
- It is characterised by the thinning of endometrium and controlled by progesterone secreted by the corpus luteum
- If the female is pregnant, metoestrus will include the early stages of embryonic development
- Progesterone levels are steadily increasing if the animal is pregnant
- In non-pregnant animals progesterone levels gradually subside with the deterioration of the corpus luteum
- In the non-pregnant animal, progesterone levels fall gradually over 30–60 days
- Pseudocyesis or false lactation can be spontaneous or may be stimulated by spaying during metoestrus, due to raised plasma prolactin levels
- It is thought that there is a less effective feedback inhibition from falling progesterone levels (progesterone reduces mammary sensitivity to prolactin)
- Alternatively this may be a throwback to ancestral origins in wild dog packs: when dominant, the bitch would have synchronised cycles with the non-breeding females and then left them to feed the puppies
- Progesterone levels are high throughout gestation until before parturition, commencing when there is a prepartum decline
- Can delay parturition by giving progesterone to females
- Corpus luteum can sustain progesterone production without any pituitary luteotrophic support (LH and prolactin) for approximately 20 days.

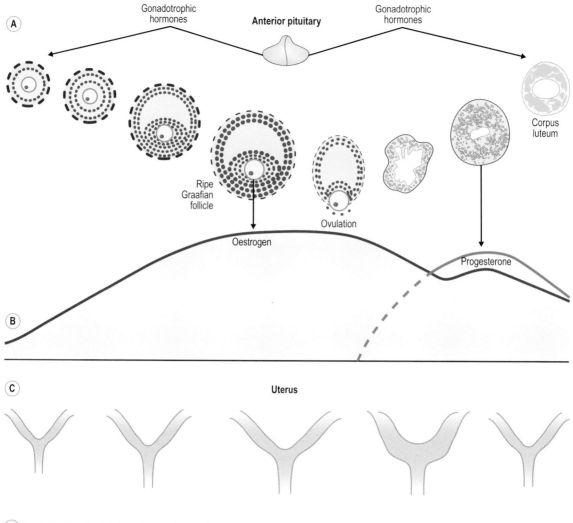

(A) Developing Graafian follicle, ovulation and corpus luteum

(B) Shows development in blood levels of oestrogen and progesterone

(C) Shows progressive development of the uterus

Figure 12.4 Diagrammatic representation of canine oestrus cycle. A, Developing graafian follicle, ovulation and corpus luteum; B, development in blood levels of oestrogen and progesterone; C, progressive development of the uterus.

Anoestrus

- In pregnant animals this is the period between parturition and pro-oestrus
- In non-pregnant animals this is the phase between the end of the luteal phase and the onset of pro-oestrus.

The queen (seasonally polyoestrus, induced ovulator)

Animals can also be seasonally polyoestrus species and induced ovulators. Examples include the cat, ferret, rabbit and mink. This means that the queen will come into season throughout the breeding season depending

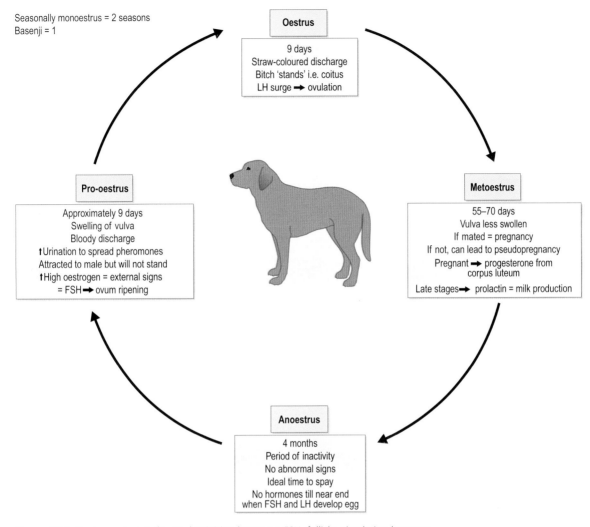

Seasonally monoestrus = 2 seasons
Basenji = 1

Oestrus

9 days
Straw-coloured discharge
Bitch 'stands' i.e. coitus
LH surge ➡ ovulation

Pro-oestrus

Approximately 9 days
Swelling of vulva
Bloody discharge
↑Urination to spread pheromones
Attracted to male but will not stand
↑High oestrogen = external signs
= FSH➡ ovum ripening

Metoestrus

55–70 days
Vulva less swollen
If mated = pregnancy
If not, can lead to pseudopregnancy
Pregnant ➡ progesterone from
corpus luteum

Late stages➡ prolactin = milk production

Anoestrus

4 months
Period of inactivity
No abnormal signs
Ideal time to spay
No hormones till near end
when FSH and LH develop egg

Figure 12.5 Canine oestrus cycle. LH, luteinising hormone; FSH, follicle-stimulating hormone.

on daylight hours (this is called photoperiodism) and ovulation is stimulated by the act of coitus. The average age of puberty varies in cats but they will usually show signs of oestrus when they have attained 2.3–3.5kg body weight depending on the time of year. The average age for the onset of puberty is 6–9 months. There is also a certain degree of breed variation, with Siamese, Burmese and other short-haired breeds tending to be precocious. The onset of puberty is seasonally influenced.

In the absence of pregnancy or in false pregnancy the cat will show repeated oestrus cycles every 2–3 weeks in spring, summer and autumn. In breeding colonies falsely controlled light can stimulate cats to remain in season. Figure 12.6 illustrates the feline oestrus cycle.

Behavioural cycle

This can be split into heat and non-heat periods.

Pro-oestrus and oestrus

- Pro-oestrus and oestrus are collectively the heat period
- Combined they have a duration of 3–10 days
- Pro-oestrus and oestrus are not as easily divided into two distinct cycles as in the bitch
- Pro-oestrus can be characterised by calling but with non-acceptance of the male
- Oestrus can be characterised by calling with acceptance of the male

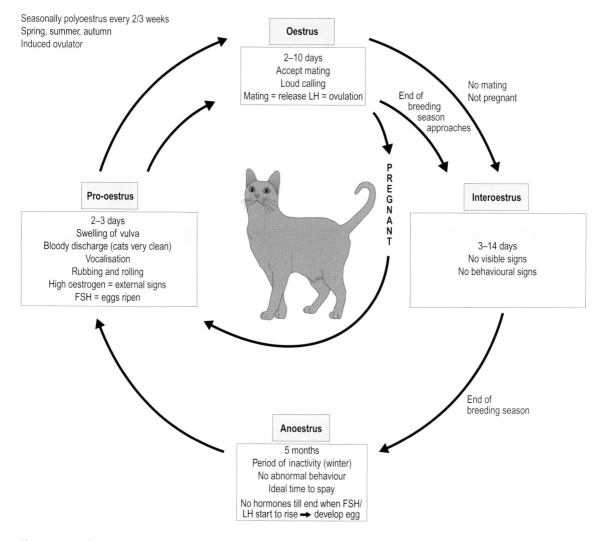

Figure 12.6 Feline oestrus cycle. LH, luteinising hormone; FSH, follicle-stimulating hormone.

- Behavioural signs include vocalisation or calling, rolling, being affectionate, rubbing, adopting the mating position and trying to escape to fulfil their wanderlust
- The mating position is for the fore-end to be crouched, the hind-end raised with the tail deflected to one side and showing paddling movements of the limbs.

Interoestrus and anoestrus

- In the absence of mating, heats will occur every 10–14 days
- There is a period between heats known as interoestrus when there are no signs of heat
- Nymphomania or prolonged oestrus may occur if the development of follicles overlaps between heats

- Anoestrus occurs when there are very short daylight hours in late autumn and winter.

Mating and induced ovulation

- An induced ovulator means that ovulation is stimulated by the act of coitus or stimulation of coitus (mating)
- Vaginal stimulation causes the release of GnRH, which causes the LH peak, leading to ovulation
- The number of follicles released and the time they are released appear to be dependent on the quantity and quality of mating, i.e. the higher the surge, the more follicles will be released
- Ovulation can be between 24 and 52 hours postcoitus

- After ovulation the heat subsides within 24–48 hours.

If pregnant

- If mated successfully, embryos develop in the oviducts 4–5 days after fertilisation
- Implantation occurs around day 12–16 postmating
- Progesterone levels are maintained by the corpus luteum and LH, then prolactin production
- If the queen ceases lactation during a breeding season there will be a brief period of interoestrus before oestrus commences; this can be within 10–15 days of weaning or kittening.

Choosing a mate

In companion animals, mating is usually planned and the breeders consider a number of variables when planning a union:

- The animals' pedigrees
- The animals' conformation
- Temperament
- Age
- Health and disease status
- Finance and convenience.

In cats, infectious diseases such as feline leukaemia, which is transmitted by mating, will need to be screened for before mating. The male and female cats are often kept in the same location to enable mating to occur once she comes into season or the owner can take the queen to the stud when the season begins. On the whole mating occurs unaided.

In dogs, timing is more critical, as the bitch is only willing to stand for a limited period of time. Prospective matings should be discussed well in advance of the event. The bitch's owner needs to watch for the first signs of her season and as soon as a bloody discharge is observed the stud dog owner should be notified and that day would be considered as day 1. Mating would normally occur between day 10 and day 12 to coincide with ovulation but individuals may vary and behavioural signs should also be considered. Indicators that can be used are a teaser, another dog on a lead or one that is castrated to prevent unwanted matings to ascertain whether she will allow the dog to mount, or scratching either side of the base of the tail and observing for lordosis. Lordosis is arching of the back, presenting the vulva and is most notably marked by the vibration and sideways movement of the tail, allowing access to the vulva. Mating is carefully monitored; the bitch and dog will be introduced with some form of restraint, e.g. collar and lead. They may wish to play for a short period before copulation and some animals can be quite shy if many people are present. The male will lick and sniff the vulva

DEFINITIONS

Gestation
Pregnancy

Gravid
Pregnant

Multigravid
Animal that has had lots of pregnancies

Primagravid
First pregnancy

then mount and penetrate the female. Once penetration has occurred the handlers should restrain the dogs and prevent excessive movement to reduce the risk of physical damage. The dog will ejaculate and dismount. At this stage the handler should aid the dog to dismount so that he ends up facing in the opposite direction. At this stage the dogs are tied; the tie is initiated by the bitch as she is holding on to the dog and can last up to 45 minutes until she releases him. During the tie, movement should be restricted and the handlers will hold the animals' head and support the abdomen. The length of the tie is considered to be linked to litter size.

Pregnancy definitions

See Box 12.3 for definitions.

Diagnosis of pregnancy

A number of diagnostic methods are available:

- Abdominal palpation
- Ultrasound examination
- Increasing body weight
- Abdominal swelling
- Behavioural changes
- Mammary gland enlargement
- Radiography: uterine enlargement, mineralisation of fetal skeleton
- Fetal heart beats via electrocardiogram
- Endocrine tests to assess progesterone levels.

COMMON DISORDERS OF PREGNANCY

A reduced packed cell volume and slight anaemia are normal physiological signs. Conception failure, embryonic absorption and fetal abortions are common in all species and in many cases will occur before the pregnancy is known. Diabetes mellitus can be compromised in gravid animals as pregnancy causes large fluctuations in glucose levels. Hypocalcaemia due to eclampsia can occur late in the pregnancy or during early lactation. Clinical signs include restlessness, panting, excess salivation, muscular tremors and pyrexia. These are caused by a low circulating blood level of calcium and if left untreated can result in death. Hypoglycaemia, low blood glucose and an associated ketosis are also common in

pregnancy due to the increased energy demands associated with it if a correct diet is not fed.

Large-animal reproduction

General advice

The selection of stock is an important variable in large-animal reproduction as breeding is often on a much larger and commercial scale (Tables 12.2 and 12.3).

Table 12.2 Large-animal female reproductive data: part 1

Species	Puberty (months)	Gestation (days)	Age to first breeding (months)	Ovulation	Monotocous/ polytocous	Cycle pattern	Oestrus cycle length (days)
Cow	6–12	282 (274–291)	14–22	Spontaneous	Polytocous	Polyoestrus	21
Mare	18 (12–29)	330 (320–360)	24–36	Spontaneous	Monotocous	Seasonally polyoestrus (long days)	21 (dioestrus at 15 days)
Sow	3–8	114 (110–116)	8–10	Spontaneous	Polytocous	Polyoestrus	21
Ewe	6–12	150 (140–160)	6–18	Spontaneous	Polytocous	Seasonally polyoestrus (short days)	17
Doe (goat)	6–12	150 (140–160)	6–18	Spontaneous	Polytocous	Seasonally polyoestrus (short days)	21

Table 12.3 Large-animal female reproductive data: part 2

Species	Oestrus cycle length (days)	Heat or oestrus length	Time of ovulation	Time to breed		Advisable time to breed after parturition
				Naturally	Artificial insemination	
Cow	21	18–20 hours	12–18 hours after end of oestrus	Heat	12 hours after first heat	60–90 days
Mare	21	4–7 days	1–2 days before end of oestrus	Day 2 and every other day	12 hours after first heat	25–35 days or second oestrus
Sow	21	2–3 days	Day 2 oestrus	Daily whilst in heat	12 hours after first heat	First oestrus 3–9 days after weaning
Ewe	17	24–48 hours	24–30 hours after onset of oestrus	Heat	12 hours after first heat	Usually next breeding season
Doe (goat)	21	24–36 hours	24–30 hours after onset of oestrus	Heat	12 hours after first heat	Usually next breeding season

Factors to consider when choosing stock include:

- Good health in males and females
- Animals that are free from disease
- Animals that are fit, not fat, utilising body scoring to assess
- Pedigrees: males and females should not be too closely related; particularly in equine reproduction pedigrees will be studied to optimise the characteristics displayed in the offspring
- Temperament of the animals: in dairy cattle milk production can be influenced by temperament
- Body size: the use of large animals with small animals can result in parturition problems
- Conformation: animals should be matched to counteract each other's faults
- Evaluation of the past breeding history for full-term pregnancies and the quality of stock produced
- Animals should be screened for hereditary disease
- Prophylactic treatments such as vaccination, parasite control and foot trimming should be considered prior to mating.

Male and female ratios should be considered. If males are allowed to cover too many females then their fertility can drop, resulting in reduced conception rates and sometimes a reduced libido.

The horse

The mare and stallion should both be in good health and not under- or overweight. Both should be vaccinated and have up-to-date parasite control. Before breeding both parties should be swabbed for equine viral arteritis and equine herpesvirus. The mare's reproductive status can be determined by rectal palpation of the reproductive system, ultrasonography, vaginal speculum examination, cultures, cytology or biopsy if required. For the stallion both testes should be descended and the quality of sperm can be evaluated for fertility, motility and abnormalities.

Horses are seasonally polyoestrus: their cycle is triggered by increasing daylight hours to 16 hours per day and the normal breeding season is March/April to September/October in the northern hemisphere, but management can expand these times.

Signs of oestrus

- When in oestrus the mare will squat her back, urinate, lift the tail and evert her clitoris (wink) at the male
- The process of squatting and urinating is known as breaking down
- No attempt should be made to kick the stallion; looking at the ear position can be a good clue as the ears should not be flat back
- The vulva is pink, moist and relaxed, and the cervix is open and oedematous (fluid-filled)

- The uterus is also oedematous and flaccid
- Ultrasonography is often employed to ascertain whether ovulation is imminent to increase the chances of successful fertilisation.

Signs of dioestrus

- After ovulation the follicular sac fills with blood to form a corpus haemorrhagicum which then matures to the corpus luteum
- Concentrations of progesterone in the blood increase within 24 hours of ovulation: this test can be used to see if an opportunity has been missed
- The behaviour of the mare will change: she will not stand for the stallion or approach him and may bite, kick, squeal, clamp and flick her tail with her ears pinned back
- The vulva has become pale, firm and dryer with the cervix closed, and uterine tone returns.

The oestrus cycle is under the same hormonal control as in small animals but in horses another hormone is important – prostaglandin $F_2\alpha$. This is produced by the endometrium (lining of the uterus) in the non-pregnant mare and triggers luteolysis (destruction) of the corpus luteum. In the pregnant horse the embryo is mobile in the uterus for the first 16 days postfertilisation and it is thought that this movement somehow tells the mare she is pregnant and inhibits prostaglandin production, thereby facilitating progesterone production from the corpus luteum and maintaining the pregnancy.

Endometrial cups

In the mare between days 40 and 120 of the pregnancy, circular areas of tissue are raised in the caudal portion of the gravid horn of the uterus (where the embryo is) and these arrange into a horseshoe pattern. They are produced in response to the trophoblastic cells of the embryo within the uterine epithelium and are known as endometrial cups. They secrete chorionic gonadotrophins or pregnant mare serum gonadotrophin. This substance acts like LH to develop extra corpus luteum to produce increased amounts of progesterone and therefore maintain the pregnancy.

The equine oestrus cycle can be manipulated hormonally. Administration of progesterone, prostaglandin $F_2\alpha$, progesterone and oestradiol combinations or GnRH are all employed to stimulate oestrus.

MATING

Mares can cause damage to often valuable stallions, so a teaser is used to ascertain if they are receptive. This is usually a pony stallion or a gelding. The mare's hind shoes are removed and hobbles or a crush may be used to prevent kicking and damage.

Pregnancy diagnosis is achieved by ultrasonography, rectal examination and hormonal assays.

Artificial insemination

This is a popular method within the equine industry, with the exception being the thoroughbred racing industry, where horses mated by this method are not eligible for registration. Artificial insemination allows access to overseas horses, reduces the risk of damage to stallions and handlers, reduces the risk of venereal disease and also enables one ejaculation to be used for more than one mare. Semen may be fresh and chilled or frozen, and is stored in 'straws'. Conception rates are generally higher with fresh semen than frozen but the process does rely on excellent detection of oestrus and careful handling of the semen. Males are trained to mount an artificial vagina to enable safe collection of semen which is subsequently analysed with sperm morphology and motility evaluated.

Embryo transfer

This is a relatively new technique, often used in female competition horses to enable them to breed and compete at the highest level. It also enables animals of high genetic merit, e.g. rare breeds, to mate more than naturally. The mare is fertilised then the embryo is washed out of the uterus of the parental mare and implanted into the surrogate to carry to term. Embryos can be frozen for future use or for transportation.

HOUSING AND MANAGEMENT

Mares due to foal should be checked at least twice daily either in the field or the foaling box. Their udders should be checked for waxing up and milk production and slackening of the pelvic ligaments around the tail. Hygiene and environmental factors should be considered and, as horses do not like to be observed giving birth, CCTV is often used to monitor the animal unobtrusively. Riding the horse usually ceases about 6 months into the gestation period. Diet needs to be adapted and a good mix or cube is often fed, with quantities increasing in the final trimester, with the aim of maintaining a body score of 2–3. Equine herpesvirus is an abortive agent; therefore it is advisable to vaccinate the mare at months 5, 7 and 9 of pregnancy and an additional flu and tetanus booster 10 months into the gestation is also recommended.

PARTURITION

The gestation period is 330–340 days but some mares will foal as early as 320 days and others as late as 400 days. Parturition in the horse is a quick process and a foal can be expected within 1 hour of the end of stage 1.

Problems associated with pregnancy

- Twins – this can lead to dystocia if allowed to go to full term; it is normal practice to abort one embryo when detected during ultrasonography during pregnancy diagnosis
- Early embryonic death – approximately 5–24% of conceptions will die in early pregnancy; there are numerous causal factors, including nutrition, climate, sire and rectal examination
- Abortion – again, there are numerous causal agents, including equine herpesvirus, equine viral arteritis, bacteria and viral and fungal pathogens.

The cow

Cattle breed all year round, with oestrus occurring at an average of 21-day intervals. In dairy cow breeding the aim is to have a calving interval of 365 days. Oestrus is relatively short, averaging a 12-hour period, but in some animals it can be as short as 4 hours. Signs include standing to be mounted, excoriation of the rump and tail head due to repeated mounting by others, the 'bulling string', a strand of mucus from the vagina, and head mounting, with the mounting cow being in pro-oestrus so she can be watched for when she stops. Behavioural signs such as restlessness, bellowing, chin resting, sniffing, licking and butting may also be seen. Metoestral bleeding, i.e. blood in the vulva, occurs 48 hours after oestrus – which is an indication that oestrus was missed!

Farmers use observation of their cows and tail paint for signs of oestrus. Teaser animals can be placed in the herd, e.g. a vasectomised bull with a chin marker to highlight activity. Bovine temperature increases by 0.1–0.3 °C during oestrus and progesterone levels in milk produced drop. Oestrus can be manipulated using hormonal devices such as a progesterone-releasing intravaginal device – a coil which is implanted in the vagina for 12 days then removed, with oestrus occurring 2–4 days later – and other variations of hormonal implants, as well as hormonal administration, as in the horse.

Artificial insemination, embryo transfer and semen analysis occur. It is likely that in the future DNA analysis and sexing of semen will also occur to reduce wastage in the industry.

The sheep

Sheep are seasonally polyoestrus but their cyclic activity is triggered by decreasing daylight hours or an increase in the production of melatonin by the pineal gland. Oestrus lasts approximately 24 hours, with ovulation occurring approximately 20 hours after the onset of oestrus. Sheep breeders aim to have groups of ewes synchronised to lamb within short time periods.

The introduction of an entire or vasectomised ram to a flock of ewes will increase LH production, causing mass ovulation approximately 3 days postreproduction, but the oestrus is silent. Progesterone sponges can be inserted into the vagina, with oestrus occurring 2 days later, or melatonin implants can be inserted for 60 days, bringing the ewes into season 6 weeks later. Pregnancy diagnosis is via ultrasound scanning and keel markers on rams, which will leave a mark on the ewes they have mated. Artificial insemination, embryo transfer and semen analysis occur.

The pig

Breeding of pigs is a tightly controlled and intensive industry. It aims to produce the maximum number of piglets per sow per year. Porcine oestrus lasts approximately 40–70 hours with ovulation occurring 38–42 hours after the onset of oestrus. Sows display an increase in vaginal mucus with a fall in pH; they become restless and have a reduced appetite. Sows are introduced to the boar when they show signs of oestrus and artificial insemination is also employed.

Health and safety note

Brucellosis, salmonellosis and other infectious agents that can be associated with large-animal abortion are zoonotic, so care should be taken around these animals.

Toxoplasmosis is dangerous to pregnant women and they should therefore avoid lambing sheep. Reproductive drugs such as prostaglandins can also cause abortion and hormonal alterations in people.

Care of the large-animal neonate

Large-animal offspring are precocial (born with their ears and eyes open) as they are required to be able to move with the herd as soon as possible to escape predators in the wild. Neonatal foals, calves, lambs and piglets are able to stand and walk within 1 hour of being born. Protocols for dealing with neonatal animals are especially important in the species where breeding has been synchronised and therefore numerous individuals will be giving birth simultaneously.

General rules to follow

- Good hygiene
- Umbilicus is a route of entry for infection
- Treat with antibacterial solution or spray
- Iodine is suitable for pigs, cattle and sheep but not horses
- Some farms will dose lambs with a prophylactic systemic antibiotic at birth.

Environment

- Clean, comfortable and meeting the five animal freedoms/needs (Chapter 9)
- Disinfect lambing, calving, foaling and pigging pens inbetween use.

Examination

- Examine the neonate for congenital abnormalities.

Observation

- All neonates should be encouraged to suckle as soon as possible after birth to ensure they receive colostrum
- Remember colostrum can only be absorbed by the digestive system for 6–8 hours after birth and it is vital to boost the neonatal immune system
- Make sure the dam has milk and is accepting suckling.

FERTILISATION AND EMBRYOLOGY

Fertilisation

The ovum is fertilised by the spermatozoa within the fallopian tube or oviduct. The sperms arrive at the ovum and begin to burrow into the corona radiata. The first sperm to enter the zona pellucida initiates the fertilisation reaction, i.e. it stops any other sperm entering the ovum. The fertilised ovum then becomes the zygote. The lifespan of sperm within the reproductive tract varies between species from a day to a week.

Fertilisation usually occurs 2–3 days after ovulation.

Zygote

The zygote continues to travel along the oviduct and undergoes various cell divisions:

1. The two cells divide to four cells to eight cells and then irregularly to form a ball of cells called the morula

2. The morula then develops a cavity, with the cell mass remaining at one end:
   ○ The cell mass is ths inner cell mass
   ○ The cavity is the trophoblast
   It is the inner cell mass which develops into the embryo
3. The inner cell mass then differentiates into three layers which will eventually form recognisable body parts:
   ○ The ectoderm: this is the outer layer – the skin and nervous system
   ○ The mesoderm: this is the middle layer – the musculoskeletal system and other internal organs
   ○ The endoderm: this is the inner layer – the lining of the gastrointestinal tract and other visceral structures
4. The mesoderm forms two longitudinal blocks of tissue at either side of the trophoblast
5. At the same time endodermal cells develop beneath the mesoderm and will eventually line the trophoblast and encapsulate the yolk sac
6. Mammalian yolk sacs contain no yolk, unlike those in birds and reptiles, where the yolk provides nourishment for the growing embryo
7. The next stage is for the mesodermal cells to produce two layers, one adjacent to the ectoderm and one next to the endoderm, forming a cavity between them
8. The inner cell mass begins to enclose the mesodermal and endodermal cells (which will become internal organs)
9. The yolk sac and trophoblast develop to form the extraembryonic membranes – the placenta, chorioallantois and allantoamnion
10. It is only now that the embryo arrives at the uterine horns and is ready for implantation.

The zygote partially destroys an area of endometrium so it can lie within it to develop securely.

The extraembryonic membranes

The extraembryonic membrane comprises:

- The yolk sac
- The chorion
- The amnion
- The allantois.

The zygote changes name to the embryo once it has become implanted within the uterine wall.

It then undergoes further stages of development (Figure 12.7):

1. The embryo (inner cell mass) curls up on itself and the yolk sac becomes narrower until the top part of

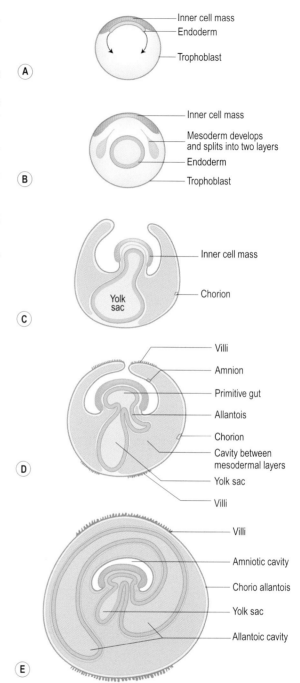

Figure 12.7 Stages in development of extraembryonic membranes. (Reproduced from Aspinall V 2006 *The Complete Textbook of Veterinary Nursing*. Butterworth Heinemann, London, with permission.)

the endoderm is pinched off and forms the primitive gut tube

2. Another diverticulum (pouch or sac) develops from within the primitive gut tube and grows out alongside the yolk sac, forming the allantois
3. The allantois will form the allantoic sac, which will hold the fetal urine
4. The yolk sac contracts as the embryo develops and the allantois increases in size and moves into the mesodermal cavity, pushing in between the two mesodermal layers
5. Simultaneously the trophoblast is expanding around the embryo until it forms a double-layered membrane encapsulating the developing embryo
6. The outer layer is the chorion and the inner layer is the amnion
7. Both the amnion and chorion consist of two layers – the ectoderm and mesoderm
8. The allantois is expanding as more fetal urine is produced until the cavity between the chorion and amnion is filled with fluid
9. The allantoic membrane then fuses with the amnion below it and chorion above it, forming two new membranes
10. The allantoamnion, which is the inner layer or 'slime-bag' of the fetus, contains the lubricating fluid for passage through the birth canal
11. The chorioallantois is the outer layer or 'water-bag' that ruptures as the fetus moves into the birth canal.

The placenta

This is the organ of exchange between the mother and the fetus. The placenta is a thickened area of extraembryonic membranes. It attaches the mammalian fetus to the endometrium lining of the uterus. The embryo/fetus receives blood, nutrients and oxygen through the placental blood supply and expels waste products from itself. The placenta also acts as an endocrine organ, providing hormones that maintain pregnancy (it produces progesterone in addition to corpus luteum). The chorioallantois within the placental areas develops villi to increase the surface area.

Marginal haematomas are areas at the edge of the placenta where there is degeneration of the maternal endothelium. The blood produced is prevented from clotting by agents secreted by the chorion and is thought to provide the embryo with iron. The marginal haematomas also give the parturition vaginal discharges their colour (green in the bitch and brown in the queen).

Table 12.4 Gestation periods of small mammals	
Dog	63 days
Cat	63 days
Rabbit	30–33 days
Mouse	19–21 days (postpartum oestrus within 24 hours)
Rat	21–23 days (postpartum oestrus within 48 hours)
Hamsters	15–18 days
Gerbil	24–26 days (postpartum oestrus within 24 hours)
Guinea pig	60–70 days (postpartum oestrus within 24 hours)

PREGNANCY AND DEVELOPMENT

Table 12.4 shows gestation periods in small mammals.

Signs of pregnancy

- Increase in weight
- Mammary gland development (not necessarily clearly seen in primigravida animals)
- Mammary glands increase in size as pregnancy develops and unpigmented teats may become pink
- Normal physiological changes, e.g. normocytic anaemia, reduced packed cell volume.

Care during pregnancy varies with species – let us look at the dog as an example.

Care of the bitch during pregnancy

Diet

- There is no need to increase food intake before the last third of the pregnancy
- The pregnant bitch should be fed a commercial gestation or growth formula
- Increase the amount of food during the last 3 weeks (start by about 10% up to 50% more than the normal amount in the final week)
- During the last 2 weeks the fetuses are becoming large within the uterus, leaving little room in the abdomen

- It is a good idea to increase the number of feeds per day to encompass the increased amount
- If a balanced diet is fed there should be no need for supplementation.

Calcium and vitamins

- These are not required if the bitch is fed a balanced diet throughout pregnancy
- Some breeders will feed bone meal.

Worming

- The bitch should be wormed before mating
- She should be wormed twice during pregnancy
- Give the last dose at 54 days to reduce the numbers of migrating *Toxocara* larvae (from the bitch to the fetuses via placenta)
- Be careful to source products which are safe to use during pregnancy.

Exercise

- Normal exercise is essential to keep the bitch fit but the owner should be sensible during the final stages and in reality the bitch should limit her own exercise during this period.

Constipation

Avoid constipation.

Vaccination

- Should be up to date before mating as many veterinary surgeons will not administer booster vaccinations during pregnancy.

General care

If a long-haired breed, the hair should be trimmed from the nipples and the vulva in the later stages or olive oil or creams can be used to keep the nipples soft and moist.

Provide a safe place as parturition approaches and ideally provide a whelping box. There are many commercial whelping products available but generally the box should be warm, easy to clean, and of an appropriate size to allow the bitch to stretch out but not too big that the puppies will get lost within it. Temperature control is required as neonates cannot control their own temperature initially; some whelping boxes have heating incorporated whilst other breeders will utilise a pig lamp (heat lamp). It is important to have a 'pig rail', a small wooden shelf, around the inside of the box to prevent

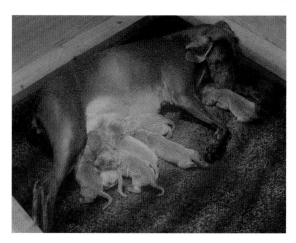

Figure 12.8 Contented litter in whelping box; the red light is due to a pig lamp being used as a supplementary heat source.

the bitch squashing the puppies when she lies down (Figure 12.8).

Interruptions to pregnancy

Natural

Abortion is defined as the premature expulsion of the products of conception, the embryo or non-viable fetus. If it occurs in the early stages of pregnancy the fetus may be reabsorbed rather than expelled. There are two types: sporadic abortion and infectious abortion.

Abnormalities of pregnancy

- Ectopic pregnancy – this is where the embryo develops outside the uterus and is rare
- Uterine rupture – this may possibly be caused by trauma, e.g. road traffic accident, or by misuse of ecbolics, e.g. oxytocin, prior to the cervix being dilated
- Uterine torsion – this can involve one horn or the body of the uterus twisting round on itself and trapping the fetus
- Inguinal hernia – where the uterus becomes trapped in the hernia.

Parturition

Gestation periods

- Bitch: 63 days
- Queen: 65 days
- Mare: 330 days.

STAGES OF PARTURITION (GIVING BIRTH)

1. Preparatory stage
2. First stage of parturition (onset of contractions)
3. Second stage of parturition (increased contractions + propulsion of fetus through cervix)
4. Third stage of parturition (passage of allantochorion, i.e. placenta)
5. Puerperium (after parturition)

Signs of parturition may include:

- Relaxation of pelvic ligaments: sunken hindquarters – this can be particularly evident in the mare
- The labia become swollen and more oedematous
- There may be a slight mucus discharge (which may not be seen, as the dam will lick it)
- Temperature changes (the bitch's normal body temperature drops by 2°C)
- The dam may refuse food
- Restlessness and nesting behaviour
- They may begin to lactate; in the mare the teats of the udder 'wax up'.

Parturition is divided into three stages (Box 12.4).

First stage

Stage 1 is characterised by intermittent, spasmodic contractions of the uterus. These will increase in strength and regularity as stage 1 progresses. The mucous plug that seals the cervix liquefies and is discharged.

The bitch will show signs of restlessness, glancing at her flanks, licking the mammary glands and vulva, shivering and panting. She may wish to be left alone or may actively seek company. She will also nest, which can include quite violent destruction of bedding materials!

The queen will show restlessness, crying, make trips to the kittening area and the litter tray, wants company, licks her flank and vulva and often purrs.

Second stage

Uterine contractions become stronger and the intervals between them decrease. The dam will begin to strain with each contraction. The first fetus passes through the cervix, stimulating a neurohormonal reflex which stimulates uterine contractions even more. The fetus is contained within two fluid-filled sacs: the inner amnion, which completely surrounds the fetus and the outer allantochorion, which forms the fetal placenta. The fluid-filled sacs help the cervix to dilate by exerting pressure on cervix tissue leading to dilation. At the beginning of the second stage the fetus is inverted with the head and limbs flexed and needs to rotate before delivery. The

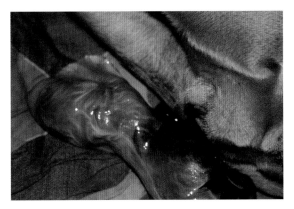

Figure 12.9 Delivery of neonate in amniotic sac.

fetus passes into the pelvic inlet, and a nervous reflex stimulates forceful abdominal contractions, helping to propel the fetus through the pelvis. The allantochorion appears at the vulva and either ruptures spontaneously or is burst by the dam. The amnion remains intact, helping to dilate the vagina. The dam continues to strain and the fetus is delivered within its amniotic sac (Figure 12.9). The dam tears open the amniotic sac and cleans the membranes from her young. Licking stimulates respiration and the dam will then bite through the umbilicus.

Third stage

The fetal membranes and placenta are expelled following the involution of the uterus. These are usually eaten by the dam. Occasionally the placenta may come out with the next offspring or it may all come at once in multiparous species. It is important to monitor the number of placentas related to the number of offspring to ensure none is left inside. Involution of the uterus is completed during this stage.

Dystocia is defined as difficulty giving birth. There are two types: maternal and fetal.

Maternal dystocia

Primary uterine inertia

- Absence or weakness of uterine contractions
- Parturition either does not start or finishes too early
- Treatment for complete primary uterine inertia is a caesarean section.

For partial primary uterine inertia and if the cervix is dilated, an ecbolic such as oxytocin may be administered by the veterinary surgeon to stimulate uterine contractions.

Secondary uterine inertia

- This occurs when there is an obstruction to delivery and the uterine muscle has become exhausted
- Treatment is to remove the obstruction, then try oxytocin or perform a caesarean section.

Nervous inhibition of labour

- Animals can inhibit labour if they are not happy with the situation or are unable to cope with painful contractions
- If the dam is unhappy with the whelping box she may prefer another location, e.g. settee, wardrobe.

Pelvic abnormalities

- May be hereditary or the result of an accident
- Narrowing of pelvic inlet interferes with delivery.

Other causes

Other causes of maternal dystocia include the following:

- Failure of cervix to dilate
- Neoplasms – tumours

- Torsion of uterus
- Hernia of the gravid uterus
- A small or infantile vulva.

Table 12.5 shows possible complications in the dam.

Fetal dystocia

Absolute oversize

- Fetus is grossly oversized
- Often occurs in small litters.

Relative oversize

- Fetus is of normal size but relatively too large for pelvis
- Can occur in breeds which have been selectively bred for small pelvis or a large head, e.g. Chihuahuas, Afenpinschers.

Other causes

Other causes of fetal dystocia include the following:

- Abnormal presentation of the fetus
- Fetal hydrocephalus – a build-up of fluid on the brain enlarging the head

Table 12.5 Possible complications in the dam		
Condition	**Clinical signs**	**Treatment**
Retention of fetal membranes	Restlessness, anorexia, slight temperature, neglects litter, vaginal discharge, straining, abdominal discomfort	Antibiotics
Puerperal metritis	Happens 3–4 days postpartum: pyrexia, anorexic, polydipsic, neglect of litter and profuse offensive reddish brown vaginal discharge	Antibiotics, cleaning dam, hand-rear litter
Mastitis	Inflammation of mammary gland. May affect one or two glands. Affected gland becomes swollen, hard, inflamed, hot and tender, often with a brown watery discharge from nipple	Hot fomentations to ease pain, antibiotics; may need to hand-rear litter
Eclampsia Lactation or puerperal tetany	Cause is low serum calcium. Causes muscle spasms, twitches. Usually occurs within 3 weeks of parturition Signs: restlessness, nervousness, panting, ataxic, progress into lateral recumbency exhibiting opisthotonus (limbs extended with head thrown back), pyrexia, can have convulsions	Intravenous calcium; remove litter for at least 24 hours; dark, quiet room; lower temperature
Hypoglycaemia	Can affect pregnant or postpartum animal. Due to reduced blood glucose levels. Easy to confuse with eclampsia. Causes weakness and possibly coma (the dam can be very aggressive towards pups)	Intravenous glucose, remove litter

- Anasarca – oedema of the fetus
- Monsters – genetic defects.

Postpartum care

This is species-specific but generally food and water are offered, discharges and lactation are checked, and the litter and dam are monitored. Temperature and cleanliness are important as the neonate is vulnerable to infection. Until the first milk or colostrum is suckled, the youngster will have no immunity so it is vital that this first suckling occurs. Also the remnants of the umbilical cord should be monitored for navel ill, signs of infections as they provide an entry route to the body for pathogenic organisms.

Feeding postpartum animals

The postpartum animal requires an appropriate amount of a balanced diet specially formulated for a lactating animal. Frequency of feeding occurs little and often and may be ad libitum. The individual species requirements should be considered.

CARE OF THE NEONATE (NEWBORN)

Initial examination

1. Record the body weight (it should increase daily by 5–10%)
2. Clean the umbilicus and check for herniation
3. Perform a respiration check: ensure breathing is regular, not noisy and at a normal rate for the species (remember that neonatal respiratory rates are normally higher than those of an adult)
4. Ensure there are no discharges in the eyes or ears
5. Examine for signs of congenital defects, particularly a cleft palette, which may interfere with suckling (Table 12.6 and Figure 12.10)
6. You may take a rectal temperature.

ENDOCRINOLOGY OF PREGNANCY AND PARTURITION

Pregnancy is maintained by the production of progesterone from the corpus luteum and the placenta. The mammary glands are stimulated to grow by the production of progesterone. Parturition is initiated by reducing levels of progesterone and the increasing production of oxytocin by the neurophysis. Oxytocin causes contractions in the smooth muscle of the uterus and opens the ducts in the mammary glands in preparation for milk

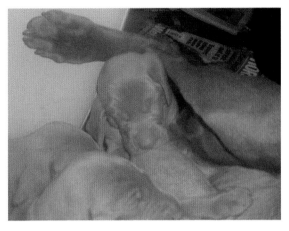

Figure 12.10 Suckling reflex.

letdown. Suckling by the newborns stimulates the neurophysis to produce more oxytocin and increases the frequency of uterine contractions. Simultaneously in late pregnancy and during lactation the adenophysis produces prolactin, that stimulates milk production. Milk letdown is under the control of oxytocin and prolactin.

Mammary gland

Mammary glands are specialised sweat glands. Their function is to produce milk in adequate quantity and of adequate quality for the litter. This ability is not dependent on the health of the dam. Mammary tissue is glandular tissue embedded within fibrous connective tissue and fat. Pregnancy causes hypertrophy of the nipples and the mammary tissue, activating it to produce mammary secretions (milk) near the end of the gestation period.

Production of milk

Milk is produced under the influence of prolactin in the glandular tissue. It passes from the glandular tissue through the gland sinus into the teat sinus, from where it will flow when there is stimulation, i.e. suckling. Milk comes from the teat sinus down the teat canal and out the teat orifice into the waiting mouth. Milk production is therefore controlled by prolactin and oxytocin, which acts to contract the smooth muscle within mammary glands to squeeze the milk out.

The first milk is called colostrum. Colostrum is an important source of maternal antibodies and it is important that the neonate receives this colostrum since it is a source of antibodies but also because the permeability of the bowel to antibodies decreases as the neonate matures. All young should ideally suckle within minutes

Table 12.6 Common congenital (inherited) defects

Dog	Hip dysplasia	Abnormality of hip joint
		Genetic and nutritional causes
		Scheme allocates a score between 0 and 53 from X-ray
		Dogs must be over 12 months of age for consideration
	Osteochondritis dissecans	Abnormality of the elbow joint
	Eye defects	Many different forms
		Schemes available, particularly for Collies, but other breeds are being tested
	Entropion	Inward-turning eyelid
	Ectropion	Outward-turning eyelid
	Cryptorchidism	Failure of one or both testes to descend
	Umbilical hernia	Protrusion of tissue through the umbilicus
	Merle	Incomplete dominant gene
		Avoid mating with white, blue-eyed dogs as these often develop glaucoma
	Scottie cramp	Autosomal-recessive
		Severe cramps brought on by exercise
		Breed-specific
	Progressive axonopathy	Degeneration of nerve fibres
		Autosomal-recessive
	Haemophilia	Failure in the clotting mechanism of blood
		Lots of different types and related conditions
		Breed societies often monitor
Cat	Manx	Autosomal-dominant
	Deafness	Due to dominant white gene
		Affects white cats with blue eyes
	Polydactyly	Extra toes on front feet
		Autosomal-dominant
	Flat-chested kitten syndrome	Affects Burmese
		Respiratory performance is compromised
	Folded ears	Incomplete dominant
		Heterozygote has folded ears
		Homozygote also has skeletal problems
Horse	Severe combined immunodeficiency	Affects Arabians
		No functional T or B lymphocytes
		The foal will die when maternal antibodies lifespan is complete – at approximately 4 months
	Atresia ani	Lack of anus
	Angular and flexural limb deformities	Can rectify given time or with veterinary intervention
	Deviation of the vertebrae	
	Patellar luxation	Common in Shetlands and miniature breeds (also seen in small breeds of dog)
	Wry nose	Skeletal deformity where the nose is twisted
	Rhabdomyolysis (tying up)	Some forms of this condition are thought to be hereditary
Generic	Heart defects	Holes in heart septum
		Patent ductus arteriosus
	Herniation	Umbilical and inguinal
	Cleft palate	The hard and soft palate fail to close, leaving communication between the naso- and oropharynx, which can lead to inhalation of milk
	Overshot or undershot jaws	Normal in some breeds

of their birth, or within 4 hours of birth or at least within 8 hours of their birth.

Milk consists of:

- Fats, proteins and carbohydrate (lactose)
- Solids, varying from <20% to >70% depending on the species
- Calcium, phosphate, magnesium, sodium, chloride and vitamins A, E, K and B.

Bibliography

Aspinall V 2006 The complete textbook of veterinary nursing. Butterworth Heinemann, London

Bourdon R M 1997 Understanding animal breeding. Prentice Hall, New Jersey

Broonan S, Legge D 1999 Law relating to animals. Cavendish, Jordan, London

BSAVA 1996 Manual of companion animal nutrition and feeding. BSAVA, Oxford

Bullied N 2001 Tailor-made proteins. Philip Allan Updates. Biological Sciences Review 2–6

Elmer T K 1982 Practical animal husbandry. John Wright, Bristol

Gregory J 1996 Applications of genetics. Cambridge Modular Sciences. Cambridge University Press, Cambridge

Hayes K 1993 The complete book of foaling. Howell Book House, New York

Kleiman D G, Allan M E, Thompson K V, Lumpkin S L 1996 Wild mammals in captivity, principles and techniques. University of Chicago Press, Chicago, IL

Moody F G 1991 Raising small animals. Farming Press, Ipswich

Palmer J 2001 Animal law, 3rd edn. Shaw, Kent

Pratt P W 1998 Principles and practice of veterinary technology. Mosby, Philadelphia

Thomas D G M 1983 Animal husbandry, 3rd edn. Baillière Tindall, Oxford

Warren D M 1995 Small animal care and management. Delmar Learning, New York

Chapter | **13** | *Jane Williams*

Terminology and management of animal collections

This chapter introduces the reader to veterinary terminology and aims to help to understand the composition of words commonly employed in the veterinary field and for animal records. The organisation of animal collections, general considerations and implementation of the five freedoms, responsible record keeping and routine monitoring processes of hospitalised animals are described in detail.

ANATOMICAL DIRECTIONS AND VETERINARY TERMINOLOGY

Tips to help get to grips with terminology:

- Break down a word and identify its parts
- Relate words to body systems
- Learn the basics
- Use diagrams, charts and webs
- Do review your progress
- *Ask* if you are unsure
- Invest in a good veterinary dictionary.

Pronunciation

Veterinary terminology includes lots of vocabulary that may have not been encountered previously. Many words can be difficult to pronounce. Some common problem areas are identified in Table 13.1. A good veterinary dictionary will include the phonetic spelling of words to enable the correct pronunciation.

Plurals

Common plurals include:

- -ae, e.g. fasciae (fascia)
- -ia, e.g. crania (cranium)
- -i, e.g. glomeruli (glomerulus)
- -ata, e.g. adenomata (adenoma).

Spelling

Be careful, as many words appear the same phonetically but are actually different, e.g. ilium and ileum.

There is far too numerous terminology utilised in veterinary science to list it all here; some useful terms are given in Box 13.1. See also Table 13.2 for the identification of word elements.

Table 13.1 Pronunciation of veterinary terminology

Letters	Pronounced
Ch	K, e.g. chronic
Ps	S, e.g. psychology
Pn	N, e.g. pneumonia
C and g Before e, i and y words	S and j, e.g. cytoplasm, generic
C and g Before all other letters	Hard sound, e.g. cardiac, gastric
Ae and ee	Ee, e.g. fasciae
I at end of word	Eye, e.g. alveoli
Es at end of word	As a separate syllable e.g. metastases would be meta-stay-seez

Table 13.2 Identification of word elements

Element	Definition
Prefix	Beginning part of a word
Suffix	End part of a word
Root	Foundation or basic meaning of the word. Can be: Prefix + root Root + suffix Prefix + root + suffix
Combining form	The root with an added vowel or combining vowel which is used to combine the original root with the suffix or another root

Anatomical directions

It is a useful tool in veterinary medicine to be able to locate precisely where, for example, a laceration is upon an animal. A number of anatomical terms are commonly used in describing the quadrupedal vertebrate (an animal that stands on all four feet) and determining direction: refer to Tables 13.3 and 13.4 and Figures 13.1–13.4.

The way an animal is positioned can also be described:

- Erect: standing tall
- Recumbent: lying down

Box 13.1

TERMINOLOGY

-atrophy
Reduced in size

Brady-
Decreased rate

-cardia
Related to the heart

Dys-
Difficulty

Haem-
Relating to blood

-itis
Inflammation of

Ophthalmo-
Relating to the eyes

-pnoea
Related to respiration

Tachy-
Increased rate; usually applies to a physiological event, e.g. breathing

-trophy
Enlarged in size

- Sternal recumbency: lying down on the abdomen (sternum)
- Lateral recumbency: lying down on one side; the side in contact with the ground gives the direction, e.g. right lateral recumbency would mean the animal has its right side in contact with the ground.

Body cavities

The animal body can be subdivided into sections or cavities. The thoracic cavity describes the chest region from the atlas to the diaphragm. The abdominal cavity is located from the diaphragm to the pelvis and can be further divided into cranial and caudal sections. The mediastinum describes the area located in the mid-thorax and which contains the heart and lungs.

173

Table 13.3 Anatomical directions	
Direction	**Description**
Cranial	Towards the cranium (head) of the animal
Caudal	Towards the rear of the animal
Rostral	Towards the nose of the animal; applies to the head only
Medial	The inner surface of the limbs
Lateral	The outer surface of the limbs
Dorsal	The dorsum or towards the back (spine) of the animal
Ventral	The ventrum or towards the abdomen of the animal
Proximal	Applies to the limbs; describes a location heading close to the body trunk
Distal	Applies to the limbs; describes a location heading away from the body trunk
Palmar	The pads/underside of the feet on the front legs
Plantar	The pads/underside of the feet on the hind legs

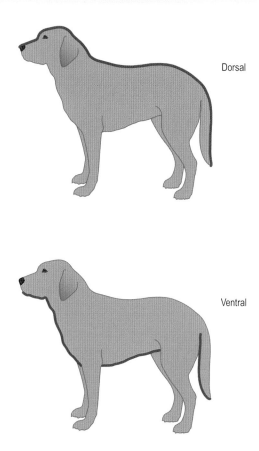

Dorsal

Ventral

Table 13.4 Anatomical planes	
Plane	**Description**
Dorsal/frontal	Section through the side of the body at right angles to the median plane – divides into ventral and dorsal sections
Median Mid sagittal Midline	Imaginary line that passes from the front to the back through the centre of the body – divides into a right and left portion
Sagittal	A section parallel to the long axis of the body or parallel to the median plane
Transverse Cross-sectional	Perpendicular transection of the long axis of the trunk, head, limb or other appendage

Cranial ←――――――――――――――――――→ Caudal

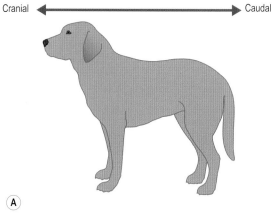

(A)

Figure 13.1 (a–c) Common veterinary directions.

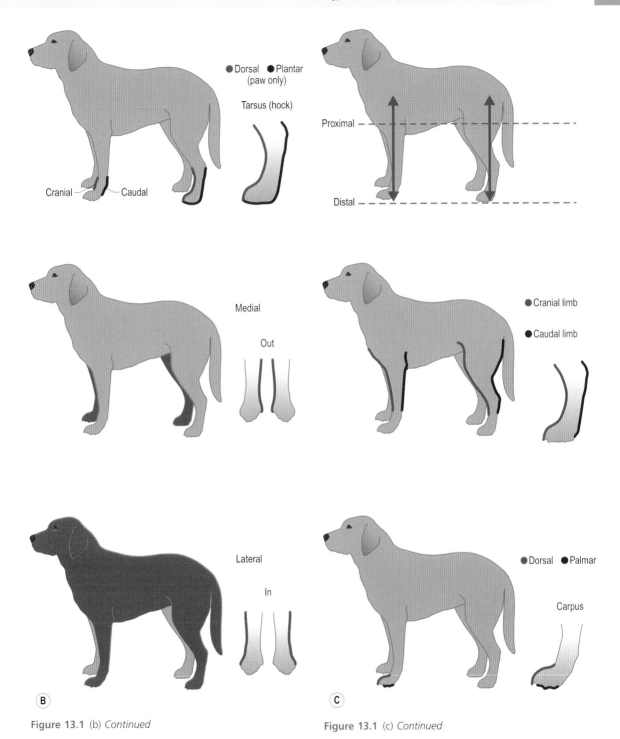

Figure 13.1 (b) *Continued*

Figure 13.1 (c) *Continued*

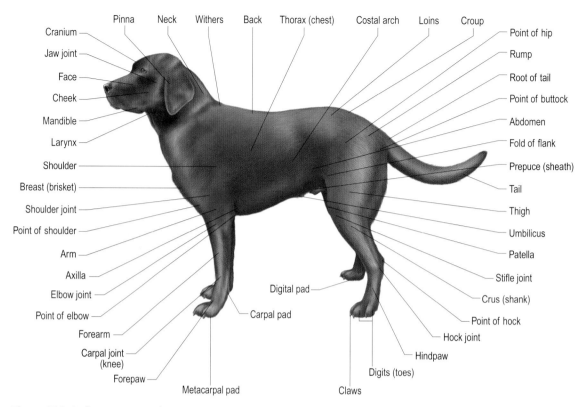

Figure 13.2 Surface anatomy – dog.

DAILY MONITORING AND HEALTH CHECKS

Assessing temperature, pulse and respiration

The daily duties of an assistant in any animal collections should involve monitoring the temperature, pulse and respiration rates of the patients under your care. Accurate and repeated recording of these variables can indicate good health or signs of illness depending upon whether they are raised, lowered or within the appropriate reference range (Table 13.5).

Frequency of recording will depend on the individual. Indications for frequent monitoring include:

- Hospitalised patients: minimum of twice daily
- History of abnormalities: as required under veterinary instruction
- Intensive care/paediatric: ideally, constant or every 10 minutes.

Table 13.5 Variations in temperature		
Pyrexia	**Subclinical/ low**	**Fluctuating diphasic**
Infection	Shock	Canine distemper
Heat stroke	Circulatory collapse	
Convulsions	Impending parturition	
Pain		
Excitement		

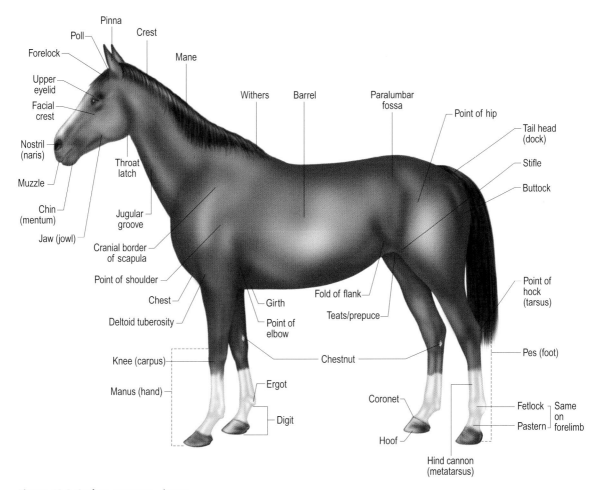

Figure 13.3 Surface anatomy – horse.

Temperature

See Box 13.2 for definitions.

How to take a temperature

1. Source an assistant to restrain the patient
2. Ensure the thermometer is clean
3. Shake the thermometer down and check that mercury is back in the bulb, above the kink
4. Lubricate the thermometer, e.g. with Vaseline, KY jelly, soap or oil
5. Gently ease the thermometer into the rectum with a twisting motion (do not force it)
6. Aim towards the upper surface of the rectum to avoid inserting it into faecal mass
7. Hold it in place for at least 1 minute
8. Remove, wipe, read (holding horizontally and rotate it until you see mercury) or wait for the beep if using a digital version
9. Record the temperature on the animal's record sheet
10. Thermometers should *not* be shared between infectious and non-infectious patients. Thermometers should be disinfected between patients.

Box 13.2

DEFINITIONS

Pyrexia
Above/raised above normal temperature range

Subclinical
Below/lowered from normal temperature range

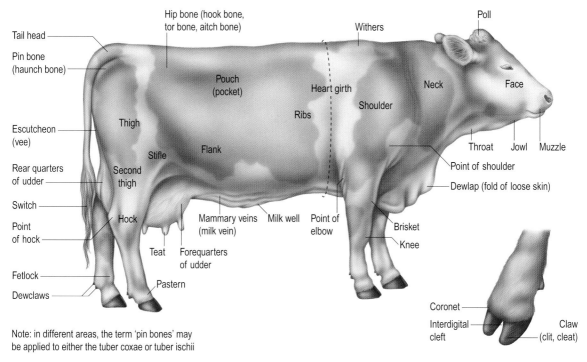

Note: in different areas, the term 'pin bones' may be applied to either the tuber coxae or tuber ischii

Figure 13.4 Surface anatomy – cow.

Table 13.6 Variations in pulse			
Raised/tachycardia	**Lowered/bradycardia**	**Weak**	**Strong and jerky**
Fever	Unconsciousness	Shock	Valvular insufficiency
Exercise	Anaesthesia	Diminished cardiac output	Congenital heart defects
Hypoxia (lack of oxygen)	Debilitating disease		
Pain			
Fear			

Pulse

A pulse is the number of pulsations (expansions) of an artery in 1 minute. Pulse corresponds to the contractions of the left ventricle.

It may be felt at any artery near the body surface. As well as recording the pulse rate, you should be recording the character of the pulse at the same time; this can be thought of as a description of what the pulse is like, e.g. thready or weak. Table 13.6 shows variations in pulse.

How to take a pulse

1. The patient should be restrained
2. Locate artery with fingers

3. Count pulsations for 1 minute
4. Record the rate and character of the pulse.

Suitable pulse sites in dog/cat (Figure 13.5)

- Femoral artery: medial aspect of the femur
- Digital artery: palmar aspect of the carpus
- Coccygeal artery: ventral aspect of base of tail
- Lingual artery: underside of tongue (anaesthetised).

In the horse the pulse is often recorded from the facial artery, located on the underside of the lower jaw bone, or the brachial artery, located just below the knee at the back of the foreleg. The digital pulse may be assessed in laminitis cases (Figure 13.6).

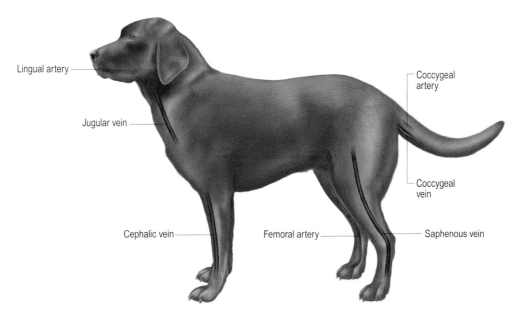

Figure 13.5 Location of major arteries and veins in the dog.

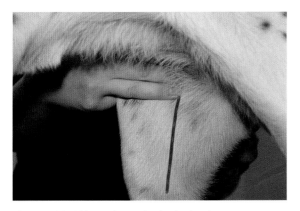

Figure 13.6 Taking a femoral pulse in the dog.

Table 13.7 Variations in respiratory rate		
Increased/ tachypnoea	**Decreased/ bradypnoea**	**Difficulty/ dyspnoea**
Heat	Poison	Inspiratory: obstruction
Exercise	Metabolic acidosis	Expiratory: bronchitis, emphysema
Pain	Sleep	Mixed: pneumonia, pneumothorax, hydrothorax, pyothorax
Poison		

A sinus arrhythmia is a pulse rate that increases on inspiration and decreases on expiration; it can be a normal abnormality in some breeds, for example Thoroughbreds. A pulse deficit describes a pulse rate that is lower than the corresponding heart rate (dysrhythmia).

Respiration

This is assessed by observing the patient or you can gently rest your hands on either side of the animal's thorax to evaluate it.

A respiration rate should be taken with the patient at rest but not asleep, whilst panting, after exercise or when the animal is stressed, as this can give falsely normal readings (Table 13.7).

How to take a respiratory rate

1. Restrain the patient gently
2. Either observe or place your hands on the thorax
3. Count either the inspirations or expirations for 1 minute
4. Assess the character of respiration, e.g. shallow, deep
5. Record on the animal's record.

Remember that the respiration rate is the number of complete breaths per minute; one breath includes inspiration and expiration. Cheyne–Stokes respiration describes alternating periods of very deep, rapid and shallow breathing followed by apnoea and often occurs just before death.

Apnoea is a cessation of breathing.

Evaluation of mucous membranes and capillary refill time

The gingiva (gums) and the membrane on the inside of the eyelids can be used to evaluate the status of the animal's circulatory system. Mucous membrane colour and feel can indicate medical problems and provide vital clues to the animal's condition. The gums are usually the easiest to evaluate by gently lifting the upper lip to observe their colour. A healthy animal should have salmon-pink gums. If the animal is experiencing respiratory problems the colour can vary from blue (cyanotic) to a grey/white colour which would indicate virtually no blood and usually means the animal is close to death. Yellow mucous membranes (icterus) indicate liver or kidney damage and brick red or congested membranes are often observed in poisoning cases. The gums should be moist and if they are tacky to the touch this can indicate some degree of dehydration.

Capillary refill time (CRT) is a simple procedure that can be performed at the same time. Using the forefinger the gum is pressed until it blanches; by applying pressure the finger is pushing the blood out of the capillaries underneath it. The finger is removed and the observer counts how long it takes for the colour to return to the area pressed; this is the time it takes for the capillaries to refill with blood. A normal CRT is 1–2 seconds and the time is increased if the circulatory system is compromised; this can be due to shock, haemorrhage or another condition which has affected the volume of circulating blood or blood pressure. Again, both the colour of mucous membranes and the CRT should be recorded on the patient's notes.

The examination

The health check examination should continue in a systematic manner either from head to tail or vice versa. A handler should restrain the animal, allowing the examiner to perform a thorough evaluation of each part of the body and record all relevant information. The head, body, limbs and tail should be checked for any signs of inflammation, fractures, wounds, haemorrhage, infection, parasites or any other abnormalities. The general position of the limbs should be ascertained to ensure there are no anatomical deformities and mobility should be checked to rule out any lameness. The behaviour of the animal should be considered as this can provide clues that it is in pain or may have neurological symptoms. The evaluation of reflex actions can be a useful tool to check brain function. Common reflexes to check are the papillary reflex, palpebral reflex and pedal reflex. Finally it should be noted if the animal has urinated, defecated, eaten, drunk or vomited. These parameters should be described in detail, giving quantities, frequencies, smells (if any), volume and a description of what they look like. Everything should be recorded on the animal's record with a time and the examiner's initials to enable follow-up as required (Figure 13.7).

Handling and restraint

Animals may require handling for:

- Grooming and bathing
- Examination of an injury, vaccination or illness
- Administration of first aid
- Administration of drugs
- Weekly health checks.

When approaching an animal for handling, you should have knowledge of its body language to enable you to take appropriate actions. Generally approach the animal in a quiet manner with confidence, talking to the animal to reassure it; it sometimes helps to lower yourself to the animal's level. Be patient and avoid trapping animals in small areas or corners where they may feel threatened. It may be necessary to employ restraint equipment to enable handling to occur.

For dogs a lead and collar combined with a calm manner and voice usually suffice. There are many different types of leads and collars available. The handler should check fit of collar, which should allow two fingers within its circumference, and should check clips and fastenings are working.

Other equipment that may be used includes:

- Muzzles: there are many different types: nylon, Baskerville, leather and cat muzzles. Care should be taken to ensure they are fitted correctly and do not damage the eyes of the animal. For animals with short or long skull shapes commercial muzzles designed specifically for these breeds are available (Figure 13.8)
- Dog catcher: a noose and pole which can be used from a distance to catch animals, including wildlife. The noose is then tightened to prevent escape and can be locked in place. A lead or other form of restraint would be used once the animal has been caught
- Cat catcher: similar to the dog catcher, but it has 'claws' at the end which grasp around the cat's neck to restrain it, and then the cat would often be transferred to a basket

Animal details						
Name:		Age:		Sex:		Colour:
Species:				Breed:		
Kennel identification:				Weight:		
Technician name:				Date/time:		

Animal health record		
		Comment
Temperature		
Pulse		
Respiratory rate		
Head		
Eyes		
Ears		
Nose		
Mouth:		
Capillary refill time		
Mucosa/gums		
Teeth		
Skull		

Right foreleg:	Comment	Left foreleg:	Comment
Nails		Nails	
Pads		Pads	
Toes		Toes	
Foot		Foot	
Limb		Limb	

Right hindleg:		Left hindleg:	
Nails		Nails	
Pads		Pads	
Toes		Toes	
Foot		Foot	
Limb		Limb	

Thorax/chest	
Abdomen	
Perineal region	
Tail	
Coat	
Behaviour	
Activity level	
Any other comment e.g. pregnant, overweight etc.	

Figure 13.7 Health check record.

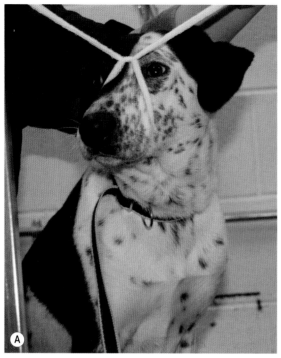

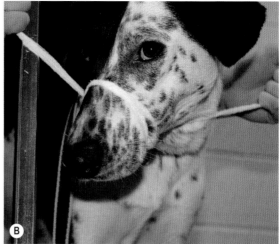

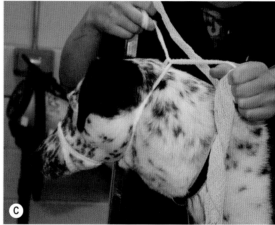

Figure 13.8 (a–c) Applying a tape muzzle.

- Cat bag: a bag designed so the body of the cat is enclosed, allowing procedures to be performed safely; they have the cat's head out and sometimes have a limb hole to facilitate venepuncture
- Crush cage: used for cats, wildlife and small animals. The crush cage is a plastic-coated wire cage which has an inner moveable wall which can be used to squash the animal against one side to prevent movement. The animal is then often injected intramuscularly with sedation to facilitate examination. One end of the crush cage can be lifted so that animals can be released quickly
- Rolled towel: simple but can be effective. The towel is used around the neck to prevent the animal from being able to turn its head and bite the handler
- Blankets/towels: these can be used to enclose the animal by wrapping them around the animal and preventing damage from claws

- Gloves, gauntlets: these are often leather or thick rubber and prevent bites and scratches; they are particularly useful in small animals. However they can be difficult to use for handling as the material is bulky and fine handling is often prohibited by it
- Chemical agents: a number of pharmaceutical agents are available for chemical restraint
- Headcollar: used in large animals, it provides the handler with control of the head, which acts as a lever for where the rest of the body moves
- Twitch: this is a metal or string device that can be applied to the nose of large animals for restraint. The nose is extended and the twitch is applied around it and tightened. The twitch must be held at all times and it is thought it may work by stimulating pressure points in the head to create a relaxed state in the animal

- Physical restraint by an assistant: scruffing the neck and holding behind the ears. A good handler can be an invaluable restraint tool.

Table 13.8 gives guidance on restraint techniques when handling dogs.

Specialist restraint

Examination of dogs

Utilise a non-slip examination area, which is escape-proof. Ensure that all potentially necessary restraint equipment and examination equipment is close to hand. Lift the animal on to the examination table and then restrain it by standing to one side of the animal, then placing the near-side hand around the animal's neck to put it in a secure head lock. The other arm holds the animal's abdomen against the restrainer's body or applies pressure on the dorsal neck region to prevent backwards movement. This is a suitable position for administration of a subcutaneous or intramuscular injection.

Examination – lateral recumbency Utilise a non-slip examination area which is escape-proof. Ensure that all potentially necessary restraint equipment and examination equipment is close to hand. Lateral recumbency examinations are usually performed on the examination room floor. Lower yourself to the side of the animal with your patient standing, place your arms across the back of the animal and grasp the off-side front and rear legs at the level of the tibia and radius. Gently pull the dog's legs upwards and back towards yourself using your knees as support for the animal's body. The dog should roll down the knees on to the floor where it is restrained when you apply downwards pressure to the limbs nearest the floor surface and use your elbows and forearms to hold down the head and body gently.

Jugular blood samples Restrain the patient in a sitting position or in sternal recumbency using an assistant to secure the rump and possibly another to secure the front legs. The first assistant holds the dog's head upright, taking care to hold the mouth shut (alternatively a

Table 13.8 Restraint techniques when handling dogs	
Restraint	**Procedure**
Muzzling	Ensure correct-size muzzle is selected and straps are adjusted to fit the dog Approach from the side or behind the patient Hold the scruff securely behind the ears; an assistant may be required to achieve this Pass the muzzle over the dog's nose and pass straps behind the head and fasten; tighten them to the required length
Applying a tape muzzle	Select an appropriate length of non-conforming bandage to fit around muzzle and the head of dog and allow tying Form a loop with a square knot Use an assistant to restrain the dog Approach from the side and place the loop of the bandage over the dog's nose with the knot at the top Tighten and cross the free ends under the lower jaw of the dog, then pass back under the ears Tie the ends in a quick-release bow around the back of the head
Lifting	Perform a quick survey to ascertain if there are any injuries – if there are, avoid them Grasp the animal around the front and hindlegs, pressing it into your own body to prevent it struggling Lift with your knees bent and your back straight For animals over 20 kg it is a health and safety requirement that another member of staff assists Smaller animals can be tucked under one arm to support the thorax, using your body to support the hindlimbs Larger dogs will require two people to lift – the first person should support the front of the dog whilst restraining the head in an arm lock, while the second person supports the hindquarters and the abdomen Always ensure the head is safely positioned away from your face to prevent the animal biting

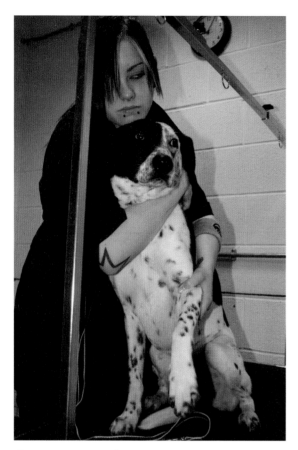

Figure 13.9 Restraint for cephalic venepuncture in the dog.

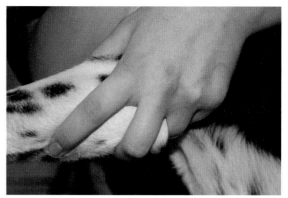

Figure 13.10 Restraint for cephalic venepuncture in the dog.

muzzle can be used) whilst the sample-taker applies pressure to the jugular region to raise the vein and obtains a sample.

Cephalic blood samples Use an assistant to restrain the patient in a sitting position. In active patients another assistant may be required to secure the rump. Ask the assistant to stand behind the animal and use the corresponding arm to the foreleg being sampled to hold the leg aloft. The hand should grasp the foreleg on either side of the point of the elbow with two forefingers at the proximal radius and two fingers at the distal humerus. The thumb is placed over the cranial surface of the foreleg where it applies downwards pressure and is rotated laterally to raise the cephalic vein (Figures 13.9 and 13.10).

Examination of cats

As cats are small animals, usually one person can safely secure a cat for examination. This can be achieved by placing one hand over the animal's thorax with the hand securing the head and neck, whilst the other arm sup-

ports the rear of the cat and holds the body into the handler's chest. If more secure restraint is required hold the cat to your body using one arm whilst simultaneously the hand will secure the animal's forelegs between the fingers to prevent scratching. The other arm and hand is used to restrain the animal's head by placing the thumb upon the caudal skull region, the forefinger on the bridge of the nose and the remaining three fingers are placed under the chin to keep the mouth shut.

Lifting cats There are very few cats which weigh over 20 kg so one person can safely lift a cat. Place one hand over the animal's thorax to support the sternum and use the other arm to support the abdomen by placing it around the side of the cat and holding the animal into the handler's chest (Figure 13.11).

Jugular blood sampling There are a number of methods used for jugular sampling in cats. One method is to hold the animal close to the handler's body, using one arm to restrain the thorax lightly and grasp the forelegs in the fingers (Figure 13.12). The other arm holds the head in extension with the hand grasping the mouth shut at the base of the jaws. Alternatively the sample can be obtained with the handler seated and holding the cat in dorsal recumbency, often enclosed in a towel. The head is extended with one hand whilst the other keeps the body secure. Although both methods can be successful it should be noted that often just raising the cat's head applying minimal restraint is the most successful technique of all.

Cephalic blood samples A very similar method to cephalic sampling in dogs is used (Figures 13.13 and 13.14). The cat is restrained in sternal recumbency with the body held against the handler with one arm, which simultaneously extends the leg to be sampled. The hand is used to raise the vein and prevent thrombophlebitis due to backwards movement during sampling. The other

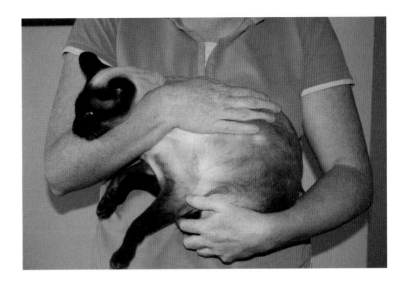

Figure 13.11 Lifting small dogs/cats.

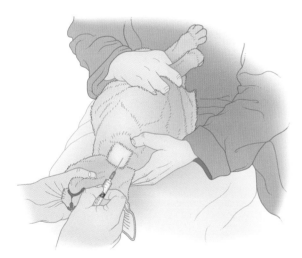

Figure 13.12 Restraint for jugular venepuncture in the cat. (Reproduced from Aspinall V 2006 *The Complete Textbook of Veterinary Nursing*. Butterworth Heinemann, London, with permission.)

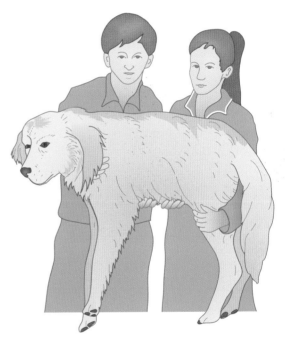

Figure 13.13 Lifting a large dog. (Reproduced from Aspinall V 2006 *The Complete Textbook of Veterinary Nursing*. Butterworth Heinemann, London, with permission.)

arm is used to restrain the head and neck, preventing injury to the person acquiring the sample.

Another problem that can be encountered in cats within the veterinary practice is removing them from their kennels. Often cats are housed with or near other animals, especially dogs, which can cause stress or fear. This can lead to aggression when the veterinary nurse attempts to remove the cat from its kennel. In this situation a towel can be used to cover the cat's head and body; then the cat can be gently scooped out or in extreme cases a cat grasper can be effective. Another method is to use a crush cage by placing it against the kennel entrance with the wire door removed, effectively trapping the cat between the kennel and the crush cage. A towel over the cage will make it more welcoming to the cat and hopefully the cat will enter the crush cage; if not, then gentle persuasion can be employed. Once the cat is in the cage, quickly replace the wire door and secure the animal. Restraint of small mammals and exotics is covered in Chapter 21, restraint of large animals

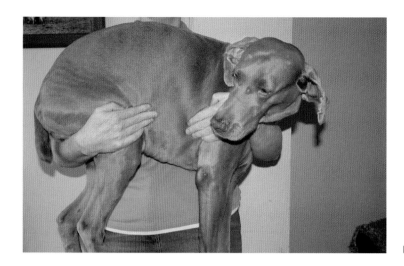

Figure 13.14 Lifting a medium dog.

is covered in Chapter 11 and restraint of horses is the dealt with in Chapter 10.

IDENTIFICATION OF HOSPITALISED PATIENTS

Possessions should be clearly labelled with the pet's name, owner's name and address (Table 13.9, Figures 13.15 and 13.16).

HEALTH AND SAFETY

The health and safety regulations play a vital role in the safe and efficient function of any animal establishment. Employers are responsible for the safety of their employees. This responsibility is written in common and statute laws to protect the rights of the individual. A safe place to work is implied by common law and can be enforced if an employee is injured because the employer has not provided a safe working environment. The main statute law that governs employers and their responsibility to their employees is the Health and Safety at Work Act 1974 (HSAWA).

Common-law health and safety duties

- Employers must take all reasonable and practicable steps to protect the health and safety of their employees
- This means that employers must assess any potential hazards and eliminate them or provide equipment to achieve this aim

- Employers are not required to provide an absolute guarantee that their employees will be safe in the workplace
- Employers are not liable for damage where the risk could not have reasonably been foreseen, e.g. an unexploded bomb was buried under the practice and went off. Another example is if you dispense a drug believing it to be harmless but in the future it is found to cause cancer
- Common-law duty is between each employee and the employer and cannot be transferred to another member of staff, for example by making that person health and safety manager for the company.

Safe premises and equipment

- Employers must provide a safe workplace for employees and visitors to the premises
- Equipment and machinery used must be safe and properly maintained
- Employers must have valid personal injury insurance for their employees under the Employers' Liability (Compulsory Insurance) Act 1966. This should be displayed on the practice premises.

Safe working systems

Employees should have guidelines that govern all aspects of their normal employment role, including:

- Working instructions
- Training
- Supervision
- Protective clothing.

Table 13.9 Monitoring of hospitalised animals

Urine	Volume Colour Smell Blood Frequency Pain Easy/difficult to pass Specific gravity		Water	Quantity consumed Frequency How the animal drinks
			Medication	Drugs being taken Quantity Frequency How taken Administration time
Faeces	Volume Colour Smell Blood Other constituents Frequency Pain Straining		Intravenous fluids	Type Flow rate Route
			Vomit	Nature Volume Smell Contents Frequency
Food	Type Quantity consumed Regurgitated Frequency How the animal eats		Staff details	Important to know who has done what Need to keep record for other staff information

Owner name:	**Case ID number:**
Address:	
Contact number:	
Animal name: Age: Sex: Colour:	
Reason for hospitalisation:	
Veterinary surgeon:	
Delete as necessary: Collar/lead/basket/toys/blanket/food/medication	

Figure 13.15 Information that should be recorded for hospitalised patients.

Owner name:						Case ID number:				
Address:										
Contact number:										
Animal name:		Age:		Sex:		Colour:				
Reason for hospitalisation:										
Veterinary surgeon:										
Delete as necessary:										
Collar/lead/basket/toys/blanket/food/medication										
Time	Urine	Faeces	Food	Water	Medication	Fluids	Vomit	Initials	Others	Comments

Figure 13.16 Hospital record form.

Competent fellow employees

- Employees have the right to expect their coworkers to be competent
- Or employees have the right to expect their coworkers *not* to be incompetent and cause danger in the workplace
- If employees are not fully competent they should only be allowed to perform certain tasks under supervision.

Health and Safety at Work Act 1974

- This is a statute law that reinforces the common law governing employers' responsibility regarding health and safety
- The main difference between common law and statute law is that the employer and employee both have a responsibility, i.e. they form a partnership to cooperate in developing safety at work
- Employers have a statutory duty of care for the health and safety of their employees
- Employees have a statutory responsibility to cooperate with the employer in meeting these obligations
- This is achieved by a written health and safety policy for the premises
- Under HSAWA legislation it is a criminal offence punishable by up to 2 years in prison if there is no written policy for the premises.

Employers have certain duties to workers and visitors to their premises:

- To develop a health and safety policy together with employees or their union representatives
- To provide safe premises, equipment and substances
- To have safe working procedures
- To provide a safe environment
- To advise of any hazards that cannot be avoided
- To prevent the emission of noxious substances, such as clinical waste.

Employees' responsibilities include:

- Taking reasonable care of themselves, their fellow workers and the public
- Helping the employer by following health and safety legislation, i.e. health and safety procedures that have been implemented in the workplace.

There is a special section of the HSAWA governing employees who work with animals in the course of their employment. Each regulation is supported by a code of practice.

Health and safety arrangements

- This covers the plans, controls and reviews of health and safety in the workplace
- Individuals must be appointed with responsibility for health and safety
- Emergency procedures must be set up and all staff provided with information about any potential hazards and how to prevent them
- A formal record must be made of all accidents (which must be analysed occasionally) – this is the accident record book
- Staff are required to warn employers of any health and safety problems
- The employer must ensure that staff are sufficiently well trained not to put themselves or others at risk
- Employees are expected to follow any health and safety instructions.

Risk assessment

- Employers are required to carry out formal risk assessments on every aspect of their work
- Therefore all potential hazards should be identified
- Each hazard is then analysed to evaluate its severity if it were to happen.

Health surveillance

- Where hazards have been identified during risk assessments, e.g. exposure to radiation, the employer should arrange medical check-ups for the employees
- Employees should inform the employer of any reactions to drugs and chemicals.

Provision and use of work equipment

- Equipment use in the workplace should be safe
- This is achieved through annual testing and protective devices
- Proper training and operator instructions and procedures must be followed
- Arrangements must be in place to ensure safe disposal of used equipment, e.g. glass and needles.

Manual handling

- Lots of injuries in the workplace arise from improper lifting
- Employers are required to set up systems that minimise injury to their employees

- Employees are required to use the equipment provided by their employer
- The maximum weight one person can lift is 20 kg, but this does vary according to the load and the relationship of where it is compared to the lifter's body.

Personal protective equipment at work

Employers must provide their staff with approved personal protective equipment (PPE) to protect them from risks such as infection from secretions, zoonotic diseases and hazardous substances. Examples include uniforms, gloves, hard hats, masks, aprons and goggles.

Control of Substances Hazardous to Health (COSHH) regulations 1999/2002

COSHH regulations are designed to protect employees from the risks of working with hazardous substances. Substances that are classed as hazardous to health will harm people, e.g. cause allergies, burns, poisoning. The most dangerous substances are classed under schedule 1 in the chemicals regulations as toxic, corrosive and irritant. A system of labelling has been implemented to help identify potential risks to the employee. Employers and employees need to carry out full risk assessments for all substances that may be hazards and when a hazardous substance has been bought it will come with a datasheet or the manufacturer should be asked to provide one. The precautions that need to be implemented should be defined to employees, e.g. protective clothing must be worn, and employees must follow precautions. If they do not, this is a disciplinary offence. Employers must monitor employees' exposure to hazards and carry out health surveillance. All staff should be trained to understand the risks and precautions in order to minimise them. All staff should be aware of the datasheets and their relevance and should be involved with developing safety procedures.

Waste disposal/clinical waste

Waste disposal is governed by the Hazardous Waste Regulations 2007. It is the legal responsibility of the employer to develop a system for safe waste disposal and to train all employees to follow this system. Waste from veterinary practices, commercial boarding kennels, commercial breeders and animal businesses would be classified as industrial waste. The industrial waste produced from these premises would be further differentiated into clinical waste. It is a legal requirement that a specifically designated area – a refrigerated room or freezer – has

been allocated for storage of clinical waste. The area must be of a suitable volume to hold the quantity and suitable for the type of waste stored there.

Hazardous Waste Regulations 2007

These were designed to reflect changes in disposal methods of waste, e.g. landfill sites and incineration. They have implemented a revised colour-coded system for the segregation of health care waste and additional waste streams such as offensive waste.

Disposal should be by an approved collector and there is a colour coding system for waste disposal:

- Black bags are collected by the local council and disposed of in landfill
- Tiger bags (yellow with black stripes) are disposed of in landfill (offensive waste)
- Sharps container: collection by a licensed waste disposal agency is permitted, disposed of in an incinerated facility
- Yellow limb bin (to be stored in the freezer) for all body parts – licensed/permitted, disposed of in an incineration facility
- Yellow rigid container – licensed/permitted, disposed of by incineration
- Orange bag (infectious) – licensed/permitted treatment facility and then landfill once hazard has been treated
- Yellow bag (infectious)– marked for incineration: hazardous waste incineration
- Yellow (infectious) and purple (cytotoxic) – sharps container/bags/rigid containers: hazardous waste – incineration
- Leak-proof containers/drums: licensed permitted facility.

Previous categories of clinical waste still apply, but these should now separate out the different categories of waste, e.g. a clinical waste bin for infectious material and one for non-infectious material.

Categories of clinical waste

- Group A: includes the following items: identifiable human tissue, blood, animal carcasses and tissue from veterinary centres, hospital or laboratories. Soiled surgical dressings, swabs and other similar soiled waste. Also other waste materials, for example from infectious disease cases, excluding any in groups B–E
- Group B: discarded syringe needles, cartridges, broken glass and any other contaminated disposable sharp instruments or items
- Group C: microbiological cultures and potentially infected waste from pathology departments and other clinical or research laboratories

- Group D: drugs or other pharmaceutical products
- Group E: items used to dispose of urine, faeces and other bodily secretions or excretions which do not fall within group A. This includes used disposable bedpans or bedpan liners, incontinence pads, stoma bags and urine containers where there is *no* risk of blood contamination.

Note: offensive waste includes dressings, plaster, casts, linen, disposable clothing which is non-infectious.

Special clinical waste containers should:

- Have a UN-type 3291 number that will specify what kind of waste it should contain
- Have a UN testing number which will show what type of waste the containers can withstand and/or weight they can hold
- Be denoted by being bright yellow or another specifically allocated colour
- State on the outside: 'Clinical waste for incineration only'.

It is illegal to put the wrong kind of waste into the wrong UN-type container. It is advised that only containers and bags stamped with a UN-type number should be used for the disposal of clinical waste, even if they are yellow.

Cadavers

- A cadaver is a dead body
- Veterinary surgeons have no legal obligation to dispose of cadavers
- This is because the owner owns the animal in law, regardless of whether it is alive or dead
- Exceptions are wildlife and euthanased strays
- Cadavers may be disposed of in several ways:
  - ○ Collection by local authority
  - ○ Commercial disposal companies licensed for this procedure
  - ○ Individually arranged – cremation/burial
- Under the Animal Health Act veterinary practices must inform the Department for Environment, Food and Rural Affairs (DEFRA) if they treat animals suffering from a notifiable disease; then disposal of cadavers is DEFRA's responsibility.

Maintenance of the hospital facilities

See Box 13.3 for definitions.

Transmission of infections requires:

- Source of pathogens
- A susceptible host
- Means of transmission for the microorganism.

> **Box 13.3**
>
> ### DEFINITIONS
>
> #### Contagious disease
> Disease that is capable of being transmitted by direct contact or indirect contact from one animal to another
>
> #### Incubation period
> The interval of time between the animal coming into contact with a microorganism and the development of the clinical signs of the disease
>
> #### Infectious disease
> Disease caused by microorganisms or microbes, e.g. Salmonella
>
> #### Non-infectious disease
> Disease not caused by microorganisms, e.g. diabetes

When considering how a microorganism has passed to an animal you have to establish:

- The routes by which an organism may have left an animal
- The routes of transmission from one animal to another
- The routes of entry into the new host.

Pathogens may be transmitted via:
- Direct contact:
  - ○ Blood
  - ○ Body fluids
  - ○ Faeces
  - ○ Urine
  - ○ Contact with clinically ill animals
  - ○ Contact with asymptomatic carriers of an infectious agent
- Indirect contact:
  - ○ Objects in the environment
  - ○ Walls, floors, doors, veterinary equipment, mucking-out equipment, feed bowls, animal feed, water or personnel.

Host resistance to microorganisms varies greatly. Host factors can affect clinical presentation, including:

- Age
- Underlying disease
- Irradiation
- Pregnancy
- Break in the body's first line of defence (intact skin, cough reflex, stomach acid), which increases susceptibility
- Vaccination
- Virulence of the microorganism.

Transmission mechanisms

There are three main mechanisms:

1. Contact: ingestion, mucous membrane exposure, cutaneous or percutaneous exposure
2. Aerosol: via air, inhalation and/or mucous membranes, coughing, sneezing, vocalising, suction, bronchoscopy
3. Vector-borne: mosquitoes, ticks, rats, humans and other animals.

Agents may be transmitted by more than one route. Transmission is affected by:

- Stability of the pathogen (labile)
- Pathogenesis of the disease
- Routes it leaves the infected host.

At this point it worth remembering that the incubation period for any disease will depend upon:

- The dose of microorganisms
- Immune status of animal
- General health of animal
- Age of animal
- Route of entry.

METHODS USED TO CONTROL INFECTION

From studying diseases we have learnt how certain microorganisms spread infection which in turn has given us ideas on how to prevent them spreading. These include:

- Avoid direct contact, i.e. isolation/quarantine
- Very high hygiene levels of animals and fomites
- Housing – reducing numbers in an area and ensuring good air movement
- Early and effective treatment
- Routine vaccination/control
- Strict import controls into the country.

Factors to consider when implementing infection controls:

- Routes of transmission
- Aetiology, epidemiology and lability in the environment of microorganisms
- Suitability of disinfectants:
  - Agent effective against pathogen
  - Dilution rates
  - Contact times
  - Organic matter
- Barrier nursing
- Isolation facilities

- Isolation equipment: clinical and mucking out, allocate to cases
- Vaccination status
- Carrier status
- Isolate all suspects
- Staff training and education
- PPE
- Practice protocols
- Routine: clean healthy animals first
- Appropriate disposal of waste, including bedding and faeces
- Clear identification of animals
- Wearing PPE for cleaning, feeding, clinical and medical procedures
- Intake: separate potential infectious cases
- Risk assessments for common infectious agents.

Protective actions for staff

- Hand hygiene
- Use of gloves and sleeves
- Facial protection
- Use of gowns, overalls, aprons
- Footwear
- Head covers
- Protocols.

Routine hygiene

All animal housing facilities should have strict hygiene protocols and these are often translated to instruction lists or schedules of work which clearly inform staff members on what cleaning protocols are in place. Schedules of work should exist to determine the order of cleaning, how to clean housing, animals, feeding utensils, use of disinfectants and to identify good practice between animals. Cleaning should occur in a logical order with the least contaminated area cleaned first. Ideally different areas will have their own equipment allocated for cleaning and feeding and perhaps different staff members. All staff should wash their hands between patients and if alcohol gels are utilised then hand washing should still occur at a frequency of every five patients. A typical cleaning regime for areas of the business should involve sweeping or vacuuming up debris, including moving furniture, cleaning with a detergent to remove organic waste, rinsing then disinfecting with a suitable product at the correct dilution which is left in situ for the correct contact time, then rinsed and dried. Animal accommodation should be cleaned at least twice a day and as required in between periods; gross contamination and bedding should be removed; the accommodation cleaned, disinfected, rinsed and dried before fresh bedding is put in place. All bowls and buckets should be scrubbed, disinfected, rinsed and dried before reuse with the same ones kept with a patient for the duration of its stay. Areas such as reception, door handles and walls should not be neglected as these often accumulate pathogens from the normal passage of clients and staff members. More thorough weekly and monthly cleaning protocols that instruct staff on a deep clean should also be in place.

Isolation

Strict controls should be in place in the isolation facility as it will house animals which are infectious or contagious or potentially so. There should be a limit to who can enter the facility and there must be strict controls between animals, i.e. no direct contact and no indirect contact. Barrier nursing should be employed by designated staff members and there must be high standards of hygiene, including designated equipment, PPE and disinfectant footbaths at entrances and exits. All barrier cases should be nursed independently and all food utensils and bedding should be treated independently. All waste should be disposed of in clinical waste as infectious material and disinfectants employed should be used at an appropriate dilution for the case (usually higher). Staff should wear an apron, gloves and mask and remove them before contact with their next patient. They should already be washing thoroughly between all patients but it is even more important for these cases.

HOUSING REQUIREMENTS OF ANIMALS

Construction of housing

When building or designing accommodation suitable to house cats and dogs, it is important to consider a number of factors. These include:

- Species/breed
- Purpose
- Budget
- Location
- Noise pollution
- Access
- Exercise facilities
- Size of units
- Ventilation
- Heating
- Cleaning
- Safety regimes
- Lighting
- Toilet/staff facilities
- Disposal of waste.

Other factors that require consideration when designing housing for individual animals include:

- Size
- Strength
- Temperament
- Breed.

Buildings must be built to building regulation standards. Planning permission may need to be obtained from the local planning office for damp-proofing, insulation and ventilation. Tables 13.10 and 13.11 provide checklists of construction standards and materials).

Table 13.10 Construction standards	
Interiors	All surfaces should be waterproof to allow cleaning and disinfection
Flooring	Should be made of impervious material (so that liquid cannot soak into it)
Walls	Should be solid to a height of 1200 mm (1.2 metres) between kennel units Should be solid to a height of 1800 mm (1.8 metres) between cattery units Materials used should be impervious or painted to waterproof to at least 1.2 metres in height Good idea to curve where the floor meets the walls – this prevents accumulation of dirt and therefore disease If not curved, all joints should be sealed with waterproof grouting
Drainage	Floors should be sloped to allow a fall of 1 in 80 (making a slight slope), which drains water/urine into a drainage channel
Wire	Catteries – use weldmesh at a minimum of 16-mm gauge to a maximum of 25-mm (size of holes prevents escapees/trapped paws) Kennels – use metal bars and frames with 10–12-mm spacings
Doors	Must be strong enough to resist impact and scratching Should be able to be secured effectively Should open inwards to secure corridor
Windows	Must be escape-proof at all times If they need to be opened for ventilation then wire mesh/fly screens should be fitted

Table 13.11 Construction materials

Material	Comfort	Hygiene	Strength/durability	Relative cost
Concrete	Cold	Easy to scrub or hose Cracks may harbour bacteria/parasites	Excellent – especially for dogs, destructive mammals, birds	Cheap
Bricks/breeze blocks	Cold	Easy to scrub or hose Cracks may harbour bacteria/parasites	Excellent – especially for dogs, destructive mammals, birds	Expensive
Wood	Warm	Difficult to clean and slow to dry Cracks may harbour bacteria/parasites	Easily destroyed by chewing or scratching	Average
Stainless steel	Cold	Easy to clean and disinfect Small cages can be sterilised	Excellent – especially for dogs, destructive mammals, birds	Expensive
Galvanised steel	Cold	Reasonably easy to clean unless it gets rust spots	Excellent – especially for dogs, destructive mammals, birds Rust spots can develop if cracked or drilled	Average
Fibreglass	Cold unless indoors	Easy to clean and disinfect	Good for small or non-destructive mammals	Average
Polypropylene	Cold unless indoors	Easy to clean and disinfect Small cages can even be sterilised	Good for small or non-destructive mammals	Average
Plastic	Cold unless indoors	Easy to clean and disinfect	Good for small or non-destructive mammals	Cheap
Glass	Cold unless indoors	Easy to clean and disinfect	Good for small or non-destructive mammals	Cheap

Environmental factors

Environmental factors that require consideration are:

- Ventilation
- Humidity
- Noise
- Heating (Table 13.12)
- Lighting.

These should be considered for all species and for internal and external accommodation.

Ventilation is necessary to:

- Ensure there is an adequate supply of oxygen
- Remove stale air
- Prevent respiratory ailments

- Reduce the spread of airborne infection
- Remove unpleasant odours
- Prevent excessive temperature.

The ventilation rate is how often the air within a building or room is changed per hour. This should be at least six changes of air per hour and in hot weather this should be doubled to 12 changes per hour.

There are two types of ventilation:

1. Passive – windows, open doors, adjustable vents
2. Active – fans, ventilation systems.

Heating is necessary to:

- Provide a comfortable environment for animals
- Reduce risk of frost damage to building
- Reduce drying time after cleaning for units.

Table 13.12 Different heating systems			
System	**Advantages**	**Potential problems**	**Safety considerations**
Hot-water/oil central heating	Clean, safe and easily controlled	May need to use extra heat in some cases	
Underfloor heating – water/oil-powered	Clean Animals benefit from heated floor	Expensive to repair Can make cleaning difficult Needs to be suitable ambient temperature	
Underfloor heating – electric-powered	Clean Animals benefit from heated floor	Expensive to repair Can make cleaning difficult Needs to be suitable ambient temperature	
Individual electric fan heaters	Can be controlled individually Heat can be directed towards animals	Noisy Encourages spread of infection Can cause overheating in animals	Small fire risk Cables can be chewed Should be waterproofed
Infrared dull emitter lamp	Good source of localised heat Controlled by adjusting distance of lamp from animal	Can cause overheating and burns No thermostatic control	Cables can be chewed Needs to be waterproofed
Electric oil-filled radiators	Clean, mobile	Surface temperature can burn animals and staff	Cables can be chewed Needs to be waterproofed

Temperature range

Healthy dogs and cats in boarding establishments:

- Sleeping area: 10–26°C
- Exercise area: same as local environment, i.e. outside.

Healthy dogs and cats in breeding establishments:

- Parturition area: 10–21°C
- Neonates (newborns): 26–29°C.

Hospitalised dogs and cats:

- Hospital cage: 18–23°C.

Large animals can withstand lower temperatures and small mammals generally require higher temperature ranges more in line with neonate values. Reptiles' and amphibians' temperature requirements vary, although they are generally higher and some form of lighting to provide heat is required.

Requirements of accommodation

Food preparation area

- Should have separate area for kennels and cattery
- Should be close for convenience
- Should be large enough to store utensils and food
- Should have a water supply/sinks/washing facilities
- Should be rodent-proof
- Should have fridge/freezer for storage.

Bedding

Bedding provides warmth, security and comfort to the animal. Bedding areas are often raised and many types of bed are available, e.g. bean bags, plastic moulded beds (Tables 13.13 and 13.14).

Table 13.13 Bedding materials for dogs and cats

Bedding	Comfort	Insulation	Absorbency	Wash/dry	Harbours parasites	Cost	Comments
Acrylic bedding/ synthetic fleece/vetbed	Reasonable for the healthy animal	Reasonable	Very good: urine soaks through	Easy care	No	Expensive initially but lasts a long time	More durable than most bedding material
Beanbags – filled with polystyrene balls	Excellent: conform (mould) to body shape	Excellent	Easily saturated	Difficult to wash and dry	Not easily	Expensive	Easily destroyed/ flatten with time
Foam-filled wedges	Excellent: conform (mould) to body shape	Excellent	Easily saturated	Difficult to wash/dry	When new no, but if damaged, yes	Good value	Easy to destroy
Duvets	Excellent: thick and mould to animal	Excellent	Easily saturated	Easy to wash in machine but take a long time to dry naturally	Potentially	Expensive	Easy to destroy
Blankets	Reasonable for healthy animals. May need several layers	Good if several layers are used	Easily saturated	Easy to wash in machine but take a long time to dry naturally	Potentially	Expensive	Easy to destroy
Towelling	Reasonable for healthy animals. May need several layers	Reasonable if several layers used	Easily saturated	Easy to wash in machine but take a long time to dry naturally	Potentially	Good value	Easy to destroy

Table 13.14 Bedding materials for small pets

Bedding	Comfort	Insulation	Absorbency	Disposable	Harbours parasites	Cost	Comments
Shredded paper	Good	Reasonable	Good (office paper not as good)	Yes	Not if changed daily	Usually free	Make sure staples are removed!
Straw	Excellent	Excellent	Not very good	Yes	Yes	Relatively expensive in small amounts	Can contain Aspergillus (mould) which may cause respiratory problems
Hay	Excellent	Excellent	Not very good	Yes	Yes	Relatively expensive in small amounts	Can contain Aspergillus (mould) which may cause respiratory problems
Acrylic/ nylon wadding	Excellent	Excellent	Not very good	Yes	No	Relatively expensive in small amounts	Can easily wrap around limbs and cut off blood supply
Polystyrene chips or balls	Reasonable	Excellent	Not very good	Yes	No	Can be free of charge	Some rodents may eat it, causing blockages

When considering what type of bedding to use you should think about:

- Species
- Weight
- Size
- Health.

Remember that all animals should be able to lie flat and turn around fully.

Emotional requirements

Remember that animals require mental stimulation and physical comfort.

Toys such as Kongs and scratching posts can prove invaluable aids to the well-being of a kennelled animal, providing environmental enrichment.

Toilet facilities

There has to be some provision for dogs and cats to urinate and defecate.

Dogs

Most will be house-trained so it is likely they will be uncomfortable about soiling their kennel. They should be taken to a toilet area at regular intervals; some may need to be let off the lead, so the area should be secure.

Cats

Cats must be provided with a clean litter tray which should be regularly cleaned and located away from their food. It is important that their usual type of cat litter is used as cats can be quite fussy about their toilet arrangements. If the cat is used to going outside then soil in the litter tray may be a successful substrate choice.

PROVISION OF EXERCISE

Benefits of exercise for kennelled animals include:

- Maintaining health and fitness
- Builds muscle

- Mental stimulation
- Play
- Weight control
- Builds owner–animal bond
- Gets owner fit!

Factors that can affect the amount of exercise provided:

- Age
- Breed
- Working/domestic status
- Health status
- Fitness
- Pregnancy/lactation
- Time available
- Location
- Safety
- Number of animals
- Sex of animals
- Temperament of animals.

Housing requirements of small mammals are considered in Chapter 21.

THE FIVE FREEDOMS/KEY NEEDS AND ANIMAL ACCOMMODATION

The design of accommodation will depend entirely on the purpose of its use. There are a few basic essentials that all of the above should have which will ensure the five animal needs are met.

Warmth, comfort and security

- Temperature should not drop below 7 °C
- Housing should be dry and draught-free
- Suitable bedding should be provided
- A darker area should be provided for sleep, especially for cats.

Mental stimulation and company

- The company of humans is essential – most of these animals are, have been or will become family pets
- The company of other animals will depend on the type of kennel and the individual situation
- Stimulation of smell, sight, sound, touch will help stop boredom and any associated problems.

Exercise

- This will depend on the age, health and individual breed of the animals
- In general dogs are easier to handle when regularly exercised

- Cats should also be given the opportunity to exercise by providing them with toys, different levels and scratching posts
- Large animals may require access to a paddock area.

Protection from disease and injury

- The housing must be unchewable with no sharp objects
- To stop the spread of infection it must be hygienic and easy to clean
- The accommodation should have its own health care policy detailing how the animals are to be kept healthy, e.g. vaccinations, worming.

Protection from fear and distress

- Usually dogs and cats are happier if they are housed away from each other
- Some individual animals may require specific housing to prevent them becoming stressed
- Large animals may be happier if housed with company, although care should be taken to avoid injury. Using pens, paddocks or stables where the animals can observe each other can be a safe alternative to housing them together.

Appropriate feeding

- Fresh drinking water should always be supplied
- Diets should not be changed from the animals' normal ones unless necessary.

Urination/defecation provision

- Both grass and a hard area should be provided and cleared up immediately
- Cats should always have a litter tray.

MAINTENANCE OF ANIMAL ACCOMMODATION

Procedures/protocols

All businesses should have designated procedures and protocols for:

- Cleaning
- Security
- Repairs
- Informing relevant persons of problems and faulty equipment.

Allocation of roles

Normally designated staff will be responsible for designated areas of a business, e.g. in a veterinary surgery the student nurses would report a faulty kennel door to their head nurse who may be responsible for arranging repairs or who may then report it to the supervisor.

If there is a problem or fault with any equipment the person who discovers it should:

- Report it to the appropriate person
- Attach/secure a label on the equipment to identify to all other users that it is faulty.

Bibliography

Aspinall V 2006 The complete textbook of veterinary nursing. Butterworth Heinemann, London

Broonan S, Legge D 1999 Law relating to animals. Cavendish, Jordan, London

Colville T, Bassett J M 2002 Clinical anatomy and physiology for veterinary technicians. Mosby, St Louis

Dallas S 2006 Animal biology and care, 2nd edn. Wiley/Blackwell, Oxford

Lane D R, Cooper B, Turner L 2007 BSAVA Textbook of Veterinary Nursing. BSAVA, Oxford

McBride D 1996 Learning veterinary terminology. C V Mosby, St Louis

Moore M 2000 Manual of veterinary nursing. BSAVA, Oxford

Pratt P W 1998 Principles and practice of veterinary technology. Mosby, Philadelphia

Simpson G 1994 Practical veterinary nursing, 3rd edn. BSAVA, Oxford

Warren D M 1995 Small animal care and management. Delmar Learning, New York

Chapter | **14** | *Jane Williams*

Principles of animal behaviour

This chapter provides a succinct introduction to a range of animal behaviour principles which can be applied to companion, domestic and wild animal species to attempt to interpret their behaviour. Ethograms are considered as a method of observing animal behaviour for research projects.

GENERAL CONCEPTS OF BEHAVIOUR

There are two kinds of behaviour – innate and learnt.

Innate behaviour

There are three major groups of innate behaviour (Figure 14.1):

1. Orientation
2. Simple reflexes
3. Instincts.

Orientation

Orientation is when an animal instinctively moves the whole of its body in response to stimuli from its surroundings (environment).

Orientation has much in common with reflex action. It is important in the natural environment as it enables organisms to move towards desirable stimuli and away from harmful ones.

There are two types of orientation behaviour:

1. Kinesis: a change in the speed of random movement in response to an environmental stimulus
2. Taxis: a directed movement toward or away from a stimulus: there are positive and negative taxes.

Simple reflexes

These are involuntary (out of the animal's control), short-lived, stereotypic (constant) responses to a given stimulus. Nervous action is restricted to the spinal cord. Where the response involves movement it happens so quickly that there is no time to modify the response (memory cannot change what is happening).

There are two types of reflex:

1. Flexion
2. Extension or stretch.

Instincts

Instincts are patterns of inherited, pre-set, stereotypic behavioural responses. Instincts develop in conjunction

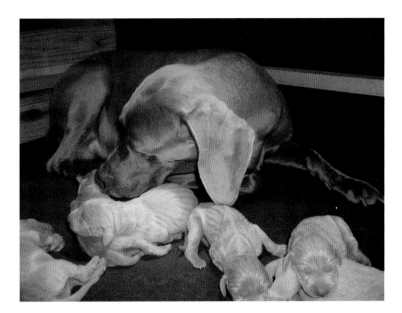

Figure 14.1 Maternal behaviour: an example of innate behaviour.

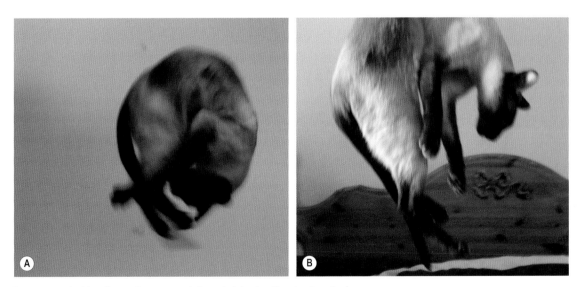

Figure 14.2 (a, b) Reflex action – a cat falls and rights itself to land on its feet.

(at the same time) with the nervous system. They do not require learning or practice to achieve successfully. They can be modified due to experience (Figure 14.2). Not all instincts are present at birth but they develop in conjunction with maturation of the nervous system.

BIOLOGICAL RHYTHMS

This is an 'internal clock' that determines when animals perform certain behaviours.

Most plants and animals are locked into a 24–28-hour biological clock or cycle, known as the circadian rhythm.

- Biological clocks are important for animals in extreme environments, e.g. deserts, for the following reasons:
  - Hibernation: the drive to reduce energy levels to survive a period of hardship
  - Migration: the drive to relocate to gather energy due to impending hardship or breeding cycles
- Bees use biological clocks to find food and follow the sun's movement to locate their hive.

Territorial behaviour

Animals instinctively desire their own territory if they are a species that is territorial. Territorial animals do not have to think about when they leave for their own home, or when they should find a mate or where the territory should be located – it is determined instinctively.

Territorial behaviour can be:

- Conflictive, involving fighting which is restrained or ritualised or unrestrained (physical contact/fighting)
- Most animals exhibit ritualised displays
- Size of territory depends upon:
  - Number of animals that inhabit it, e.g. single or groups
  - Resources it contains, e.g. water, food, shelter
- Territory needs to be of a sufficient size to support the group/individual and be successfully defended against intruders
- Territories benefit animals and are defended in many ways, e.g.:
  - Humming bird
  - Sticklebacks
  - Ants
  - Baboons
  - Dogs
  - Giraffes
  - Peacocks.

Learnt behaviour

There are seven major types of learnt behaviour:

1. Habituation
2. Exploratory behaviour or latent learning
3. Observational learning
4. Imprinting
5. Trial-and-error learning
6. Classical conditioning
7. Insight.

Animals exist through both innate behaviour (not learnt) and learnt behaviour.

Why do they need learnt behaviour?

The environment we live in is constantly changing. At present we are the top predator, but imagine if aliens invaded and started killing humans. As animals we would have to learn from our experiences and those of others to enable us to survive. Animals learn from exploring their environment, watching their parents and siblings and watching other animals.

Habituation

When animals are subjected to repetitive stimuli they gradually cease to respond if the stimulus does not produce a harmful reaction. This saves valuable energy in the natural environment.

Often the initial stimulus would be fear-inducing, for example:

- Horses may be scared of umbrellas
- Crows may be scared of a scarecrow.

Exploratory behaviour/latent learning

This type of learning happens by accident and so is considered 'hidden' learning.

Animals explore areas of their environment when there is no direct need or reward (i.e. there is an absence of reinforcement) but to gain information for a later date. For example, it would be advantageous for a rabbit to know possible escape routes around its warren before it met a fox. In the early 20th century a scientist, Tolman, studied this behavioural phenomenon using rats and a prefabricated maze. The study is described below.

Method of Tolman's study

- The maze had two arms which the rat could not see until it reached X or Y. One box was white and the other was black
- In experiment 1, both boxes contained food
- In experiment 2, the white box A contained food, but box B gave the rat an electric shock
- In experiment 3, both boxes contained food again.

What do you think happened?

The rats learnt to go to box A and to avoid box B, even when both boxes contained food.

Observational learning

Young animals usually observe their parents and copy their behaviour, e.g. sheep which are hand-reared with no contact with adult sheep won't eat grass and may starve at weaning. Animals can also copy from other animals in their social group, siblings or in their environment. Practice is usually needed to refine skills. Traits are not inherited but the ability to learn is.

Imprinting

When animals are born they fit into one of two categories depending on their development:

- Precocial animals: born with their eyes and ears open, and able to run within a few hours of birth
- Altricial animals: born with their eyes and ears closed and the nervous system not fully developed; normally born within dens where they continue to mature.

Young animals, especially precocial ones, associate and identify with their parent/s. This process is known as imprinting. It can affect a wide range of behaviour, particularly if the first object with which the animal associates is not its mother. Scientific studies in imprinting were carried out by Konrad Lorenz on geese. Lorenz demonstrated imprinting to humans, cardboard boxes and tractors. His studies showed filial imprinting:

- Was a period of rapid learning
- Occurred within the first 8–12 hours.

There is a second kind of imprinting, sexual imprinting, which is a longer process occurring from several weeks of age until maturity or adulthood is reached. Sexual maturity 'shows' an animal what species it should mate with.

Both kinds of imprinting are irreversible once established.

Trial-and-error learning

Trial-and-error learning is also known as:

- Operant conditioning
- Instrumental conditioning.

This aspect of behaviour was studied using a Skinner box, named after the scientist who invented it. A Skinner box is a problem box where the animal has to solve the puzzle through trial-and-error learning, e.g. a lever has to be pressed, then a food reward will be given. An animal's spontaneously generated behaviour is instrumental in obtaining a reward. Animals learn by association and link the reward to the stimulus.

Classical conditioning

This is classic learning by association and was first advocated by a Russian scientist, Ivan Pavlov. Pavlov was studying how much saliva dogs produced when presented with food and started to think about associations. He rang a bell when he fed the dogs; eventually just ringing the bell made the dogs salivate (Figure 14.3).

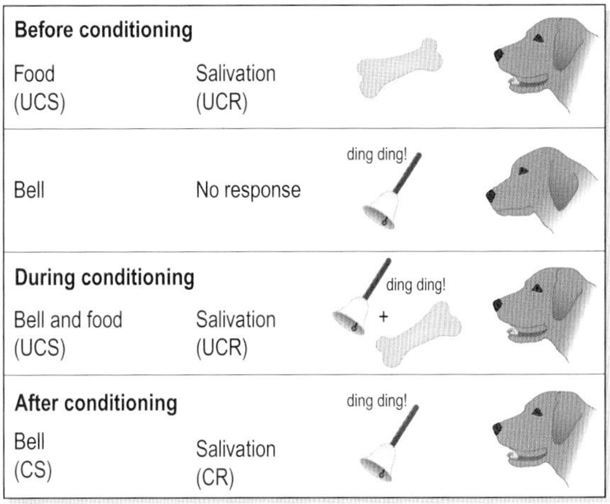

Figure 14.3 Classical conditioning. UCS, unconditioned stimulus (food) (the UCS is also referred to as the reinforcer); UCR, unconditioned response (salivation to food); CS, conditioned stimulus (bell); CR, conditioned response (salivation to bell).

Insight

This is the highest form of learning and the most difficult to interpret. It is also known as problem-solving. Learning is based on information previously learnt by other behavioural activities.

Studies in this field were completed by Kohler, a German scientist, using chimps. He put the chimps in a room with bananas hanging from the ceiling and boxes and left them, observing to see if they could figure the problem out.

ETHOLOGY VERSUS EXPERIMENTAL PSYCHOLOGY

Ethology

- Natural environment
- Design and mechanism of behaviour (Figure 14.4).

Experimental psychology

- Unnatural environment
- Mechanism of behaviour (Figure 14.5).

Evolutionary behaviourists

- Functional accounts of behaviour/design.

The founders of modern ethology are considered to be Konrad Lorenz and Niko Tinbergen. Both laid the foundations of modern ethology and how behaviour is

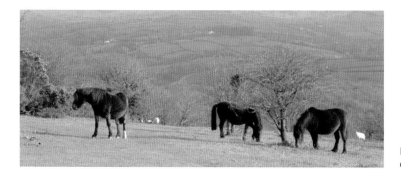

Figure 14.4 Ethology study – observing equids in their natural environment.

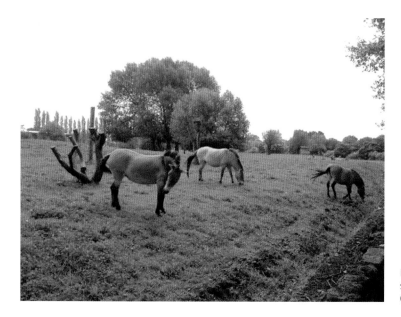

Figure 14.5 Experimental psychology study – observing equids in captivity (zoo).

studied and evaluated. Both advocated the importance of straightforward observation of animal behaviour under natural conditions. Lorenz explored the concepts of instinct and imprinting: he produced numerous theories in these areas which have had a great influence on his field. Tinbergen was an exceptional field biologist whose work surrounded numerous observations in the natural environment and subsequent papers. Tinbergen is probably most noted for his four questions which ascertain why an animal behaves in a certain way.

Tinbergen's questions

What is the causal explanation?

This looks at the causes of behaviour – external (environment) and internal (chemical levels in the body) (Figure 14.6a).

What is the developmental explanation?

How has the behaviour developed in the animal? Was it always present in the animal or was it learnt (Figure 14.6b)?

What is the functional explanation?

What is the purpose of the behaviour? How does it affect the survival and reproduction of the animal?

What is the evolutionary explanation?

Like other traits, a large proportion of an animal's behaviour is inherited, and evolved from an earlier ancestor – so is this current behaviour inherited?

These four questions effectively try and evaluate the animal's motivation for specific behaviours. Lorenz went

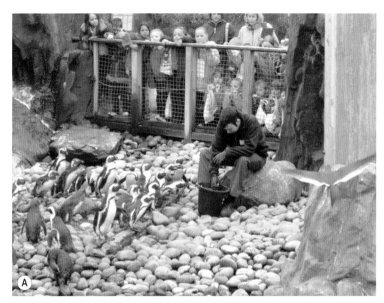

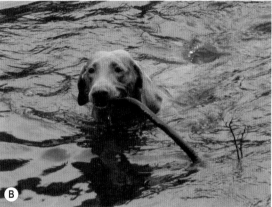

Figure 14.6 (a) Consider Tinbergen's questions: what are the motivation and explanation for the penguins' behaviour? A causal explanation could be captive breeding and hunger drivers. (b) What is the motivation for this gundog to swim and retrieve? Is it genetics or learnt behaviour?

on to develop a psychohydraulic model for motivation. This theorises that causal factors must accumulate to motivate an animal to perform a behaviour.

Ethologists are concerned with:

- Identifying and describing species-specific behaviours under natural conditions
- Understanding evolutionary pathways through which the genetic basis for behaviour came about
- Using ethograms – a descriptive documentation of their observations
- Discovering fixed-action patterns, sign stimuli and innate releasing mechanisms
- Defining instinct.

Experimental psychologists

- Also known as behaviourists
- Trained in psychology

- Reject the notion of instinct
- Interested in the flexibility of behaviour shown by individuals rather than evolutionary basis
- Interested in understanding the environmental requirements for the development of behaviour in the young
- Studied how new behaviours are learnt (usually using rats, pigeons)
- Experimented under laboratory conditions
- Formulated general laws of behaviour that could be applied to all species, including humans.

Tension exists between the two schools, and this is epitomised by the debate of nature versus nurture.

Nature

- Instinctive behaviour
- Innate behaviour

Table 14.1 Problems with viewing behaviour as either nature or nurture

Instinctive	Learnt
Genes are inherited but it could be argued that behavioural patterns per se are not	Learning is a process that changes preformed behaviour – chicken-and-egg situation
Genes do affect behaviour but animals develop within some form of environment	Studies of preparedness and learning predispositions contradict the idea that through the process of reward and punishment any stimulus can become associated with response
'Sameness' of behaviour in a species: cannot rule out that all members have learnt it	
Deprived experiments still take place in an environment so not truly valid	
It is logically impossible to test behaviours in all environments	

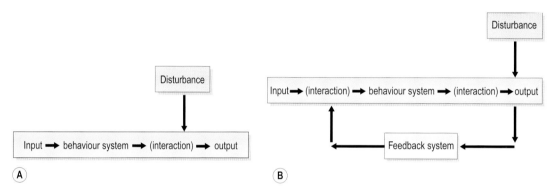

Figure 14.7 (a) Simple open-loop control systems. (b) Closed-loop control systems.

- Inherited behaviour
- Genetic bases of behaviour.

Nurture

- Acquired behaviour
- Learnt behaviour
- Environment.

The ideal of nurture in development is mainly credited to an American psychologist, John Watson. He famously wrote:

> Give me a dozen healthy infants, well formed, and my own specified world to bring them up in and I'll guarantee to take any one at random and train them to become any type of specialist I might suggest – doctor to thief, regardless of his talents, penchants, tendencies, abilities, vocations and race of his ancestors.

In reality it is generally assumed that behaviour is a combination of nature and nurture. More recent evaluation concentrates on behavioural development and how the environmental factors interact within this (Table 14.1).

INFLUENCES ON ANIMAL BEHAVIOUR

Homeostatic control

Homeostasis in the animal body concerns all the metabolic systems and their actions to keep everything in status quo or balance. In behavioural terms homeostatic control concerns feedback loops. There are two types of control systems, as follows.

Simple open-loop control systems

(Figure 14.7a)

In this system the output is affected by disturbance and no correction takes place.

Closed-loop control systems

(Figure 14.7b)

In the closed-loop system the results of the disturbance feed back to affect the input to the behavioural system.

Example: stretch reflex

Output (state of tension in the muscle) is affected by a disturbance (stretching in other muscles) and a feedback mechanism (muscle spindle) records the change and feeds back to change the input (motor nerve) and restores the original input.

or

An animal feeding is disturbed by a possible predator. A feedback mechanism records this information and changes the animal's input so it stops feeding and moves away. The animal feeds back the change in situation and restores the original input, i.e. it starts feeding again.

Fixed-action patterns

A behaviour that is independent of environmental stimuli for its form is known as a fixed-action pattern. It is slightly complicated by the concept that an environmental stimulus may be responsible for the fixed-action pattern being performed correctly.

Example: territorial display

Animals will posture and use audible signals to defend their territory. These actions are fixed-action patterns; however, they will not display these signals unless an environmental stimulus is present, i.e. an intruder is trying to invade their territory.

Fixed-action patterns are instinctive behaviours. They are usually stereotypic and species-specific but may be confused with learnt behaviours. For example, bird song is not instinctive but learnt; however, captive birds will sing, but the song pattern/content is different from that of their wild relatives. Experiments which deprive animals of parental/species interaction have been undertaken to distinguish between a fixed-action pattern behaviour and learnt behaviour.

Care must be taken when performing deprivation experiments as the lack of expression of a behaviour may merely mean the requisite stimulus has not been presented. Stimuli that act as forerunners for the expression of fixed-action patterns are known as releasers. But fixed-action patterns also may not be exhibited if the animal is not in the appropriate physiological or developmental stage, e.g. courtship behaviours will only be shown in mature animals.

The identification of fixed-action pattern is associated with Konrad Lorenz (of imprinting fame). He theorised fixed-action patterns as instinctive responses that would occur reliably in the presence of identifiable stimuli (signs or releasing stimuli). These could then be compared across species.

Imprinting

Lorenz also initially theorised the concept of imprinting via experiments on young geese and chickens. These spontaneously followed their mothers from almost the first day after they were hatched, and Lorenz discovered that this response could be transferred to an arbitrary stimulus if the eggs were incubated artificially and the stimulus presented during a critical or sensitive period. The process of imprinting has since been evaluated in many species, with many displaying some version of it, and in humans it has evolved into the concept of developmental psychology. The idea of a sensitive period, particularly in mammalian imprinting, has developed into a more transient concept with complex social imprinting taking years rather than hours to imprint.

Natural selection

The concepts of natural selection and how Darwin arrived at his theory have been expanded to demonstrate phenotypic and genotypic adaptations in species. Behaviour does have a genetic basis and has been shown to evolve akin to physiological and anatomical characteristics. Behaviour evolves to adapt an individual to reproduce, to capture resources and to avoid predators. Reproductive behaviour of males and females is related to their anatomy and physiology; males have excess gametes so try and inseminate as many females as possible whereas females produce fewer gametes and are selective about their mates – sexual selection.

Natural selection enables species to adapt and survive in their environment or to develop into related but distinct second species through evolution or to become extinct.

Elective selection

This is a form of natural selection but instead of the environment highlighting adaptations that may be advantageous or detrimental, a third party, i.e. humans, has performed the selection process.

Domestication is a prime example of elective selection. Early humans would have bred from wolf puppies that had a behavioural adaptation which enabled them to remain in human company (placid, more tolerant) by selecting individuals which exhibited this behavioural phenotypic trait. Over many years it has become established as a genotypic trait in today's domestic dog population.

Elective selection can also be used in conservation programmes to increase the gene pool or to pass on an advantageous genotypic trait.

Effect of captivity on behaviour

Animals in a captive environment may exhibit natural behaviours but also may not.

In captivity the stimuli are often not present due to enforced environments which would act as triggers to display their natural behaviour. Similarly, unnatural behaviours may be seen as the animal adapts to its current environment, whether that be a zoo, safari park or somebody's house.

Stereotypies, fixed sequences of behaviour, may develop in captive animals. These are patterns of behaviour that are repeated over and over again and are thought to be related to stress due to environmental conditions.

Stereotypies can be observed across species, e.g. pacing in zoo animals, or may be specific to individuals within a species, e.g. one pig may show stress by pacing and rubbing against bars but another may show stress by only rubbing its nose.

There are problems when evaluating the cause of stereotypies in animals. They are associated with welfare issues but some behaviourists advocate that these may be coping mechanisms and perversely could be advantageous to the animal involved. Also they may be exhibited after the welfare issue is removed. For example, ex-battery chickens still display pacing backwards and forwards, even when removed from their cages.

Another dilemma is the ability to categorise natural behaviour in the domestic species. For example, normal behaviour is significantly different for the domesticated dog from that of its wild ancestor. Stress is also attributable to pleasurable situations, e.g. in humans a passionate kiss can give the same physiological stress response as an electric shock!

Another problem in captive wild species can be improper imprinting, particularly by hand-reared young, which can lead to socialisation and reproductive problems in later life. Attempts are made to avoid this by using elaborate models that resemble the natural parental species.

Neural control

Hormones and how they affect the nervous system also have a profound impact on animal behaviour. Hormones are chemical messengers that can trigger neurotransmitters that subsequently inhibit or excite neurons (nerve cells), producing some form of reaction.

Example

Oestrogen is a female hormone. In dogs it stimulates ovulation during the oestrus cycle, and therefore the female is receptive to fertilisation. It also alters the bitch's behaviour: she will have a swollen vulva and a sanguineous discharge (full of pheromones), she will urinate frequently to spread the pheromones and she will only accept a dog mounting her after the peak of oestrogen levels, i.e. when she has ovulated.

Group interaction

Many species of animal have evolved complex social hierarchies or social systems which affect their interaction within the social group and with other groups, or within a population. This can occur both intra- and interspecies.

Social interaction is a huge subject, ranging from why animals group together in herds and how they find and defend territories, to what mating system they have.

Social groups differ widely in their complexity and the types of interactions that animals have with each other.

Eusociality is a system where some individuals are sterile and where the society has developed into castes with specific roles, e.g. insects such as bees.

Social organisation in vertebrates

- Lot of variety
- Often depends upon nature of food supply, density of population, age, sex structure
- Territorial systems
- Some have a solitary existence, some are monogamous and others polygamous
- Social organisation can vary in different seasons.

Social structures tend to develop from established behaviour between individuals in a relationship, whether this be a monogamous pair or a family group. Behaviours become established in set situations, e.g. when food is available do the animals gorge themselves or share out the food?

Dominance is a concept that affects social hierarchies. It can be sex-linked in males or females, or both. Different species exhibit different social structures.

Ethogram production: describing behaviour

Behaviours can be described either by their structures or by their consequences. In everyday conversation we tend to describe behaviours by their consequences, e.g. 'Oh, look, it's feeding!' when we see a starling repeatedly inserting its beak into the ground.

Often it is better to describe a behaviour by its structure, because this stops one assuming what the behaviour is for. After all, the starling might simply be searching for food rather than actually feeding. So describing this behaviour as 'inserts beak into ground' is safer than describing it as feeding.

Before beginning a study, observe your subject and familiarise yourself with the range of behaviours exhibited. Formulate unambiguous categories of behaviour, ensuring they are clear enough for someone else to use, even perhaps illustrating them with a drawing.

Keep in mind what effect you, the observer, have on the animal's behaviour. This should be kept to a minimum unless you are deliberately acting as a predator, for example. If the animal is in an artificial environment, e.g. a cage or a zoo, think about what effect this will have on its behaviour.

Types of measure

Once you have identified your behaviour categories and clarified the focus of the study, you need to think about how you will measure the behaviours you observe. Four types of measure are commonly used in behavioural studies: latency, frequency, duration and intensity.

Latency

Latency is the time interval from a specified event to the onset of the first occurrence of the behaviour. Its units are those of time, e.g. seconds or hours.

Frequency

Frequency refers to the number of occurrences of the behaviour per unit time. Its unit are those of time, e.g. min^{-1} or /minute.

Duration

The duration of a behaviour is a measure of how long a behaviour lasts. Its units are those of time, e.g. seconds or minutes.

Sampling rules

You will need to decide how you are going to sample. Four main methods are used: ad libitum, focal, scan and behavioural.

Recording rules

Three main approaches are used: continuous recording, instantaneous sampling and one-zero sampling.

Continuous recording

Here, as the name suggests, you record continuously. This is really only possible if:

- You select just one individual (focal sampling)
- You have only a small number of behavioural categories, which you can accurately remember without having to take your eyes off the animal
- The animal changes behaviour only infrequently.

Instantaneous sampling

In instantaneous sampling, a signal goes at a regular interval (say every minute). The signal might be an electronic beep, or you might work in a pair, with one of you keeping an eye on a watch with a second hand, telling your partner, who is recording, whenever it is time to record. In either case, whenever the signal is given or the beep is heard, you record your observation.

One-zero sampling

Here a beep goes, or a signal is given, at regular intervals. You then record whether or not a particular behaviour has occurred since the last beep. If it has, you record a 1. If it hasn't, you record a 0 (hence the name one-zero sampling). One-zero sampling is most often used with focal sampling for recording occasional behaviours which don't last long, such as a bout of grooming or play.

One-zero sampling can be combined with instantaneous sampling, so that you record whatever the animal is doing when the beep goes (or signal is given) and you record whether or not certain behaviours have occurred since the last beep or signal.

Constructing an ethogram

An ethogram is a careful description of all the behaviours that a species of animal exhibits. It is obtained by many, many hours of careful observation of the animals, preferably in their natural habitat as well as possibly in a laboratory environment. The descriptions may be made by means of drawings or words or both.

Summary: how to observe behaviour using ethograms/checklists

1. Think language – give scientific and specific descriptions of what you actually see
2. Research your subject's normal behaviour
3. Undertake a preliminary study – familiarise yourself with the behaviour of the study group/individual
4. Be unambiguous – be specific with details and make notes containing clear categories of behaviour
5. Produce a key to behaviours – written descriptions and/or pictures
6. Think about how you influence the animals' behaviour whilst you are studying them
7. Think about how the location and environmental conditions influence the animals' behaviour whilst you study them
8. Define the focus of the study and stick to the point
9. Identify how long the study will be, how often you will observe the animals, when you will do it and any factors which influence these choices

Date of study:	Time of study:	Comment on dam e.g. location, activity at commencement:	Comment on environment:
Recorder's ID:	Individual pup ID:	Sex of pup:	Length of observation:

Behaviour:	Duration (seconds):	Comment:

Figure 14.8 (a) Canine neonatal social behaviour ethogram: individual study. (b) Canine neonatal social behaviour ethogram: key to behaviours. (c) Canine neonatal social behaviour ethogram: key to individuals.

10. Define the intensity of behaviour you observe – a jump could be barely off the ground or 2 metres
11. What type of sampling – ad libitum or focal or scan sampling?
12. What type of sampling – continuous or instantaneous?
13. Does my checklist/ethogram work? Try it out with a trial run.

Example checklist

The behaviour of individuals within the group was recorded using ad libitum, focal sampling techniques whilst ascertaining an overall impression of group behaviour. Instantaneous, scan sampling methods were employed. A key to behaviours exhibited is included in Figure 14.8.

DARWIN AND EVOLUTION

- Evolution has both a general and a behavioural definition
- Evolution is a change in the frequencies of different alleles in a population or species over the course of generations.

Behaviour	Description
SN	Suckling at nipple (number should be recorded where possible)
RR	Rooting reflex
FN	Feeding at nipple (number should be recorded)
CD	Crawling over dam's body
SV	Suckling dam's vagina
SL	Suckling littermates (ID pup if possible)
SNO	Sleeping – no leg or eye movement
SLM	Sleeping – rapid eye movement, leg movement
LNS	Lying still not asleep
CM	Crawling – movement across environment using body as primary motor and not legs
W	Walking – movement across environment using body as primary motor (or attempting to)
V	Vocalisation (detail)
PS	Play – solitary
PO	Play – object directed
PL	Play – littermate directed
PD	Play – dam directed
POT	Play – other
UD	Urination – dam induced
UI	Urination – independent
DD	Defecation – dam induced
DI	Defecation – independent
OT	Other

Figure 14.8 (b) *Continued*

Individual	Sex	Distinguishing features	Eyes open date
1	M	Silver grey, no white	10 days
2	M	Silver grey, 'Y' white on thorax	11 days
3	M	Silver grey, white line left of midline on thorax, short tail	10 days
4	F	Silver grey, white patch in square on thorax	11 days
5	F	Silver grey, no white	12 days
6	M	Silver grey, no white, runt approx. half size of littermates	13 days

Figure 14.8 (c) *Continued*

Evolution can lead to:

- Minor modifications in a population
- Speciation: larger changes which result in a new species.

Darwin had no concept of genes but realised via observational and knowledge evidence that traits were inherited by the offspring from their parents.

Darwin had travelled the world for 5 years on HMS Beagle as a naturalist and during this time he formulated his hypothesis or theory of natural selection. These original ideas have been integrated into the science of genetics. Darwin's observations are phenotypes because he wrote about what he saw.

Basic principle of natural selection

Certain members of a population or species possess specific phenotypic traits or adaptations which may, or may not, equip them to be better able to survive. This is called phenotypic adaptation.

Over time, if this adaptation gives the animal an advantage, the genes coding for it will become more plentiful and the genotype for the adaptation will increase in frequency. This is called genotypic adaptation.

Different parameters are utilised to measure a population's or species' ability to survive. These include the following.

Reproductive success

Organism's production of offspring

- Number of offspring born
- Number of offspring that survive to weaning
- Number of offspring that survive to mating.

'Selection' is perhaps a misleading word to quantify the process; it implies that animals choose the path to evolve. In reality phenotypic traits that lead to an increased survival rate will enable these individuals to mate and thus pass on that trait.

Fitness

- Probability that an organism with a particular genotype and phenotypic make-up will reproduce
- Can be short-term or long-term.

Short-term fitness

- Potential for each genotype to be reproduced in the next generation.

Long-term fitness

- Potential of genotypes to be reproduced in the gene pool in subsequent generations.

Remember that the relative fitness of genes will vary depending upon existing environmental factors.

- Ecological niche: location and functional role in the ecological system.

Niche factors include:

- Nest sites
- Food habits.

Competition is when there are limited resources that are necessary for survival and reproduction of animals in an area. If the resources are required by animals of different species, this is called interspecific competition, whereas if resources are required by animals of the same species, this is called intraspecific competition.

Remember that competition does not necessarily indicate direct conflict between individuals. Cooperative and altruistic behaviours are often adaptive and exhibited by mated pairs or related individuals.

Causes of evolution

Natural selection

Genetic mutations give rise to new phenotypic traits that confer advantages to individuals or increased fitness to their genetic make-up.

Mutation pressure

This is dependent on the ratio of one allelic form to another and the resulting frequencies of these alleles within the population, e.g. A : a frequencies of 0.45 : 0.55 (always measured out of 1 and males and females are often considered separately). If one individual changes, the ratio becomes 0.5 : 0.5, and so on over many genera-

tions. Eventually, over thousands of generations there may be an overall phenotypic effect on the species.

Gene flow

- Animals moving from one population to another result in new alleles entering the gene pool
- This can cause a shift in allele frequencies
- Not thought to be a major contributory factor in evolutionary change.

Genetic drift

- Variation in allele frequencies through random fluctuations
- Happens in all populations to a small degree
- Has a big effect in small populations
- Occurs due to chance mating.

Evolutionary behaviour

Theory of evolution is the single most important conceptual framework for developing hypotheses about the ultimate forces that shape the traits of organisms. Behavioural traits can evolve just like anatomical and physiological traits.

We use the knowledge of evolutionary theory to formulate hypotheses about, and how to design experiments to prove, the adaptive significance of behaviour. This questions the relationship between proteins, genetic code and the behaviour of animals.

Structural proteins control how the cell functions, e.g. proteins found in the neurilemma can control the reaction of the neuron to different neurotransmitters. Enzymes play a role in the synthesis of biologically active molecules, e.g. pheromones used by many species to attract a mate and mark territory.

Example

If neck length in an animal is determined genetically, by studying two animals we can identify their phenotype by sight alone and their genotype by applying their phenotype to what we know about their genes or we have to perform breeding experiments to establish it.

If phenotype is a description of the trait, we look at the animal and describe what it looks like with respect to the characteristic.

- Animal A phenotype has a short neck length
- Animal B phenotype has a long neck length.

If we know that long neck length is dominant over short neck length in our animals and we assign neck length as N for dominant allele and n for recessive allele, then we can theorise the animals' genotype.

- Animal A genotype is nn
- Animal B genotype is Nn or NN.

BEHAVIOURAL STRATEGIES

Animals use numerous strategies to ensure their survival in the natural environment. We shall discuss the prey–predator relationship and then evaluate some of the other mechanisms used to counteract each other's presence.

Prey–predator relationships

In the natural environment there are many examples of the complicated behavioural relationships that exist between prey and their predators (Figure 14.9).

Predators must be able to:

- Recognise their species' chosen prey
- Locate their prey generally and an individual victim
- Communicate the location of their prey
- Establish successful hunting strategies – individual or communal.

In contrast, prey must learn or have innate behaviours that allow them to:

- Survive to reproduce
- Protect their offspring
- Recognise their predators.

A proportion of the behaviours exhibited by both groups are innate whereas other behaviours are learnt from observing their parents and/or family groups.

Prey animals have a number of survival mechanisms:

- Herds – large family groups, often with members on guard duty
- Communication behaviours, e.g. foot stamping, warning calls, to alert all the group to danger
- Moving in large numbers creates a wall to predators who must try and separate an animal (usually a weak, ill member or a youngster)
- Some species keep their young in the middle of a group, thereby giving them protection
- Camouflage techniques are employed to hide individuals or youngsters
- Mimicry of poisonous species is often seen in butterflies or animals may exhibit visual signals/colours to warn of danger
- Some animals have the capacity to lose their toes or tails to ensure survival if caught
- Attach mechanisms and use of spines and shells make it difficult or impossible for an animal to be eaten and frighten off an attacker

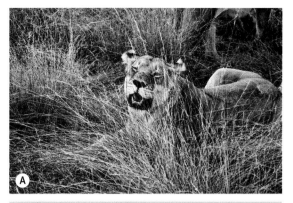

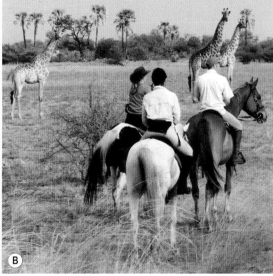

Figure 14.9 (a, b) Predator–prey relationships. (a) Lion. (b) Giraffes can be approached on horseback as both species are prey animals; however the presence of the lion pictured in (a) would cause panic.

- Recognition of predator odours, e.g. rainbow trout and pike
- Recognition of predator outlines, e.g. hawk outline.

Predator mechanisms are often the opposite mechanism to counteract the prey behaviours. These include:

- Camouflage to enable stalking or to entice prey
- Vocal communication to ensure successful hunting
- Learning how to be successful at hunting specific species
- Highly developed senses to locate and capture prey
- Ambush techniques
- Cooperation between species in extreme cases, e.g. seen in the ocean between sharks, dolphins and sea lions with shoaling mackerel.

Examples

The Viceroy butterfly is edible for jays. Monarch butterflies are toxic to jays, inducing vomiting as the caterpillar stage feasts on poisonous plants. Once they have encountered a couple of Monarchs, birds will learn not to eat them. The Viceroy mimics the markings of the Monarch which gives it protection from jays, as they also avoid the Viceroy because of its markings.

Many species of butterfly, moth and caterpillars will expose eye spots on their hind wings when startled by birds. This posture is designed to startle their attacker and researchers have found it is quite effective.

Mobbing behaviour

This can occur when an individual invades another's territory, whether intentionally or not. It can also be an effective hunting behaviour. The group of animals will strategically mob the intruder, attacking it until it is driven out.

This behaviour is seen in rookeries, especially when there are young present, and in other bird species to prevent predatory birds, e.g. kestrels and hawks, from attacking youngsters. It is also seen in tamarin monkeys against predatory snakes.

Cryptic behaviours

These are behavioural strategies which centre on some form of deceit in the animal species using them. Mimicry is the classic cryptic behaviour. It can take many forms, including mimicry of markings or coat coloration, mimicry of attacking mechanisms of predators or adoption of a posture designed to intimidate the predator. Mimicry is not only prey behaviour and examples are also seen in predatory species.

Antidetection behaviours

Camouflage is a very effective form of antidetection behaviour seen in animals. Animal coats and/or markings enable them to blend with their natural environment to make it hard for their prey or predators respectively to spot where they are located. This mechanism is often used by young animals, which are particularly defenceless.

Other antidetection behaviours include stalking whilst hunting where slower movements are used to prevent individuals being spotted by their targets. Hunting or movement at dawn and dusk can also decrease the likelihood of certain animals being seen. Another antidetection mechanism often used where young are involved is hiding them in or near to a den. Mothers will often skirt around the area surrounding their den before going back to it to prevent exposing it to predators. Youngsters will often employ static behaviour, i.e. keeping perfectly still in the nest or their environment, to avoid detection from predators.

Remember the study of behaviour fits into a number of different view points:

- Psychologists are interested in mechanisms that control behaviour
- Evolutionary biologists are interested in why the mechanisms came to be as they are
- Ethologists believe that the distinction between mechanism and design is fundamental to the study of animal behaviour.

Example

In some species of woodpecker, male birds will throw eggs fertilised by another male out of the nest to encourage the female to lay more and therefore pass on their own genes. Ethologists believe that the birds are designed by natural selection to behave in this way, because the behaviour fulfils a certain function which is important to their survival and reproduction.

Adaptive behaviour

If we look at how animals have adapted to changes in their environment we can appreciate the ethological viewpoint.

Adaptive behaviour in two ways

- Genotypic adaptation: genetic adjustment occurs through evolution (natural selection)
- Phenotypic adaptation takes place within the individual animal on a non-genetic basis.

Genetic or evolutionary adaptations occur over a long period of time. For example, a bird nests in a varied habitat containing both cliffs and fields. Some birds will nest in both places; however, the birds that choose cliff nest sites have more surviving young. These young birds will return to their nesting grounds and subsequently have more surviving young of their own. Over time the species will adapt to all nests on the cliffs as a result of natural selection.

Phenotypic adaptations involve learnt behaviour, maturation and temporary physiological adjustments. An example of phenotypic behaviour could be seen in the same species of bird. If, whilst nesting, an individual bird adjusts its position on its clutch of eggs to maintain the temperature, e.g. on a hot day it sits slightly off the eggs to allow them to cool, this would increase their success of hatching.

Territorial behaviour or territoriality

Territorial behaviours are common in the animal kingdom. Many animals will defend areas of land against intruders. Successful territories will provide individuals or family groups with:

- Adequate food supply
- Adequate water supply
- Nesting/breeding sites
- Safety
- Lack of competition
- Quality of resources available
- Mates.

Territorial defence can result in posturing, vocalisation and general display behaviours designed to intimidate the competitor. This will often degenerate into aggressive behaviour if the resource is valuable enough.

Competition for resources occurs in two main ways:

1. Exploitation
2. Exclusion.

Exploitation

- Exploitation of resources in a habitat will result in all the resources being depleted
- There may be some regeneration of the resources
- But overexploitation results in fewer resources
- What happens is an animal arrives at a super new territory, followed by another and another. There is no aggression as there is lots of food available. However, numbers of animals arriving continue to grow until a point is reached when one animal arrives and there are not enough resources to meet its needs. The result is that this animal and those following it will move on to a new territory.

Exclusion

Competition by exclusion occurs where an animal or group of animals successfully defends a resource.

They usually use a variety of keep-out signals:

- Scent marking
- Vocalisation
- Posturing
- Display
- Aggression.

Example: Mongolian gerbils

Social units consist of multi-male, multi-female age-structured groups, thought to be families. Group size varies from 2 to 17 animals. Non-overlapping territories are defined by clustered distribution of burrows, by common areas of activity in group members and by chases across the border zones between the areas used by each group. Territory size correlates to group size ranging from 325 to 1555 square metres. It varies according to group size, food availability and, most importantly, the body weight of the largest male gerbil. Within each group, differential social status is indicated by dominant as well as subordinate character. Males range more widely and are more active than females. Males defend the territory by chasing and marking the border lines – this behaviour increases when the females are in oestrus. The dominant male utilises all the territory, whereas juveniles stay near burrows and females wander about less.

Orientation behaviour

There are three kinds of orientation behaviours:

1. Migration, including migration routes
2. Homing instincts
3. Photoperiodism.

Migration

Migration is the regular seasonal movements between breeding regions and wintering regions.

In temperate zones and arctic latitudes there are marked changes in the distribution of resources between the summer and winter. Birds and animals living in these climates have three survival methods:

- Migration – move to a favourable area
- Residency – evolve adaptations for tolerating the harsh conditions
- Hibernation – store reserves whilst resources are abundant and wait it out.

There is fossil evidence of migration in birds which suggests that current migratory paths have probably evolved since the last ice age.

Other types of migration

Partial migration

- Some of the population migrate, some remain resident
- This may be an interim stage of a fully migratory habit
- It could be established if numbers of full migrants survive and reproduce better than those animals and birds that remain resident.

Differential migration

- Different portions of the population migrate different distances
- Often linked to sex and/or age of the participants.

Irruptive migration

- Some species only migrate certain years and the distances travelled vary
- Irruptive species behave as normal migrants except that they stop migrating once an abundant food source is located.

Timing of migration

Precise arrival and departure dates are an important aspect of migration to maximise the survival and reproductive success of the migrating birds.

Internal rhythms govern the timing of migration. Zugunruhe is a restlessness that indicates species preparing to migrate.

There are different types of control over timing:

- Ultimate control – long-term climate trends, tracked by photoperiods
- Proximate controls – immediate weather conditions, either poor or good; extremes of weather may inhibit migration
- Migratory fattening – migrants store reserves of fat (to be used as fuel for migration) which will be depleted when they know have enough fuel to make their journey.

Physiological adaptations associated with migration

- Fat deposition
- Increased reliance on fat/lipids as a fuel source in comparison to other seasons
- Fat mobilisation/enzymatic activity is increased in the animal's body
- Mass-specific aerobic capacity – the capacity for the body tissues to use oxygen to produce energy (adenosine triphosphate) increases at the time of migration
- Flight muscle hypertrophy leads to increased total aerobic output and power output
- Capacity for heat production can be increased, e.g. shivering increases to produce heat as climate cools as migration progresses.

Distances travelled during migration vary, with birds being the farthest travellers: distances of up to 13 000 km (one-way) have been recorded for arctic terns. The longest non-stop flights in birds can reach up to 3000 km; however most species fly shorter distances and stop to refuel before recommencing their journeys.

Speeds in migratory birds can vary between 30 and 40 km/hour for passerines to 50–80 km/hour in ducks and shore birds. Altitude in migratory birds also varies, with nocturnal migrants typically flying higher.

Homing instincts

For successful migration animals and birds must be able to find their way to the correct breeding and wintering grounds. This is achieved using a number of methods, including:

- Directional orientation: orientation of migratory flights in the proper direction, e.g. south in autumn/north in spring, appears to be genetically predetermined as even inexperienced members are successful
- Navigation: finding their way back to a specific locality, thought to involve previous experience (learnt behaviour).

Species may migrate during the day – diurnal migrants – or during the night – nocturnal migrants.

Types of navigation
Visual orientation

- Use of geographical landmarks, e.g. rivers, coastlines
- Diurnal migrants often follow such signs.

Sun compass

- Birds particularly appear to be able to use the position of the sun to provide information of proper migratory direction
- Birds also compensate for the changing position of the sun in the sky (about 15° per hour) by using their photoperiod clock or internal clock to adjust their orientation.

Celestial navigation

- Nocturnal migrants use the position of the stars as cues for orientation.

Geomagnetism

- Geomagnetism is use of the earth's magnetic field for orientation.

Example: homing instinct: pigeons Pigeons can find their way back to their home territory relatively easily. However experiments were performed where the birds had small magnets attached to their backs to see if this would affect their orientation skill. The results showed that on sunny days pigeons still found their way home but on overcast days they did not. This suggests that homing instincts and navigation skills are a combination of the above methodologies.

Photoperiodism

In most latitudes there are seasonal changes in the length of the photoperiod – changes in the length of the day.

- Photoperiods are measured as light:darkness ratios (L:D) in hours
- Only at the equator are L:D ratios recorded as 12:12 all through the year
- Because day lengths change seasonally it is advantageous to animal species to be able to anticipate and adapt to the concurrent environmental changes that occur
- For example, animals will breed in the spring to take advantage of warmer climate and increased food resources.

Most seasonal events are triggered by a photoperiod of a certain length – this is referred to as the critical day length or critical photoperiod. The critical photoperiod differs between species and between different latitudes. Some species will be triggered into action as the photoperiod falls, i.e. the days are shorter, whereas other actions will be triggered by longer days or photoperiods.

Reproduction in animals is often triggered by a critical photoperiod. In male animals testis size is affected by photoperiod. In hamsters the testes are small on short days and dramatically enlarged on long days as sperm production increases (the critical photoperiod for the hamster is 12.5 hours for reproduction). Female hamsters have a similar critical day length which triggers oestrus, therefore coordinating the breeding cycles of both sexes.

The control of photoperiodism in animals is thought to be by clock genes and clock-related genes. These have evolved circadian and circannual rhythms in animals to generate daily and seasonal rhythms.

ABNORMAL BEHAVIOUR

Abnormal behaviour differs in pattern, frequency or context from that shown by most members of the species in conditions which allow a full range of behaviours.

- In order to recognise that behaviour is abnormal, the person observing must be familiar with the range of normal behaviour of that species, i.e. individual idiosyncrasies
- For some abnormalities, recognition depends upon knowledge of the behaviour of that particular individual
- A difficulty may arise if many of the animals show the same kind of abnormal behaviour, for example it could be thought that bar biting is normal in sows
- Animals need to be studied, not necessarily in the wild, but in complex environments that allow them the opportunity to show the full range of their behaviour

- Abnormal behaviour typically occurs in situations of confinement and isolation.

Stereotypies

In stereotypies a sequence of movements is repeated several times with little or no variation.

Examples

- Caged animals will pace a route over and over
- Caged birds will fly or hop from perch to perch following a route
- Caged monkeys will rock backwards and forwards for long periods
- The behavioural repertoires of animals include many examples of repeated actions, e.g. walking, flapping flight and various displays that are not stereotypies. To distinguish these, thought must be paid to an apparent lack of function of the stereotypy.

Self-directed and environment-directed abnormal behaviour

Some animals show behaviour that is mostly normal in pattern but is abnormal in respect of the object to which it is directed or the extent to which it occurs.

Typically this occurs in situations of confinement and isolation, i.e. poor housing.

Examples

- Vigorous body friction or flank biting in horses
- Young calves housed in individual crates lick parts of their body they can reach, ingesting vast quantities of hair
- Caged parrots pluck their own feathers
- Recently weaned (usually early) calves and piglets will suck and/or lick the walls of their pens
- Confined grazing animals will eat litter, earth or dung. Grazing would normally be a major occupation and confinement stops this, so the animals graze on whatever is available.

Abnormal behaviour addressed to another animal

- Usually normal behaviours inappropriately directed
- Sometimes animals treat each other, or parts of each other, as if they were objects to be investigated, obtained or eaten
- Usually in this instance the space is so confined the other animal cannot move away. Such behaviour includes wool pulling, feather and body pecking, anal

massage and ingestion of faeces (pigs) and tail biting.

Animals treated as a sexual partner

Many farm animals are kept in single-sex groups, never encountering the opposite sex. There are therefore many homosexual interactions. It may follow that when presented with the opposite sex these animals will not behave in the usual fashion, e.g. cows riding the backs of other cows.

Animals treated as a mother

Young mammals weaned at an early age from their mother often show teat seeking and sucking directed towards inanimate objects or pen mates. Sometimes this behaviour persists into adulthood. Cats should not be separated from their mother until they are 12 weeks old. They require 6 weeks until weaning and a further 6 weeks suckling their mum for confidence building.

Animals treated as rivals

Some aggressive behaviour will protect the individual or young. When this becomes intense or frequent, welfare problems may occur. Again, husbandry and housing are at fault.

Some aggressive behaviour may be shown towards people, e.g. kicking, biting, goring, rearing.

Failure of function

Conditions imposed on some animals, especially farm animals, lead to abnormalities of sexual behaviour, parental behaviour and basic body movements.

Inadequacies of sexual functioning

Silent heat, quiet ovulation, suboestrus

* The physiological changes of oestrus occur without the behavioural changes accompanying it
* These animals are capable of being artificially fertilised and their fertility levels are quite normal
* This problem usually occurs with individuals at the bottom of the social hierarchy
* If animals are managed in very large groups there is constant social confusion, leading to instability of the social group, creating social stress which in turn leads to oestrus suppression.

Male impotence

* Generally, among farm animals the males and females are together for such short periods of time that the males often don't know how to react to the female

* This can be such a problem that males may be culled.

Parental behaviour

Problems in parental behaviour are largely maternal – the male function is usually just to protect. Animals are generally not bred for their maternal ability.

Problems

* Neonatal desertion
* Neonatal aggression
* Maternal failure
* Stealing young
* Killing young and maternal cannibalism.

Basic movements

Some housing prevents movements occurring or being carried out easily.

* Wing flapping – battery hens
* Walking – calves in crates
* Walking – sows in stalls
* Lying down on slippery floors – especially hoofed animals.

Anomalous behaviour

Anomalous behaviour involves either very high or very low levels of activity and responsiveness. Usually it is due to an inadequacy in the rearing or housing conditions.

Prolonged activity

* Lying, sitting, standing for great lengths of time.

Tonic immobility or state of hypnosis

* Submissive inertia
* Response to fear, e.g. a hen will freeze in the presence of a hawk
* Unless in a normal situation, consider abnormal.

Hyperactivity

* Sometimes normal but can result in injury, e.g. stampedes
* Is due to the flight-or-fight response, which is fear-induced
* Fear is a reflex.

Hysteria

- Extensive alarm reaction, especially in poultry
- Again, flight-or-fight response
- Occurs more often where animals are kept in high densities
- A good stockman will knock before entering the barn.

SOCIAL BEHAVIOUR

The study of social behaviour and group living tends to be grouped under the heading of behavioural ecology. Behavioural ecology is a branch of evolutionary biology. Behavioural ecologists consider an individual's success at survival and reproduction by evaluating its behaviour and the effects of natural selection.

Group living

In most animal species some form of investment is required by parents to ensure successful rearing of their offspring to adulthood. To achieve this, communication and cooperation behaviours are utilised to some extent.

Sexual and parental behaviours can be considered as basic forms of social behaviour. Indeed, these may be the only forms of social behaviour exhibited by solitary species.

However it is not right to assume that a large group size is indicative of highly social groups. Sometimes large numbers may merely be due to defensive strategies or a particularly valuable resource.

Advantages of group living include:

- Increased vigilance
- Dilution effect of predatory attack
- Group defence against predators
- Group hunting
- Enhanced offspring viability via cooperative breeding.

Disadvantages of group living include:

- Disturbance effect of prey
- Optimum group size – environment
- Decreased reproductive opportunities.

Bibliography

Avey R, Cuthill I, Miller R et al 1994 The five kingdoms and behaviour. Nelson Thornes, Cheltenham

Beaver B V 1994 The veterinarian's encyclopaedia of animal behaviour. Iowa State Press, Iowa

Haupt K A 1998 Domestic animal behaviour for veterinarians and animal scientists, 3rd edn. Manson Publishing, London

McFarland D 1999 Animal behaviour, 3rd edn. Longman, London

Pierce J M 1999 Animal learning and cognition, 2nd edn. Psychology Press/Routledge, New York

Ridley M 1995 Animal behaviour, 2nd edn. Blackwell, Oxford

Toates F M 1980 Animal behaviour. John Wiley, Chichester, West Sussex

Chapter | **15** | *Jane Williams*

Behaviour of common species

This chapter describes the normal and abnormal behaviour of a range of companion animals and livestock species to enable the handler to apply these principles to promote health and welfare.

NORMAL CANINE BEHAVIOUR

The Latin classification for the domestic dog is *Canis familiaris*.

It is a member of the order of Carnivora and is classified as a predatory species. The link between humans and dogs is thought to have arisen from a predatory link between the species.

Dog is a member of the family Canidae, along with the:

- Wolf
- Coyote
- Jackal
- Fox
- Cape hunting dog.

Carnivora have evolved a social structure related to the size of prey, i.e.

- Solitary orders: small prey
- Groups: larger prey.

Darwin theorised that the wolf, coyote and jackal were the ancestors of the domestic dog. Konrad Lorenz theorised that some domestic dogs were evolved from the wolf but the majority evolved from the Golden Jackal. Today, it is generally considered that the domestic dog has multiple ancestors which themselves originated from common ancestry.

There is also documented evidence that domestic dogs have successfully bred (i.e. have produced fertile offspring) with wolves, jackals and coyotes. All the species have a virtually identical chromosome number.

Evidence that suggests the wolf is the main ancestor of the domestic dog is displayed in complex social groups and hierarchal order observed within the wolf and the dog.

Domestication

Approximately 40 000 years ago Ice Age humans and wolves would have been competing for the same prey of large animals. Humans would have warmth provided by cooking fires in a cold climate and around the fires scraps of animal meat, bones and hides would prove a strong draw to a hungry wolf. It is surmised that wolves learnt that there was food available near to humans and humans learnt that the presence of wolves alerted them to the presence of other predators. The relationship evolved as early humans took wolf puppies from the den and 'cultivated' them. The pups would be selected from the more timid animals which had established a scavenging relationship with humans. It is thought that due to the strong social order evident in wolf hierarchy, if humans could become established as the dominant pack member the wolf pups should remain tame. In time the tame wolf pups would have undergone selective breeding by mating the more adaptable and quieter individuals to develop traits that were desirable.

The domestic dog dates to 12 000 years ago and from 10 000 years there is evidence from archaeological finds that the partnership was firmly cemented.

Original roles of dogs in human society include:

- Scavengers, to act as dustmen
- Guards
- Hunting tools
- Protect crops
- Herd crops
- Used in war – the mastiff
- Haulage.

Selective individuals would have been bred to accentuate advantageous traits for the ecological niche.

Domestication has disconnected the biology of modern breeds from environmental selection pressures and allowed forced evolution to occur, which has resulted in the vast array of breeds we have in the modern world.

Behavioural development

It is often debated whether behaviour in dogs is nurtured or genetically based. Certain behavioural traits must be genetic or we would not have specialised groups, e.g. pointers. But it is apparent through study that a combination of genetics and the environment will determine the behaviour exhibited.

It is widely recognised that there are five phases of development of canine behaviour:

1. Neonatal period
2. Transitional period
3. Socialisation period
4. Juvenile period
5. Adulthood.

Neonatal period

- First 2 weeks of life
- Completely dependent upon mother
- Many reflex responses are present:
  ○ Extensor dominance
  ○ Rooting reflex
  ○ Defecation/urination

- Sleep and feed
- Vocalisation skills vary between breeds.

Transitional period

- 2–3 weeks
- Period of rapid development
- Starting to gain independence from the dam
- Development of the neurological system and the sense organs
- Eyes and ears open, which results in the pup beginning to respond to stimuli
- Locomotory skills begin as the pups learn to crawl then walk then lope.

Socialisation period

- 3–10 weeks (4–8-week period is the most vital for social development)
- This phase corresponds to maturation of spinal cord and central nervous system, providing the necessary neurological skills to enable interaction with the environment
- Play is initiated and the early manifestations of adult behaviour are observed:
  ○ Biting
  ○ Barking
  ○ Sexual behaviour
  ○ Dominance
  ○ Submission.

Juvenile period

- From 10 weeks until sexual maturity
- This phase is breed-dependent with the smaller breeds maturing quickest
- Basic behaviour patterns remain but undergo improvement as the pup's motor skills mature
- Puppies learn the relevance of behaviours
- Up to 4 months the animals learn quickly but after this period behaviours already learnt appear to interfere with new behaviours and the rate of learning slows down
- They are still immature with short attention spans
- Pups raised in an external environment will explore the outside of the den from 12 weeks of age, which suggests that rehoming at this age should be less stressful in domestic canines
- Males begin the adult male urination pattern as they use olfactory marking to establish their own territory.

Adulthood

- Puberty and sexual maturity are reached
- Animals are still continuing to learn about their environment

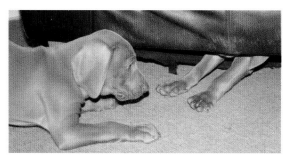

Figure 15.1 Play behaviour in littermates.

- Different breeds will show different rates of learning and different behaviours.

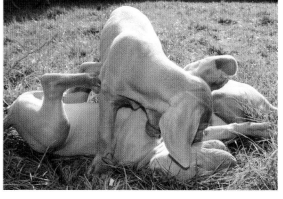

Figure 15.2 Intra-litter play fights help establish dominance hierarchies.

The influence of the environment

Animals are learning from the moment of their birth. They will copy behaviours from the dam, e.g. if she exhibits fear of humans they will.

Hierarchy is first encountered within the litter during the social phase of development when initial primary social relationships are formulated. Play develops essential social skills to enable an individual to integrate successfully into the social order.

In wolf litters, dominant pups will become the dominant adults in the pack. In the domestic dog it is more complicated and varies with breed. Behaviourists have concluded that dominance shown in early play is not necessarily an indicator for adulthood but may often be copied behaviour. However, if no social contact occurs during the critical period between 3 and 8 weeks, then it has been observed that pups find it difficult to forge primary social relationships, including those to humans, one particular sex, e.g. men or women, or to strangers. In domesticated canines homing of litters usually occurs at 8 weeks of age, though some behaviourists would advocate slightly earlier, taking advantage of the increased learning capacity to the environment which occurs during the critical period.

Play

Dogs' desire to play has often been cited as the reason humans have domesticated them. It is thought that in play animals develop communication skills through 'safe learning' as play gestures indicate that behaviour displayed is not for real and therefore poses no social threat (Figure 15.1). Wolves and jackals have been observed at play during their early developmental stages akin to their domestic cousins. It has been hypothesised that social species of animal have an innate need for play (Figure 15.2) and problems such as tail chasing observed in solitary individuals could possibly be self-directed play in the absence of a play partner.

Social behaviour in the dog

Wolves are classified as type 3 carnivores: this translates to a pack establishing a strong social order or hierarchy. This is usually related to the ages of individual members and the inherent dominant hierarchy among the male and female members of the group. There is a dominant alpha pair who will normally be the only pairing to produce young while the rest will assist in care and defence of the youngsters. The pack participates in group hunting, with coordinated hunting behaviours observed, and pack size is relative to the size of the prey available, e.g. mainly deer packs will consist of approximately seven members. If a territory has a plentiful food supply the pack does not grow bigger but individuals may leave to establish their own breeding colonies. Hierarchy within the pack is maintained through social contact and exists in both male and female ranks.

Feral dog populations

In some areas of the world where there are stray dog populations it has been observed that dogs will form social packs. The sizes of these packs are dependent upon the resources, e.g. food available. Within these small social units an unprovoked hierarchy has been documented, supporting the wolf as domestic dog's ancestor and placing dogs as a type 3 carnivore.

Domestic dogs

In domestic dog populations many of their wild relatives' social behaviours can be observed, although

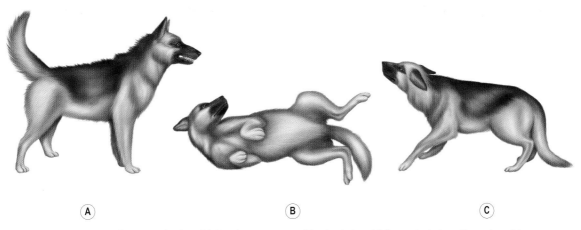

Figure 15.3 Canine visual communication. (a) Dominant posture; (b) submission; (c) fear submission. (Reproduced from Aspinall V 2006 *The Complete Textbook of Veterinary Nursing.* Butterworth Heinemann, London, with permission.)

selective breeding by humans has had an influence. Communication tends to be via olfaction, vision, auditory means and physical contact. Figure 15.3 illustrates canine visual communication.

Dominant postures include standing tall, holding the tail high, head up with the ears erect and making direct eye contact.

Submissive postures include keeping the body low, in extreme cases lying on the back and presenting the inguinal region, often in conjunction with urination, extreme tail wagging, nuzzling, licking, ears back and drooped and often with a grinning expression of the mouth, known as the 'submissive smile' (Figure 15.4).

The range of postures is utilised to reflect 'emotions' and as such can be important indicators of temperament.

Aggression can be categorised by one or all of the following:

- Baring the teeth
- Raising coat hair (hackles up)
- Standing with a dominant or submissive posture: animals in pain or that are fearful often take a submissive position but care must be shown as they can still display aggression.

The position of the ears and the degree that the eyes are open plus the position of the lips can indicate:

- Anxiousness
- Excitement
- Fear
- Playfulness.

Interference by humans may have resulted in domestic dogs relying more on olfaction than on visual communication.

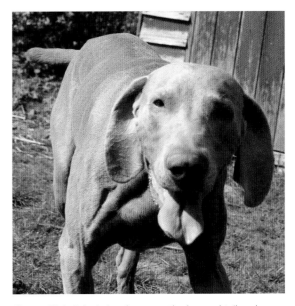

Figure 15.4 Submissive dog; note the lowered tail and lowered and back ears.

Olfaction

Olfaction or the interpretation of scents is an important communication tool in canines. Scents dwell in the environment, providing a reliable marker for territories and communication with other individuals.

Faeces, urine and glandular secretions are all utilised in olfactory communication.

Faeces

In wolf packs it has been observed that faeces are used to mark territories and that the frequency of defecation increases if alien faecal matter is encountered within a wolf's territory. Domestic dogs tend to defecate at an increased frequency when off the lead with no owner present, perhaps indicating that humans have interfered with inherent communication methods.

Urine

Urination is the bane of many dog owners' lives! Urine marking is a common behavioural problem observed in entire male dogs. Cocking the leg or raised-leg urination is displayed by the majority of male animals; subordinate individuals can be late starters, but there is an increased frequency in dominant individuals. The volume of urine passed can determine whether the act is for elimination or for scent marking. Male dogs will often show the raised-leg display without actually urinating, suggesting a communicative role for this action. Many males and some females will scratch and kick their back legs after urination and/or defecation; this is theorised to spread scent, even though they often miss. Another theory for this action is that it is to leave scent from the sebaceous glands or interdigital glands in the feet, or it could it be a visual communication.

In wolves, double marking of male-on-female urination cements pair formation and improves courtship success, which is another behaviour that can be observed in their domestic cousins. Overmarking is common practice in packs but not in lone animals, suggesting territorial marking. Raised-leg display is often repeated after urination and is thought to affirm dominance.

Urine is also an important medium for communicating the readiness of a bitch to mate and the frequency of urination increases during the oestrus period.

Anal glands

These are present in all species of Canidae. Glandular secretion analysis shows differences between groups and individuals. The glandular secretions are secreted on the faeces.

General odours

These are used by all species of Canidae for communication. Glands in the facial region, tail, perineum and anal region secrete social odours. There are two types of gland: the sebaceous glands, which produce oily secretions, and the suderiferous glands, which produce watery secretions and are used more commonly in social communication. The anal region in wolves is utilised for postural communication: the wolf will sniff the base of another's tail. The dominant wolf will present the anus to a subordinate and then it will check the other animal's anus. In very subordinate animals the anal region will be withdrawn, i.e. the animal will clamp its tail to prevent examination, and if both members are of the same rank each will present the anus for examination and check the other member's. This is more commonly seen in male animals but females do exhibit the behaviour during oestrus. Domestic dogs exhibit a similar behaviour between unfamiliar individuals and follow the same sequence of behaviours or a fixed action behaviour pattern:

Example: dogs in the park

- Inspect head and anal region (Figure 15.5)
- Females tend to approach the other animal's head and males the bottom
- Irrespective of the other animal's sex, both try to reduce inspection by clamping
- Is this evidence of retained inherited social behaviour?

Vocal communication

There are advantages for using this method, including:

- Long-distance communication
- Ability to communicate if visually impaired, e.g. night/dense cover
- Allows pinpointing of individuals' locations.

This behaviour is more common in the domestic dog than its ancestors and a broad repertoire of sounds have developed (Figure 15.6). Wolves howl when seeking company or trying to contact or to recall the pack after hunting. Dogs have developed numerous sounds, e.g. a growl can be defensive, a warning or a threat. One belief is that selective breeding by humans has resulted in the broader communication repertoire.

Reproductive behaviour

Domestic dogs are capable of mating any time whilst their wild relatives only produce sperm seasonally. The

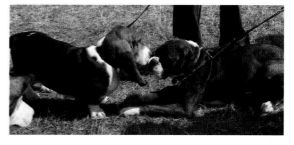

Figure 15.5 Meeting behaviour in the dog.

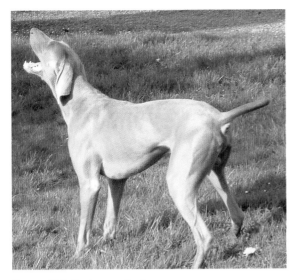

Figure 15.6 Canine vocalisation.

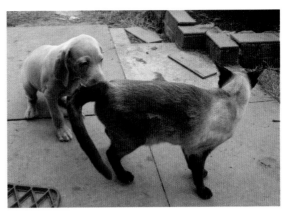

Figure 15.7 Investigative play will enable puppies to socialise with new species.

bitch (in domestic and wild species) is seasonally mon-oestrus. During the oestrus period the bitch displays visual signs of her season, including a swollen vulva and olfactory signals via vaginal discharges and an increased frequency of urination. Bitches may develop a preference for specific mating partners and appear to prefer animals with which they are already familiar. Mating behaviour includes precopulatory play, which is seen particularly in inexperienced pairings. This is followed by explor-atory sniffing and licking by the male, mounting and the resultant tie.

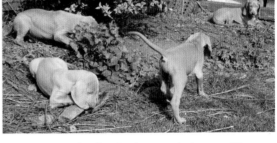

Figure 15.8 Exploration develops puppies' personalities.

Maternal behaviour

When near to term the bitch will try to roam and be restless. The pregnant bitch is often disobedient, tears up bedding and affectionate animals can become aloof. They will try and locate a secluded area to nest, mirroring the feral animal where the bitch will leave the pack and look for an abandoned hole (similar to wolf behaviour in finding a den). It is preferable to provide the bitch with a whelping box before her due date to allow her to acclimatise before the first stages of labour commence.

Developing social behaviour

Social behaviour is practised and established during play (Figures 15.7–15.9).

Behaviourists believe that dominance hierarchies are established by 8 weeks of age, then retained into adult-hood, which has been substantiated in research on wolves. Yet research within the domestic dog population has demonstrated fluidity within the hierarchal structure

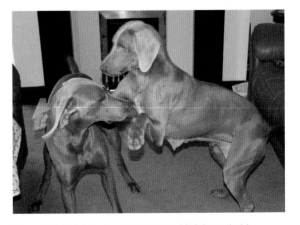

Figure 15.9 Adult play serves to establish household hierarchies.

in the litter, suggesting that for domestic dogs social relationships are not fixed until adult life.

Human influence

How do humans fit in?

Hypothesis: Humans are simply other dogs to domestic dog breeds

If no social contact is given to humans during the critical period, dogs will demonstrate a fear response to human stimulus. However, socialised dogs use adaptations of dog behaviour to communicate with people; for example, a raised paw is indicative of a dog requesting play behaviour from another dog. Puppies in new homes only experience anxiety when isolated from human company and not on leaving their 'pack' or litter. Domestication could have increased the dog's dependence upon humans, as humans have selected animals with an increased capacity to be trained. Dogs look at humans as an extension to their social order or pack, providing:

- Leadership
- Security
- Food
- Control
- Exercise
- Defined sleep areas and patterns
- Praise: social rewards.

All these behaviours act to reinforce human dominance and problems only occur when canine individuals challenge the status quo.

The competition theory

Canine behaviour can also be thought of in terms of competition for resources. All animals have a need for food and water to survive; they will seek to reproduce and to establish these vital parameters will often require a territory or migratory strategy to acquire them.

Domestic dogs may exhibit inappropriate behaviour to other animals or humans if there is competition for what they view as resources. For example, food on your dinner plate would be desirable for your pet dog as well as yourself, or your bed would be a comfortable and secure sleeping area. Competition problems tend to arise in situations where the dog would consider itself in a favourable position to win the competition, for example when a new pet has been introduced, a new partner moves into the house or the family has a baby. Alternatively, dogs which have not had social hierarchies established may be more prone to competition behaviour as they may be able to improve their social rank via this behaviour.

DOMESTIC CAT BEHAVIOUR

The Latin classification for the domestic cat is *Felis catus.* The domestic cat is thought to link its ancestry to:

- *F. silvestris silvestris* – European wild cat
- *F. silvestris libyca* – African wild cat.

The main evidence points to the African wild cat being the main ancestor. There have been attempts to mate domestic cats with European wild cats but these have produced infertile offspring and one has never been successfully tamed.

Domestication

This was first achieved by the Ancient Egyptians in approximately 3000 BC. There is evidence of cats with collars on in hieroglyphics dating to 2600 BC and from 1600 BC there are lots of paintings, effigies and archaeological evidence of the domestication having been successful.

Although mainly speculative, it is thought that because Egypt was based upon an agricultural economy, i.e. there were lots of grain crops, there was a large vermin problem. This would have attracted wild felines and, as with the domestic dog, a mutually advantageous relationship began. Natural selection of the wild felid population would have led to tamer cats becoming more amenable to human contact due to increased food availability. This, combined with human influence via selective breeding for temperament but not for breed type, led to the domestic cat.

Development of breeds

The main role for cats in the human world was rodent control; cats had already evolved naturally to be excellent rodent hunters and killers. Therefore there was no need for selective breeding for type, only temperament, to make the breed more amenable to humans. Breeds developed related to geographical location and climate; for example, the British breeds are stockier with dense coats whilst Asian breeds have a slender frame and thinner coats. Until recently there were only basic genetic differences amongst the breeds but an explosion – genetically speaking – occurred when humans decided to engineer different breed types and coat colours due to the pet market.

Behavioural development

The cat has a less structured behavioural development pattern than the dog. The same stages are apparent but are less developed.

Neonatal period

- Birth–2 weeks
- Eat/sleep
- Dependent on mother.

Transitional period

- Begin to gain independence
- 2–3 weeks.

Socialisation period

- From week 3–9/10: some behaviourists believe up to 14 weeks
- Increase in social play
- Not as vital as similar period in dogs
- Human contact during this period is important for cats to accept humans in later life.

Juvenile period

- Sexual maturity reached
- Breed-dependent
- Behaviour patterns show no significant difference
- Motor skills develop further and are enhanced
- At maturity they display independence.

Senses

Thermoregulation is partially developed at 3 weeks but fully developed by 7 weeks. Olfaction is partially developed at birth but fully by 3 weeks and hearing is developed partially at birth but fully at 4 weeks. Vocalisation is limited and sight does not begin to develop until the third or fourth week.

Motor skills

Flexor dominance is apparent until adolescence when it is replaced by extensor dominance, i.e. the ability to land on all four feet. Motor control is fully developed at 11 weeks. Before this kittens display both rooting and suckling reflexes. Social play is seen primarily until weaning when object play becomes more apparent as the kittens practise essential killing techniques. In feral populations mothers will introduce prey from 4 weeks of age, progressing from dead to injured to uninjured. Initially the mother will kill prey in front of her young, allowing the behaviour to be learnt until eventually they can kill unassisted. Predatory behaviour is instinctive in cats, and animals, regardless of whether they have encountered rodents or not, will show predatory behaviour towards them from 6 months of age. However other hunting skills are evidently learnt as cats living in populations which catch fish will learn this skill but cats which have not encountered fish by 6 months will not be able to do so.

Play

In cats play activities are present but not in the same way as dogs, where play appears to have a purely fun element. Cat play is a safe way to practise the essential skills required to hunt and to hone social skills. There are three types of play exhibited in felines:

- Locomotory
- Social
- Object play.

Locomotory play can be social or solitary in nature and involves running, rolling, jumping and climbing. Object play essentially focuses upon an object and again it may be solitary or social in nature. Social play includes wrestling, rolling, biting and fighting and can occur with cospecifics, e.g. a human hand that responds as a kitten would. Vocalisation often occurs during play and early social play is rough but this decreases as the concept of pain is learnt. Behaviour is modified to remove the final attack sequence and the kittens will run then abort, jumping away at speed with their back curved. From 8 weeks of age stalking and hiding are displayed. Play can occur with adult cats but the frequency is reduced – the behaviour is primarily observed between kittens.

Individuality

Cats are noted as being great individuals – this appears to be a combination of genetic factors and environmental influence.

Organisation

Feline territories are divided into two areas: a core area and a home area. An individual will defend the core area against intruders whereas the home area is a shared resource which can incorporate a number of cats' hunting grounds.

Cat populations vary from single individuals to groups and areas range depending on food availability and distribution. Generally there will be a smaller cat population in territories where food is sourced via hunting and an increased population in areas where scavenging complements the prey available. It is theorised that cats that survive entirely on caught prey do not live in groups.

Generally it has been observed that two broad types of social structure exist in feline populations and these are dependent upon food supplies. These are female social groups and solitary cats.

Solitary cats

- Ranges overlap
- Female ranges will be overlapped by larger male ranges
- Thought to be food-dependent
- Male territories are bigger than female territories – male cats need more food.

Groups

- Occur where there is sufficient food to sustain all
- Males are usually loosely attached to the group
- Comprise adult females and their kittens
- Cooperative kitten rearing/nursing
- Structure is maintained by antagonism – strange females are ousted and progeny is recruited (akin to lion behaviour).

Pet cats

- Often forced to live in a group
- This is usually tolerated well
- Still have territories and ranges
- Male areas are approximately 10 times the size of female areas.

Communication

Cats utilise olfaction and visual communication methodologies. Faecal and urine marking are commonplace. Visual signals include facial and body posturing, with the position of the ears and eye shape indicating mood (Figure 15.10). Clawing and scratching is a combination of visual and olfactory communication, and is seen in pet, feral and farm cat populations. This behaviour leaves a very visual sign of their activity and probably also a deposit from the pedal glands whilst maintaining good claw condition, which is a sign of dominance.

Vocalisation occurs in the queen and tom during the breeding season, with the queen calling and the tom howling. Purring is classically associated with contentment but cats are also known to purr when in pain or frightened. Hissing and growling are also heard in fear situations.

Tactile communication includes body rubbing on items and with co-specifics such as the hands and legs of owners. This is also thought to be a form of olfactory communication, with secretions being released from glands in the cheeks. In groups it has been observed that rubbing cheek glands occurs from subordinate animals to dominant ones, which could help to reaffirm social position.

Olfaction is often used as a means of communication as it is long-lasting and, as cats hunt when vision is impaired, can be used effectively at these times. It is thought to have a major role in establishing and maintaining territories. Observed cats in hunting ranges will avoid confrontation and will let another cat pass (often just sitting down until the other has gone). Clashes only occur if there is a surprise meeting. Evidence to reinforce this view includes the fact that on their home ranges cats cover faeces but leave them uncovered in their hunting ranges. Urine is also used to confirm territories.

Urine can help cats distinguish between different groups and individuals, as in canines.

It is theorised that sprayed urine contains anal secretions and plays a more important role in olfactory communication than in excretion of urine. Urine also plays a role in oestrus with males exhibiting flehmen behaviour when they sniff it.

Reproductive behaviour

Females are seasonally polyoestrus and the beginning of the breeding season is determined by day length. Toms show increased activity during spring months and this then declines as the daylight hours decrease.

Maternal behaviour

Cats do not tend to build nests but improvise and whilst some may seek solitude others crave attention. Infanticide has been observed by male cats (in a mirror of lion behaviour) and in feral colonies communal dens and nursing among related females have been observed.

Neutering

Neutering causes behavioural changes in both sexes; females no longer exhibit oestrus and males show a reduction in spraying, odour of urine decreases, and roaming and fighting should lessen. In addition castrated cats live longer than entire male cats (there is probably a link with the incidence of feline immunodeficiency virus and feline leukaemia virus).

Social interactions

Normal meeting behaviour begins with cats nose to nose with no touching. Then the head and neck are extended with the body slightly crouched to enable a quick retreat. The cat will attempt to sniff along the neck of the other to the flank and on to the anus whilst preventing the other cat from examining its own anal region. If one cat is submissive or dominant this ritual breaks down. If one of the cats is a dominant animal the approach will persist until one desists or an attack is provoked. Cats also respond to model cats as with normal cats and humans

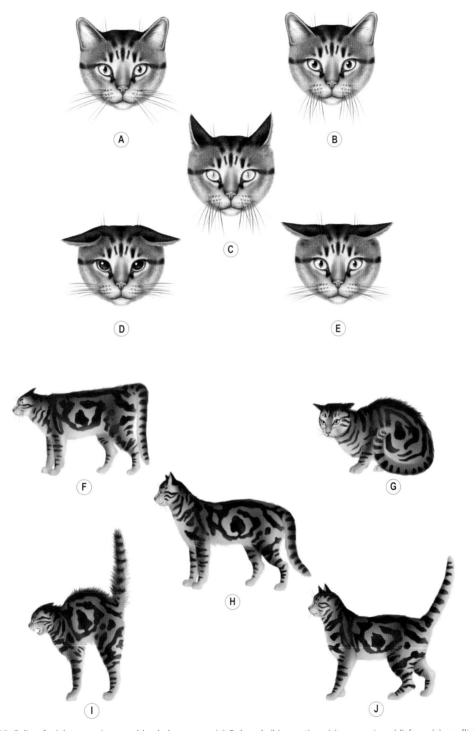

Figure 15.10 Feline facial expressions and body language. (a) Relaxed; (b) greeting; (c) aggression; (d) fear; (e) conflict; (f) aggression; (g) conflict – the cat may attack if cornered, as frightened; (h) relaxed posture; (i) fear; (j) greeting posture. (Adapted from Aspinall V 2006 *The Complete Textbook of Veterinary Nursing*. Butterworth Heinemann, London, with permission.)

can trigger the greeting behaviour by using an outstretched finger to substitute for the nose.

In social colonies individuals indulge in lots of social contact. Aggression is rarely seen except to strange females and young males.

Cat–human bond

Factors that influence it

- General housing conditions, including number and quality of cats and humans
- Owner behaviour
- Cat behaviour.

Most humans rate their relationship with their cat as near to ideal!

EQUINE BEHAVIOUR

The domestic horse can be dated back 5000–6000 years to the end of the Neolithic period. Horses historically have an important role in human development as a food source, for transportation, for haulage, to work the land, for war and for pleasure.

Communication

Horses have laterally set eyes giving a wide field of vision (as do most large animal herbivores). This enables them to spot predators as they are grazing – a vital survival strategy. Research suggests they see in colour vision but only a limited range of colours is distinguishable. Eye position also plays a role in communication in social hierarchy via direct and indirect eye contact.

Vocalisation

Equids use a range of vocalisations during communication. Some common examples are:

- Neigh (or whinny):
  - Neigh is a greeting/separation call
  - It appears to have a role in herd cohesion
- Nicker:
  - Care-giving: epimeletic call
  - Care-soliciting: et-epimeletic call
  - Occurs between mare and foal when rejoined
  - Animal-specific
  - Also seen when mare in oestrus/stallion
  - Can occur between owner and horse and is usually food-associated
- Both the nicker and the neigh will elicit replies

- Other sounds observed include:
  - Snorts
  - Squeals
  - Roars
- Short snort signifies alarm
- Prolonged snort/sneezing expresses frustration.

Greetings

Horses live in social groups or herds and establish social relationships within these. Greeting behaviour occurs by animals putting their muzzles together nostril to nostril. Their nostrils flare but there is no apparent or perceptible accompanying vocalisation, although this is often followed in submissive group members by a squeal in defence.

Emotions

- Ears/eyes are important, as with dogs/cats
  - Alert: ears forward
  - Aggression: ears back/flattened
  - Submission: ears turned outwards
  - Champing/tooth-clamping with the lips retracted (licking and chewing): no danger, usually observed in juveniles
  - Mare in oestrus: swivelled-back ears and loose lips
- Stallions exhibit flehmen in response to urine
- A food anticipation expression has been identified
- Ears tend to signal direction of vision (Figures 15.11 and 15.12).

Posture

A relaxed horse will exhibit quiet behaviour as it is secure in its environment. Conversely a nervous animal will exhibit movement as it prepares for a flight reaction. Aggression is demonstrated by threatening behaviour which can include biting, kicking and lashing the tail. When frightened equids will tuck their tail to the rump and stand with all feet close together. Muscle guarding is often exhibited in anticipation of pain and may be seen in animals prior to exercise. Frustration is thought to be displayed by pawing the ground – some believe this to be displacement behaviour from feeding in the wild during winter when a horse would need to move snow by pawing it to access grazing.

Olfaction

- Important role in sexual behaviour
- Stallions exhibit flehmen when they smell urine
- Frequency increases with proximity to oestrus
- Stallions overmark urine

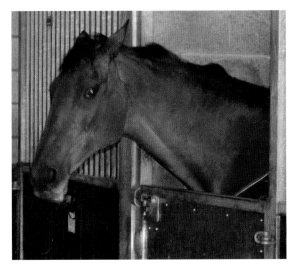

Figure 15.11 Discontented horse; note the position of the ears.

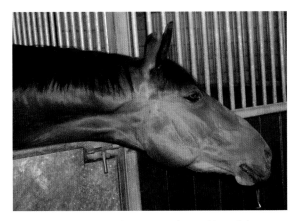

Figure 15.12 Attentive horse: note the position of the ears.

- Flehmen is also exhibited in response to the unknown, e.g. medicine, food.
- It is thought that wild stallion mark their territory with manure piles
- This behaviour is observed in domestic stallions who manure pile, whereas mares/geldings move on an outwards circle, spreading manure further afield from the original site.

Social structure

Free-ranging

- One stallion to 2–20 mares, average of 6
- Alpha female leads the herd in flight, rest, new grazing (usually an older/larger mare)
- Stallion drives from behind, only coming to the fore if a potential threat appears
- Mares choose a stallion and herd at puberty and will often leave their birth herd
- Mares that do stay within their birth herd show reduced fertility rates
- Age appears to be the main factor linking to dominance and social status of mother
- Mares exhibit aggression to newcomers but stallions will protect them
- Aggression in feral horses is most commonly observed over competition for resources, especially water
- At water holes the herd conforms to a strict drinking order:
  - ○ Stallion → Mares → Juveniles
- Juveniles are the only members that another group will usurp
- Stallions defend their harem, not their territory
- When stallions meet:
  - ○ Sniff, have nostrils flared and prance
  - ○ Defecate and investigate each other's manure
  - ○ Vocalisation – subordinate stallions have shorter, lower-frequency calls than dominant ones
  - ○ Seldom there is a confrontation – they fight.

Domestic

- Remain stable in groups
- Linked to food dominance as often not true social groups as would be seen in wild
- No apparent link between dominance and size or length of residency
- Dominant mares have dominant daughters
- Horses less than 3 years are never dominant
- Mares appear to have preferred associates with whom they share resources without competition
- These are often related individuals of similar social rank
- Dominance is determined by temperament and mother's social rank.

Aggression

- Many manifestations, e.g. kicking, biting, neck wrestling, chasing
- Often seen in play behaviour
- Eye/ear position crucial
- Stallions' aggressive behaviour includes:
  - ○ Arched neck display
  - ○ Faecal pile display
  - ○ Head bowing
  - ○ Threatening to bite
  - ○ Squealing
  - ○ Snorting
  - ○ Prancing

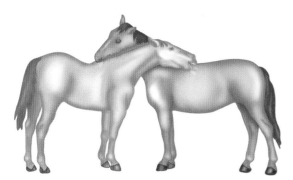

Figure 15.13 Sites of mutual grooming in the horse. (Reproduced from Aspinall V 2006 *The Complete Textbook of Veterinary Nursing*. Butterworth Heinemann, London, with permission.)

- ○ Pushing
- ○ Levade
- ○ Rearing and boxing
- ○ Balk in defence
- When establishing social order it is essential that the horses involved have the opportunity to flee to prevent injury.

Horses exhibit mutual grooming. They stand shoulder to shoulder and nibble withers and back (Figure 15.13):

- Normally occurs between individuals close to each other's social rank in hierarchy.

Development of behaviour

Foal

- Suckling reflex within first few minutes
- Stands within 15–60 minutes
- Responds to tactile, visual and auditory stimuli within 1 hour
- Nickers within 1 hour
- Walks within 1 hour and is proficient within 3 hours
- Defecates within 1 hour
- 2 hours: successful sucking (in a larger breed it takes longer)
- 2–3 hours: lies down and sleeps
- 3 hours: grooms and gallops
- 1 day: plays, urinates, exhibitis flehmen, grazes, communicates, suckles: it is a fully functional mini horse
- Feeding behaviour
- Play can be social or solitary: exclusively solitary within first 2 weeks and by 8 weeks virtually exclusively social
- Flehmen is exhibited with more frequency in colts than fillies: investigative behaviour.

Behavioural problems

Equine aggression

Equine aggression occurs towards people and towards other horses.

Towards people

- People in the stable encounter problems when dealing with a dominant horse
- Dominance over horse can be re-established from the ground
- Methods include:
  - ○ Free-lunging
  - ○ Preventing the horse entering your space
  - ○ Hobbling – tie the horse's leg for 5 minutes then release it and allow the horse to walk, then repeat until the horse learns you control its movement; this method is not often utilised in modern equine establishments!
  - ○ Reward animals when they display no aggression or punish aggression – you need to have quick reflexes and successfully identify behaviours
  - ○ In severe cases isolate the horse in the dark with no resources and with humans providing for all its needs: continue until the horse seeks human company, demonstrated by vocalisation; again, this method is not often considered in modern equine establishments
  - ○ Pharmacological methods: succinylcholine, an immobilising agent except for respiration: exert dominance while the horse is on the ground (used when the alternative is euthanasia).

Towards other horses

- Change in management
- Reduce competition between horses
- Try hormone therapy – progesterone is thought to inhibit the aggression centres within the brain
- Tryptophan triggers release of serotonin and reduces aggression displayed
- Shock collars as with dogs (the horse will need to acclimatise) – negative reinforcement – not indicated for use in the UK.

Split/prolonged oestrus

- Oestrus should be 5–7 days but in some animals it can last up to 90 days!
- Seasonally polyoestrus
- Oestrus is often accompanied by aggressive behaviour
- Drug therapy
- May be due to abnormal number of ovarian cysts producing abnormal fluctuations of reproductive hormones (polycystic ovaries).

Box walking/weaving

- May occur as displacement behaviour for herd-rejoining behaviour
- Attempt to increase contact with other equines
- Can be due to claustrophobia
- Stereotypy: frustration/stress/pain
- Try introducing stimuli, e.g. toys, or increase space
- There is some evidence that it is inherited.

Pawing

- Displacement behaviour for frustration
- Wild horses would paw the ground to remove snow to get at grass.

Stall kicking

- Usually associated with food
- Kicking can be with the feet or with the hocks: potential injury risk
- Frustration
- Inadvertent conditioning by owner, e.g. titbits
- Retrain owner and horse.

Loading

Failure to load can be due to:

- Dark inside
- Hollow noise of hooves: insecurity
- Instability of vehicle: insecurity
- All of the factors above trigger innate fears
- Fear is learnt from bad experiences
- Hitting the horse is not recommended: the association with pain reinforces the negative feeling, as will injuries received when the horse avoids loading
- Some horses do suffer motion sickness
- Retrain: train the horse to move forward by touch from behind (using a lunge whip wrapped in cloth so it is not painful): begin with a few steps, and progress to up to the trailer but don't allow the horse in: next, go in and then go out again: repeat until the horse is able to progress to short journeys
- Desensitisation – this is prolonged therapy: leave the trailer open in the field together with the horse and feed the horse in the trailer; this usually requires more than 1 month so is not a short-term answer
- Parelli training: teach the horse to follow an object rather than to move away from one
- Clicker training has also been used.

Head shyness

- Due to poor management
- Progressive desensitisation
- Positive reinforcement and counterconditioning.

Ridden problems

- These include bucking and napping
- Physical problems must be ruled out first
- Counterconditioning and positive reinforcement work well
- They require a patient and uniform approach.

BOVINE BEHAVIOUR

Little is known about bovine behaviour in comparison to other species discussed, even though there has been a close relationship with humans for a long period of time. Cattle do vocalise to identify group members, during play, during mating and to signify safety or that danger is approaching. Aggression is more commonly seen in cows than in bulls and there is a dominance hierarchy in place which can be observed by positioning within the herd.

Bulls exhibit a hierarchy with no requirement for overt aggression. Determinants of dominance appear to be height, weight, age, sex and the presence or not of horns.

Dominant cows do not need to win all interactions, only the majority, to maintain their position. When moving as a herd the submissive cows are driven first but the dominant animals will be first to food. Dominance increases when in oestrus and decreases during pregnancy. Breed dominances are observed; in bulls more aggression is seen in dairy breeds than in beef cattle.

Mutual grooming does occur, usually between age mates and kin, and there is an association between grooming and milk production (older animals display increased grooming). Maternal aggression is often observed.

PORCINE BEHAVIOUR

Communication by vocalisation is important; 20 pig calls have been identified, including grunt, bark and squeal. The grunt is the familiar sound used when rooting or excited. Sounds are often used in sequences to display mood. Vision does not appear to play an important communicatory role. Tail position is an indicator of good health if it is curled and can also indicate mood:

- Elevated curly tail: greeting/competition over food/mating/chasing
- Straightened tail: sleep, relaxed.

Group behaviours are observed; for example, piglets huddle to increase temperature and adults also huddle, as pigs have poorly developed thermoregulatory mechanisms. Olfaction is used: boars and sows utilise pheromones in urine (sows are better at detecting).

Free-ranging pigs

- Live in groups of 8 (3 sows and offspring)
- Males are solitary for most of the year but may form all-male groups during the winter.

Confined pigs

- Teat order determines hierarchy when young
- Piglets are often very violent and use their needle teeth to achieve the best position (at the anterior pair of nipples)
- Hierarchy formation also occurs within mixed groups
- Fights can take place but most hierarchies are determined within 24 hours, although they may take as long as 3 days to establish
- Females take longer than males
- Breed dominance is observed
- Hierarchal status is maintained by threatening behaviour
- Most aggression is food-related
- To prevent aggression it is a good idea to group pigs according to sex and body size after weaning
- Tranquillisers, shelters (to hide heads in) and pheromones are also often used to reduce aggression.

Tail-biting

- Often seen in captive, penned pigs
- Thought to be due to a lack of oral stimulation; normally pigs would root for 7 hours a day
- When the tail begins to bleed because a pig has sucked it due to displacement behaviour for rooting, this turns into a stimulus for aggression and may lead to biting
- One solution is to give pigs corn on the cob to play with
- Also check iron levels as a deficiency can stimulate this behaviour.

Grooming

- Subordinate pigs groom dominant ones
- The dominant pig will lie on its side and let the subordinate pig groom its belly (nibbling)
- In confined pigs behaviours such as scratching replace natural behaviour.

EXOTIC ANIMAL BEHAVIOUR

Exotic species encompass small mammals, birds, reptiles and amphibians. The range of behaviour displayed is vast and thorough research should be undertaken to evaluate what would be considered normal and abnormal. It is important to consider whether species would be housed individually or live in groups. Consider the impact of same-sex and mixed-sex groups, biological rhythms and whether animals are nocturnal or diurnal.

Many animals in this group will exhibit stress in captivity unless they become habituated to handling usually from an early age; hand rearing can be problematic, especially in parrots which imprint and subsequently rely on human contact; when it is removed they may feather pluck. Neutering can also be beneficial in species such as rabbits to reduce aggression. Enrichment of animal housing is important to meet the key needs, allowing these animals the capacity to express normal behaviour.

HUMAN–ANIMAL INTERACTION

History

It has been previously discussed how cats and dogs evolved into companion animals for human beings. Establishment of the human–animal bond is one of the factors which make human society's relationship with pet animals unique.

Historic role

- Scavengers
- Protect crops
- Hunting
- Working/genetic manipulation of breeds
- Pest control
- Pets/companions.

Remember that the status of different species and breeds varies worldwide depending upon local customs. For example, British people revere the dog yet Korean people will class them as a food species.

Main reasons to have pets

- Companionship
- Child substitutes
- Working role
- Aid for disabilities
- Guard.

Pets and children

- Teach responsibility
- Develop character
- Used as therapy for problem children
- Improve social and emotional development
- Thought to improve cognitive development due to bonding
- Develop parenting skills
- Develop life skills – marital skills, social networking.

Pets and geriatrics

- Companionship
- Security
- Reduce stress and increase well-being
- Allow independence
- Provide socialisation opportunities
- Increase exercise.

Physiological effects

- Pets As Therapy (PAT) dogs/cats used as therapy during rehabilitation from illness – promote well-being
- Research has found that pets:
  ○ Reduce stress
  ○ Increase well-being
- A study of cardiac patients suffering from coronary disease found that 5.7% of people with pets and who had recently had been hospitalised due to problems died compared to 28.2% of people without pets.
- Animal uses in therapeutic medicine are increasing:
  ○ Guide dogs
  ○ Hearing dogs
  ○ PAT dogs
  ○ Dolphins and dogs in autism
  ○ Seizure-alert dogs
  ○ Dogs for the disabled
  ○ Hippotherapy.

DRUG USE IN BEHAVIOURAL THERAPY

Drugs have their place in treating problem behavioural cases and in some instances can prove an invaluable aid during counterconditioning. Drug prescription must follow UK legislation. Newer drugs are less addictive, cause minimal sedation and are of low toxicity.

Table 15.1 Neurotransmitters and their actions

Neurotransmitter	Action
Amino acids Glutamate Gamma-aminobutyric acid (GABA)	Rapid point-to-point action Primary excitatory Primary inhibitory
Acetylcholine	Excitatory
Catcholamines/ indoleamines	Arousal of autonomic nervous system Depletion leads to depression
Dopamine	Depletion leads to depression Increase may be associated with stereotypic disorders
Noradrenaline (norepinephrine)	Parasympathetic effects Drugs that inhibit production used to treat depression
Adrenaline (epinephrine)	Sympathetic effects Drugs block production and reduce fear
Serotonin	Sleep–wake cycle control, mood and emotion control

Indications for drug therapy

- As an adjunct to behavioural therapy:
  ○ Treatment of separation anxiety, fears and phobias
  ○ Allow problem to be resolved quicker or in a safer manner
  ○ Concurrent retraining is necessary, otherwise problem may recur when drugs are stopped
  ○ Drug-aided desensitisation, controlled flooding and counterconditioning
- Where the behavioural problem is unlikely to be resolved by retraining alone:
  ○ Urine marking
  ○ Compulsive disorders, e.g. tail chasing
- When an underlying medical condition is the cause of the behavioural problem:
  ○ Cystitis, hyperthyroidism etc.
- Drugs therefore form a critical part of therapy.

Prior to treatment the following should be considered:

- Complete medical exam and diagnostic tests
- Accurate behavioural diagnosis
- Institution of an approved behavioural programme

- Individuality in response to psychoactive drugs
- Side-effects
- Cost.

The drugs used within the behavioural remit tend to concentrate their action on the central nervous system. A knowledge of the functions of neurotransmitters is essential (Table 15.1). With this knowledge, we can manipulate an increase or decrease in neurotransmitter frequency, which in turn will influence the response to stimuli.

Bibliography

Aspinall V 2003 Clinical procedures in veterinary nursing. Butterworth-Heinemann, Oxford

Aspinall V 2006 The complete textbook of veterinary nursing. Elsevier, London

Avey R, Cuthill I, Miller R et al 1994 The five kingdoms and behaviour. Nelson Thornes, Cheltenham

Beaver B V 1994 The veterinarian's encyclopaedia of animal behaviour. Iowa State Press, Iowa

Haupt K A 1998 Domestic animal behaviour for veterinarians and animal scientists, 3rd edn. Manson Publishing, London

Landsberg G, Hunthauzen W, Ackerman L 2005 Handbook of behavioural problems in the dog and cat, 2nd edn. Elsevier, Oxford

McGreevy P 2005 Equine behaviour. Saunders, Philadelphia

Pierce J M 1999 Animal learning and cognition, 2nd edn. Psychology Press/Routledge, New York

Ridley M 1995 Animal behaviour, 2nd edn. Blackwell, Oxford

Thorne C 1999 Waltham book of dog and cat behaviour. Butterworth Heinemann, Oxford

Toates F M 1980 Animal behaviour. John Wiley, Chichester, West Sussex

Chapter | **16** | *Jane Williams*

Grooming

This chapter considers the importance of grooming to maintain health in animals. The basic equipment used to facilitate the grooming process is discussed and basic grooming routines are provided.

Grooming is employed to improve the appearance of animals, for contact to build the human–animal bond and to promote health. Grooming can remove dead hair, thin thick hair, shorten long hair, trim nails, pluck hair, remove matted hair, massage the skin to promote circulation and skin tone and make the animal easy to clean. It also provides a valuable opportunity to health check the animal.

In the UK, there are 209 pedigree dog breeds recognised and classified by the Kennel Club into different groups according to the purpose they were originally bred for. Breed standards are available for each individual breed which outline the physical characteristics and behavioural attributes that quantify a specific breed.

There are seven groups:

1. Hound group
2. Gundog group
3. Terrier group
4. Utility group
5. Working group
6. Pastoral group
7. Toy group.

Cross-breeds are dogs whose parents were a combination (usually half and half) of pedigree breeds. These dogs often display a mixture of their ancestors' traits and examples include Lurchers and Labradoodles.

CANINE COAT TYPES

There are a number of different canine coat types:

- Wire
- Silk
- Wool
- Double
- Smooth.

There are three main types of hair. Guard hairs are thick, long and stiff and form the outer layer of the coat: their function is to make water run off the body. Wool hairs are thinner, softer and wavier than outer hairs; they lie close to the skin and act as an insulating undercoat. Sinus hairs comprise the whiskers and are found around the eyes, nose and mouth; they are very coarse and adapted to sense movement and contact. Some breeds have dense over- and undercoats, e.g. Husky, whereas others have no undercoat, e.g. Weimaraner. Consideration of the individual dog's coat type is essential before grooming to enable the correct products, equipment and techniques to be employed.

Wire coats

Examples of wire-coated breeds are the Dachshund and the Schnauzer. Wire coats are characteristically harsh with a dense topcoat and a softer undercoat. They can be long or short. The topcoat is harsh and wiry and the undercoat is dense. The exception is the coat of the jaw, the eyebrows, the chin and the ears; there is a beard on the chin, the eyebrows are bushy but the hair on the ears is almost smooth. The legs and feet are also well covered with a harsh coat.

Silky coat

Examples of silky-coated breeds are the Pekingese and the Afghan. Silky coats are characteristically long and straight with a very fine texture on the ribs, fore- and hindquarters and flanks. Hair is long from the forehead backwards, with a distinct silky 'topknot'. On the foreface the hair on the face is short but the ears and legs are well coated.

Wool or curly coats

Examples of wool-coated breeds are the Poodle, Burlington Terrier and the Irish Water Spaniel. Wool coats are characteristically profuse and dense with a harsh texture and have thick, curly hair.

Double coats

Examples of double-coated breeds are the Rough Collie, the German Shepherd, the Old English Sheepdog, the Samoyed, the St Bernard, the Lhasa Apso and the Shih Tzu. Double coats are characteristically made up of a dense soft undercoat concealed by a longer topcoat. The coat is profuse, of good harsh texture, not straight, but shaggy and free from curl, with an undercoat of waterproof pile.

Smooth coat

Examples of smooth-coated breeds include the Boxer, the Weimaraner and the Pointer (short and fine-haired smooth coat) and the Labrador and the Corgi (long and dense smooth coat). Smooth coats are tight to the body. Short smooth coats are characteristically short, flat and coarse to the touch with slightly longer hair under the tail. Long smooth coats are characteristically short and dense without wave or feathering, giving a fairly hard feel to the touch and with a dense undercoat.

FELINE COAT TYPES

Feline coats can be described as:

- Long
- Short
- Hard
- Soft
- Silky
- Coarse
- Thick
- Wavy.

In pedigree breeds coat type is an integral component of the breed standards and these are regulated by the Governing Council of the Cat Fancy. Generally for grooming a cat's coat is considered to be short-haired, long-haired or semi-long-haired, Burmese, Oriental and Siamese, although in the USA only short- and long-haired coats are recognised. Table 16.1 provides categorisation of feline coat according to breed type.

GROOMING EQUIPMENT

There is a vast range of grooming equipment available designed for use in a range of animal species (Figures 16.1 and 16.2). Dogs, cats and horses are the species in which grooming commonly occurs.

Slicker brush

These are used to remove dead hair from the coat in medium- and long-haired dogs. The hair is brushed following the natural direction it falls. Avoid using this brush in areas where there is little hair cover, e.g. hocks and elbows, and be aware that excessive pressure or use can result in 'brush burns'. Care should be taken especially with new brushes whose pins will be sharp; positioning the fingers one on either side of the handle and the middle finger on the back of the brush can monitor

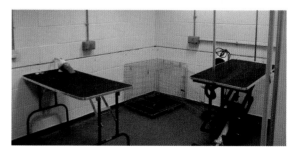

Figure 16.1 Grooming tables: with and without restraint frame.

Table 16.1 Feline coat categorisation

Coat type	Breeds	Characteristics
Long hair	Persian	Double coat: long overcoat and soft undercoat Prone to matts
Semi-long hair	Birman, Turkish Van, Ragdoll	Coat is long but not as long as the Persian and not double with a finer or shaggier texture, therefore less prone to matts forming
Short hair	British Short Hair, Manx, Foreign Abyssinian, Russian Blue, American Shaded Silver, Red Tabby	Dense coats which are easy to care for
Short curly coat	Cornish Rex, Devon Rex	None or very short guard hairs with lots of curly down hairs
Short, wire coat	American Blue Wirehair	Thick, woolly, wiry coarse coat It looks crimped, ringlet or curled in appearance
Hairless	Blue Sphynx	Appears bald but has some hairs present – fine covering of down hairs
Burmese	Burmese	Short
Oriental	Oriental Black, Blue and Havana	Short
Siamese	Siamese, Balinese	Short

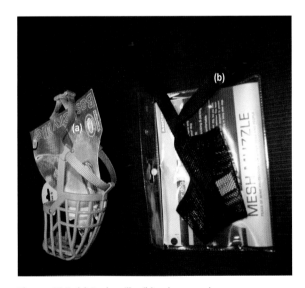

Figure 16.2 (a) Baskerville; (b) nylon muzzle.

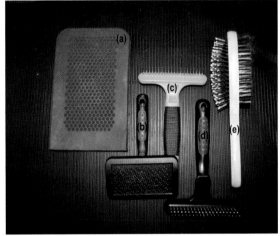

Figure 16.3 Selection of grooming brushes. (a) Hound mitt; (b) slicker brush; (c, d) grooming rakes; (e) combination pin and bristle brush

pressure. A pin brush is a type of slicker but with longer pins, used in long-haired dogs (Figure 16.3).

Dematting tools

Matt breakers come in many varieties: matt rakes, matt combs, single blades and comb kings. These can be used to remove large matts; often they have sharp blades and care should be taken not to cut the animal. The matt comb cuts through the matt but preserves the coat underneath. Blades require regular sharpening to maintain their efficacy. Comb kings are particularly useful for thinning double coats and aid hand stripping; they also have blades which are replaceable.

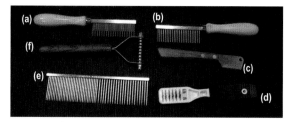

Figure 16.4 Selection of grooming combs. (a, b) Mixed-width combs; (c) undercoat stripper; (d) coat thinner; (e) wide-toothed comb; (f) comb king.

Stripping tools

Hand stripping is used on wire coats and silky coats to maintain the correct coat texture and colour by removing the dead topcoat and dead undercoat. Hand stripping can be achieved using the thumb and forefinger to avoid cutting the animal; the skin must be kept taut to prevent damage and reduce pain. Stripping knives are available.

Toothed combs

A wide variety of toothed combs are available with different spacing between the teeth to suit the coat type they are designed for. Choice will depend on the density and thickness of the hair to be groomed. Wide-toothed or long-toothed combs are used for thick coats and long-haired breeds. Narrow-toothed or short-toothed combs are used for short-haired breeds. Flea combs have very finely spaced teeth designed to remove fleas or flea dirt from the coat. When using combs, care should be taken to avoid pulling on coats as this can damage the hair. Combs need to be kept sterilised and should be regularly checked for broken teeth (Figure 16.4).

Scissors

A range of scissors are available for cutting and trimming coats. Double-edged thinning scissors are designed for thinning hair and blending the coat. Single-edged thinning scissors are used to remove hair. Carbon steel straight cutting scissors tend to be used for trimming whilst carbon steel curved cutting scissors are also used for trimming hair but particularly that of the feet. Heavy-duty scissors may be necessary to achieve straight cuts on the feathers of the leg (Figure 16.5).

Curry combs

Curry combs are used on smooth-coated animals. They remove dust and loose and dead hair and enhance shine. There are two main types: the rubber curry comb is con-

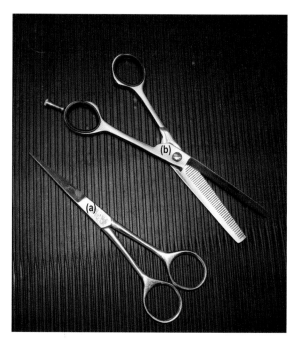

Figure 16.5 (a) Straight scissors; (b) thinning scissors.

structed from moulded plastic with pronounced points designed to groom and massage skin. Hound gloves or mitts are made from moulded rubber with short points and fit over the groomer's hand to groom and massage the skin in hound breeds.

Nail clippers

These are designed to cut the animal's nails. There are two types: guillotine and pliers-type. Guillotine clippers cut at a 90° angle to the nail and the pliers-type cuts on the bias. Both require regular cleaning including disinfection and maintenance of the hinge joint with oil (Figure 16.6).

Coagulants

These are products which make the blood clot. They are used when clipping nails to stop haemorrhage. Commercial products are available such as Quik Stop, potassium permanganate and silver nitrate pencils.

Clippers

Many different types are available to suit different jobs. They can be rechargeable or mains-operated with integral or interchangeable blades. The blades require regular disinfection and oiling. When clipping, the blade should be laid flat against the grain of hair. In dogs most clip-

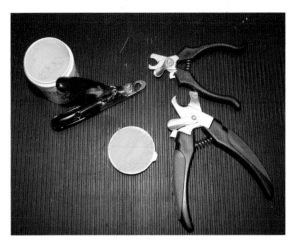

Figure 16.6 Equipment for nail clipping.

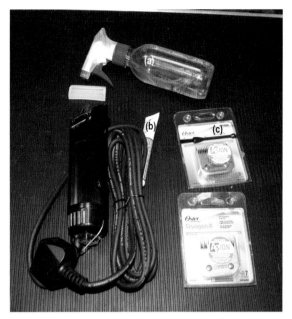

Figure 16.7 Clipping equipment. (a) Clippercide; (b) oil; (c) blades.

ping is done following the direction of coat growth whereas in horses the coat is clipped in the opposite direction to the lie of the coat. Avoid cutting or digging into the skin and avoid overheating as this can result in clipping burns from hot blades or fidgety animals and ultimately can burn out the motor.

Clippers can have snap-on plastic combs which guide the length of hair and produce a more uniform cut. Blade sizes vary according to use but generally high numbers translate to closer clips and lower numbers leave more coat. During clipping clippercide or clipper spray should be used regularly to disinfect and lubricate the blades. It is good practice to have a number of blades available for use to reduce the risk of overheating. Blades will require resharpening at regular intervals as blunt blades pull at the hair and spoil the overall effect (Figure 16.7).

Grooming tables

These should have a non-slip surface and ideally should be of adjustable height to enable the groomer to work at a comfortable height. They should incorporate some form of restraint apparatus: the most common is an overhead bar to which the dog's lead, belly and leg straps can be fastened, allowing the groomer to work independently.

The bath

Bath design should incorporate height adjustment, considering both the groomer and the animal, as lifting a heavy wet dog from a height could prove problematic. Some baths are hydraulic, whereas others incorporate a door to enable the animal to walk in and out. A shower

unit is often used to provide a flexible and adjustable-temperature water source (Figure 16.8).

Blasters

Blasters are commercial dryers that are used to remove or blast water from the animal's coat. The hose can be used with heat to dry the coat. They often come mounted on a stand which is height-adjustable to enable all breeds and table sizes to be used in conjunction with them (Figure 16.9).

Hair dryers

Commercial hand-held heated dryers are used to finish drying the coat and may be better tolerated around sensitive areas.

THE GROOMING PROCESS

1. Restrain the animal,
2. Place the animal and table at the correct height for the groomer and restrain it (Figure 16.10)
3. Begin grooming the rear legs to ascertain temperament away from the teeth
4. Groom out the entire coat by brushing with the grain (in the same direction) as the coat, using appropriate equipment

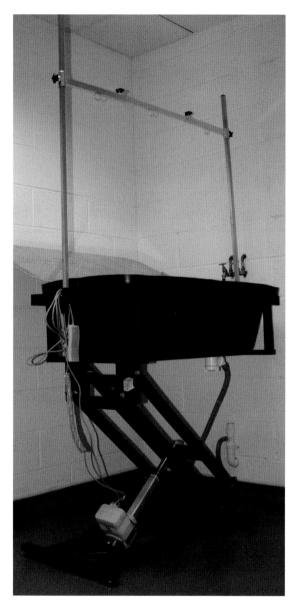

Figure 16.8 Hydraulic grooming bath. The use of hydaulics can prevent back strain in the handler.

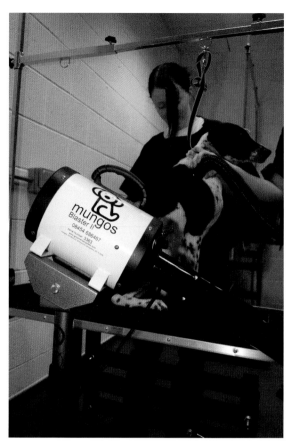

Figure 16.9 A blaster, used to remove excess water from the coat.

5. Dematt if required using clippers or a matt stripper
6. Use a comb in the matt and cut against the comb to reduce the risk of cutting the animal
7. Comb through the coat to check all matts are removed
8. Long-haired breeds may require feet and ears to be trimmed or plucked
9. Check ears, nails and anal glands.

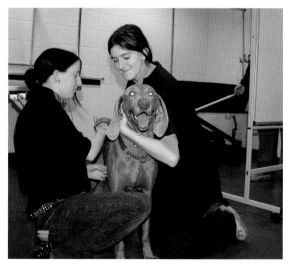

Figure 16.10 Grooming a large dog on the floor for safety.

The bathing process

1. Place a non-slip mat in the bath
2. Test water temperature; ideally aim for body temperature
3. Collect all equipment that may be required and have it to hand, e.g. shampoo, conditioner, sponge and towels (at this stage the ears may be plugged with cotton wool)
4. Brush-out of the coat and any clipping should be performed before the animal is wet
5. Restrain the dog and place it in the bath and restrain it again
6. Adjust the bath to the groomer's height
7. Check dog is secure and then wet the coat thoroughly using a plastic jug or shower, leaving the head till last
8. Apply shampoo and lather well; work into the coat, not forgetting stomach, elbows, toes, pinnae and urogenital area
9. Rinse thoroughly until water runs clear: when doing the head, take care to avoid water getting into the animal's eyes and ears
10. Squeeze out excess water with the hands, wrap the dog in a towel and remove it from the bath.

The drying process

1. Restrain and rub the animal dry with absorbent drying cloths and towels
2. A blaster or hair dryer can be used to dry the coat
3. Check the temperature of the dryer before use and throughout the drying process to prevent the animal getting burnt or overheating
4. If the dog is not used to the blaster, begin at the rear on a low setting to allow the animal time to adjust
5. Keep changing the area and distance of the dryer so no area is being dried for long periods at a time
6. In dogs with medium/long coats, try using a slicker brush to brush the hair in all directions to ensure it is dried down to the roots
7. Brush through the entire coat to check it is dry and ensure there are no knots, matts or debris.

Figure 16.11 provides an example of a grooming plan that could be used to record the grooming process.

Ear care and plucking

Ears should be cleaned using a commercial ear cleaner solution or wipe. Do not poke your fingers into the vertical canal; gently remove excess dirt and debris from the external canal using an ear wipe. Holding the pinna upright, insert a small quantity of ear cleaner into the canal, then massage the base of the ear to distribute the cleaner. Use another wipe to wipe the external canal gently to remove any debris that has been dislodged.

Very hairy ears may be plucked or trimmed using thinning scissors or forceps but beware, as the dog may object to this process.

After drying you can finish off by regrooming the dog and making any final adjustments.

Shampoos and conditioners

Properties of an ideal product would include:

- Hypoallergenic
- Non-toxic
- Non-irritant
- Cheap
- Easy to use
- Lathers well
- Removes dirt without stripping oils from coat
- Easy to rinse
- Pleasant smell
- Parasiticide, antibacterial and fungicidal.

There is a wide range of products available to suit coat types, conditions and owner preferences. Products include shampoos, conditioners and coat enhancers. Shampoos clean the coat, conditioners serve to replace essential oils lost during bathing, coat enhancer applies gloss and replaces oils and detangler sprays enable tangles to be brushed out more easily during grooming. Table 16.2 outlines factors which affect shampoo choice.

Table 16.2 Factors that influence shampoo choice	
Coat type	**Products matched to type of coat**
Owner preference	Products chosen by the owner, e.g. smell/perception
Salon-approved	Products recommended by professional groomers
Medicated	Products that clean and contribute to the treatment of animals, e.g. fleas, eczema, mites
Veterinary-prescribed	Products that treat conditions which are prescription-only, i.e. dispensed by vet
Coat enhancers	Products which make coat smoother and shinier

Name of groomer:		
Date:		
Client name:	Contact telephone number:	
Dog's name:	Age:	Sex:
Colour:	Possessions:	Special notes:
Client instructions:		
Dog's prior experience of grooming:		
Kennel number:	Water:	Food:
Toilet opportunity:	Urine:	Faeces:
Preliminary examination:		
Coat type:		
Coat condition:		
Skin condition:		
Parasites:		
Nails:		
Anal glands:		
Dental health:		
Ears:		
Eyes:		
Behaviour:		
Grooming plan - to be completed prior to grooming		
Start time:	Finish time:	
Review of grooming:		
Client information:		
Client contacted by:	Dog to be collected at:	

Figure 16.11 A typical grooming plan.

Table 16.3 Shampoo types

Shampoo type	Recommendations	Comments
Hypoallergenic	Suitable for all coat and dog types	Does not cause allergies
Parasiticidal	Kills parasites – fleas and lice	Veterinary-prescribed Medicated shampoo
Antibacterial	Kills bacteria – suitable for skin conditions	Veterinary-prescribed Medicated shampoo
Fungicidal	Kills fungi and yeasts – suitable for skin conditions	Veterinary-prescribed Medicated shampoo

There are five main types of shampoo (Table 16.3):

1. Cleansing: these shampoos contain a strong active ingredient that acts against grease and dirt
2. Mild: these remove grease and dirt, leaving in some of the natural oils
3. Medicated: these shampoos contain mild antibacterial products that act on the skin
4. Veterinary: prescribed by vets for particular skin conditions
5. Insecticidal: kill parasites.

When choosing a shampoo one should consider the following:

- Frequency of washing
- Age of animal
- Allergies
- Age of animal
- Cost
- Owner allergies
- Groomer allergies
- Level of dirt/contamination, e.g. Swarfega is used for oil contamination
- Ease of use
- Products can be bought ready for use or requiring dilution
- Dilution: follow manufacturer's instructions.

Use of conditioners

Regular washing can remove the natural oils from the coat. Applying a conditioner can replace lost essential oils and aims to restore the coat to its natural state. Using a mild shampoo can be important to reduce the risk of stripping the coat of its natural oils, especially in dogs which require a waterproof or insulating coat.

Conditioners also promote the client's perception that groomed dogs should smell nice and have a soft, glossy coat. Conditioner should be matched to the dog's coat and the shampoo used and care should be taken not to leave any in the coat as it will become greasy.

Clipping nails

Clipping nails is a relatively straightforward procedure. Good restraint is essential and there are a number of commercial products available. Nail clippers come in a variety of shapes and sizes to suit all nail types. The nail should be clipped so it is in line with the associated pad and care should be taken to avoid cutting the quick, which is the nail's vascular and nervous supply. If haemorrhage does occur then styptics or haemostats such as potassium permanganate or silver nitrate can be applied to promote coagulation and stop bleeding.

Procedure for clipping nails

1. Collect all equipment required and have restraint equipment ready for use if required
2. Recruit a helper to restrain the dog and prevent the dog's leg from moving
3. Clip the nail in a quick, decisive manner in line with the base of the pad
4. Apply haemostat if required!

For wrigglers use your helper to prevent movement. With black nails apply the golden rule 'less is more'. All equipment should be checked to see if it works before you start and if bleeding does occur then apply haemostat but don't panic, as the bleeding will usually subside quickly.

GROOMING HORSES

Horses in work are usually groomed at least once per day to promote a healthy appearance, to remove dirt, debris and sweat residue from the coat and to build up a relationship between the horse and its handler or rider. Grooming equipment is organised into a grooming kit which is allocated to an individual animal to prevent the spread of disease. It may be kept in a grooming tray or box and should be regularly disinfected. The horse may be groomed inside or outside the stable and should be tied up using a quick-release knot via a piece of string before starting the process. The handler should wear a hard hat, gloves and steel toe-capped boots to prevent injury. Individuality should be considered as not all horses will tolerate the same rigour of grooming or may be temperamental in certain areas.

The grooming kit should contain:

- Dandy brush: a hard bristle brush used for removing mud and sweat. Avoid its use in clipped horses and those with sensitive skin
- Body brush: a soft bristled brush used for brushing out the mane, tail and sensitive areas
- Curry comb: constructed from metal or plastic, the body brush is passed over the grooves of the curry comb to remove dirt and dust which is then collected in the curry comb; tapping the curry comb on the floor will remove the debris from it. Rubber curry combs can also be used to massage the coat and improve circulation
- Sponges: used to bathe the eyes, nostrils, genitals and udder; a separate sponge should be used for each area to prevent cross-contamination
- Mane comb: a metal or plastic comb used to brush and remove knots from the mane and tail
- Wash brush: used during bathing, often to wash mud and dirt from the hooves
- Hood pick: metal or plastic versions are available; they have blunt ends which are used to remove compacted mud and debris from the indentations on either side of the frog in the hoof
- Stable rubber: a soft cloth used at the end of the grooming process to polish the coat and give it a healthy shine.

Bathing the horse is a similar process to that described for the dog. However there are not many baths big enough for use! Hose pipes or buckets are commonly employed to carry water; ideally the water should be at body temperature. The horse should be secured using a quick-release knot or by an assistant. The head is usually washed and dried first, taking care not to get water in the eyes or ears; head collars are available which have a detachable throat lash to enable a sponge to be used underneath them whilst maintaining a degree of restraint. The coat, mane and tail should be thoroughly wet then shampoo applied and massaged into them. All areas should be rinsed thoroughly to ensure all shampoo residue has been removed, then excess water is removed using a sweat scraper and the horse is walked, rugged up or placed under heat lamps to dry the coat.

Clipping horses

Clipping is commonplace in the equine industry, particularly during the winter months when horses grow a thick winter coat for insulation which results in profuse sweating during exercise. There are a variety of different clips performed to suit the individual horse and owner. The process is similar to that described for dogs, obviously taking care to prevent injury to the handler or the animal. As horses are large a number of blades are needed to prevent heat generation during the clipping process.

Bibliography

Aspinall V 2006 The complete textbook of veterinary nursing. Butterworth Heinemann, London

Dallas S 2006 Animal biology and care, 2nd edn. Wiley/Blackwell, Oxford

Dallas S, North D, Angus J 2006 Grooming manual for the dog and cat. Wiley/Blackwell, Oxford

Lane D R, Cooper B, Turner L 2007 Textbook of veterinary nursing, 3rd edn. Butterworth-Heinemann/BSAVA, Oxford

Moore M 2000 Manual of veterinary nursing. BSAVA, Oxford

Pratt P W 1998 Principles and practice of veterinary technology. Mosby, Philadelphia

Simpson G 1994 Practical veterinary nursing, 3rd edn. BSAVA, Oxford

Warren D M 1995 Small animal care and management. Delmar, New York

Chapter | **17** | *Hayley Randle*

Research methods

This chapter examines common ethical issues and practices in modern research for animal management students and staff. It is likely that research studies focusing on animal health will rely on laboratory-based experiments whereas those examining welfare will tend to utilise field-based studies. It is the intention that this chapter will provide a basis for both types of study.

Regardless of the nature of the research study undertaken the experimenter must be familiar with the principles of experimental design and able to apply them properly. A poorly designed study can, at best, only generate poor-quality data. Whilst the assumption that the 'more data the better' may be true in a general sense, a data set comprising a smaller number of good-quality data points is always preferable to one made up of a larger quantity of poor-quality data points. There is nothing worse than being presented with a mass of data which are effectively meaningless, especially when this situation could have been easily avoided by more thorough planning at the experimental design stage. Even the most simple and apparently straightforward research project is becoming increasingly costly to implement, therefore steps must be taken in order to ensure the best use of the available resources (i.e. time, money and staffing). Furthermore, the comprehensive application of the principles of experimental design is crucial to the ability to maximise the data output of the piece of research being undertaken.

This chapter will cover the main principles of experimental design in relation to animal-based studies and provide an introduction to basic statistics. The intention of the statistics section of this chapter is to enable the reader to make sense of the mass of statistical terminology that appears in scientific publications such as journal articles. For example, what is the meaning of $P < 0.05$? This chapter is not intended to provide a step-by-step guide to statistics; there are plenty of excellent books in use already, including Zar's *Biostatistical Analysis* (1996) and Eddison's (2000) *Quantitative Investigations in the Biosciences Using MINITAB* (a commonly used entry-level statistics package).

WHAT IS SCIENTIFIC RESEARCH?

Before focusing on animal-based research in detail it is necessary to consider what research – in particular, scientific research – is actually about. A scientist will typically make statements such as: 'I shall try an experiment', 'I have a theory that …' and 'I will treat this question scientifically'. Key terms frequently used include 'science'/'scientific', 'experiment'/'experimental', 'theory'/'theorise'. Definitions of these terms are provided in Box 17.1.

It can be seen that there is considerable overlap in the definitions of the terminology associated with research. It is therefore no coincidence that the authors of published academic texts frequently use these terms interchangeably. All of the key words presented form part of 'research' which itself is defined in terms of 'the system-

Box 17.1

DEFINITIONS OF SCIENTIFIC TERMS

Experiment (noun)

A procedure undertaken to make a discovery, test a hypothesis or demonstrate a known fact

Experiment (verb)

To explore, to investigate, to probe, to sample, to search, to test

Experimental (adjective)

Based on or making use of an experiment

Science (noun)

1. A branch of knowledge involving the systematised observation of and experiment with phenomena. 2. A systematic and formulated knowledge, e.g. of a specified type or on a specified subject

Scientific (adjective)

1. (a) (of an investigation) According to the rules laid down in an exact science for performing observations and testing the soundness of conclusion; (b) systematic, accurate. 2. Used in, engaged in, or relating to (especially natural) science

Theorise (verb)

1. To evolve or indulge in theories. 2. To consider or devise in theory

Theory (noun)

1. A supposition or system of ideas explaining something, especially one based on general principles independent of the particular things to be explained. 2. A speculative view. 3. The sphere of abstract knowledge or speculative thought. 4. The exposition of the principles of a science

Definitions taken from Thompson D (ed.) 1996 Oxford compact English dictionary. Oxford University Press, Oxford.

atic investigation into and study of' … 'discovery' … and 'critical investigation' (Thompson 1996). It is imperative, then, that researchers ensure that the studies they design adhere to the core principles of research evident from the terminology outlined in Box 17.1.

Imagination- and evidence-driven research

Imagination-driven research, also known as 'pure research', requires complete freedom to undertake an investigation simply for the sake of it. This is the kind of research that most researchers can only dream about

being able to do and would enable all of the 'what if' ideas/musings to be investigated. In reality, funding is simply not available to support such curiosity-led research ideas and the majority of published research falls into the latter category. Evidence-driven research, also referred to as 'applied research', is undertaken in order to examine specific questions for a precise purpose. There is a strong expectation of evidence-driven research to produce firm, statistical conclusions that have immediate application within the allied industry. Furthermore, proponents of evidence-driven research/science maintain that conclusions can only be published if they are supported by 'hard evidence'. Conclusions written along the lines 'it appears that' or 'there was a trend that suggested' are considered to be inadequate, and instead findings must refer to objectives, hypotheses, test statistics and probabilities.

It is worth noting that in reality, however, the two approaches are to some extent reconciled. The imagination-driven scientist may have the idea for the research, whereas the evidence-driven scientist designs the experiment and tests the idea. Clearly there is a potentially interesting overlap between science and art here. Those who have had responsibility for the feeding of animals will know that, although an individual animal's diet can be rationed according to scientific principles (which are likely to involve calculations based on factors such as live weight, production requirements and the constituents of the feedstuff), it is often an 'artistic tweak' such as the adding of a 'bit' of 'this' and a 'spot' of 'that' that produces the required output. These additions are based solely on knowledge and experience and are rarely quantifiable (as evidence-driven science requires!). In summary, a good scientist should be driven by both imagination and evidence, be able to apply scientific principles rigorously in order to produce viable data from a comprehensively designed experiment/study, whilst remaining open-minded. Needless to say this can be quite a tall order, but as Barnard et al. (2007, p. 1) state: 'science is simply formalised speculation backed up (or otherwise) by equally formalised observation and experimentation. In its broadest sense most of us "do science" all of the time.'

THE RESEARCH PROCESS

Uncontrolled and controlled research

Research can be further categorised into uncontrolled and controlled studies (Manly 1992). Uncontrolled studies are where the experimenter is essentially just looking to see 'what is going on', and the underlying processes of what he/she is observing are not necessarily understood. The objectives of such studies are likely to contain wording such as 'exploration' and 'investigation'. Data may also be subjective (i.e. depend very much on the individual observer's view and interpretation of what is being seen). It can be seen in Figure 17.1 that the starting point is the 'uncontrollable events' where all that the experimenter can do is simply observe what is happening. At some point there may be a change in what is being seen. At this point the experimenter can ask: 'what caused that change?' Based on any previous knowledge (don't forget that all good research projects will have been preceded by a thorough review of the literature), the experimenter will be able to investigate more deeply by making further changes to the experimental set-up (for example, removing some animals from a group, manipulating environmental temperature) and recording any further changes in what is being seen or recorded as a result of the intervention. It should be remembered that with uncontrolled research there may not be a spontaneous visible change (also referred to as a 'perturbation') in what is observed. In this case the experimenter will manipulate the population, i.e. apply an intervention, with the intention of effecting a change in what is being observed. Any consequent changes (or not) will be recorded. With the latter scenario it may simply be a case of the experimenter inventing different things to look at, for example dividing the population into different samples (by age or by gender) and doing comparisons. Whilst the options are endless, they can lack focus. As can be seen in Figure 17.1, subsequent analysis can be of simply descriptive or a more complex analytical nature.

Figure 17.2 illustrates controlled research in which the observer/experimenter identifies the variables that are going to be examined and measured before the study commences, and retains full control over the design of the study, the form of the data collected and therefore the outcome of the work. Three main types of experimental design are used in controlled research: one-off, unreplicated studies; replicated studies (where a series of identical studies are undertaken); and studies undertaken in order to gain information upon which to form a model. (This last type is popular in clinical drug trials.)

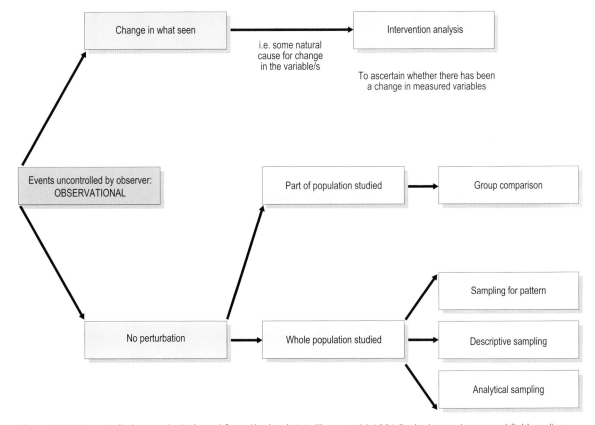

Figure 17.1 Uncontrolled research. (Adapted from Eberhardt L L, Thomas J M 1991 Designing environmental field studies. Ecological Monographs 61:52–73.)

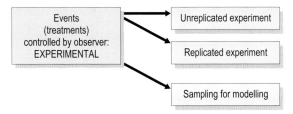

Figure 17.2 Controlled research. (Adapted from Eberhardt L L, Thomas J M 1991 Designing environmental field studies. Ecological Monographs 61:52–73.)

Clearly the experimenter has more responsibility for, and ownership of, the design of the study and consequently the data that are obtainable in controlled research than in uncontrolled research.

It is worth noting that in reality research of an uncontrolled general exploratory nature is usually much more difficult to assess and analyse than research which relies on a controlled experimental design and set-up. Although controlled research appears to be more labour-intensive in terms of setting up, it is much easier to implement and to deal with the data that have been generated and results in conclusions that can be usefully and rapidly applied.

Induction and deduction

Before commencing any data collection it is important to remember the importance of the continual cross-referencing of what is currently under investigation with what is already known (i.e. laws and theories). It is crucial to find out what is already known about a particular area before conducting your own research. Figure 17.3 illustrates the relationship between the philosophies of induction and deduction, and the uncontrolled and controlled approaches to research. In summary, induction will permit the acquisition of facts (which may be of a baseline nature) and often depends on the use of an uncontrolled research approach, whereas deduction allows prediction and explanation of facts based on the use of controlled research approaches.

Researchers must be aware that research is an ongoing process and cyclical in nature. An experiment designed to answer one specific question typically generates many more questions. The trick is for the experimenter to remain focused on the question in hand and not to go off at a tangent until the initial research has been conducted. The ability to remain focused to achieve successful completion of a research project is what I consider to be the difference between a 'butterfly-brain' researcher who flits about all over the place never reaching a useful endpoint and one who is not!

Any piece of research will rely on the identification of clear objectives, such as 'This study will identify …'. Each

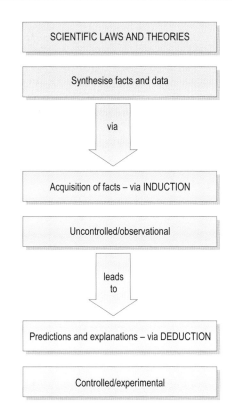

Figure 17.3 Synthesis of induction and deduction.

objective will have associated with it hypotheses which are integral to the statistical analysis process. The relationship between induction, hypotheses and deduction, illustrated in Figure 17.4, indicates the iterative nature of research whereby the acquisition of new facts (through induction) and explanation and prediction (through deduction) leads to the modification of hypotheses and the expansion of the original research question.

SIX STEPS TO A GOOD RESEARCH STUDY

It is essential to follow a prescribed format when setting up a piece of research, whether a small student project or a full-scale postdoctoral project. The six main steps are:
1. Generation of the research question
2. Formulation of hypotheses
3. Designing the experiment
4. Data collection and collation
5. Data analysis
6. Reaching statistical conclusions.

Each of these steps will be addressed in turn.

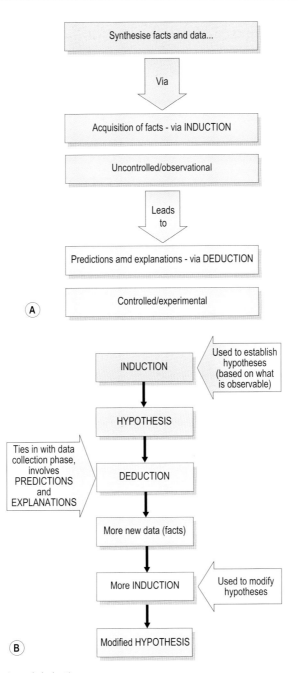

Figure 17.4 Induction, hypothesis and deduction.

Generation of the research question

Remember that the researcher is responsible for producing outcomes that are useful and applicable within the allied industry, for example the development of drugs for treating animal illness or the modification of husbandry practices to improve welfare. One of the first steps in any research project is to conduct a comprehensive review of the existing academic literature. Literature reviews can be an onerous task in their own right, therefore a useful tip is to focus on the desired endpoint. A useful analogy is one of a funnel, whereby the literature that is reviewed starts broadly and then narrows down to the objective of the proposed study. If a research project has attracted funding then a comprehensive review of the published literature will normally have been conducted in order to assemble the necessary application paperwork. It is crucial to be aware of all of the work that has been done in your area, not least to avoid literal replication and to help inform the construction of your alternative hypothesis/hypotheses. A useful tip is to look at the introduction sections of academic papers published in animal health/welfare journals; these are relatively short (in scientific journals introductions rarely exceed 1000 words), sharply focused (despite in the region of 30 references typically listed at the end of the paper) and usually end with a statement of the objectives of the study that is reported in the paper.

Formulation of hypotheses

Hypotheses are fundamental to scientific research and are broadly defined as 'a statement of belief about how the real world behaves'. Hypotheses must produce predictions which can be falsified by experimentation.

Hypothesis construction

Hypotheses come in opposing pairs. Consider the following example: One group of dairy cows are fed on a normal dairy ration, A, whilst another group of cows are fed on a new dairy ration, B, that is claimed to alter the butter fat percentage of milk. The hypotheses would be written as follows:

- Null hypothesis (H_0): There is no significant difference in the butter fat percentage of cows on dairy ration A and the butter fat percentage of cows on dairy ration B.
- Alternative hypothesis (H_a): There is a significant difference in the butter fat percentage of cows on dairy ration A and the butter fat percentage of cows on dairy ration B.

Significance testing and probability

Hypotheses are meaningless without significance and probability. It is therefore necessary to be able to apply the method for determining which hypothesis is going to be accepted and which hypothesis is going to be rejected. Although statistical analysis is very much based on numbers, at this point it is useful to be able to think outside the box as it is necessary to understand probability. Every single statistical analysis will generate a probability (P) value which will be between 0.0001 and 1.0. (Note that a P-value can never equal zero, despite some of the output that statistical packages may return!) Statistics refers to 'the probability that the observed result arose by chance'. In order to understand what this means, consider the following: 'Suppose we repeat an experiment 100 times: how many times would you get the same result?' For the dairy ration study, suppose the study showed that ration B resulted in a higher milk butter fat content than ration A. If the study was repeated on 99 more occasions, how likely are we to get the same result (i.e. that ration B resulted in a higher milk butter fat content than ration A)?

There are three standard critical probability levels – 0.05, 0.01 and 0.001. A P-value of 0.05 is the same as $5/100$ (= $1/20$), which means that there is a 5 in 100 (1 in 20) chance that the observed result occurred by chance and therefore cannot be relied upon to be repeatable. In other words, there is a 5 in 100 chance that the opposite result would be obtained (i.e. that ration A resulted in a higher milk butter fat content than ration B). It has become accepted that as long as the result is 95% probable (i.e 95/100) then the result is acceptable and can be relied upon.

Similarly, a P-value of 0.01 (1/100) means that there is a 1 in 100 chance of different result occurring, but 99 in 100 that the same result will occur. Likewise a P-value of 0.001 (0.1/100) means that there is a 1 in 1000 chance of a different result occurring. The general rule is that as long as the P-value is less than 0.05 (i.e. $P < 0.05$), the result is reliable and can be used. Furthermore, the lower the P-value (i.e. closer to zero), the more reliable and repeatable the result is.

Once a probability value has been obtained it is possible to reach a statistical conclusion using the following rules:

If $P < 0.05$, the result is significant, the H_0 is rejected and the H_a is accepted. The conclusion is then reached that there is a significant difference in the butter fat percentage achieved between rations A and B. (Further analysis will be needed to investigate the direction of the differences.)

If $P \geq 0.05$, the result is non-significant, the H_0 is accepted and the H_a is rejected. The conclusion is then reached that there is no significant difference in the butter fat percentage achieved between rations *A* and *B*.

Hypotheses, samples and populations

Populations and samples

It is rarely possible to gain information from an entire population and in reality the best that can be achieved is to study a part of the population (i.e. a sample).

Figures 17.5 and 17.6 illustrate simple plots of two data samples. In Figure 17.5 it can be seen that the data from the two samples overlap and appear to come from the same population, whilst those in Figure 17.6 do not.

It is likely that the plot in Figure 17.5 represents a situation where the H_0 (that there is no significant difference) is likely to be accepted, whereas the plot in Figure 17.6 represents a situation where the H_a (that there is a significant difference) is likely to be accepted.

Normal distribution and tails

Any sample of data will conform to some kind of shape such as that of normal distribution, which is typified by a bell-shaped curve (Figure 17.7).

In normal distribution around 95% of the values cluster around an average value. The remaining 5% of the values are split between those that are less than the majority and those that are more than the majority. These sit in the tails of the distribution. Tails are linked to the formulation of the alternative hypothesis. Bearing in mind that the H_a states that there is a difference, then there is an option simply to 'sit on the fence' and just state simply that 'there is a significant difference' without specifying a direction – this is known as a two-tailed test and this approach should be adopted in most situations. However, if, and only if, the experimenters are confident that they know everything there is to be known about the subject area, they may wish to formulate a one-tailed alternative hypothesis. This would typically state that 'there is a significant difference' and ration *B* will result in higher milk butter fat than ration *A*, i.e. the direction of the difference has been stated. One-tailed hypotheses are best used with caution as an unexpected result may be returned where the difference is in the unanticipated direction, and therefore cannot be explained. It is also more difficult to achieve significance with one-tailed tests.

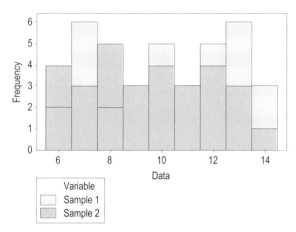

Figure 17.5 Histogram plot of two samples of data from a single population.

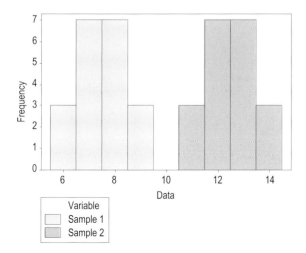

Figure 17.6 Histogram plot of two samples of data from two different populations.

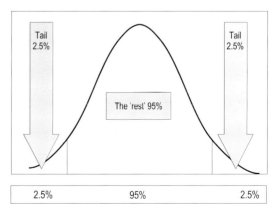

Figure 17.7 Example of a normal curve.

Designing the experiment

There are many texts devoted purely to experimental design, for example Manly (1992). This chapter seeks only to provide some guidance. When designing experiments it should be remembered that the crux of statistical analysis is the ability to ascribe variation correctly to different sources. Within a set of data variance may be identifiable, i.e. attributable to the variables under investigation, or non-identifiable (often referred to as residual or error variation). Residual or error variation comprises all of the other factors that are going on, but are not being investigated explicitly. For example, when examining the effect of enclosure temperature on activity levels by a group of small primates kept in an indoor enclosure in a zoo, other possible influences, for example wind strength and direction, effect of visitors and time since last feeding, are ignored and combined to form error or residual variation. The majority of statistical tests rely on the comparison of identifiable and non-identifiable (error/residual) variation. The point of most experiments is to examine the effect of changing one variable (the independent variable, IV) on one or more other variable(s) (dependent variables, DV), whilst keeping all other experimental conditions (and independent variables) constant. It is imperative to clarify which of the variables involved are independent (i.e. those being investigated or manipulated by the experimenter) and which are dependent (i.e. those which generate the information required about the IV) during the experimental design phase before the commencement of the data collection period. In the primate example above, the IV is the enclosure temperature (this can be manipulated by the experimenter) and the DV is the activity level (which may be influenced by enclosure temperature). A further example follows. In a study of the effect of feeding a particular neutraceutical on equine lameness the researcher would use an IV, feed type (which may comprise two treatments – treatment 1, feed only and treatment 2, feed plus neutraceutical). The DV would be the information that is recorded as an outcome of the experiment, and would be something like 'lameness score'.

The importance of a correctly designed experiment cannot be overemphasised. A frequently cited example of how a badly designed experiment can lead to wrong conclusions follows. Sir Ronald Fisher gave an example in which three human subjects (*A*, *B* and *C*) were each given a large drink consisting of half an alcoholic short and half water (subject *A* had half gin, half water, subject *B* had half whisky, half water and subject *C* had half brandy, half water). All subjects became drunk. Since the common element in all three drinks was the water, the conclusion was reached that water causes drunkenness!

Experimental design

There are five recognised characteristics of a well-designed experiment: clearly defined hypotheses, experimental treatments, IVs and measures (DVs) and experimental units (subjects). There will also be replication (to ensure variability is measurable for subsequent statistical analysis) and randomisation in order to avoid bias. These characteristics are best demonstrated using an example (Box 17.2).

The experimental design described can now be assessed in terms of the five characteristics of a well-designed experiment (Table 17.1), in addition to the identification of the IV (treatments X and C) and the DV (number of midge bites).

Why replicate?

Without replication it is impossible to measure the inherent variability among the experimental units that are treated alike. It is also possible to assess the extent of the difference between treatments in relation to the inherent variability between the subjects (experimental units) within a treatment. In other words, the extent of the difference between horses on the same treatment and the two groups of horses on the different treatments is important. It can be seen in Table 17.2 that horses on compound X vary from 3 to 6 bites, whilst horses treated with compound C vary from 5 to 9 bites.

Box 17.2

EXPERIMENTAL ASSESSMENT OF THE EFFECTIVENESS OF COMPOUND X AS A MIDGE REPELLENT IN HORSES

An experiment was planned to test a new preparation as a repellent against the sweet-itch-causing midge (*Culicoides* sp.) for horses. The active ingredient, compound X, is dissolved in alcohol and applied topically to the skin on the body, as the test treatment X. Treatment X is to be compared with a control treatment C (comprising only alcohol, also applied topically). The null hypothesis states that there is no significant difference in the number of midge bites received by horses treated with X and horses treated with C. The alternative hypothesis states that there is a significant difference in the number of midge bites received by horses treated with X and horses treated with C. There are eight subjects in all: four are selected at random to have treatment X applied and the remaining four to receive treatment C. All horses are then turned out into the same field at dusk for 30 minutes. The horses are then taken indoors and the number of midge bites received by each horse recorded

Table 17.1 Assessment of how well the experiment has been designed

Characteristic	Assessment
Clearly defined hypotheses	The null hypothesis is that there is no significant difference in the number of bites between X and C. The alternative hypothesis is that there is a significant difference in the number of bites between X and C
Clearly defined experimental treatments (IVs) and measures (DVs)	There are two experimental treatments: X and C. The IV is drug preparation for topical application. The DV (measured data) comprises number of midge bites
Clearly defined experimental units	There are eight experimental units, i.e. eight horses
Replication	Each treatment was replicated four times. Four horses had compound X applied and the remaining four had compound C applied
Randomisation	The horses were randomly selected for each treatment

IV, independent variable; DV, dependent variable.

Table 17.2 Number of midge bites received by subjects on either treatment X or C

	Experimental Unit (Horse)							
	1	2	3	4	5	6	7	8
Treatment	X	X	C	C	X	C	X	C
Data (bites)	3	6	5	8	5	9	4	6
Totals	Total bites treatment X= 18; total bites control treatment C= 28							

In total 18 bites were received by horses on treatment X (average $18 \div 4 = 4.5$ bites per horse) and 28 bites were received by horses on treatment C (average $28 \div 4 = 7$ bites per horse). This means that 10 fewer midge bites were received by the horses treated with X than by the horses treated with C (an average of $10 \div 4 = 2.5$ bites per horse).

Why randomise?

When allocating the treatments to the experimental units randomisation is necessary in order to avoid the occurrence of bias. Table 17.2 showed that the group of 4 subjects on treatment X received fewer midge bites than the group of 4 subjects on treatment C. The key question is: could this difference (2.5 bites/subject on average) be indicative of a real treatment effect (i.e. X versus C) or simply be caused by the variation between individual experimental units (horses) receiving the same treatment? Statistical tests will enable us to answer this question – as stated above, the majority of tests rely on the examination of the treatment variation in relation to the residual/error variation.

Box 17.3

ADDITIONAL EXPERIMENTAL DESIGN CONSIDERATIONS FOR THE HORSE MIDGE EXAMPLE

- Have each of the experimental units (horses) been equally exposed to midge attack?
- Is eight experimental units (horses) sufficient?
- Should a third treatment, application of no alcohol, be included?
- Some of the experimental units (horses) appear to be more susceptible to midge bites than others (Table 17.2, horses 4 and 6). How can this be controlled for?
- The experimental units (horses) comprised males and females. Should gender be taken into account? If so, how?
- What was the condition of the skin before the application of the treatment?
- Should this be controlled? If so, how?
- If X does result in fewer midge bites, what should be the next steps of the investigation?

More aspects of experimental design to consider for the midge example

Box 17.3 lists a number of additional questions that should be considered about the design of the midge experiment.

Further features of a well-designed animal-based experiment

There are a number of additional features of animal-based experiments that require careful consideration during experimental design.

Controls and confounding factors

The horse–midge example relied upon the use of a control treatment; however, there could have been an experimental confound because of the handling of the horses and the compounds used in the treatment. Furthermore, compound X was dissolved into alcohol, which itself could have had an effect on the number of midge bites received by the individual horses. When designing experiments, awareness of all the possible confounding factors is imperative if valid and reliable results are to be obtained.

Experimenter (and owner) bias

There are many points during an experiment when the experimenters' expectations can influence the outcome of the study, including when administering the treatments, when recording/measuring the data and when analysing the data. However, bias can be controlled by means of blind (where the person who is responsible for recording the data does not know which treatment the animal has been on until the experiment is completed) and double-blind experiments (where neither the experimenter nor the subject, or subject's owner, knows which treatment the animal has been allocated to until the experiment is completed). Double-blind experiments are particularly common with clinical drug trials.

Replication (between studies)

In addition to replication within an experiment there can also be replication between studies. However, given resourcing difficulties frequently experienced today, literal replication (where identical conditions, procedures and measures are used) is best avoided in favour of constructive replication which attempts to build upon existing work (e.g. through the use of a different procedure, condition or species).

Order effects

Order effects are particularly common in studies involving animals and therefore the treatment and observation of an individual on successive occasions must be avoided, due to the 'dulling' of the subject's sensitivity and potential blanketing of any other results arising from the treatment itself. It may be possible to overcome order effects by carefully presenting treatment to groups in different orders, but this is unlikely to be successful.

Independence of data points

In any experiment there is the assumption that individual data points or measurements are independent of each other, but in animal-based research this is often violated due to one (or more) of the following: the pooling fallacy, litter and other group effects and independence of categories.

The pooling fallacy is caused by treating successive measurements from subjects as if they were independent. As Martin and Bateson (2007) point out, taking additional measurements from the same subjects is not the same as increasing the number of subjects in the sample. To clarify, it is commonly believed that if repeated measures are taken for a single subject they should be averaged to give a single score per subject, and that the sample size, n, should equal the number of subjects, not the number of data points/measurements obtained.

Litter and other group effects

Problems of independence also occur when subjects have much in common, such as being litter mates. If within-litter relations are ignored then the statistical differences between groups are likely to be overestimated. The existence of litter effects can be investigated by examining both the within-litter variation and the variation between the litters. If the variation within the litter is significantly smaller than that between the litters then there is a litter effect (since the measurements between litter mates are not statistically independent) which is confounding the experimental/control comparison. Litter (group) effects can be designed out of the experiment by only taking measures from one randomly selected individual from each litter/group, using the litter/group average as the measure or incorporating a possible litter effect into the statistical analysis.

Independence of categories

Problems with independence may also occur if categories or measures are not independent of each other. Two variables may be related, either because there is an association between the two, or because the two variables are measures of the same thing. This experimental error is frequently made when using both frequency and duration as simultaneous measures of behaviour.

Data collection and collation

The importance of developing an organised and methodological approach to data collection cannot be over-emphasised since the data collected must enable the experimenter to fulfil the objectives of the study. Animal-related studies tend to generate substantial amounts of information rapidly, so it is essential to deal with all of the data effectively. Most animal researchers will download or transfer data into a spreadsheet before transferring it to a dedicated statistical package for analysis. Regardless of which software package is used, it is important to deal with data efficiently on a regular basis. This will not only allow the early identification of any errors but also prevent tedious data-inputting overload at the end of the data collection period.

Preliminary data collection/pilot studies

No matter how well planned a study is, it is always worth conducting a pilot study in which a small amount of data are collected and analysed, in order to allow the researcher to ascertain whether the methodology used is really appropriate and if the data required to fulfil the objectives of the study can be generated effectively. Any inadequacies can be identified and dealt with at this stage with minimal data wastage at worst.

Reliability and validity

Reliability

Reliability is a key feature of data collection and is often referred to as 'goodness' and reflects the extent to which a measurement is repeatable and consistent, i.e. free from random errors. Any measure that is recorded comprises two components: a systematic component representing the true value of the variable and a random component caused by (inevitable) imperfections in the measurement process. In an ideal world your measures would be perfect, only measuring what you are intending to measure. However, when dealing with animals, this is less likely to be the case, therefore we need to ensure that any measure taken has as small a random component as possible.

Four factors have been identified to determine how reliable or good a measure is. First, precision indicates how free the measurement is of random error (a 100% precise measure will be totally free of random errors). Second, sensitivity indicates how changes in the value will result in changes in the measure being taken (a sensitive measure will always reflect a change in the true value). Third, resolution indicates the ability of the measure to detect change in the true value (a measure with a high resolution will be able to detect the tiniest change in the true value). Fourth, consistency indicates the ability of the measure always to measure the same thing, i.e. to return the same value (a consistent measure will always produce the same results when taken repeatedly). Figures 17.8 and 17.9 show the weighing of a 16 hh horse using a proprietary weigh tape/band and a

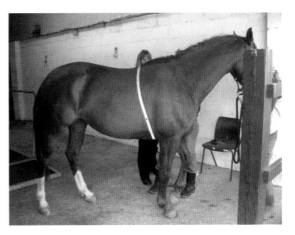

Figure 17.8 Weighing a 16 hh horse using a proprietary weigh tape/band.

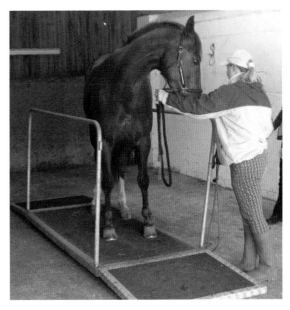

Figure 17.9 A horse being weighed using a weighbridge.

weighbridge. The weigh tape underestimated the weight of the horse by 46 kg (approximately 10% of the actual body weight!) and is therefore not a reliable measuring tool.

Validity

Validity reflects the extent to which a measurement actually measures what it is supposed to be measuring, and may also be referred to as rightness. Both accuracy (how well the measured values correspond with the true values) and specificity (how focused the measure is on measuring what it is supposed to be measuring) contribute to the overall validity of a measure. Clearly then the reliability and validity of the measures to be used should be assessed prior to the main data collection period.

Determining how to sample the population

Populations and samples are fundamentally important in data collection, since the parameters of a population are estimated using a sample of items from the population, assuming that the sample provides a true reflection of the population. Eddison (2000) describes four main reasons for using samples instead of entire populations as follows: first, when there is an unknown population size; second, when there are limited resources; third, to minimise disruption to populations; and fourth, when sampling may be more accurate than using the whole population (transcription errors increase with increasing sample size). There are problems with populations as they possess inherent variability and often comprise a number of subgroups which may be very different from one another.

How many samples?

Up to a point the more data collected the better, since statistical power is improved by increasing the sample size. But data collection is always constrained by time and money, and even if not, eventually the returns in terms of increased statistical power for collecting masses of data are diminished. It is therefore essential to know the point at which sufficient data have been collected for data analysis.

Types of data

Broadly there are two types of data: those that result in the counting of units (counts) and those that result in data that can be measured on a numeric scale (measurements). Together these result in four levels of measurement. Count data are nominal, whilst measurement data may be – in ascending order of strength of measurement – ordinal, interval or ratio.

Nominal data can be classified according to mutually exclusive categories or classes, such as male/female or type *A*/type *B*/type *C*. When dealing with counts the sampling units are typically the space, volume or time interval in which they are observed, or all or part of an organism. Examples include: number of larvae/m^3, number of eggs laid per minute, number of parasites per host. Ordinal (ranking) data can be classified according to mutually exclusive categories or classes, and also ranked according to a common property, for example where $A > B > C > D$ and so on. Interval data can be classified according to mutually exclusive categories or classes, which are ranked according to a common property, and also the distance between two points on the scale is meaningful. The zero point and units of measurement are arbitrary. For example, body temperature is measured on an interval scale.

Finally ratio data can be classified according to mutually exclusive categories or classes, which are ranked according to a common property, or the distance between two points on a defined scale is meaningful. For interval data, the zero point and units of measurement of ratio data have a true zero point. This means that the ratio of any two measurements is independent of the units of measurement. Looking at, for example, time, the ratio between any two data points is the same whether they are measured in seconds, minutes, hours or days.

When dealing with measurements of characteristics the sampling units are defined in terms of groups, individuals or parts of individuals. Examples include mean pulse rate for an animal, the daily energy requirement of a sheep, or the speed of a nerve impulse in a primate. In these examples the sampling units would be the humans, the sheep and the nerves, and the populations that they would be drawn from would be all of the relevant individuals that could have been sampled (other humans, sheep, primate nerves).

Box 17.4 lists eight fundamental properties of sampling units.

Sampling units must be independent of one another in order to avoid creating bias. Indeed, independence is a critical assumption of most statistical analysis, but is very often violated due to either multiple measurement or association. Multiple measurement occurs when an individual (data point) is counted more than once, or contributes more than one measurement to the end data set, and is often mistaken for replication. Association occurs when the subjects being selected are closely associated with each other, and is very common in animal behaviour studies using individuals which should actually be grouped such as litter mates.

Entire populations and statistical populations/sampling frames

Sampling units are drawn from a population. However, in some cases, the whole population may be so large (such as the population of humans) that it would be impossible for every individual in that population to be chosen in theory. Therefore the sampling process itself is often constrained in that is only possible to select samples from a subsection of the entire population. The subsection of the entire population is known as the statistical population or sampling frame. For example,

Box 17.4

FUNDAMENTAL PROPERTIES OF SAMPLING UNITS

- All sampling units in the population have an equal chance of selection (to avoid bias)
- The unit must be stable (any changes would result in invalid comparisons)
- The proportion of the population found in an area must remain the same throughout the sampling period. If changes occur then the sampling regime must be altered in order to accommodate these changes
- If the sampling units are counts/frequencies, the unit of area, volume or time interval must be clearly specified
- The sampling unit must be clearly identified in practice; for example, double counting of hosts should be avoided (in other words, the overlapping of sampling units which would result in multiple measurement must be avoided)
- The sampling unit must be a reasonable size
- The size of the sampling unit must be relatively large compared to the size of the organism being counted (this is to avoid errors due to edge effects, since bias can be introduced if many organisms are found on the edges of a sampling unit)
- The size of sampling unit used to study animal subjects should be at least the same size as their range of movement (in order to avoid movement of individuals from one sampling unit to another, resulting in double counting and therefore multiple measurements)

when taking measurements on a herd of goats the herd is a subset of the entire population of goats (worldwide). The statistical population/sampling frame may well be goats living in the UK.

Using sampling techniques

The two most common sampling techniques used in animal-based research are simple random sampling and stratified random sampling.

Simple random sampling is used when each member of the sampling frame has the same probability of being selected, the population is uniformly dispersed and does not contain subgroups. The statistical population should be homogeneous, not heterogeneous, in composition and dispersion. The method is best explained using an example. A researcher wants to compare the growth rates of two groups of lambs fed on creep feeds X and Y. A total of 200 individually numbered lambs of similar ages and weights are available. Twenty are to be selected and allocated to the two different creep feeds. During the study all 20 animals will be kept under identical conditions, apart from feed type.

There are a number of possible methods for making random selections, from 'low-tech' methods such as picking numbers from a hat to 'high-tech' methods such as using random number tables or a list of random numbers generated by a computer. (Note: these 'random' numbers are not truly random, since they will repeat themselves after hundreds of thousands of numbers, and should be thought of as pseudorandom numbers.) The numbers from the list of random numbers are selected in a methodical pattern in order to maintain the randomness of the numbers in the table. Random number lists in tables are usually laid out in a series of rows and columns. The first number (fixed point) should be selected (randomly) and from there selections made by moving on in a fixed direction. Once the required number of random numbers has been selected, the finishing point on the table should be marked, to start at this point next time. (Note that using the same starting point on subsequent occasions introduces systematic errors into the selection procedure.)

Stratified random sampling is used when it is known that one or more factors influence the dispersion (or heterogeneous nature) of the individuals within the statistical sampling population. The variability due to the heterogeneity of the population is taken into account in the sampling regime by the division of the area to be sampled into several strata according to the factor causing the variation. Simple random samples are then taken from each stratum. If the stratification of the sampling population involves different-sized strata, more samples are taken from the larger strata, whilst fewer samples are taken from the smaller strata, using proportional allocation. For example, an experimenter wants to assess the effectiveness of a tick treatment on a population of dogs homed in a rescue centre. A sample of 20 dogs is to be selected. The sampling frame comprises 6 Terriers, 8 Border Collies, 8 Labradors and 10 Greyhounds. There are then four strata from which samples need to be taken and it is necessary to take more samples from the larger strata than from the smaller strata. The number of dogs to be taken from each stratum (here breed/type) is determined as follows using proportional allocation.

The statistical population (sampling frame) comprises 32 dogs in total. Stratum A/Terriers comprising 6 dogs accounts for $6/32 = 0.20$ of the total sampling population. Similarly, stratum B/Border Collies account for $8/32 = 0.25$ of the total, as does stratum C/Labradors, whereas stratum D/Greyhounds accounts for $10/32 = 0.30$ of the total. To sample 20 dogs from the four different strata/breed types proportionally the following calculations are used: stratum A/Terriers accounts for 0.20 of the total sampling frame therefore $0.20 \times 20 = 4$ Terriers should be selected. Likewise stratum B/Border Collies and stratum C/Labradors each accounts for 0.25 of the total sampling frame, therefore $0.25 \times 20 =$

5 dogs of each type should be selected. Finally stratum C/Greyhounds accounts for 0.3 of the total sampling frame, therefore 0.30 × 20 = 6 Greyhounds should be selected.

Determining how much data to collect: estimation of necessary sample size

It is always sensible to work out how much data to collect as there is no point in overdoing it. It is possible to calculate (the estimated) sample size needed to give a sample mean which is within specified limits of the true (population) mean value using some pilot measurements which have already been obtained to give an estimate of population standard deviation.

To summarise, three pieces of information are needed in order to estimate a necessary sample size (n):

1. An estimate of the population standard deviation (s)
2. The level of statistical significance required to be attached to the estimate (a)
3. The maximum acceptable difference (D) between the sample mean (0) and the true/population mean (m); (where $D = |0 - m|$).

The minimum sample size required (n) can be calculated using the equation below:

$$n = \frac{s^2 z^2}{D^2}$$

where z = the critical value of the cumulative normal variable (z) at the $a/2$ level of significance.

For example, an ethologist wishes to estimate the mean frequency with which infant rhesus monkeys approach their mothers. A pilot study was carried out, consisting of six 1-hour observation periods in which the number of approaches made was recorded as follows: data: 9, 12, 7, 15, 13 and 4 approaches per hour.

The following estimate was calculated.

The estimate of population standard deviation (s) = 4.10 h^{-1}

The following were set:

The level of significance (a) = 0.05

The maximum difference (D) = 2 h^{-1}

(This means that the ethologist wishes to be 95% confident that the sample mean will be within 2 approaches per hour of the true value.)

The sample size (n) is calculated using the equation:

$$n = \frac{s^2 z^2}{D^2}$$

Therefore:

$$n = (4.10^2 \times 1.96^2)/2^2$$
$$n = 16.1$$

This means that $n = 17$ (note that n is always rounded up) and that at least 17 measures of approach rate are required in order to be 95% confident that the measured (sample) mean rate is within 2 approaches per hour of the true (population) mean value.

Determining whether sufficient data have been collected

The two most commonly used methods for assessing whether sufficient data have been collected are assessing internal consistency and split-half analysis.

Internal consistency is a crude but efficient method in which the data collected to date are randomly split into two equal sections and the resulting two halves are analysed separately. If both sets of data generate clear conclusions that are in agreement it can be assumed that enough results have probably been accumulated. If, on the other hand, one or both of the separate data sets generates poor conclusions, or the two sets of data produce conflicting conclusions, then it can be assumed that the number of results obtained are insufficient and that more data are required.

Split-half analysis is a more sophisticated method, often used in behaviour studies, in which the data for a particular category of behaviour are split randomly into two halves and correlation coefficients calculated between the two sets of data. If the correlation coefficient is suitably high (over 0.7, at least) then it can be said that the data set is reliable and that enough data have been collected.

Data analysis

It is important to remember that statistics is simply a tool to help answer questions, not vice versa, and to take care not to become either obsessed with statistical techniques or cavalier with the use of statistics. It can happen.

Data analysis comprises exploratory data analysis (EDA) and confirmatory data analysis (CDA).

Exploratory data analysis

EDA is also known as descriptive analysis and involves collating and summarising data in preparation for subsequent CDA, and plays an important role in deciding which statistics to apply in order to test the hypotheses stated at the outset of the experiment.

EDA examines the distribution of measurements and includes measures of central tendency, dispersion and the shape of distributions. The results of EDA can be presented by graphical and tabular means.

Measures of central tendency

Various measures of central tendency exist, which are commonly referred to as averages. The mean is most commonly used in parametric statistical testing, whilst the median (the middle value in a numerically ordered data set) is commonly used in non-parametric statistical testing. The mode (the most frequent value in a data set) is rarely of any use in statistical testing. The example below illustrates how sometimes the three values are similar.

Example set of values:

$$2, 3, 4, 4, 5, 5, 5, 6, 6, 6, 7, 7, 8, 9$$

Mean = 5.5
Median = 5.5
Mode = 5.5

The (arithmetic) mean is the most stable of the three averages and is also closely related to some important measures of variability, and can be calculated from the equation:

$$\text{Mean } (\bar{x}) = \frac{\sum x_i}{n}$$

where $\sum$ (sigma) means 'sum of'; x is the data value and n is sample size.

Care must be taken to ensure, first, that the distribution of data for which the mean is being calculated is symmetrical (since the means of skewed distributions are not very accurate or useful) and second, that there are no extreme values or outliers (the mean is greatly influenced by these).

The median is the middle datum point in the data set (which has been organised into ascending, or descending, order. If there is an even number of values in the data set then the median is halfway between the two middle values.

The median is particularly useful if the frequency distribution is not symmetrical – where the mean is influenced by extreme values. This is demonstrated by the example data set above where the middle datum point falls between 5 and 6 and is therefore averaged to 5.5.

The mode offers a quick and easy method of gaining an impression of the central tendency: the most frequent value. However, it is the least useful measure and can also have more than one true value, resulting in multimodal distributions.

Measures of dispersion

There are several measures of variability, some of which are closely related to each other (and also to the mean).

The range is a straightforward measure of the spread of the data points, being the difference between the maximum and minimum values in a data set. Although it may be influenced by extreme values, it remains a particularly useful measure of dispersion where the frequency distribution is asymmetrical. There is no loss of information, but there is the potential for bias.

The interquartile range attempts to overcome some of the deficiencies of the range. This measure is the difference between the maximum and minimum values in the data set after the top and bottom quartiles (or quarters) have been excluded. This reduces the influence of extreme values, but it does remove data from a data set in an arbitrary manner irrespective of whether there are extreme values or not. There is a loss of information.

The variance is the root of probably the four most important measures of dispersion. The variance measures the difference between each value and the mean, as shown in the equation:

$$\text{Population variance } (s^2) = \frac{\sum (x_1 - \bar{x})^2}{n}$$

where $\sum$ (sigma) means 'sum of'; x represents data value; $\bar{x}$ is the mean and n represents sample size.

When a population parameter is estimated by a sample statistic, there is generally some error (that is why we study statistics). The significance of this error decreases with sample size. This is logical because, with very large sample sizes, the sample approximates to the population. At small sample sizes, this error becomes more important. Hence, for sample statistics, a modified version of the variance is used. It takes into account this error due to sample size. The formula for the sample variance is given by the equation:

$$\text{Sample variance } (s^2) = \frac{\sum (x_1 - \bar{x})^2}{n - 1}$$

where x is a data value, $\bar{x}$ is the mean and n is sample size.

Note that the effect of $(n - 1)$ will be greatest when the sample size (n) is small.

For computational purposes, these two formulae are not particularly convenient. The following two versions of these formulae, shown in the equations below, are much easier to use:

$$\text{Population variance } (s^2) = \frac{\sum x^2 - \frac{\left(\sum x\right)^2}{n}}{n}$$

$$\text{Sample variance* } (s^2) = \frac{\sum x^2 - \frac{\left(\sum x\right)^2}{n}}{n - 1}$$

*This is the equation that is always used to calculate variance.

The standard deviation is closely related to the variance but is used instead of the variance to describe the variability present in a data set (the spread of a distribution), because it is expressed in the same units as the mean. Standard deviation can be calculated using the equation:

$$\text{Standard deviation } (s) = \sqrt{\text{Variance}}$$

The coefficient of variation is used to express the dispersion of a data set (the standard deviation) relative to the average of the data set (the mean). For example, a spread of 10 in 100 is clearly more important than a spread of 10 in 10 000. The coefficient of variation is derived using the equation:

$$\text{Coefficient of variation (CV)} = \frac{\text{Standard deviation}}{\overline{x}}$$

The coefficient of variation is often expressed as a percentage by multiplying the above formula by 100.

The standard error is closely related to the standard deviation and variance, and used extremely frequently. If a series of samples are drawn from a population, then their means will form a normal distribution around the population mean. The variance of that distribution will increase as the number of samples increases. This relationship is described by the equation:

$$\frac{s^2}{n}$$

where s^2 = the population variance and n is sample size. We have already seen that, in terms of descriptive statistics, by being measured in the same units as the mean, the standard deviation (note that standard deviation is the square root $(\sqrt{})$ of the variance) is more useful than the variance. Taking the square root of the equation above results in the equation:

$$\text{SEM} = \frac{s}{\sqrt{n}}$$

This standard deviation of this sampling distribution of the means is called the standard error of the mean (SEM). The SEM is extremely useful because it allows for the error in estimating the population mean using the sample mean. As the sample size increases, the standard error will decrease, as the error in the estimation decreases with larger sample sizes.

The SEM or standard error is typically expressed as a ± value around the mean.

The normal distribution

All data sets conform to some kind of distribution, that is, there is variability around an average value. Most data collected by scientists conform to a normal distribution.

Data that have been collected can be put into classes and plotted as a histogram. As the amount of data collected increases (i.e. sample size increases), and providing that the data are not biased, the histogram becomes a continuous distribution, as illustrated in (Figure 17.10).

Characteristics of normal distributions and probability

The shape of the normal distribution is defined by its mean and standard deviation.

Probability is measured on a scale of 0 (an impossibility) to 1 (a certainty).

If we took a sample of, say, 1000 individuals' heights the data would conform to a normal distribution. If we selected one of the 1000 individuals at random then the probability of selecting one whose height is between the minimum and maximum heights (1.4 and 2.1 metres) would be 1 (i.e. certain). Similarly, the probability of selecting an individual whose height falls between two heights, 1.6 and 1.8 metres, would be proportional to the area under the curve between those two points.

A standardised normal distribution is a normal curve where the x-axis is measured in standard deviations (standard normal variates/z-scores). This leads to the general rule shown in Table 17.3.

As a general rule, if a variable is normally distributed, approximately 68% of its scores will fall within one standard deviation of the mean, 95% of its scores will fall within two standard deviations of the mean, and 99.7% of its scores will fall within three standard deviations of the mean.

Confidence intervals

Confidence intervals are used to estimate population means precisely, using the following relationships:

* If many samples are taken the distribution of the sample means is normal
* The standard deviation of the distribution of sample means is the SEM
* 95% of the area under a normal curve will fall between −1.96 and +1.96 standard errors either side of the mean.

Therefore, a range of 1.96 standard errors above and below the mean of this distribution of sample means will include 95% of the sample means. If 95% of all of the sample means are within 1.96 standard errors of the population mean, then the probability that the population mean is within 1.96 standard errors is also 95%. There is a probability, of 95%, that this range (mean ± 1.96 standard error) – the confidence interval – includes the population mean. The upper and lower limits of this

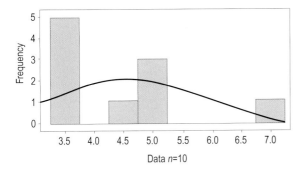

Data *n*=10

Table 17.3 Relationship between percentage of area under standard normal curve and number of standard deviations (limits) above and below the mean

Percentage of area under the curve	Number of standard deviations above and below the mean
50	0.674
90	1.654
95	1.96
99	2.576
100	3.09

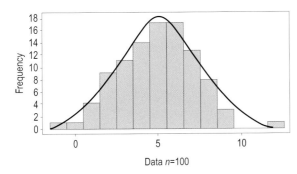

Data *n*=100

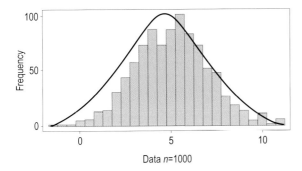

Data *n*=1000

Figure 17.10 Histogram of data with (a) *n* = 10; (b) *n* = 100; (c) *n* = 1000.

confidence interval are the upper and lower confidence limits, and can be calculated using the equation:

$$\text{Confidence interval} = \text{mean} \pm (1.96 \times \text{SEM})$$

Dealing with non-normal data: data transformation

Moderate deviations from a normal distribution are not too serious, but in some cases the distribution is clearly not normal and the data require transformation in order to become approximately normally distributed. The three most commonly applied data transformations are:

1. The square root transformation
2. The arcsine square root transformation
3. The logarithmic transformation.

The square root transformation is used on count data, such as frequencies, which tend to follow a Poisson distribution. The original data values (x) are converted by taking the square root of x. If there is a 0 in the data set, then 0.5 is added to each x-value before taking the square root. The arcsine square root transformation is used when data are in the form of proportions (or percentages). Each value (p) is transformed by taking the arcsine of the square root of p, where $0 < p < 1$. As a general rule, if the values of p fall between 0.3 and 0.7, the transformation is not necessary. The logarithmic transformation is used either when the mean and variance of a data set are positively correlated (i.e. as one increases, so does the other) or when the frequency distribution is skewed to the right. The log of the original data values (x) is taken. If the original data set contains a 0 then a value of 1 is added to each of the original x-values before taking the log.

263

Presentation of the results of EDA

The results of EDA can be presented either in a graphical (Figure 17.11) or in a tabular (Table 17.4) format.

Types of confirmatory data analysis

There are two main types of statistical test: parametric and non-parametric.

Parametric tests

Parametric tests are so called because they make assumptions about the parameters of the population from which the sample data set originated. The parameters that the assumptions are based on are the mean, variance and frequency distribution. Parametric tests assume that:

- The data follow a normal distribution – the assumption is of normality
- Samples of the data set (or subgroups of the data set) possess equal variances – the assumption is of homogeneity of variance
- The data are measured on an interval or ratio scale
- The effects of different treatments or conditions are additive – the assumption is of additivity.

Non-parametric tests

Non-parametric tests tend to be less powerful than their parametric equivalents; however, since they are free from the assumptions of the parametric tests they are less dependent upon assumptions of normality and as a result tend to be more robust (especially with large sample sizes). Non-parametric tests can analyse ordinal data, whilst some tests, such as the chi-squared test (used to investigate associations between two variables) can even analyse nominal data. The two main advantages of non-parametric tests over parametric tests are that they are easier to perform manually and can cope with small sample sizes.

The exact statistical test employed depends on a number of factors, including:

- The type of data – nominal, ordinal, interval and ratio
- The distribution of data and whether data are parametric or non-parametric
- The question being asked – for example, is the question about differences, or relationships? Different statistical tests are used in different situations

Reaching statistical conclusions

The final step of the scientific method is to reach conclusions that clearly relate to the aims and objectives of the experiment and have immediate application within the wider industry.

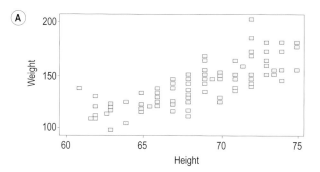

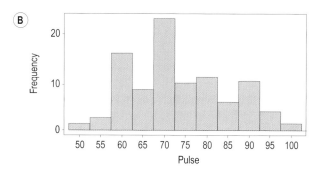

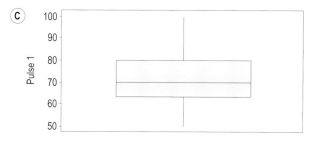

Figure 17.11 Presentation of the results of exploratory data analysis in a graphical form. (a) Scatter diagram of weight against height; (b) histogram of pulse rate data (pulse 1); (c) boxplot (box-and-whisker plot) of pulse rate data (pulse 1).

Table 17.4 Examples of tabular presentation of exploratory data analysis (EDA) including simple frequencies and/or percentages: cross-tabulations showing frequencies and more complex formats

(a) Summary of descriptive statistics of pulse rate data

Variable: Pulse Rate (Pulse)	
Descriptive statistic	**Value**
n (sample size)	92
Mean	72.87
Median	71.00
Variance	121.22
Standard deviation (sd)	11.01
Standard error of the mean (SEM)	1.15
Minimum	48.00
Maximum	100.00
Range (maximum – minimum)	52.00
First quartile (Q1)	64.00
Third quartile (Q3)	80.00
Interquartile range (IQR) (Q3 – Q1)	16.00

(b) Simple frequencies (tallies/counts) and percentages of participant gender data

Variable: gender	Count	Percentage
Male	57	61.96
Female	35	38.04
Total	92	100.00

(c) Cross-tabulation of participant data: frequencies of gender by drug treatment

		Columns: Drug Treatment		
		Drug A	**Drug B**	**All**
Rows: gender	Male	20	37	57
	Female	8	27	35
	All	28	64	92

(d) Cross-tabulation of gender by drug treatment displaying mean pulse rate

		Columns: Drug Treatment		
		Drug A	**Drug B**	**All**
Rows: gender	Male	75.600	76.027	75.877
	Female	95.125	84.222	86.714
	All	81.179	79.484	80.00

THE ETHICS OF ANIMAL USE IN RESEARCH

Any research using animals must have gained ethical clearance. The statements made by Marshall Hall in 1831 (Box 17.5) were influential in the ultimate production of legislation covering the use of animals in experimental research. The main points of the 1986 Animals (Scientific Procedures) Act are summarised in Box 17.6. Ethical considerations play a fundamental key role in experimental design, making a substantial contribution to the determination of sample size. Clearly there is no need to use more individuals than is necessary in order to gain a reliable result in the study.

As Barnard et al. (2007, pp. 7–8) stated, since animals are sentient beings, due consideration must be given when using them in experiments. Concern must focus on both the living organism itself and also those remaining in the population from which it was selected or removed. Specific questions must be asked about suffering (itself a difficult term to define) and issues such as whether it is permissible for an individual or small number of species to suffer in the name of scientific research for the good of the whole species (or, indeed, the good of a different species) clearly need to be

Project title and proposed start date	Insert short and focused title here
Principal investigator	This must be your Research Project Tutor
Other investigator/s	This is you, the student
Project objectives	Insert up to 3 (no more than 3) clear objectives for your study
Species	State in Latin please
Numbers of animals involved	Insert the precise number of animals to be involved Once you have gained approval you cannot use more animals than stated here
Experimental techniques to be used	Home Office-regulated procedures: Y / N? If yes, Project licence number: Detail personnel carrying out each activity, confirming competence **Insert statement:** No Home Office-regulated procedures will be used (Students will not be allowed to undertake these kind of activities)
Duration of experience of animals	(State the length of time that the animals will be involved in the study, from the start to the end of each day)
Destination of animals after investigation	Usually the animals stay in their existing husbandry system after the study has been completed This is good practice and you should do your best to design your study in this way
Housing during investigation	It is always advisable (preferable) to retain the animals involved in your study in their normal housing system If they are not, you need to state clearly how they are to be housed, and why it is necessary to keep them in a way that is different from their normal housing system

Final statement (max. 500 words)

Scientific (and production system) outcomes:

State what the desired outcomes for your study are. (These should be clearly related to your earlier-stated objectives)

Pain, distress or lasting harm:

Insert a statement such as 'The animals will not be exposed to pain, or suffer distress or lasting harm, during the course of the proposed study'

Replacement:

Replacement refers to the use of non-animal alternatives if possible, for example tissue culture rather than laboratory rodents
However, in the types of study that you are likely to want to do, this is not possible

State that it is not possible to replace live animals with a substitute if the proposed study is to achieve its objectives

Reduction:

Reduction refers to minimising the number of animals involved in the study to a number that is necessary to achieve the stated objectives of the proposed study. Care also needs to be taken not to reduce the numbers of animals involved to such a level that the study becomes useless as it fails to generate useful (and statistically analysable) information

State that the minimum number of animals needed to generate sufficient data for analysis in order to address the objectives will be used

Refinement:

Refinement refers to the modification of methods used so that the adverse experience of the animals is reduced as much as possible
For example, social species should not be socially isolated during the study

State that efforts have been taken in the designing of the study to refine the husbandry conditions (if necessary) in order to avoid causing the animals any undue distress and suffering. If you have to change their husbandry system in order to carry out your study, explain how efforts have been made to make it as good as possible in terms of the welfare of the individual animal

Figure 17.12 The animal (vertebrate) ethics project submission and report forms used by the University of Plymouth.

Box 17.5

MARSHALL HALL'S (1831) STATEMENTS ON THE USE OF ANIMAL-BASED EXPERIMENTS

They should never take place if the necessary information could be obtained by observations

There should always be a clearly defined and obtainable objective

Scientists should be well informed about the work of their predecessors and peers in order to avoid unnecessary repetition of an experiment

Justifiable experiments should be carried out with the least possible infliction of suffering (often through the use of lower, less sentient animals)

Every experiment should be performed under circumstances that would provide the clearest possible results, thereby diminishing the need for repetition of experiments

Box 17.6

KEY POINTS FROM THE 1986 ANIMALS (SCIENTIFIC PROCEDURES) ACT

It is illegal to carry out experiments or procedures on any vertebrate which may cause it pain, suffering, distress or lasting harm and the Act regulates the use of animals in research

The Act also regulates work on free-living animals as well as on laboratory animals

A project licence and personal licence (issued by the Home Office) are required for 'regulated procedures'

The Code of Practice for the Housing and Care of Animals Used in Scientific Procedures publications produced by the Home Office must be complied with

Project title	
Proposed start and end dates	
Principal Investigator	
Other investigators	
Project objectives	
Species (involved in sampling)	
Number of individuals involved (approx)	
Sampling technique/s used (Give brief description)	
Perceived effect on remaining population Outline any actions planned to minimise disruption	
Perceived effect on habitat invertebrates removed from Outline any actions planned to minimise disruption	
Approval given (signature and date)	

Figure 17.13 The invertebrate ethics form used by Duchy College.

addressed. These considerations are not the scope of this chapter. Good sources of information include Midgley (1983); Clarke (1987); Rolston in Regan and Singer (1989); Singer (1995); Gilland et al. (2002) and Sandøe et al. (1997) and Armstrong and Botzler (2003).

More recently, guidelines for the treatment of animals in behavioural research and teaching were published in *Animal Behaviour* (ASAB 2006). It is an expectation that all academic organisations supporting any animal-based research (remember that this need not be the traditional laboratory-based research that typically comes to mind when we think of 'animal research') will have set procedures and auditable paperwork for the granting of ethical approval for any research involving animals. Petrie and Watson (1999) made a good point that it is much easier to conduct an experiment on humans than on animals, as essentially all that is required is informed consent paperwork from the participant or the parent/guardian of the recipient. However, it is the role of the keepers and animal research scientists to be involved in the research.

Figure 17.12 illustrates the animal (vertebrate) ethics project submission and report forms used by the University of Plymouth, whilst Figure 17.13 illustrates the invertebrate ethics form used by Duchy College. The boxes in these forms are annotated in order to provide an explanation of their function.

Bibliography

Armstrong S J, Botzler R G (eds) 2003 The animal ethics reader. Routledge, London

ASAB 2006 Guidelines for the treatment of animals in behaviour research and teaching. Animal Behaviour 71:245–253

Barnard C, Gilbert F, McGregor P 2007 Asking questions in biology – a guide to hypothesis-testing, experimental design and presentation in practical work and research projects, 3rd edn. Pearson, Prentice Hall, Essex

Clarke S R L 1987 Animals and their moral standing. Routledge, London

Eberhardt L L, Thomas J M 1991 Designing environmental field studies. Ecological Monographs 61:52–73

Eddison J C 2000 Quantitative investigations in the biosciences using MINITAB. Chapman and Hall, CRC, London

Gilland A, Matfield M, Regan T et al. (eds) 2002 Animal experimentation: good or bad? Hodder & Stoughton, London

Manly B F J 1992 The design and analysis of research studies. Cambridge University Press, Cambridge

Martin P, Bateson P 2007 Measuring behaviour: an introductory guide, 3rd edn. Cambridge University Press, Cambridge

Midgley M 1983 Animals and why they matter. Penguin Books, London

Petrie A, Watson P 1999 Statistics for veterinary and animal science. Blackwell Science, Oxford

Regan T 1984 The case for animal rights. University of California Press, Berkeley

Regan T, Singer P (eds) 1989 Animal rights and human obligations. Prentice Hall, Englewood Cliffs, pp. 23–24

Sandøe P, Crisp R, Holtug N 1997 Ethics. In: Appleby M C, Hughes B O (eds) Animal welfare. CABI, Wallingford, pp. 3–17

Singer P 1995 Animal liberation, 4th edn. Pimlico Books, London

The code of practice for the housing and care of animals used in scientific procedures. Available online at: www.homeoffice.gov.uk/docs/hcasp5.html

Thompson D (ed.) 1996 Oxford compact English dictionary. Oxford University Press, Oxford

Zar J H 1996 Biostatistical analysis, 3rd edn. Prentice-Hall International, London

Chapter | **18** | Lisa Yates

Complementary therapies

This chapter considers the expanding field of complementary therapy, its applications and the legislation that applies to the practice of the different techniques involved.

Complementary therapy is a generic term encompassing a variety of techniques that aid the holistic healing of animals. These techniques differ from medical techniques because they concentrate on the cause of the illness as well as the symptoms. The aim of complementary therapy is to treat the emotional, mental, spiritual and physical components of an animal and therefore attempt to heal the whole body.

Many techniques are available within complementary therapy and the majority come under these five headings:

1. Bodywork therapy
2. Herbal therapy
3. Homeopathy
4. Energy therapy
5. Communication therapy.

These five therapies, the techniques involved, the areas in which these techniques are utilised and the laws governing their use will be discussed within this chapter.

BODYWORK THERAPY

Bodywork is a term used within complementary therapy to describe therapeutic and healing techniques which involve a hands-on approach through touch, exercise or physical manipulation.

Techniques used within bodywork therapy include:

* Physiotherapy – equine sports massage
* Bowen technique
* Equine touch technique
* Trigger point myotherapy
* Craniosacral technique
* Chiropractic
* Osteopathy.

Physiotherapy

Physiotherapy involves using physical techniques, either on their own or combined within a regime, to treat injury and movement dysfunction. Physiotherapy is often used in rehabilitation following an accident or surgery to assist the animal back to full health. Physiotherapy can also be used to prevent injuries occurring and this is especially utilised with performance or working animals. Physiotherapy can be used, with varying degrees of success, in most small and large animals. This is particularly the case for horses, dogs, cats and valuable livestock.

Techniques used within physiotherapy include effleurage, pétrissage, friction, tapotement, passive joint mobilisation and active joint mobilisation.

Effleurage

Effleurage is an introduction to massage using light strokes to warm up and mobilise the soft tissue. This is followed by heavy strokes to aid drainage of the lymph system.

Pétrissage

This is the compression of muscles from side to side using hands in a gentle motion. This is used to relax muscles and tendons, reduce adhesions and enhance blood circulation.

Friction

Friction is combined with other techniques to aid the healing process after an injury. The scar tissue or adhesion is massaged by hand in small, circular motions whilst it is under tension. This is used to loosen the tissue and aid collagen formation.

Tapotement

This involves using both hands in a tapping motion. If the hands are cupped this is called cupping and if the hands are straight this is called hacking. Tapotement is carried out to stimulate underlying tissue and is useful in physiotherapy to aid in the recovery of injuries which cause muscle wastage.

Passive joint mobilisation

This involves putting a recovering joint through its normal range of movement whilst supporting by hand. It is very important that the joint has been warmed up before this is attempted or further damage could occur. Figure 18.1 shows passive joint mobilisation in horses.

Active joint mobilisation

This involves the animal taking part in voluntary exercises that encourage weight-bearing. This will need to be supported at first until muscle tone has increased and the animal can carry its own weight.

As governed by the Veterinary Surgery (Exemptions) Order of 1962, physiotherapy is one of the only therapies that can be given by a non-veterinarian to an animal. This is only if the animal has been diagnosed by a veterinary surgeon and the surgeon has decided that a physiotherapist can treat the animal under the surgeon's direction. The term 'animal physiotherapist' is not protected by law but qualified practitioners will be a member of a professional body and recognised by the Royal Veterinary Society.

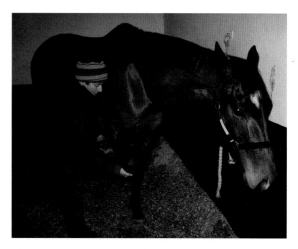

Figure 18.1 Passive joint mobilisation involves moving the joint after warm-up whilst supporting the limb at all times.

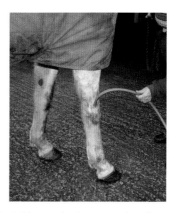

Figure 18.2 Cold-water hosing can reduce heat and the onset of swelling.

Modern techniques are also available which use physiotherapy equipment to aid the healing of the patient. These include hydrotherapy, hot and cold therapy, phototherapy, ultrasound, muscle stimulation and magnotherapy.

Hydrotherapy

This is the treatment of animals using various techniques, all of which involve water. The most common types of hydrotherapy are hosing, swimming and spas. Hosing can be carried out by the owner, normally after instruction by a veterinary surgeon, using either cold or hot water depending on the injury. Applying cold water to the affected area will help to reduce inflammation, heat and pain from new impact injuries which cause cuts and bruising (Figure 18.2). Hot water should not be used because it could increase the inflammatory response.

Hot-water hosing will increase the blood circulation and is used to increase blood volume at sites of injury, relieving stiff joints and muscles.

Swimming is another form of hydrotherapy which is becoming increasingly popular. Swimming is often used as part of a rehabilitation programme by physiotherapists after instruction from a veterinary surgeon for horses and dogs that have had moderate to severe back or limb injuries. Animal swimming pools are either round with the handler in the middle or straight with a handler either side. Swimming helps the animal to start exercising the injured area without the concussive effects. Following on from this, training regimes for sports animals often now involve swimming exercises or the use of a water walker to aid the increase in fitness and muscle tone (Figure 18.3).

Hot and cold therapy

Cold therapy involves cold packs being applied to a trauma site to reduce swelling and heat. Hot therapy involves hot packs being applied to a trauma site to relieve stiff joints and muscles. Ice packs and hot/cold boots are available to carry out these techniques (Figure 18.4). These are often used in stabled horses to reduce swelling of the limbs during periods of inactivity. A contrast of the two is used when cold therapy will no longer work. By using a cold pack for a period of time, switching to a hot pack and alternating, circulation will be increased and swelling reduced.

Phototherapy

This involves using low-level infrared or blue laser lights over an affected area. The red-light technique penetrates the skin and is absorbed within the tissues to increase cell metabolism, blood flow and collagen formation. This speeds up the healing process by reducing heat, pain and swelling and reducing scar tissue formation. Infrared laser treatment is also used to relieve muscle spasm and for general relaxation. Blue lasers inhibit bacteria and are used on animals to eradicate bacteria from a wound and therefore aid the healing process. Laser treatment is often

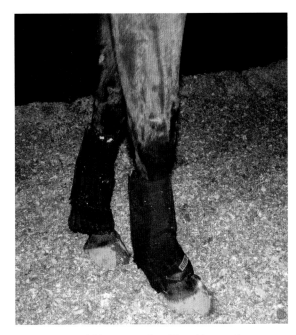

Figure 18.4 Cold boots are placed in cold water for a period of time before applying to the horse to reduce the onset of heat and swelling during periods of inactivity.

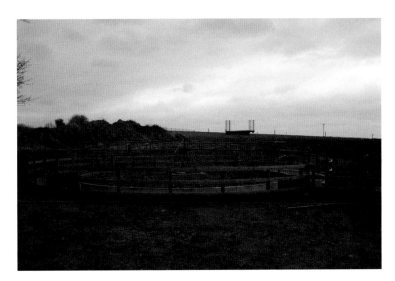

Figure 18.3 A water walker involves the horse walking knee-deep in water for a specified length of time to promote muscle tone and fitness.

used within physiotherapy on horses and dogs. This type of treatment can only be given by a veterinary surgeon or physiotherapist on the surgeon's instruction.

Ultrasound

This requires specialist equipment that, using a conductive medium gel, sends a soundwave through the skin to stimulate the tissue cells. The sound sent is at such a high frequency that it cannot be heard by humans and animals. Ultrasound is used on muscles, tendons and ligaments to treat swelling and tissue damage. The ultrasound waves massage the area, increasing blood flow and therefore speeding the healing process. This aids reduction in swelling and repair of damaged tissue and softens scar tissue. Ultrasound is often used by physiotherapists rehabilitating horses and dogs after injury. This type of treatment can only be given by a veterinary surgeon or physiotherapist on the surgeon's instruction.

Muscle stimulation

This involves using specialist equipment to treat muscle conditions (neuromuscular electrical stimulation (NMES)) or promote pain relief and relaxation of muscles (transcutaneous electrical nerve stimulation (TENS)).

Neuromuscular electrical stimulation

NMES uses high-voltage electrical impulses and can only be carried out by a qualified physiotherapist after diagnosis by a veterinary surgeon. NMES is used during rehabilitation of animals, mainly horses and dogs, after injury or disease that results in muscle wastage or dysfunction. NMES involves using a device that is attached to the animal via electrodes which are placed either side of a specific muscle group. These electrodes transmit an electrical signal to the group, stimulating the nerves in the muscle with electrical impulses. Impulses are a natural function of the healthy muscle and stimulate the muscle groups to contract and relax. This is simulated through NMES, causing the muscle to contract and relax, building muscle function and tone. NMES is also used with performance animals to help improve the health of damaged muscle after extensive training.

Transcutaneous electrical nerve stimulation

TENS uses low-voltage electrical impulses and therefore can be used by the animal owner after strict instructions from the physiotherapist and veterinary surgeon. TENS is used on animals as a drug-free form of pain relief, as a muscle relaxant and to aid in the treatment of muscle, joint and bone problems. It is thought that TENS works either by the mild electrical impulses blocking the pain signals that are received by the brain or because electrical stimulation of the nerves induces the body to produce the natural painkillers, endorphins, which block the perception of pain. Neither theory has been proved. Either way, it has been shown that animals do gain a relief from pain with the use of TENS machines but further research is required to evaluate its true effectiveness.

Magnotherapy

In magnotherapy the animal's body is stimulated with a magnetic field to relieve pain and aid natural healing. Magnotherapy can be performed with either permanent magnets or pulsed electromagnetic field magnets. The animal's body has a natural electric current running through it caused by the electrically charged particles of a cell (ions). Ions affect the metabolism, or working, of the cell. By using magnets, a weak electrical signal is transmitted to the affected area by the magnetic field which interacts with the ions, increasing the blood flow and therefore the productivity of the cells. This leads to an increase in oxygen utilisation and nutrient transport within the cells. This increase in utilisation of the cells within the injured area means that healing time and pain are reduced. Magnotherapy can be used to treat sore backs and muscles, stiff arthritic joints and inflammation of tendons or tendon sheaths in all animals. It is mainly used in horses and companion animals.

Permanent magnets

Permanent magnets are the weakest form of magnotherapy. Permanent magnets are taped on to the animal over the injured area or inserted into blankets, boots, rugs or collars. The magnet gives out a very weak magnetic field and for this reason the animal needs to wear the permanent magnet for long periods of time for it to have an effect. Although equipment containing permanent magnets can be bought off the shelf, a veterinary surgeon's advice should be sought before application.

Pulsed electromagnetic field magnets (PEFM)

PEFMs require equipment that has a pulsing current running through a coil of wire to make the magnetic field. The resulting electric current is stronger than in a permanent magnet, meaning that it will work a lot quicker and penetrate deeper into the animal's body. PEFMs are mainly used by veterinary surgeons and physiotherapists after diagnosis but can be used by the owners under instruction.

Bowen technique

Bowen technique was invented by an Australian named Tom Bowen. This technique was originally utilised on greyhounds and racehorses to improve performance. Since then it has become popular with humans, as well as canines and equines of all disciplines.

Bowen technique is identified by the Royal College of Veterinary Surgeons as a manual therapy and therefore can be performed by non-veterinary surgeons after diagnosis and instruction under the Veterinary Surgery (Exemptions) Order 1962. Although there is no legal requirement to be trained in Bowen technique to practise it, there is an industry requirement that all animal Bowen therapists are trained in human Bowen therapy and specialise. Qualified Bowen therapists can be found on the Bowen Therapists European Register and it is recommended that only registered therapists should be used.

Animal Bowen technique can be used on horses and dogs. Bowen technique is a non-intrusive, gentle, hands-on technique which involves the therapist using a rolling action with fingers and thumb over specific muscles, tendons and ligaments. This movement is said to stimulate the body to rebalance itself and promote healing and pain relief and increase energy levels. On horses Bowen technique can be used to treat conditions such as:

- Poor lymphatic system response
- Low immune system
- Poor circulation
- Respiratory problems
- Inflammation of limbs
- Stiffness and pain in the neck and back
- Muscle conditions such as atrophy, underdevelopment and stiffness leading to lameness or poor performance
- Kinetic abnormalities, including uneven stride length, not bending properly and leaning on one rein.

The rolling motion of the Bowen technique is performed on the animal at set trigger points over the whole of the body and not just at the injury site. This gives a holistic approach to heal the whole body. The therapy lasts for approximately 45 minutes with several intervals in between the hands-on application. This is so that the animal has the chance to readjust and so the body can respond to the treatment. During the treatment it is often seen that the horse will relax. This is due to the movement aiding the release of endorphins, stimulating a relaxed feeling.

On dogs the treatment is very similar. The technique is used to promote relaxation, healing and pain relief. Treatment is especially successful with:

- Behavioural problems
- Improving blood circulation
- Improving lymphatic drainage
- Improving the function of the digestive tract

- Treating muscle, tendon and ligament injury resulting in lameness and pain.

The technique involves using fingers and thumbs in a light rolling movement over the whole of the dog's body to soften the tissue and treat the symptom.

Bowen technique is becoming increasingly popular as an alternative therapy in treating animals. Encouraging results have been seen with both horses and dogs.

Equine touch technique

Equine touch is a technique that was developed by Jock Ruddock in 1997. The technique uses a holistic approach which balances the whole body rather than treating a particular area. Equine touch is carried out by firstly gaining information from the owner and veterinary surgeon and observations. When the area of concern is diagnosed then pressure is applied at certain soft-tissue points on the body in a particular pattern. The points used vary from insertion points of muscles and tendons to opposing muscle groups and energy meridians. These activities of pressure are interspersed with rest periods to give time for the cells to realign. Stretching is often carried out after these phases to relax areas that have been manipulated. Carrying out the technique aids blood circulation, lymphatic drainage, relaxation and pain release and encourages muscle tone.

Equine touch is not classed as a therapy to heal but more of a way to relax and rebalance the horse. Equine touch is also used in conjunction with other therapies to complement treatment. Equine touch should only be carried out by a qualified practitioner after diagnosis and advice from a veterinary surgeon.

Trigger point myotherapy

Trigger point myotherapy is a muscle therapy which involves using compression over muscle trigger points to relieve stiffness and pain and enhance muscular function. A muscle trigger point is a tight band or knot that develops in a muscle that is overstretched or damaged. This area can either have localised pain or be the cause of pain in other associated areas of the body. Trigger point myotherapy involves putting pressure via fingers, knuckles and elbows on the trigger point for several seconds. Although this will temporarily relieve the pain, it will be short-lived if the therapy is not reinforced by passive stretching exercises to relax the muscle and frequent stretches and exercises to promote flexibility and strength within the area.

Trigger point myotherapy is utilised in dogs and horses. In dogs it is used following injury to relieve pain, stiffness and swelling and for maintenance to enhance muscle and joint function, promote body tone and improve movement. In horses trigger point myotherapy is used to treat a variety of conditions, including cold-backed, abnormal gait, unbalanced or refusing to perform, as well as injuries from accidents and trauma.

Trigger point myotherapy should only be performed by a qualified practitioner under instruction from a veterinary surgeon.

Craniosacral therapy

Craniosacral therapy is a technique that treats horses and dogs by improving the function of the craniosacral system using a gentle hands-on approach. The craniosacral system consists of the bones of the back and head, the associated membranes and cerebrospinal fluid. The function of the craniosacral system is to protect the nerves, brain and spinal cord. When an animal has head trauma, hind-end lameness, breathing problems, behavioural or emotional problems, it can become tense, feel pain and show impaired performance. This is associated with a reduced flow of cerebrospinal fluid. This reduction leads to a build-up of toxins which can cause pain and distress. The cerebrospinal fluid moves in a wave-like motion called the cranial rhythm. The cranial rhythm cannot be seen and can only be felt by trained practitioners. When the animal is tense this cranial rhythm is impaired and needs to be rectified to aid the health of the animal. Craniosacral practitioners do this by locating the cranial rhythm and very gently palpating an identified area of concern (Figure 18.5). This aids the flow of the cerebrospinal fluid, dispersing the toxins and improving the function of the body.

Craniosacral therapy should only be performed by a qualified practitioner under instruction from a veterinary surgeon.

Chiropractic

Chiropractic therapy revolves around the musculoskeletal system and primarily the spine, pelvis and the nervous system. It can be utilised on any animal but is common practice for horses and dogs. All animal chiropractors must have trained and qualified in human chiropractic before specifying their technique on animals and be registered on the General Chiropractic Council, although qualifications in animal manipulation can be gained. Completing a postgraduate diploma in animal manipulation is used to become a McTimoney practitioner. This type of manipulation does not require previous chiropractic qualifications and is recognised by veterinary surgeons. Chiropractic and McTimoney treatments can only be carried out under instruction after diagnosis from a veterinary surgeon and should be followed up by a full written report.

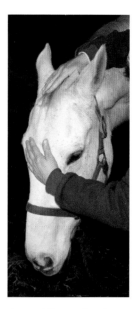

Figure 18.5 Craniosacral therapy involves gentle palpation of the cranial rhythm to relax the horse and relieve pain.

Chiropractors or McTimoney practitioners are used for various back and limb disorders. On dogs these include:

- Stiff joints leading to difficulty walking or climbing stairs
- Reluctance to go for walks
- Crying out when attempting to move or after exercise
- Signs of distress when handled.

Musculoskeletal disorders of the horse include:

- Limb lameness
- Uneven gait
- Sore or cold back
- Unbalanced when ridden
- Uneven muscle development
- Irrational behaviour
- Other unexplained lack of performance.

The manipulation therapy used by chiropractors and McTimoney practitioners involves assessing the animal before treatment, manipulating specific areas to alleviate pain and giving exercise advice to maintain health. The assessments carried out include watching the animal walking and trotting in a straight line and on a circle for abnormality in the gait or lameness, observing the animal whilst stationary to look for an abnormal stance and checking hoof and shoe wear for unevenness. Chiropractic is used to treat the whole animal and the manipulation technique involves palpating the muscles either side of the spine and pelvis area to identify any incorrectly aligned joints. These are usually identified by the presence of muscle spasms, swelling or hot/cold spots. If any are found then an adjustment is carried out: this involves using the hands to give a precise, rapid movement over the misaligned joint. This is done so quickly that the muscles do not have the chance to react or contract against the manipulation and therefore the joint can be realigned. After treatment it is advised to let the animal rest or have light exercise for a period of time. This is because aligning the joints can be uncomfortable in the first few days. After this has settled down, stretching exercises will be advised to keep the animal flexible and prevent further injuries.

Osteopathy

Osteopathy is a manipulation technique similar to chiropractic. The main difference is that chiropractic mainly works on the joints of the spine and pelvis and associated nervous system, whereas osteopathy puts equal importance on all joints and surrounding muscles, tendons and ligaments. Osteopathy should only be performed by a qualified animal osteopath under instruction from a veterinary surgeon. The osteopath should also provide the veterinary surgeon with a written report after treatment.

An osteopath can be used on most domestic animals and is commonly used on dogs and horses. Animals that require osteopathy include those that have stiff joints, lameness, difficulty moving and jumping, sore backs, reduced performance and those needing rehabilitation after injury.

Osteopathy treats animals through a range of techniques, including stretches, the manipulation of bones, joint rotation and massage techniques. After instruction by a veterinary surgeon, an osteopath will first find out the history of the animal from the person responsible. The history will include any injuries or operations, change in behaviour, the animal's normal daily routine and nutritional status and any other information about its general health. The osteopath will then examine the animal's movement, making note of any lameness, abnormality within the gait, stiffness, reluctance, unusual head carriage or any other indications that there is something wrong. After assessment the osteopath can make an informed decision on what treatment is required. The whole animal will be treated with various techniques, including stretching, joint mobilisation and rotation, manipulation if required to realign joints and massage techniques to soften the tissues and reduce tension. After treatment it will be advised that the animal has a period of time for relaxation before continuing with normal daily routine. Exercises may also be advised to reinforce the initial treatment. Through these osteopathy techniques, increased mobility and flexibility can be achieved. Also blood circulation and lymphatic drainage can be improved to reduce swelling and stiffness and improve the overall health of the animal.

HERBAL THERAPY

Herbal therapy involves the use of plant materials and plant extracts to assist with holistic healing and maintenance of health. The plant materials frequently utilised include leaves, roots, flowers and extracted oils. These materials are used orally as a feed supplement, through the nose in the form of an inhaler or as a topical application to the skin.

Techniques used within herbal therapy include:

- Herbal remedies
- Aromatherapy
- Bach flower.

Herbal remedies

Herbal remedies are an alternative natural form of conventional pharmaceutical medicines. Herbal remedies involve using specific herbal roots, leaves, stems and flowers to assist healing. Herbal remedies can be used to treat specific illnesses or dysfunctions or can provide a holistic effect, promoting health and vitality to the whole animal. Unlike conventional medicine, herbal remedies need to accumulate within the animal's body before they can take effect. A period of 7 days or more is normal before any improvement is seen. Herbal remedies come in a variety of forms, from topical applications of creams and gels to oral applications produced as tablets and capsules. Herbal remedies should be given in specified quantities recommended by a veterinary surgeon.

Table 18.1 shows a variety of herbal remedies, their mode of application and use.

Aromatherapy

Aromatherapy is the use of essential oils to treat and prevent specific disorders and dysfunctions. Essential oils are extracted from the leaves, flowers, roots, stems and fruit of plants. Essential oils are very potent and should not be given orally or used without being diluted with a carrier oil or water-based gel. Three drops to 5 ml is the highest recommended dilution. Diluted essential oils can be offered to the animal to smell or used topically during massage. All usage of essential oils should be agreed with a veterinary surgeon before treatment.

Essential oils can be useful in the treatment of large animals, particularly horses and dogs. Some can be used on cats if diluted well but are not recommended for smaller animals. Essential oils are highly volatile and are

Table 18.1 Herbal remedies, their mode of application and medicinal use

Herb	Application	Use
Basil	Orally, diluted in water	Antiseptic/antibiotic properties. Also an expectorant to aid respiratory disorders
Garlic	Orally as food supplement or tablet	Antibacterial, antifungal and antiviral given in capsule form. Also used to protect against parasites and as an expectorant to treat respiratory disorders
Seaweed	Orally as food supplement	Good source of vitamins and minerals. Can also improve coat condition
Nettles	Orally as food supplement	Diuretic effect for use in liver and kidney disorders. Also a natural stimulant to increase energy levels
Dandelion	Orally as food supplement	Diuretic effect for use in treating liver and kidney disorders
Chickweed	Orally as a food supplement and also topically as a cream	Rich in vitamins and minerals. Expectorant effect to treat respiratory disorders. Also a laxative. Cream is used for skin conditions
Aloe vera	Orally as a food supplement or capsules. Also topically as a cream or gel	Antibacterial, antiviral and anti-inflammatory actions. Used orally as a laxative or to treat ailments such as intestinal disorders or headaches. Used topically as a wound ointment for wounds and skin irritations
Elderberry	Orally as food supplement	Promotes the immune system
Valerian	Orally as food supplement	Treats insomnia, anxiety and nervousness

therefore easily absorbed into the blood stream via the nose and brain or the skin. Larger animals have the ability to cope with the chemicals within the blood stream whereas this would cause detrimental effects on smaller animals.

Animals should never be forced to smell essential oils. The animal should be offered the choice of smelling but allowed to turn away if not interested. This is called self medication. A number of diluted oils can be offered to an animal for it to choose which one it would like to smell. If the animal is interested it will smell the oil with enthusiasm, lick its lips, try and lick the bottle and follow the smell around. The diluted oil should be offered daily until the animal decides it is no longer interested. At this stage the treatment would be complete.

For topical application the diluted oil should be applied to a very small area to begin. This is to make sure no reaction is going to occur. The oil can then be rubbed in the specified area as instructed by a veterinary surgeon.

Essential oils can be used for a variety of disorders or dysfunctions and work well alongside other bodywork and energy techniques.

Table 18.2 shows some of the essential oils that are available for animals and their uses.

Bach flower

Bach flower remedies were developed by Doctor Edward Bach. The remedies are natural and used to help animals with a range of emotional difficulties. Bach flower remedies can be used to treat any animals and are particularly utilised with horses and companion animals. Bach flower remedies can be given straight from the bottle or by adding to feed or water. 4-5 drops is the normal recommended dose. Bach flower remedies can be given without veterinary advice but it is advised to speak to a veterinary surgeon to make sure there are no underlying issues.

There are 37 Bach flower remedies and each has a specific use. The Bach flower remedies can also be combined to help multiple difficulties at the same time. The most common combination that is used is called rescue remedy. Rescue remedy combines Clematis, Impatiens, Rock rose, Cherry plum and Star of Bethlehem. This combination provides an emergency remedy that can be used in traumatic situations to calm and de-stress the animal. Rescue remedy can also be used in normal situations to help calm overanxious animals.

The 37 Bach flower remedies and their uses are shown in Table 18.3.

Table 18.2 Essential oils used in aromatherapy and their uses

Essential oil	Use
Benzoin	Aids respiratory disorders and can be used as a muscle rub
Bergamot	Enhances the immune system and has antiseptic properties
Black pepper	Muscle relaxant and helps intestinal dysfunction. Also good as a muscle rub for arthritic animals
Chamomile	Stress-relieving and has anti-inflammatory properties
Citronella	Calming effect and can be used as an insect repellent
Eucalyptus	Decongestant for respiratory disorders and can be used as an insect repellent
Frankincense	Helps stress-related respiratory and intestinal disorders and has antibacterial properties for use with wounds
Grapefruit	Relieves stress
Lavender	Relieves stress, shock and depression. Also helps to eliminate scar tissue
Lemon	Has detoxifying and antibacterial properties. Can be used to help eliminate warts
Peppermint	Stimulates the body and aids intestinal disorders. Also can be used to soothe sprains and strains
Pine needle	Aids respiratory disorders and can be used as a muscle rub for arthritic animals
Rosemary	Aids concentration and improves coat condition
Sweet marjoram	Can be used as a mild sedative or to relax muscles
Tea tree	Enhances the immune system and used in the treatment of parasite and fungal skin conditions

HOMEOPATHY

Homeopathy is the use of specific herbs, plants, minerals and animal extracts to treat a disease. The choice of homeopathic remedy is matched to the symptoms the animal is showing. A remedy can then be found that would give similar symptoms in a healthy animal. The homeopathic remedy then acts on the animal's body systems in a similar way to the disease but in a more powerful form to increase the immune system and fight off the disease. As the choice of remedy is decided by the symptoms of the individual a different group of remedies may be required for the same disease in different animals. This means the treatment is unique to each animal. The decision of remedies can only be decided by a veterinary surgeon. It is against the law for anyone else to prescribe homeopathic treatment.

Homeopathic remedies are made from potent extracts that have to be diluted in water and alcohol before use. After dilution the solution is shaken vigorously before diluting again. This procedure is repeated over and over until it is at a safe dilution to be used. As a result, homeopathic remedies are non-toxic, give no side-effects and are safe to use. If a wrong remedy is given it will not work but will also have no detrimental effects.

Homeopathic treatment can be used on all animals. Homeopathic remedies can be given orally or used topically and can be used on a variety of ailments from coughs, colds, asthma and behavioural problems to wounds, inflammation and arthritis. Homeopathic remedies can be used on their own or in combination to treat a variety of symptoms at the same time. Tonics can also be produced for regular use to treat the whole animal and improve vitality and health.

A list of common homeopathic remedies and their uses is shown in Table 18.4.

ENERGY THERAPY

Energy therapy techniques involve using mechanical vibrations and electromagnetic forces. These are set at specific wavelengths and frequencies to heal an animal by stimulating the body's electrical system.

Techniques involved in energy therapy include:

- Shiatsu
- Acupuncture
- Crystal technique
- Reiki.

Table 18.3 The 37 Bach flower remedies and their uses

Bach flower remedy	Use	Bach flower remedy	Use
Agrimony	To relieve stress and associated disorders in animals that hide their troubles from themselves and others	Larch	To improve confidence and determination in animals who lack self-esteem
Aspen	To stop the onset of unknown fear in animals that frighten easily	Mimulus	To make animals with known fears more confident
Beech	For animals that are intolerant to other animals, people and situations	Mustard	To reduce the effect of a sudden onset of depression and make the animal happier with life
Centaury	Used to make timid and submissive animals more brave and dominant	Oak	To relax an energetic animal between bouts of activity
Cerato	To improve concentration in easily distracted animals	Olive	To restore strength and vitality on overexhausted animals
Cherry plum	To prevent the onset of aggression and self-harming in animals that easily lose self-control	Pine	To build self-confidence
Chestnut bud	To break unsuccessful behaviour problems and help the animal learn from mistakes	Red chestnut	To stop animals being overanxious when separated from owner or companion
Chicory	To control possessive and territorial behaviour and make the animal more loving	Rock rose	To calm animals who become panic-stricken with the onset of extreme fear
Clematis	Makes animals that are inattentive and easily distracted more active and interested in life	Rock water	To make a stubborn animal more responsive
		Scleranthus	Can be used to improve balance and make animals more decisive
Crab apple	To stop animals obsessively cleaning and to treat skin conditions	Star of Bethlehem	Helps animals recover from trauma and shock
Elm	To restore confidence in animals that get easily overwhelmed with situations	Sweet chestnut	To calm animals suffering from anxiety
Gentian	Restores confidence in animals getting over a trauma	Vervain	To calm highly strung animals
Gorse	To help animals recover from disease and increase motivation	Vine	To make dominant animals more accepting of instruction
Heather	Used to settle animals that are vocal if left on their own	Walnut	To help animals deal with new situations
Holly	To calm aggressive and jealous animals	Water violet	To make aloof animals more sociable
Honeysuckle	Used to calm animals who have problems dealing with a change in lifestyle	White chestnut	To calm anxious animals
		Wild oat	Restores sense of purpose in depressed animals
Hornbeam	To improve vitality and enthusiasm in lethargic animals	Wild rose	To increase energy levels in uninterested animals
Impatiens	To improve patience in irritable nervous animals	Willow	To stop animals being destructive

Shiatsu

Shiatsu, meaning 'finger therapy' in Japanese, is an old therapy that treats the animal by rebalancing the flow of energy. It is believed that energy flows through a series of paths around the body, called meridians. This energy needs to be flowing smoothly to keep the body in balance. If the energy flow becomes unbalanced then a disease or illness will occur. There are 12 primary meridians and these work in pairs. The pair, or yin and yang relationship, means that they oppose but complement each other. To do this effectively they must be in balance. If they are not then the energy flow will not be balanced, leading to undesirable symptoms. Table 18.5 shows the 12 primary meridians and the function they have within the body.

The technique of shiatsu is mainly carried out on horses but can also be utilised on dogs and cats. Shiatsu involves using pressure applied by finger, thumb, palm, forearm and elbow on the acupressure points of the meridians to rebalance the flow of energy. The pressure is of a gentle nature and the animal dictates how long a session will last. A series of sessions may be required to succeed in improving the health of the animal.

Shiatsu is recognised by the Royal College of Veterinary Surgeons as a form of physiotherapy and therefore according to the Veterinary Surgery (Exemptions) Order of 1962 it can be administered by a non-veterinary surgeon after diagnosis and under instruction.

Acupuncture

Acupuncture is similar to shiatsu by balancing the flow of energy via the 12 meridian pathways (Table 18.5). In acupuncture needles are inserted into acupuncture pres-

Table 18.4 Common homeopathic remedies and their uses

Remedy	Use
Aconite	Shock
Arnica	Bruising
Arsenicum album	Gastroenteritis
Cantharis	Cystitis
Hepar sulph	Abscesses
Hypericum	Crush injuries
Ledum	Insect bites
Phosphorus	Haemorrhage and vomiting
Rhus tox	Injury
Ruta gray	Tendon injury
Silica	Foreign bodies

Table 18.5 The grouping of primary meridians and their functions

Group	Primary meridians		Function
	Yin	Yang	
Wood	Liver	Gallbladder	Healing of joint and ligaments Reduce stiffness Reduce arthritic pain
Fire (primary)	Heart	Small intestine	Treat shock and trauma, fear and distress
Fire (secondary)	Triple warmer (immune system)	Heart protector (pericardium)	Reduce overexcitement and relieve chest tension
Earth	Spleen/pancreas	Stomach	Treat digestive disorders Soothe colic Ease muscle aches, promote muscle tone
Muscle	Large intestine	Lung	Treat respiratory abnormalities Improve blood oxygenation Regulate bowel function Improve skin disorders
Water	Kidney	(Urinary) bladder	Relieve exhaustion Treat sore back Reduce stress

sure points located along the meridian lines to relieve pain and treat disease. Acupuncture is an invasive treatment and can only be performed by a veterinary surgeon. It is an offence for anyone other than a veterinary surgeon to perform acupuncture on an animal. Acupuncture is utilised in animals varying from small mammals such as rabbits, dogs and cats to large mammals such as horses.

Acupuncture is carried out with very thin stainless-steel needles. The acupuncture points become tender when in need of stimulation and the needle will enter the skin without force. If force is required then the incorrect acupuncture point has been found. The needle should cause no pain to the animal and should be left in for approximately 10 minutes.

According to Chinese medicine a disorder or dysfunction is due to a disruption in the energy flow through the body. The acupuncture points used are found along the meridian pathway and correlate to the condition that needs treating. For example, swelling and heat need cooling; therefore a water acupuncture point would be used. By placing needles at this point the flow of energy is unblocked, leading to a balance of the system and improved health of the animal.

Scientists also have their view on what acupuncture does. They believe that the needles stimulate trigger receptors within the body. These send signals to the brain to release natural pain-killing hormones called endorphins. Scientists therefore believe that acupuncture is a form of pain relief rather than treatment.

Although there is a difference in opinion as to the use of acupuncture it has become an increasingly popular alternative therapy.

Crystal therapy

Crystal therapy is the use of crystals or minerals to relax an animal and promote energy balance. Crystals work by stimulating the animal's electromagnetic energy field which surrounds the body. By stimulating this field physical, emotional, mental and spiritual problems can be addressed. Crystals are a non-invasive, natural treatment which can be used on any species of animal. Crystals are not an alternative to proper veterinary advice. This should be sought if abnormalities occur with an animal.

Various crystals can be used in crystal therapy and all have their own specialism. In general, warm-coloured stones – red, orange and yellow – stimulate energy flow, and cool colours – blue, green and violet – calm overactivity. The crystals are applied on the animal's body, in the animal's bed or accommodation, placed nearby, added to a collar or held in the hand. The way the crystals point also has an effect on how well they work. If the point is away from the animal, energy is moved away

from that area and if it is pointing towards the animal the body is recharged. Care must be taken if adding a crystal to an animal's bed or accommodation that it is not placed in a way such that the animal can injure itself.

Crystals are said to be beneficial for many ailments including anxiety, depression, muscle injuries, trauma and digestive dysfunction. Their main use is to relax the animal and this is shown by the animal yawning and going to sleep when the crystals are used.

Reiki

Reiki is a Japanese technique which reduces stress and induces relaxation. Reiki is a non-invasive gentle therapy that works on balancing the energy within the body by stimulating the seven energy centres. Reiki complements other forms of conventional medicine or alternative therapies but should never be used as an alternative to veterinary care in ill animals. Under the Veterinary Act of 1966 it is illegal for anyone other than a veterinary surgeon to diagnose an illness and recommend treatment.

Reiki can be used on all species of animals, whether healthy, ill or dying. Reiki is beneficial for healthy animals because it can keep an animal relaxed and maintain overall well-being. In ill animals reiki can assist conventional medicine by keeping the animal calm and assisting with the healing process. Reiki has been proven to enhance the release of natural endorphins within the body and this works as pain relief and gives a 'feel-good' factor. Dying animals also benefit from reiki because it relieves fear and anxiety by relaxing the animal until the time comes to pass away.

Reiki is performed by a healer who initially stands away from the animal. The energy is transmitted at a distance through the hands and it is up to the animal to move towards the healer. Some may move further away or others will move towards the healer for a hands-on approach. Either way, the energy can still be passed on. Treatment can be repeated as many times as required to heal the animal or on an ongoing basis to maintain health.

COMMUNICATION THERAPY

Animal communication means communicating with an animal via telephony. Telephony involves the exchange of images, thoughts, words, emotions and feelings from animal to communicator. The communicator can then translate the information gained and tell the owner what the animal is thinking.

Communication can be used on any species of animal to assist the owner in the following areas:

- Behavioural/emotional: the communicator will be able to tell the owner why the animal is aggressive/submissive and what can be done to change this emotional disorder
- Health: the communicator will be able to determine how the animal feels and if any pain is experienced. This could be useful to tell to a veterinary surgeon but is no substitute for a veterinary surgeon's diagnosis and advice on treatment
- Environmental: the communicator will be able to find out what the animal feels about its environment and what it would like improved.

Animal communication is used to bring an owner and an animal closer together and assist in maintaining well-being.

Evaluation of the field of complementary medicine demonstrates the wide variety of alternative therapies available. Most can assist in the treatment of animals in some way but none can replace proper veterinary diagnosis and treatment. An animal's health and well-being are of paramount importance and the best possible care must be given at all times. It is also a legal requirement under the Veterinary Surgery Act of 1966 that all animals have an assessment and diagnosis by a trained veterinary surgeon before treatment. Treatment should also be carried out by a veterinary surgeon or a person instructed by a veterinary surgeon, as outlined in the Veterinary Surgery (Exemptions) Order of 1962. Alongside this stipulation alternative therapy can complement conventional medicine to improve and maintain animal health and vitality.

Bibliography

Bird C 2002 A healthy horse the natural way: a horse owner's guide to using herbs, massage, homeotherapy, and other natural therapies. Lyons Press, Connecticut

Boldt E Jr 2002 Use of complementary veterinary medicine in the geriatric horse. Veterinary Clinics of North America: Equine Practice 18:631–636

Brennan M L, Eckroate N 2006 Complete holistic care and healing for horses: the owner's veterinary guide to alternative methods and remedies. Kenilworth Press, Shrewsbury

Bromiley M W 1994 Natural methods for equine health. Blackwell Science, Oxford

Bromiley M W 2007 Equine injury, therapy and rehabilitation. 3rd edn. Blackwell, Oxford

Fleming P 2002 Nontraditional approaches to pain management. Veterinary Clinics of North America: Equine Practice 18:83–105

Fougere B, Wynn S G 2006 Veterinary herbal medicine. Elsevier Health Sciences, Oxford

Gomez Alvarez C B, L'ami J J, Moffat D et al. 2007 Effect of chiropractic manipulations on the kinematics of back and limbs in horses with clinically diagnosed back problems. Equine Vet Journal 2: 153–159

Habacher G, Pittler M H, Ernst E 2006 Effectiveness of acupuncture in veterinary medicine: systematic review. Journal of Veterinarian International Medicine 20:480–488

Hektoen L 2005 Review of the current involvement of homeopathy in veterinary practice and research. Veterinary Record 157:224–229

Janssens L A 1992 Trigger point therapy. Problems in Veterinarian Medicine 4:117–124

LinksBuchner H H, Schildboeck U 2006 Physiotherapy applied to the horse: a review. Equine Veterinarian Journal 38:574–580

Porter M 2005 Equine rehabilitation therapy for joint disease. Veterinary Clinics of North America: Equine Practice 21:599–607

Ramey D, Rollin B 2003 Complementary and alternative veterinary medicine considered. Blackwell, Oxford

Williams C A, Lamprecht E D 2008 Some commonly fed herbs and other functional foods in equine nutrition: a review. Veterinary Journal 178: 21–31

Xie H, Preast V 2005 Xie's veterinary acupuncture. Iowa State University Press, Iowa

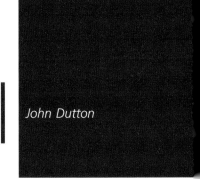

Principles of ecology

CHAPTER CONTENTS

This chapter aims to provide an overview of ecology with a brief introduction to its links with the conservation of biodiversity, species and habitats.

Ecology as a science is one of the least understood of the natural sciences, in comparison to biology, botany or zoology. There are numerous definitions of ecology which have been used since this science was first defined by Ernst Haeckel in 1866. One of the most recent is that of Townsend et al. (2003), according to whom ecology is 'the scientific study of the distribution and abundance of organisms and the interactions that determine distribution and abundance'.

Ecology is therefore the study of organisms in relation to the environment in which they live; that is both the living or *biotic* and non-living, physical or *abiotic* (e.g. water, nutrients, sunlight, topography) parts of the environment. The science of ecology can be summed up as examining '*where* organisms are found, *how many* occur there and *why*' (Krebs 1985).

It is often helpful to think of the environment in which an organism occurs as a large jigsaw. In this the organism is represented by a segment which interlocks with numerous other segments representing the organism's requirements for survival (e.g. food, shelter, nest/den, territory) and conflicts with other organisms and species, and the weather. Changes to any one of the segments can have an influence – albeit indirect on some – on the other segments.

SCALES IN ECOLOGY

Ecology operates on a number of scales. It is important to have an appreciation of these scales, their impact on an ecological understanding of organisms and systems and their relations to each other.

Spatial scale is perhaps the easiest to grasp; no area is too large or too small to have an ecology. At one extreme there is small-scale or 'microecology' which, for example, exists within the community of bacteria and protozoa within the gut of insects. The array, number of species and complexity of interactions can be comparable to more familiar, larger-scale habitats such as tropical rainforests. At the other extreme there is 'megaecology' which includes such relationships as those between ocean currents, climate and habitat occurrence, or between forests and downstream flooding. Probably the most familiar megaecology at present is the global ecosystem which has been highlighted, as the issues connected to the so-called greenhouse effect, global climate change and increased atmospheric carbon dioxide are discussed extensively in the media.

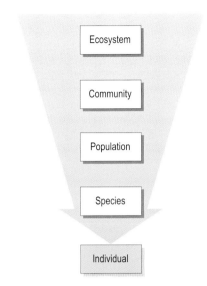

Figure 19.1 Inverted-triangle arrow showing the decrease in complexity and decline in the number of interactions at the different ecological scales.

The understanding of ecology at such extremes of scale is vastly incomplete. The complexities of the inter-relationships and difficulty of study at such scales mean that the principal ecological knowledge and understanding are found in medium-scale ecology. It should be noted that even at this scale ecological knowledge is incomplete and new information is being discovered all the time.

The second scale is that of timescale. The human lifespan, the largest scale to which humans normally relate, does not easily fit with ecological process and the lifespans of other organisms. Some species will have lifespans which can be measured in days, e.g. species in the Gastrotricha phylum (minute aquatic animals) have lifespans of about 3 days, whereas others have lifespans much longer than those of humans – giant tortoises have been known to live approximately 177 years (in captivity). Plant species are known to live even longer: individuals of the common or pedunculate oak *Quercus robur* have been recorded as approximately 1500 years old, the Huon pine *Lagarostrobos franklinii* is known to live for 3000 years and on a Tasmanian mountain there is a stand which is considered to be all one tree due to matching DNA and is thought to be over 10500 years old.

It is not only lifespan that is of importance but the timescale over which ecological processes can occur. The precisely synchronised mass spawning by reef corals occurs on one night a year, the mating display of the female glow worm *Lampyris noctiluca* only lasts a few weeks until mating, whereas the adjustment of habitats

to the end of the last ice age (approximately 10 000 years before the present) may still be taking place. Such time-scale differences need to be considered when examining ecological processes and relationships to ensure that long-term relationships and impacts are not missed.

A third scale in ecology, and that on which this chapter focuses, is that of biological scale. The science of biology tends to deal with the 'within-organism' scales such as cells, tissues and organs. Ecology then is involved with the next levels: individuals and species, populations, communities and ecosystems. The levels of complexity and number of interactions increase with higher level or scale (Figure 19.1).

INDIVIDUALS AND SPECIES

For many ecologists the individual organism of a particular species is the smallest ecological unit that is of interest. For some groups of species, e.g. birds, mammals, insects, reptiles and amphibians, individuals of a particular species are easy to identify. They are a specific shape – for example, a shrew has a long nose, two eyes, two ears, four legs and a tail – and thus are easily distinguished from one another as they are independent; each is a single unit and is determined genetically as such. As such they are termed *unitary* organisms.

Conversely, with *modular* organisms, such as trees, shrubs and corals, it can be far more complex to identify an individual among the masses. Growth is by repeated production of modules (e.g. leaves, tubers, polyps) and their form or shape is not necessarily predetermined but indeterminate and often depends on the prevailing conditions which might affect their shape, e.g. trees on exposed coasts take on a shape streamlined by the prevailing wind.

Although how an individual organism survives and copes with its environment and how it competes with other individual organisms can be of great interest, it is often of more value to examine such interactions at the species level.

Species definitions

The simplest definition of a species is that which when individuals reproduce their offspring, they are viable, i.e. that they themselves can produce offspring, and so on. This is known as the reproductive species concept and focuses on the idea that species exist and maintain their genetic uniqueness because they do not interbreed with other species. The classic example which highlights this is when a male donkey *Equus asinus* and female horse *E. caballus* interbreed to produce mules which are (normally) infertile. As horses and donkeys are separate, distinct species, when they do interbreed their offspring cannot produce further offspring and thus the original species' distinctiveness is maintained. Such species have also been termed biospecies.

However, recently ecologists have come to realise that such a definition is overly simplistic. As a result other concepts of species have been proposed: the biological species concept and the recognition species concept.

The biological species concept views a species as a group of natural populations that interbreed and are reproductively isolated from other such groups. A species therefore consists of many individual organisms which share a common gene pool, which is separate from other distinct individual organisms which belong to another species, with its own gene pool.

This concept even allows species which are indistinguishable morphologically to be classified as separate species if they do not interchange genes. The separation of species under the biological species concept is maintained by what are termed reproductively isolating mechanisms, first defined by Dobzhansky in 1970. Such a mechanism is any property that prevents genes from being exchanged between species and as such can maintain the genetic uniqueness of species even if they exist in close proximity. A number of mechanisms, both pre-mating and postmating, which would act in such a way have been described (Table 19.1).

The recognition species concept considers species to be groups of organisms with common ways by which they recognise and respond to mates, which are unique to their species. Such methods of mate recognition have been termed specific mate recognition system and

encompass all aspects of mating, from courtship behaviour and song, to pheromones and compatibility of reproductive organs and gametes. In contrast to the biological species concept this species concept highlights the factors that attract organisms from one species together rather than how separate species are isolated from one another. The recognition concept considers the reproductively isolating mechanisms to be an incidental result of divergence among specific mate recognition systems rather than an active cause of species formation.

Classification of species

The debate as to exactly what defines a species is all well and good. However, the practicality of distinguishing one species from another is perhaps more valuable. Traditionally species have been classified and distinguished taxonomically using morphological or structural features, i.e. what they, or parts of them, look like. This can be extremely useful when identifying species from one another, as long as the distinguishing features are clearly visible. For many lesser-known and especially small species, such as insects, this is not the case and they are often lumped together under family names. Beetles are a group of insects which have the largest number of species, with currently about 350 000 species identified; over 100 beetle families are known to occur in the UK.

The taxonomic system which is universally accepted by the scientific community is based on that devised by Carl Linnaeus and is known as *Linnaean taxonomy*. In this

Table 19.1 Dobzhansky's classification of reproductive isolation mechanisms

Premating mechanisms

Ecological or habitat selection	The species concerned occurs in different habitats within the same general region
Seasonal or temporal selection	Mating or flowering times occur during different seasons
Sexual isolation	Attraction between the sexes of different species is weak or absent
Mechanical isolation	Physically the shape of genitalia or flower parts prevents copulation or the transfer of pollen
Isolation by different pollinators	Flowering plants of related species may be specifically adapted to attract different pollinators
Gametic isolation	In species with external fertilisation, male and female gametes may not be attracted to each other
	In species with internal fertilisation the gametes or embryos of one species may be non-viable in the physical environment of the other species

Postmating mechanisms

Hybrid inviability	Hybrid zygotes have reduced viability or are non-viable
Hybrid sterility	The first-generation hybrids of one sex or of both sexes fail to produce functional gametes
Hybrid breakdown	The back-cross hybrids have reduced viability or fertility

Modified from Mackenzie et al (2001).

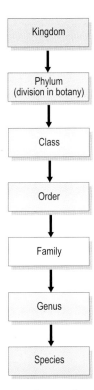

Figure 19.2 The Linnaean taxonomic system.

system all species are classified or grouped in a ranked hierarchy showing how species are related and at what level (Figure 19.2). All groups, at whatever level, are referred to as *taxa* (or *taxon* in the singular). Currently there are considered to be five kingdoms, Monera (one-celled organisms with no nucleus), Protista (one-celled organisms with nuclei), Fungi, Plantae (plants) and Animalia (animals). At present viruses do not fit within any of these kingdoms.

The most important aspect of the Linnaean system is the use of *binomial nomenclature*, the combination of the genus name and single specific name to identify the species uniquely – the species name. For example, the European hare is *Lepus europaeus*, where *Lepus* is the genus and the unique species name is *europaeus*. This scientific name is unique to this species and is not interchangeable with any other species. As a result, even if local or common names differ, the scientific community can ensure it is referring to the same species by always using the scientific name, at least when first mentioning a species in a report or research paper. The genus *Lepus* contains 23 species found as far afield as Africa, Asia, Europe, the USA, Tibet and Japan. As long as the European hare is at first referred to alongside the scientific name of *Lepus europaeus* then everyone will know to which exact species this refers. It is perhaps worth noting

that for those required to write scientific names it is convention to put these in italics (when word processing/typing) or underlined (when handwriting).

It is also worth noting here that there is an alternative classification system, although as yet not widely accepted or widely used. *Cladistic classification* refers to the phylogenetic relationships between species and employs the recency of common ancestry alone for grouping taxa.

Evolution of species

Natural selection and adaptation by individuals within a population can lead to the evolution of species, known as speciation. There are three hypotheses by which species may evolve via natural selection: allopatric, parapatric and sympatric speciation.

Allopatric speciation is where new species evolve in geographical isolation from the species from which they originate. Over time the geographical range over which a species occurs becomes subdivided, isolating different populations of the species from one another. As different selection pressures occur on these different populations natural selection and adaptation may favour different genotypes, leading to a divergence in the genetic composition of the different populations to such an extent that if these populations were to inhabit the same range again they would not be able to breed and as such would be separate, distinct species.

Such speciation takes place more readily in small populations, on the extreme edges of a species range. If the isolated population contains few individuals it is known as *peripatric speciation*. In peripatric speciation the genotypes may already be distinctly different from the species as a whole. Such *founder effect*, whereby the original individuals of a new population may have a high proportion of uncommon or rare alleles, can play an influential role in speciation. The existence of over 170 species of cichlid fish in Lake Victoria, Africa, has been attributed to allopatric speciation where changes to the river drainage feeding the lake caused population isolation and subsequent natural selection.

Parapatric speciation is thought to occur in species where populations are contiguous and only partly geographically isolated and the populations can meet across a common boundary during the process. A species occupying a huge geographical range may become adapted to different environmental conditions in the different parts of its range. Intermediate populations or hybrids will be found through the range but the large distances involved allow speciation to occur so that when those populations at the extremes of the range meet they are distinct and separate species.

The herring gull *Larus argentatus argentatus* and the lesser black-backed gull *Larus fuscus graellsii* are two distinct species which have evolved from a common ancestry. As the species colonised and encircled the northern hemisphere these two species diverged and where they occur together in northern Europe they do not inter-breed and are clearly distinguished as separate species. However, throughout their range they are clearly linked by a number of freely interbreeding intermediate populations or subspecies.

Sympatric speciation is perhaps the speciation hypothesis which is most contentious. There is no geographical isolation and all individuals are, theoretically, able to meet. It is suggested that within populations of a species there is a change in, for example, host, food or habitat preference by which the populations become reproductively isolated and as such there is no gene exchange between the populations. By becoming reproductively isolated subsequent generations show preference for a particular food or plant, reinforcing the isolation and leading to eventual speciation.

Although contentious, there is some evidence of at least an intermediate stage of sympatric speciation. Such an example is that shown by the ermine moth *Yponomeuta padellus*, the caterpillars of which feed on either apple or hawthorn trees. Mature females prefer to lay their eggs on the species on which they were raised, caterpillars also show a preference for the tree species on which their mothers were raised and adult moths show preference in mating with individuals from the same tree species. Although the apple and hawthorn types are not isolated it can be seen that such preferences may be leading to eventual speciation.

Species niche

To understand that a species is distinct due to its genetic construction or its physical form is relatively easy. However, species can also be separated by the *niche* that they occupy.

The concept of a species niche always seems difficult for some to understand. However, it is simply the position an organism fills in its environment, comprising the conditions under which it is found, the resources it uses and the time it occurs there. Contrary to the belief of many, niche is not a place but the space in which a species exists, the food it eats, its nesting requirements, in what sort of climate and weather, at a particular time of year.

The niche is a multidimensional volume where each variable which affects the organism is regarded as a single axis or dimension within which there will be a range (minimum to maximum) in which the organism can survive or occur. By considering a number of such variables it is possible to refine the picture of a species niche. Theoretically it would be possible to incorporate every dimension of variables and their interrelationship to define an ecological niche fully for a species or a

species' lifestage. It would, however, be nearly impossible to be sure all variables had been included.

It is perhaps worth noting here that a species habitat differs from its niche. A *habitat* is the locality, site or particular type of local environment occupied by an organism, or more simply where it lives. Niche, in contrast, is a (detailed) summary of the tolerances and requirements of species. Typically a habitat contains many niches and as a result supports many different species; a wetland habitat will support a wide variety of species – those which occur in open water, shallow water, emergent vegetation, invertebrates, amphibians – all of which have different niches. Thus a habitat can be seen as an area which supports the occurrence of all the factors which make up a species niche. The *habitat requirement* of a species, therefore, is linked to the existence of all such factors within a specific habitat.

If species are adapted to use resources differently due to natural selection there is normally little *interspecific competition*, i.e. there is little competition between different species. For example, this may be that they feed on different-sized invertebrates, or at different heights in woodland, or perhaps that one species is diurnal whereas another species may be nocturnal. Whatever the separating factor, and to humans this may be difficult to identify, species are thus separated by their niche.

It is worth noting that competition within individuals of the same species, *intraspecific competition*, can be very high, e.g. the great tit *Parus major* competes for the best nest sites within oak woodland as opposed to poorer-quality nest sites in hedgerows. As individuals within a species are all trying to use the same resources it has been suggested that a species could also be defined as a group of genetically related organisms whose members compete more with their own kind than with members of other species.

In the absence of interspecific competition or predation a species may be able to occupy a broader niche using a wider range of resources or under a wider set of environmental conditions, e.g. wider temperature range. Such a *fundamental niche* allows a species to take advantage of unoccupied niche space. However, when exposed to factors such as interspecific competition or predation a species may occur in a more restricted niche, the *realised niche*. The European wild rabbit in the UK, where predation is relatively low, will graze in open grassland areas great distances from the cover of thick vegetation. However, in the Iberian peninsular where the number of predators is far higher, the rabbit will not graze further than 20 metres from the cover of vegetation.

Where two species compete in a stable, homogeneous environment either one species will exclude the other or both species will coexist. The *competitive exclusion* principle states that they will only coexist in such environments if there is some form of niche differentiation; if they had identical requirements one species would out-compete the other.

Autecology

Autecology is the ecology of individual organisms or single species; it could be equated to the natural history of a species. The compilation of autecological information is a very useful exercise, although to compile a full picture of the ecology of an individual species may be excessively time-consuming and may require input from different disciplines. A key use for such information is for informing decisions for species of conservation concern. Space limitations prevent a case study being presented here but some of the key areas of information which might be incorporated into such a study include: distribution, climatic and weather constraints/requirements, habitat requirements, nutrient and food requirements, lifecycle, population dynamics, life expectancy, predators and home range and territory size.

POPULATIONS

A population is defined as a group of organisms of the same species occupying a particular ecological area. Population ecology still involves the study of individual species but now in a population context, i.e. the way in which individuals of the same species interact with each other.

The population size for unitary species, such as birds and mammals, is the total number of individuals within a given area. For modular organisms, such as corals or plants, things are slightly more complex. In these cases the number of segments (or ramets) or the number of shoots (modules) may give a more meaningful picture of abundance.

Populations generally have a structure which incorporates different numbers of individuals at different ages. Such *age structure* is described as the number of individuals in each *age class* as a ratio of one class to another. Age classes may be defined as either specific categories, e.g. years, or life history stages, e.g. eggs, seeds, larvae, pupae. The statistical study of the size and structure of populations, such as age and sex distribution, and changes within them is known as *demography*. The use of *age pyramids* is common practice when displaying demographical data; the width of the layers represents the numbers in each age classes, and the ratio of males to females is shown by the different widths on either side of a central line.

A population where the ratio of one age group to the next remains the same is said to have a *stable age distribu-tion*; the shape of the age pyramid does not change over time. Such a population could also be seen to have a *stationary age distribution* as it is neither increasing nor decreasing, i.e. the birth and death rates for each age class are constant, as is the overall population size. Those populations that are growing are characterised by a large number of individuals in the youngest age classes, giving the pyramid a broader base. Populations with a high number of individuals in older age classes are usually declining. It is worth noting that populations which are either increasing or decreasing can still have a stable age structure as long as the ratio of one age group to the next remains the same.

If a population's age distribution is disrupted by some form of temporary event such as flooding, starvation or disease, the pyramid may show low, or even a lack of, affected age class. In such cases the age composition will gradually be restored when conditions allow the birth and death rates to return to normal.

For those species where age class may only show a limited picture of the population, e.g. insects with larval stages, the number of individuals at each stage – the *stage structure* – may be valuable in describing the population structure. In addition, the use of age classes has limited application for many plant species. As growth rates are indeterminate, the size of individual plants of the same age and species can show large differences. As an alternative the use of *size classes* such as mass, area coverage, amount of branching or (in trees) diameter at breast height may be more useful.

Population dynamics

Perhaps the most important area of population ecology is that of *population dynamics*, the study of factors that influence the size, form and fluctuations of populations.

The factors which affect populations are wide-ranging and varied. However, the key factors that influence population dynamics are births, deaths, immigration and emigration. Where births and immigration equal deaths and emigration the population will be stable; where births and immigration are greater than deaths and emigration there will be population growth – the population will be increasing in size; and where births and immigration are less than deaths and emigration there will be population decline – the population will decrease in size.

Birth is perhaps a misleading word to use as it implies actual 'birth' occurring. A more accurate term would be *natality*, which means the production of new individuals, be it by birth, hatching, germination or fission. In contrast, the *fecundity* of an organism (or population) is its potential reproductive capacity. This can be measured by the number of gametes or asexual propagules (buds or spores).

Natality rate is the number of individuals produced per female per unit time; this is dependent on the type of species. Some species breed less than once a year, some breed once a year, some several times a year and others breed continuously. The number of offspring produced in each breeding period is also highly variable, with some species producing thousands, e.g. spawning fish, whereas others produce fewer than 10, such as many mammals, with many only producing one or two offspring per period. In contrast, *fertility* is the reproductive performance of an organism (or population) measured as the number of viable offspring produced per unit time.

Successful reproduction per female over a period of time is referred to as *realised natality*. Realised natality reflects the seasonality of breeding, the number of broods per year, the size of broods and the length of gestation. The condition of the individual female will have a large influence, as will the amount of resources available. Realised natality is often density-dependent (see below).

Food resource availability and quality are critical for successful reproduction; breeding is even suspended or terminated if such resources are insufficient. The timing of the onset of breeding in European wild rabbits has been shown to relate to food quality and availability: milder winters prompt earlier breeding and milder climates result in prolonged breeding seasons and, in some years, renewed breeding in the autumn period.

The natality rate will often vary with the age of the parent individual. The *age-specific birth* (or natality) *rate* is the number of offspring produced per unit time by females in different age classes. Such age-specific rates may be due to the experience of the individuals, their fecundity or fertility.

The number of deaths or *mortality rate* is the number of individuals of a population dying within a specific period of time divided by the average population size over that time period. As with natality rates, mortality rates can be calculated either for populations as a whole or for specific age classes within populations to produce *age-specific mortality rates*. An example would be a population of European wild rabbits with a size of 1000 at the start of the time period, which is reduced to a population of 600 at the end of the time period. The average population was thus 800 individuals with a mortality rate of $400 \div 800$, which is 0.5.

Immigration and emigration are factors of the type of species. In some species emigration can be low: juveniles may join the same population in which they were born and remain within its bounds for their whole life. In contrast, some species exhibit high levels of dispersal once they reach specific stages in their lifecycle. Such

dispersal or emigration can be shown in either both males and females or in just one sex; this is species-specific. When such dispersing individuals join new populations they can be said to be immigrants into this new population. In the European wild rabbit it is predominantly the juvenile males which disperse from their natal group. Such juvenile males can disperse or emigrate some distance from their parent population. When immigrating into a new social group they have to be accepted by the existing individuals, especially the males, which may take some time.

Survivorship and life tables

Instead of examining mortality it is often of greater interest to examine the number of survivors within a population: *survivorship* therefore is the converse of mortality. This is often expressed as *life expectancy*, i.e. the average number of years still to be lived by population members of a specific age. Data on survivorship for a particular population can be presented on a *survivorship curve*, with the curve showing the proportion of survivors through each phase or stage of life (normally using a log scale).

Life tables are an exceedingly useful tool for understanding populations. They summarise the fate of a *cohort*, i.e. a group of individuals born at roughly the same time, from birth to the end of the lifecycle. Such *cohort analysis* shows the number of individuals within each age class or life stage (similar to age pyramids) along with age-specific survival and mortality rates. Life tables may also give age-specific mortality rates, life expectancy and fecundity. Life tables can also be presented in a more diagrammatic form than the table form.

The proportion of individuals surviving to the start of the next stage is the *age-specific survival rate*. The use of a proportion of the original number of individuals allows the comparison of different studies undertaken at different times involving different numbers of individuals. By examining a series of life tables for cohorts from successive years it is possible to examine at which stage mortality has the greatest influence on the size of the population. That is the *key factor* which contributes the most; this is known as *k-factor* analysis. In brown trout *Salmo trutta* in the Lake District, UK, the key factor from 17 years of data and mortality identified at six life stages was found to be mortality in the alevin stage; fluctuations in the mortality of alevins were reflected in population fluctuations.

Population growth and density dependence

In population terms density is an important factor. Density can be defined as the number of individuals per unit area, per unit volume or even per unit of habitat. Depending on the species concerned, density can vary enormously. For larger mammal predators this could be one or two per 10 km^2 to hundreds of thousands per square metre for soil invertebrates.

The density of a population can influence the birth and death rate of that population; such a relationship with density is said to be *density-dependent*. Birth and death rates not influenced by density are said to be *density-independent*.

In the early stages of population growth resources are abundant, mortality rate is minimal and reproduction is as rapid as possible. The population size increases geometrically until some upper limit is approached where the growth rate declines to zero as the population becomes more dense and stabilises at the maximum that the environment can support. This upper limit or equilibrium density is constant for a particular set of variables in a particular habitat and is referred to as the *carrying capacity*. In the great tit the size of clutches and the number of pairs producing a second brood are affected by density.

LIFE HISTORY STRATEGIES

The life histories of different species will show vast variations as species will be adapted to optimise their niche spaces. However, two life history strategies which occur at either end of the life history continuum have been described. Those species, which are adapted to maximise the rate of population growth, are termed *r-selected*. *K-selected* species, at the other extreme, exist in populations at or near the carrying capacity (see below) and are considered to be more competitive. The characteristics of these two strategies are summarised in Table 19.2.

Although it is recognised that on close investigation the *r-* and *K*-selection strategies do not fit many real species perfectly, they have some merit. General patterns across taxa show that large mammals and woodland trees have many of the *K*-selected characters whereas many annual plant and invertebrate life histories reflect many of the *r*-selected characters. Perhaps the imperfect fit of these theoretical strategies to real examples usefully highlights that, despite the ecological explanations for the interrelationships between species and abiotic factors, there are frequently exceptions which do not follow the rules.

Population fluctuations

Populations rarely remain constantly at their equilibrium density or carrying capacity but frequently fluctuate around this point. A population with density-dependent growth might overshoot the carrying capacity and then show diminishing fluctuations around it until such time as the population growth stabilises at the carrying capacity.

Table 19.2 The main characteristics of r-selected and K-selected populations

| Character | Continuum | |
	r-strategy	K-strategy
Population size	Variable Usually below the carrying capacity Emigration common Recolonisation high	Constant In equilibrium Near the carrying capacity Recolonisation uncommon
Mortality	Often high Variable Not density-dependent	Often regular Density-dependent
Survivorship curve	Type III	Type I or II
Reproduction	High energy allocation to reproduction Many, small offspring	Low energy allocation to reproduction Few, large offspring
Population development	Rapid	Slow
Competition	Poor competitors	Good competitors
Lifespan	Short	Usually more than 1 year to very long
Environment	Unstable	Stable or variable but predictable

289

However, in some cases the cycle around the carrying capacity can persist in what is known as *delayed density dependence*. The larch bud moth *Zeiraphera diniana* larvae emerge in spring at the same time as the larch flushing; their feeding alters the physiology of the larch and leads to a reduction in needle size, and hence their food quality, in the following year. High larval density causes poor food quality in subsequent years which results in the crash of the larch bud moth population. The larch can recover due to low larval numbers which in turn lead to an increase in food quality and an increase in larval numbers. Such delayed density dependence can persist indefinitely within a population.

Such delayed density dependence can also cause cycles in predator and prey abundance. The classic, oft-quoted, predator–prey cycle is that of the Canadian lynx *Lynx canadensis* and the snowshoe hare *Lepus americanus*. Snowshoe hare abundance is reduced by predation when lynx numbers are high, which in turn causes a reduction in lynx numbers in subsequent years (due to lack of prey). As the lynx numbers decline predation pressure is reduced, allowing hare numbers to recover. The resulting cycle is roughly on a 10-year basis. This cyclic relationship is not quite so simple as to involve only the lynx and snowshoe hare. As with the larch bud moth larvae, high hare numbers have a detrimental impact on the quality of their food plants, causing reduced reproductive potential in the hares. As a result this classic predator–prey cycle contains a third interacting component in the form of the plants.

Changes in environmental conditions, such as weather or flooding, can also cause fluctuations in population numbers around their carrying capacity. Such environmental influences can lead to good years and bad years and are not predictable. Large, long-lived species are more tolerant of such environmental variation as any short-term implications can be absorbed within their life history. Small, short-lived species are more likely to show significant fluctuations in numbers and may, in extreme cases, become (temporarily) locally extinct. Events such as the unseasonal flooding of the River Severn in July 2007 in the Gloucestershire area of the UK will have had a serious, although perhaps short-term, impact on those species which utilise the valley meadows for breeding.

Metapopulations

A population is a group of organisms of the same species occupying a particular ecological area. A *metapopulation* consists of a number of populations linked by the immigration and emigration of individuals. As such it is important to consider the interrelationship of populations which form a metapopulation, especially in the context of conservation.

Communities

Ecological communities have been defined as either a group of interacting populations, or an assemblage of species populations which occur together in space and time. Communities are essentially the biological or biotic part of ecosystems, i.e. excluding the physical or abiotic environment. The complex properties of, and patterns within, communities, the *community organisation*, arise from the interaction between individuals and species, competition, predation, parasitism and mutualism.

The number of different species within a community and their abundance will influence *community composition* and *community structure*. Community composition depends on *species richness*, i.e. the number of species it contains or its *species diversity*. The relative abundance of the species within a community will heavily influence its structure. A community in which the species are roughly in equal abundance will show evenness, whereas where one or a few species are in greater abundance than all the other species, the community will exhibit *dominance*. Those communities showing dominance will have a lower overall diversity than those communities showing evenness. The community structure will be greater with a greater number of species present and as species number increases the *community complexity* also increases. A number of factors influence the species richness within communities, and these are summarised in Table 19.3.

Community boundaries

As the distribution of communities is strongly controlled by abiotic factors it is obvious that as these factors change the communities will also change. The boundaries or transitional zones between adjacent communities are known as *ecotones*. Such ecotones may have an abrupt change where there is no overlap between species of adjacent communities, there may be a gradual change with the distribution of species changing at approximately the same time, or there may be a gradual change with the distribution of species being different and a continuum existing.

The steeper the environmental gradient the better defined the edges of species distribution. It is relatively rare to see abrupt changes, although these exist on cliff edges, between terrestrial and aquatic communities. It is more usual to see a gradual change as different species phase out and in due to the changing controlling factor. The characteristic changes in forest communities up an altitudinal gradient show a gradual but distinct change within specific altitudinal bands. Some ecotones can be 10 km wide as one dominant tree species gives way to

Table 19.3 The principal factors that affect species richness and thus also structure within communities

Physical or abiotic factors
Size of community
The larger the area of a community, the greater the number of species populations that it can support. For example, a garden pond will contain a limited number of small organisms whereas a lake is able to support populations of many species of varied size

Spatial patchiness within a community
Spatial patchiness within a community allows organisms with differing requirements to coexist. For example, a rock pool with a smooth surface will support a lower species diversity than a rock pool of equal size that has cracks and crevices within the rock and a sandy bottom. More microhabitats will support a greater number of niches

Harshness of a community
The harshness of a community will affect the number of species able to survive within that community. For example, exposed rocky shore communities which are exposed to severe storms will support fewer species in lower numbers than rocky shore communities in more sheltered locations

Predictability of change within a community
If changes within a community are predictable, e.g. cyclic, different species will be able to utilise the community space at different times of the cycle. In deciduous woodland the spring ground flora are able to thrive on the woodland floor whilst light availability is good before the leaves of the trees grow. When the leaves shade out the light from the woodland floor the shade-tolerant species can use the same woodland floor space

Disturbance within a community
Disturbance, either occasional but severe, or low-level but frequent, will affect the population size within a community. If population sizes are kept low or are reduced periodically there will be room within which other species can become established. Trampling by livestock within grassland communities can create bare soil areas which might be exploited by new species not currently present

Isolation of the community
The greater the distance between similar communities, the less likely species are to be able to immigrate and emigrate between them. Thus fewer species are likely to be able to colonise a community in which they are absent

Biotic factors
Age of the community in evolutionary terms
Species within communities evolve together so the longer they have occurred together, the more interrelationships will have evolved. Oaks have been in the British Isles for approximately 9000 years and are associated with 284 insect species; the hawthorn *Crataegus monogyna* and Midland hawthorn *C. oxyacantha* (7000 years) are associated with 149 species. In contrast, introduced species such as the sycamore *Acer pseudoplatanus* (in the UK for 650 years) and horse chestnut *Aesculus hippocastanum* (400 years) are associated with 15 species and four species respectively

Age of a particular community at a site in time
Recently developed communities at a particular site will contain fewer species than those that have been established at a site for a long period

Primary productivity within a community
The higher the primary productivity, the greater number of herbivores a community can support without competition between the herbivores. The more herbivores within an area, the more carnivores which can survive

Community structure
The greater the structure within a community, the greater its complexity and the greater the number of niches that are available to be exploited by species and thus a greater number of species present. Woodland provides nests for birds, a large leaf and bark area for insects, ground cover for small mammals. Many of these niches would not be available in habitats such as grasslands

Competition within a community
Some species are highly competitive, e.g. for space or food. Highly competitive species such as bracken, *Pteridium aquilinum,* can exclude other species, reducing the species richness

another dominant tree species but within the ecotone both species occur in mixed abundance.

Ecotones in man-managed landscapes are rarely naturally occurring: the community boundaries, i.e. between woodland and pasture or pasture and agriculture, exist due to human intervention. Normally these boundaries are very abrupt, within the width of a fence or hedge. However, narrow boundaries between adjacent communities can be utilised by species which show a preference for such zones rather than those formed by the communities either side – this is known as the *edge effect*. The narrow edges between woodland and open areas or woodland tracks are specifically used by a number of butterflies which are of conservation interest, such as the pearl-bordered fritillary *Boloria euphrosyne*. Without appropriate management of these ecotones the existence of the butterflies would be at risk.

Community interactions

As the first definition of a community highlights, the interactions between populations within communities are critical. These interactions can be horizontal, such as competitive interactions between species at the same *trophic level*, or vertical as *trophic interactions*, e.g. between plant and herbivore or prey and predator. Trophic levels can be seen as different energy levels or the positions within a community at which species feed, or obtain their energy.

At the basic level the *autotrophs* or *producers* are those species which can feed themselves, i.e. those which can synthesise complex organic substances from basic inorganic substrates. Generally these are *photoautotrophs*, species that by photosynthesis convert carbon dioxide and water using the sun's energy into carbohydrates with oxygen as a waste byproduct. Most plants are photoautotrophs; exceptions include insectivorous plants such as the pitcher plants and sundews, or parasitic plants such as broomrapes. In contrast there are a relatively small number of *chemoautotrophs* which obtain energy by oxidation in the absence of sunlight, e.g. bacteria at deep ocean volcanic vents.

The next levels are made up of *heterotrophs*, species which need to ingest organic compounds from their environment. At the first level of heterotrophs are the *primary consumers* or *herbivores* that consume plants and vegetative matter. Above the herbivores are the *consumers*, which are most often *carnivores*, although they could also be *omnivores*. Carnivores are meat or flesh eaters and prey on other species whereas omnivores eat a mixed diet of both plant and animal material. Finally there are the *detritivores* or *decomposers* which feed on dead organic matter.

Heterotrophs can be either *generalists* or *specialists*. Generalists benefit as they are able to consume a wide variety of food or prey and thus will not be food-limited at any time. Specialists are those species which are adapted to specialise on one or a few food or prey types. Although specialists face the risk of being unable to locate sufficient food because they have specialised, they are more efficient at extracting energy from their food, giving them an advantage over the generalists. Omnivores, by definition, are generalists.

The simplest set of trophic interactions can be depicted by *food chains*. A food chain is a sequence of species on successive trophic levels within a community through which energy is transferred by feeding. Conventionally food chains are drawn with the producer at the bottom with successive trophic levels being interconnected by arrows, and the direction of the arrows indicating the direction of energy transfer. The highest carnivore in a chain is sometimes referred to as the *top carnivore* or *top predator*. Top carnivores can also be labelled *keystone species* if they have a significant and disproportionate effect on the community, e.g. the northern sea otter *Enhydra lutis*. However, the term has also been applied to species whose disappearance from a community would have a significant effect on its structure. Decomposers are rarely included within food chains, although their importance to the functioning of communities should not be underestimated.

It is rare for food chains to have more than five levels. As there is a loss of energy at each level it has been proposed that for fourth- and fifth-level carnivores to exist they would need to have a huge range in order to obtain sufficient to eat. An alternative explanation is that the longer the chain, the more unstable it will become; if lower levels were somehow to become significantly reduced in numbers those species higher up the chain would be at risk of dying due to lack of food.

Although food webs are useful they are not particularly accurate at depicting the real interactions which occur in communities. *Food chains* provide more realistic pictures of community trophic interactions. Food webs are effectively a collection of food chains showing the pattern of energy or nutrient flow throughout a community: again, all interactions are depicted by arrows whose direction shows the flow of energy. Although food webs are more realistic than food chains, i.e. they can depict omnivores where food chains cannot, they do have disadvantages. By purely examining the interactions depicted by the arrows it is not possible to get an idea of the importance of different interactions: one arrow may represent 90% of an organism's diet and another 10%, but this is not clear. In addition it is difficult to summarise all the interactions in a web, even if they are known and species may be grouped together for convenience or as a reflection of the interests of the scientists who compiled them.

Neither food chains nor food webs give a quantitative picture of the interactions within communities. In an attempt to rectify this Charles Elton devised the *pyramid of numbers* whereby the numbers of individuals at each trophic level are depicted by a horizontal box, whose width indicates the relative numbers of the organisms at each level. If the existence of parasites is taken into account this often results in an inverted pyramid of numbers as a great number of parasites can exist on one or two carnivores. Inverted pyramids also often result when producers are included; a single tree supports many other smaller organisms. An alternative to pyramids of numbers are *pyramids of biomass*, calculated by determining, for a given unit area, the biomass at each trophic level.

ECOSYSTEMS

Ecosystems are units representing the interaction of all living (biotic) and non-living (abiotic) components in a particular locality. In the previous sections the main biotic components have been outlined and the important interactions highlighted. Even in those sections it is clear that it was not possible to outline community interactions, for example, without mentioning the involvement of some abiotic components. It is best to accept that the biotic and abiotic components are inextricably linked and thus cannot easily be separated for convenience.

Ecosystems can be of any size, depending on the communities with which they are connected; aquatic ecosystems may be as small as a garden pond or as extensive as a lake or ocean system. *Biomes*, divisions of major global community types characterised by specific climate conditions, can be thought of as 'super ecosystems'. Although the influence of every abiotic component is important within an ecosystem, modern ecologists tend to view ecosystems in terms of energy and carbon flow and nutrient cycles.

Energy flow and efficiency

The bodies of all living organisms within an ecosystem form a standing crop of biomass, either expressed as energy, e.g. J m^{-2}, or dry organic matter, e.g. tonnes ha^{-1}. The majority of biomass in ecosystems is formed by the plants; the *primary productivity* of an ecosystem is the rate at which biomass is produced per unit area by the plants, again expressed as either energy, e.g. J m^{-2} day^{-1}, or dry organic matter, e.g. kg ha^{-1} year^{-1}. The total amount of energy produced by the plants is known as *gross primary productivity*. As a proportion of this is lost during respiration by the plants, the *net primary productivity* represents the rate of production of new biomass available for consumption by the heterotrophs. The rate of production of biomass by the heterotrophs is termed *secondary production*.

The energy available to the herbivore populations is limited to that which is produced as net primary productivity. However, to utilise this energy requires a transformation from plant carbohydrate to animal carbohydrate. Such an energy transformation cannot be 100% efficient (the second law of thermodynamics states that there will be a reduction of free energy at every transformation) and thus the animals will have less energy and will therefore be in fewer numbers than the plants on which they feed. Such energy loss continues through the trophic levels and as a result the animals within each become progressively fewer in number. It must be noted that energy is not only lost through transformation wastage between the trophic levels: plants and animals consume energy to survive.

The proportion of net primary production that flows through the trophic levels is dependent on *transfer efficiencies* in the manner energy is used and passed from one level to the next. The percentage of total productivity available at one level which is consumed by the next level is referred to as *consumption efficiency*. In the case of the first-level carnivores it is the percentage of herbivore productivity eaten by carnivores; the remainder is waste and enters the decomposer chain. Herbivore consumption efficiencies are very low, e.g. 5% in forests and 25% in grasslands, reflecting low herbivore densities or more usually the difficulty of utilising plant material. Carnivore consumption efficiencies are less well known: vertebrate predators may consume 50–100% of production from vertebrate prey but as little as 5% from invertebrate prey. Invertebrate predators are more efficient at consuming invertebrate prey, with as much as 25% of production being consumed.

The percentage of food energy ingested into the digestive systems of consumers which is assimilated across the digestive system walls and becomes available for growth or used as energy for living is referred to as *assimilation efficiency*. The remainder is lost as faeces and enters the decomposer chain. Carnivores achieve high assimilation efficiencies, up to 80%, whereas herbivores and detritivores have low assimilation efficiencies, 20–50%. The composition of plant materials, e.g. cellulose and lignin, means that animals cannot effectively digest them. However, plant seeds can be assimilated with an efficiency of as high as 70% and leaves up to 50%.

The percentage of assimilated energy which is incorporated into new biomass is referred to as *production efficiency*. The remainder of the assimilated energy is lost to the ecosystem as respiratory heat. Production efficiencies show distinct taxonomic variation: invertebrates have high production efficiencies, 30–40%, losing little energy as respiratory heat. Ectothermic vertebrates have intermediate values of efficiency, around 10%, whereas endotherms, with high energy expenditure associated with maintaining a constant body temperature, convert only 1–2%.

From analysis of the net primary production and transfer efficiencies it is possible to formulate an idea of the pathway of energy flow at different trophic levels within different communities. In a computer-modelled grassland system, the results of which closely match field observations, 29% of net primary production was consumed by herbivores but only 2% of secondary production was based on this. The significant finding was the critical importance of the decomposer system: of every 100 J of net primary production, 55 J flow into the decomposer system per year, with less than 1 J going into secondary production. A method of depicting the flow of energy from one trophic level to the next is *pyramids of energy*.

Nutrient cycles

The fundamental difference between energy transfer and nutrient transfer is that the pattern of nutrient transfer is cyclic. The elements forming the molecules which make up organisms are unalterable under natural conditions. As a result they remain in circulation when molecules pass from one trophic level to the next. In contrast, a proportion of energy is lost at each change in trophic level. An understanding of the major nutrient or biogeochemical cycles is thus critical in understanding how these nutrients are available for organisms to utilise.

The global *carbon cycle* is driven by the two opposing processes of photosynthesis and respiration. It is chiefly a gaseous cycle with carbon dioxide as the main component passing between the atmosphere, hydrosphere and biota. The carbon held in the lithosphere has only become available in recent centuries due to human activities such as fossil fuel extraction. Terrestrial plants use atmospheric carbon dioxide as their source of carbon for photosynthesis whereas aquatic plants utilise dissolved carbonates. Exchanges of carbon dioxide between the atmosphere and the oceans link these two subcycles. Inland aquatic systems and the oceans obtain carbon via weathering of calcium-rich rocks such as limestone and chalk, although this process is exceedingly slow – the turnover time of a carbon atom in rock has been estimated to be 100 million years. Respiration by plants, animals and microorganisms releases the carbon locked in the products of photosynthesis back into the atmosphere and hydrosphere.

Nitrogen is one of the two elements which, if lacking, most often limits plant growth. The atmospheric phase of the *nitrogen cycle* is critically important. Nitrogen fixa-tion occurs in plants with root nodules, or mycorrhiza, containing nitrogen-fixing bacteria or fungi. Nitrification – bacterial oxidation of ammonium to nitrite and then to nitrate – occurs naturally following the natural formation of ammonium ions or following their addition as fertiliser. Denitrification – the reduction of nitrate to nitrogen dioxide, dinitrogen oxide, nitrogen monoxide or nitrogen by anaerobic bacteria – is also important in making nitrogen available to the biotic component of ecosystems. There is evidence that nitrogen from geological sources may be significant in productivity in both terrestrial and freshwater communities.

Phosphorus is the second element which most often limits plant growth if it is in insufficient quantities. Principal reserves of phosphorus are found in rocks and ocean sediments as well as soil water, rivers, lakes and oceans. The *phosphorus cycle* can be described as a sedimentary cycle due to the tendency for mineral phosphorus to be transported from land to the oceans where it eventually becomes incorporated into sediments. Phosphorus is released from rock by chemical weathering and may enter the terrestrial community for an indefinite period before it enters an aquatic system and eventually progresses into the ocean sediments.

Natural biogeochemical processes release sulphur into the atmospheric part of the *sulphur cycle*. These are sea-spray aerosols, anaerobic respiration by sulphur-reducing bacteria and volcanic activity (a minor contribution). Bacteria release sulphur from waterlogged bog and marsh communities and marine tidal-flat communities, although oxidation of sulphur compounds to sulphate reverses the flow from the atmosphere. Weathering of rocks results in approximately half of the sulphur flowing off land into aquatic systems; the remainder comes from atmospheric sources. A proportion of the sulphur is cycled within plant–decomposition interrelationships but in comparison to nitrogen and phosphorus a smaller fraction is involved in such internal recycling. As with phosphorus there is a continual loss of sulphur into the ocean sediments.

The principal source of water for the *hydrological* or *water cycle* is the oceans. Evaporation into the atmosphere as a result of radiant energy allows water to be distributed around the globe by the winds. Precipitation brings water back to the earth's surface where, if this is over land, it can be temporarily held in soils, lakes and icecaps. Losses occur from terrestrial systems due to evaporation and transpiration or via freshwater streams and rivers or groundwater aquifers, eventually returning to the oceans. The oceans contain the majority of water (97.3%), polar ice caps and glaciers account for 2.06%, groundwater aquifers, 0.67% and freshwater rivers and lakes, 0.01%. The amount in transit at any one time is very small, equalling about 0.08% of the total, which includes the water draining though the soil, flowing in rivers and present as clouds and vapour in the atmosphere.

Succession

The factors which dictate the species within a community or ecosystem, the species richness and the community/ecosystem structure rarely remain constant indefinitely. Over time, and this may be a considerable timeframe, communities at particular locations will change. Such community change has been termed *succession* and is due to the changing abiotic conditions and the responses to these changes by the biotic components. The *classical model* of succession defined it to be a continuous, unidirectional, sequential change in species composition of a natural community. The sequence of communities is termed a *sere* and the distinct successional stages within a sere are known as *seral stages*.

In early successional seral stages the community will consist of pioneer species with a low biomass that can survive in low nutrient environments. Mid-successional seral stages have high biomass, high organic nutrient availability and high species diversity; often community complexity peaks at such mid-successional stages. The final seral stage is formed by a *climax community* which is that community which occurs at the end of a successional sequence under a particular set of environmental conditions. It was originally thought that only one climax community would appear for a specific geographical region to which all successional processes led – the *monoclimax* community.

Succession is a self-driven or *autogenic* process. Changes in the abiotic components of the environment occur as a result of the interaction between species and between species and their environment. As a result of such changes species in the following seral stage can become established and ultimately outcompete those species which were present in the previous seral stage. For those communities that start on newly formed substrate, e.g. glacial moraines, volcanic lava flows or alluvial deposits, where there is no presence of organic material or occupation by any organisms, the succession is called *primary succession*. In contrast *secondary succession* is that which occurs following disturbance to pre-existing communities by fire, flood or human activity.

There are three processes which have been shown to have a strong influence on succession. *Facilitation* is the term given to the changes in the abiotic conditions that are driven by the developing community, the pioneer species altering the condition of the substrate so that subsequent species can invade, e.g. mountain avens and alder on boulder clay (Figure 19.3). The resistance of species of one seral stage to invasion by species by later successional species is termed *inhibition*. Establishment by invading species is only possible therefore following

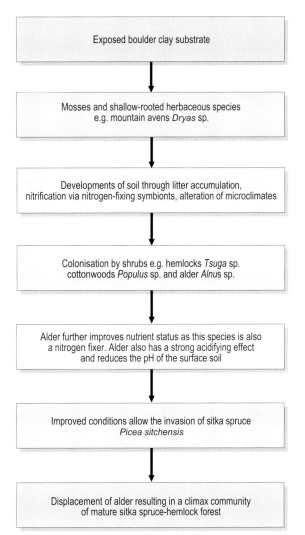

Figure 19.3 Serial stages and successional processes on boulder clay deposited by retreating glaciers at Glacier Bay, Alaska.

disturbance or replacing them as they die, i.e. when gaps within the community occur. The late successional species can invade as they have *tolerance* to lower resource levels and can outcompete earlier species for limited light and space, e.g. in abandoned field succession.

The timeframe over which succession occurs can vary enormously. Some successional stages can be very short, often depending on the particular environment in which they are occurring. Primary succession to woodland can take in excess of 100 years. *Allogenic succession*, the serial replacement of species as a result of external environmental factors, such as the response following the last ice age, took place for thousands of years, and it could be argued is still occurring. Allogenic succession is not autogenic and following the retreat of the Pleistocene ice sheet the climate warmed and allowed the establishment of communities, initially of easily dispersed species such as pines and birches, followed by slower-dispersing shade-tolerant species such as oaks.

Allogenic succession also occurs over shorter periods such as where sediments are accreting, e.g. on sand dunes or in estuaries. Silt accretion in estuaries can cause salt marshes to extend seaward and the land communities to invade the landward limits of the marsh, e.g. at the Fal estuary, Cornwall, UK.

A final form of succession is *degradative succession* which refers to the autogenic primary succession of dead organic matter. Here dead organic matter is colonised and decomposed by different species, each invading and disappearing in turn as the degradation uses and exhausts some resources and makes others available.

The classical model defines succession to be unidirectional and sequential. However, the sequence and even direction of change are not guaranteed. Changes in abiotic components may not always favour particular seral stages, and the invasion by species will depend on their availability. The biogeography of species, where they occur and their mechanisms of dispersal will dictate the availability of species to new areas. A sere may have a typical sequence but the availability of species and the success of any invasion may alter the direction of the sere from this sequence. If the conditions change the succession may reverse, with previous communities reappearing under previous abiotic environmental conditions.

SPECIES RARITY AND CONSERVATION

Nature conservation of rare species and habitats is an idea and activity which has been in the public arena for many years. However, the lack of understanding of the underpinning causes, concepts and science is perhaps the cause of much misunderstanding. *Rarity*, the state of being uncommon, or rare, occurs naturally in some species. Rabinowitz (1981) identified seven types of rarity based on the combination of three characteristics:

1. Size of geographical area (large versus small)
2. How specific are the habitat requirements (wide versus narrow)
3. Local population size (high versus low).

This classification gives eight character combinations and shows that the rarity of a species does not solely rely on whether it only occurs in small populations or is highly specialised in its habitat requirements. Those species occurring in a large geographical area, with the

ability to occur in a wide variety of habitats and having a high population, are those that are not rare and can be considered *common species*. All other combinations of the three characteristics describe the different types of rarity, e.g. the New Guinea harpy eagle *Harpyopsis novaeguineae* is rare due to its occurrence at low densities, despite having large home ranges and occupying a wide habitat range; the osprey *Pandion haliaetus* is widespread but only feeds on fish and thus has specific habitat requirements and is also rare.

Over 50% of the species on earth are found within tropical forests which are considered to be the most diverse of the terrestrial ecosystems. However, the density of individual populations can be very low, with some having densities of less than one per hectare. Such rare species have highly specific habitat preferences and niche requirements, such as particular light regimes occurring within forest gaps of a particular age. *Endemic species*, those which are restricted to particular, often small, geographical locations, are frequently found in tropical forests and on remote oceanic islands where the species have evolved in isolation.

At different scales species can show different levels of rarity, e.g. at local, national and international levels. As a scarce summer visitor to the UK the nightingale *Luscinia megarhynchos* is at the northernmost limit of its breeding range and has very specific habitat requirements, and yet in continental Europe this species is far less specialised in its habitat requirements and is far more tolerant of disturbance. It used to be a source of confusion when one county wildlife trust claimed a specific site was critical for the continued survival of a particular species when the very same species was more abundant several counties away.

More recently the term 'biodiversity' has come to prominence, mainly as a result of the International Convention on Biological Diversity which was part of the Earth Summit held in Rio de Janeiro in 1992. Biodiversity encompasses the genetic variants within species, the diversity of species and diversity of habitats or ecosystems. The misunderstanding of biodiversity is that many feel that it is about maximising biodiversity everywhere, however inappropriate, whereas in fact it is more about ensuring that there is somewhere for everything, every species, every habitat to exist.

Nature conservation is focused on the conservation of rare species and habitats. The threats or rarity status of species and habitats of conservation concern are normally as a result of anthropogenic, or human-induced, influences rather than a naturally occurring rarity. However, for those species which are naturally rare under one of the seven categories, human activities can exacerbate such rarity. The main focus of nature conservation is to prevent species *extinction*, the disappearance of a species from an area or habitat, and retain sufficient numbers of species, or sufficient areas of habitat, to ensure long-term population or habitat viability. Extinction can be either local or regional, with the potential for recolonisation from other areas, or a species can become *extinct*, when there are no individuals of that species living anywhere. One of the best-known examples of an extinct species is the dodo *Raphus cucullatus*.

The harvesting of species at an unsustainable rate in comparison to natural reproduction and mortality rates, *overexploitation*, has resulted in significant species decline and thus causes concern to conservationists. The decline in whale populations is well publicised; similar threats are current in shark populations, whereby hunting for sport, for making shark fin soup and as accidental bycatches of commercial fishing all contribute to the estimated 200 million shark deaths per year.

Habitat destruction, where habitats have been destroyed to make way for urban and industrial development, farming, mining or timber extraction, leads to threats to those species requiring these habitats for their survival. Almost 100% of the USA's natural grasslands have been lost and since European settlement in New Zealand approximately 90% of the country's wetlands have disappeared. Global forest destruction has been estimated at 170 000 km^2 per year with the loss of tropical forests being estimated to be 1% per annum or greater; more than half the wildlife habitat has been destroyed in tropical countries. Such habitat destruction is not a new occurrence, nor restricted to tropical regions. Most of Europe's native woodland has been destroyed; the destruction of the native British forests was begun by Neolithic man, approximately 6000 years before today.

Development of land for agriculture and industry can also cause *habitat fragmentation*. When a large area of the habitat is fragmented the effect is to reduce the overall area and increase the distance between the remaining fragments. The quality of the habitat of the remaining areas will also deteriorate: the areas will be small with large boundaries, or edge, and may become dominated by edge communities which favour the junction between the two. Areas of undisturbed interior habitat will become scarce and as a result the species which need such conditions to survive will be susceptible. In the Amazon forests it is the raptors and large fruit-and nectar-feeding birds that disappear first as the habitat becomes fragmented. Dispersal and immigration between patches of similar habitat can be difficult or impossible depending on the intervening habitat or land use.

The loss or reduction in population size of just an individual species can also result in *habitat degradation*. The extinction of the single insect pollinator of an endemic silversword (a succulent) species in Hawaii will lead to the eventual extinction of this species. Thus a single or a few species can have a disproportionate effect on other species or communities if they themselves become scarce or extinct.

The introduction of *alien* or *introduced species* to areas where they did not previously occur has had a significant impact. The list of species which have been transported around the world is quite extensive and includes both those introduced for specific reasons, as well as accidental or unintentional introductions. Domestic livestock, pigs, goats and cattle were all introduced to new areas as European countries explored new lands. At one time the British Royal Navy among other navies even had a policy of releasing domestic animals on to uninhabited islands to ensure there was a recognisable food source for any shipwrecked sailors. The list of impacts in different geographical locations is extensive: some may have gone unrecorded as the botany and zoology of many areas had not been explored before such introductions.

Domestic cats *Felis catus* have been one of the worst perpetrators when introduced to new areas, often becoming feral. Inevitably in areas with no predators the resident species were not adapted to avoid predation, e.g. ground-nesting birds. A number of local and total extinctions in New Zealand and its offshore islands have been attributed to the cat, such as the Stephen Islands wren *Xenicus lyallii*. At present the Durrell Institute continues to control feral cat populations actively in parts of Mauritius to prevent excessive predation of the Mauritius pink pigeon *Columba mayeri* and Mauritius kestrel *Falco punctatus*.

Of the inadvertently introduced alien species the rats, the brown or Norway rat *Rattus norvegicus* and black rat *R. rattus*, have probably had the most impact. Rat-induced catastrophes are most frequent on temperate islands. The earliest well-documented case took place on Lord Howe Island when, a few years after the first invasion by black rats from a grounded steamship, five species of endemic forest bird had become extinct – 40% of the indigenous land bird species. Rats are known to prey on eggs and fledglings and well as seeds and other animals and once rats have become established in new areas, especially on islands, they are difficult to eradicate.

Although the majority of work on introduced species focuses on introduced animals, the introduction of plant species can also have a detrimental impact. In the British Isles the introduction of rhododendron species for horticultural purposes led to the establishment of this species in the countryside. The habitat it creates is species-poor and as it is invasive it outcompetes native vegetation and causes habitat degradation. The hottentot fig *Carpobrotus edulis* is currently a cause of concern for conservation managers as it smothers native vegetation, causing significant habitat degradation.

The introduction of non-native species has also caused issues with preservation of the genetic uniqueness of species. It is generally accepted that a species is a species because its offspring is viable – if individuals from different species interbreed, their offspring are not viable. However, by introducing species from different geographical regions the native and introduced species may not have established reproductive isolating mechanisms and thus if they interbreed they may be able to produce viable hybrid offspring. An example is that between the introduced ruddy duck *Oxyura jamaicensis* and the white-headed duck *O. leucocephala* in Spain. The ruddy duck was introduced into the British Isles as an ornamental species from North America. They escaped and formed free-flying populations, some of which emigrated to Spain, where they are breeding with the white-headed ducks. Without management it is feared that the population of white-headed ducks will be lost and replaced by ruddy–white-headed hybrids.

Pollution can have a detrimental impact on both species and habitats. Pollutants come in many guises – agricultural pollution such as slurry, fertilisers, pesticides and herbicides, industrial pollutants such as heavy metals, atmospheric pollution caused by industrial and domestic emissions of carbon dioxide, sulphur dioxide, oxides of nitrogen, oil spills from tankers. The scale of the impact of pollution can range from local to global. The pollution of aquatic habitats by slurry and fertilisers can cause *eutrophication* and *algal blooms*, where the growth of algae and aquatic vegetation is excessive. Such growth can clog watercourses and when it dies can lead to oxygen depletion due to decomposition.

Bioaccumulation or *biomagnification* of pesticides has also been recorded within species. Pesticides such as organochlorines are ingested by organisms at the base of the food chain. When these are consumed by a predator which fails to excrete the pesticide it becomes accumulated within the individual. As more lower-level organisms are consumed, the pesticide becomes bioaccumulated and biomagnified. If the predator is subsequently consumed by a higher-level predator the pesticide passes up the food chain and greater accumulation and magnification occur. As a result, top predators can accumulate extremely high doses. The biomagnification of DDT (now banned) in peregrine falcons *Falco peregrinus* was established as the cause of thin eggshells, resulting in a significant egg breakage and a decline in their numbers. It should be noted that not all pesticides are bioaccumulated; some are easier for species to metabolise and excrete and therefore will not accumulate within the body.

Atmospheric pollution has resulted in a number of issues for conservation. In the 1970s and 1980s *acid rain* was a result of the emission of sulphur oxides and nitric oxide from industrial and power generation processes, which reacted in the atmosphere to produce sulphur dioxide and nitrogen dioxide. Acidification of freshwater aquatic systems resulted in fish die-offs, as well as leaching of toxic metals due to the acidification of soils. Direct impact on forests was also recorded. Currently *global warming*, or the *greenhouse effect*, is high in the public consciousness. The cause of global warming is contentious, although it is generally accepted to be partly as a result of industrial and vehicular emissions, especially of carbon dioxide as well as methane, nitrous oxide and ozone. The exact impact of global warming is as yet unknown but it is predicted that as global climates alter, the distribution, ranges and abundance of species will change.

These anthropogenic changes are more likely to affect some species than others. In addition to those species that are already ecologically rare, species with poor dispersal ability or sedentary behaviour are more likely to be susceptible. Any species which has declined in numbers will suffer a loss of genetic diversity and as a result its long-term survival is questionable as its ability to adapt to changing environmental conditions is reduced. The *minimum viable population* is that which is required to ensure that long-term genetic variability is maintained within a population. Although detailed ecological study is required to identify such a minimum population for a species, the best estimate of 250–500 individuals is accepted to avoid inbreeding. However, many endangered populations are already below this level, e.g. Amur leopard *Panthera pardus orientalis*, of which only 35 are currently estimated to remain in the wild. Frequently the protection of habitats and the prevention of species extinction are the priorities and overshadow any concerns over genetic diversity.

It is worth noting that no one factor is necessarily solely responsible for species decline. It is often a combination of a number of factors, e.g. habitat destruction and fragmentation making sites more vulnerable to pollution or to disturbance by introduced species, which leads to species becoming of conservation concern.

CONSERVATION ACTIONS

The issues outlined above may make depressing reading. However, measures are being taken to reduce and even reverse the impact of the anthropogenic factors on wild populations and habitats. Initially the identification of species and habitats of conservation concern, i.e. those at risk, is critical so that some form of prioritisation can be instigated. The International Union for Conservation of Nature Species Survival Commission Red List of threatened animals is one such method which utilises well-considered criteria by which to categorise species into priority groups: extinct in the wild, critically endangered, endangered, vulnerable, near-threatened. The Zoological Society of London has used different criteria to identify a conservation priority list of species – their Evolutionarily Distinct and Globally Endangered (EDGE) of existence programme.

Habitats and regions of conservation priority have also been identified. Priority ecoregions have been identified by using features such as species richness, endemic species, unusual or evolutionary phenomena and global rarity of habitats, with the Global 200, the priority 238 ecoregions, consisting of 142 terrestrial, 53 freshwater and 43 marine ecoregions. Plantlife has a set of criteria for identifying the world's most important plant areas and Birdlife International identifies important and endemic bird areas for priority conservation action.

Such priority lists can then be the focus of efforts by both governmental and non-governmental conservation efforts. International conservation organisations use such listings to promote their work and identify those areas and species which are most in need of their resources. Such efforts may be in situ, within the country or area in which the species exists, or ex situ, i.e. captive breeding in zoos. Although ex situ conservation measures are vital for some species, the effort and money required for successful species reintroduction are immense. It is therefore generally considered that in situ conservation of species, by habitat protection and removal of threats, is the better option, although ex situ measures for some species are essential as their rate of decline, and the causes of such declines, may not be able to be resolved before the species is lost.

These priority categories are global in their context and there is still much national and regional focus. Within the UK biodiversity action plans identify 1149 species, including the water vole *Arvicola terrestris* and spreading bellflower *Campanula patula*, and 65 habitats, such as lowland heathland, which are listed as priorities for conservation action. Most countries have a network of nature reserves, from the small local reserve to large national parks, incorporating key habitats and landscapes. It is increasingly recognised that managing such areas in isolation, particularly the smaller areas, is unsustainable, in terms of species viability, in the long term. As a result attention is being given to landscape scale ecology and management. In the UK payment schemes, such as Environmental Stewardship (previously Countryside Stewardship), are designed to promote management of agricultural land for the benefit of wildlife. Even simple measures such as providing interlinking wildlife corridors to allow species to disperse and move from one area to another, and the provision of wildlife areas to encourage the occurrence of, for example, invertebrate prey, can improve wildlife prospects. Many conservation organisations are actively working on landscape scale projects, e.g. the Severn Vale Biodiversity Project in Gloucestershire has the long-term aim of creating a network of wildlife-rich parishes connected by wildlife corridors within its 47 km^2 area in order to assist wildlife population movement and support metapopulation dynamics.

International and national legislation has its role to play. It provides legal protection and mechanisms by which action is taken once priorities have been identified. The array of legislation is extensive and ranges from international conventions which protect by controlling trade in endangered species, the Convention on International Trade in Endangered Species of Wild Fauna and Flora (CITES), those which protect specific habitats, e.g. the Convention on Wetlands, or the Ramsar Convention, and those that protect particular species such as the Convention on Migratory Species (Bonn Convention), to European legislation such as the European Council Directive 92/43/EEC on the conservation of natural habitats and of wild fauna and flora (the EC Habitats Directive) and national legislation such as the UK Wildlife and Countryside Act 1981 or the Countryside and Rights of Way Act 2000 (CROW). Currently the Kyoto Protocol, which requires signatory countries to reduce greenhouse gas emissions by specified amounts, is under scrutiny as some notable countries have yet to ratify this protocol.

Nature conservation measures are undertaken by both statutory and non-governmental organisations. In the UK statutory organisations include the Department for Food and Rural Affairs (DEFRA), Natural England, Joint Nature Conservation Committee, Scottish Heritage and the Countryside Council for Wales. The statutory organisations are supported or supplemented by non-governmental organisations such as the Royal Society for the Protection of Birds (RSPB), Mammal Society, British Trust for Ornithology (BTO), the county wildlife trusts, Wildfowl and Wetland Trust (WWT). The activities of these organisations include owning and managing land, undertaking research and lobbying governments for further conservation action. UK-based international organisations, those which have an international nature conservation outlook, include the World Lands Trust and Birdlife International.

Although there is a large amount of information by which to manage and improve nature conservation, both nationally and internationally, there is a need to work on an evidence-based approach. The understanding of ecological relationships in particular areas and the impact of management activities require investigation and monitoring, and management strategies need to be adapted if research findings identify more appropriate management activities.

AND FINALLY

This chapter only gives a brief overview of the principles of the science of ecology and its links with conservation. Space has precluded the inclusion of more detail and a broader coverage of the topic and readers are encouraged to refer to the texts in the bibliography suggested as further reading.

Ecology is fundamentally an applied science and as a result it is important to obtain an understanding of the ways in which ecology and ecological relationships can be studied in the field.

Therefore not only are teaching or learning the strategies and methodologies by which to select and collect ecological data important, but also the practicalities of doing so in field situations. It is rarely sunny and warm when undertaking fieldwork. Being properly prepared, with suitably designed and prepared record sheets, photocopied on to waterproof paper and perhaps comb-bound to prevent them being blown away in the wind, ensures that despondency will not occur as the field notes which have taken hours to collect are either destroyed by a heavy downpour or blow away across the countryside! Proper planning and preparation, facilitated by good communication between group members (if appropriate), are thus critical for fieldwork to be successful.

Bibliography

Gurnell J 2006 Live trapping small mammals: a practical guide, 4th edn. The Mammal Society, Southampton

Henderson P A 2003 Practical methods in ecology. Blackwell Publishing, Oxford

Krebs J C 1985 Ecology: the experimental analysis of distribution and abundance, 3rd edn. Harper & Row, New York

Mackenzie A, Ball A S, Virdee S R 2001 Instant notes in ecology, 2nd edn. Bios Scientific Publishers, London

Rabinowitz D 1981 Seven forms of rarity. In: Synge H (ed.) The biological aspects of rare plant conservation. Wiley, Chichester, pp. 205–217

Sutherland W J (ed.) 2006 Ecological census techniques, 2nd edn. Cambridge University Press, Cambridge

Townsend C R, Begon M, Harper J L 2003 Essentials of ecology, 2nd edn. Blackwell Publishing, Oxford

Williams G 1991 Techniques and fieldwork in ecology. Collins Educational, Glasgow

Chapter | **20** | *Rachel Rayers*

Exotic species

This chapter explores the expanding range of animals that are now kept in captivity and identifies good practice in husbandry and management methods. Although as current as possible, husbandry techniques improve all the time and up-to-date research should be undertaken regularly to maintain high standards of welfare.

WHAT IS AN EXOTIC?

Any non-native animal is technically an exotic, from hamsters to honey gliders and skinks to snakes. Since common names and definitions of what constitutes an exotic can be vague, correctly identifying animals scientifically ensures that research of health and welfare needs is species-specific.

GENERAL CARE

Research the species

Not enough emphasis can be placed on thorough and accurate research. It is the carer's responsibility to gain the knowledge required to provide care that meets and, indeed, exceeds the five key needs (Chapter 11). It is vital to investigate several routes of research, including books, the internet, experts in the field and reputable breeders and suppliers. However, bear in mind that some information may be anecdotal, so check accuracy.

The reason why research is needed is to identify the environment the animal inhabits in the wild and the range of normal behaviours that are usually exhibited. This will allow the recreation of suitable conditions in captivity to ensure the animal has as high a quality of life as possible. It also assists with the identification of the species, including its scientific name, ensuring the correct information is obtained. This is an important consideration in the import and export of exotics as some species have specific legislative concerns.

Accommodation
Small-mammal set-up

Housing design has to take into account species-specific needs. Table 20.1 describes more detailed needs of the most commonly kept small mammals.

Small-mammal substrates and dust bathing material

Most enclosures require a substrate of some kind; the choice depends on the species, cost and availability.

- Straw can be eaten; it allows urine to pass through to newspaper
- Hay provides fibre in the diet
- Shavings: avoid sawdust as it can lead to eye and respiratory problems
- Shredded paper: avoid toxic inks

- Newspapers: avoid toxic inks; can also stain fur/hands
- Presterilised peat can allow fossorial species to dig but there is a risk of humidity problems – should be pathogen-free if presterilised

Table 20.1 Housing small mammals

	Social grouping	Accommodation
Rabbit	Pairs or small groups with neutered males	Size: three times the length of the prostrate rabbit with a depth of one rabbit length Height allows standing on hindlegs Raised off floor Separate sleeping quarters Access to run and grass in summer Grass underlain with wire mesh to prevent escape Temperature not above 26–28°C or below freezing
Rats and mice	Rats: pairs or small groups with neutered males Mice: all female groups or single males	Wire cages with a solid, plastic bottom to prevent chewing Glass tanks are not as ventilated and rats and mice have high ammonia content in their urine: excessive ammonia build-up can occur Temperature 18–26°C: above 28–29°C will result in hyperthermia and death Accessories include tubes: solid wheels, climbing platforms/branches, sleeping area and wooden chewing blocks
Hamster	Nocturnal and solitary in the wild. House individually	Enclosed housing with complex tunnel systems as hamsters have large territories in the wild Avoid high levels Temperature 18–26°C: lower than 5–6°C results in hibernation; above 29–30°C results in hyperthermia and death Accessories include: solid wheels, extensive tunnel system, sleeping area and wooden chewing blocks
Gerbil	Singly, female pair or neutered male pair	Glass tanks with a deep substrate (10–15 cm) allow this semifossorial species to bury to its heart's content Temperature 20–25°C Accessories include: tubes and wooden chewing blocks
Guinea pig	Mixed social groups of neutered males or females	Hutch design similar to rabbits but smaller Access to grass recommended: as they cannot dig, only enclosed sides are needed Guinea pigs are tolerant of a wide temperature range but let common sense dictate – move into sheltered area during weather extremes Accessories include: large-diameter tubes and wooden chewing blocks
Chinchilla	Will form pairs – breeding or neutered	Active climbers: need tall enclosures in access of 2 m³ with areas to hide in Wire is recommended with solid or mesh base Temperature not to exceed 20–22°C due to thickness of coat Accessories include: large-diameter tubes, branches, nest box, appropriate dust bath and wooden chewing blocks
Degu	Same-sex pairs or small groups with neutered males	Follow guidelines for chinchilla set-up Dimensions. should be no less than 70 (length) × 70 (height) × 44 (width) cm Semifossorial, so deep layer of suitable substrate should be provided in a container large enough to allow small-tunnel construction

Table 20.1 *Continued*

	Social grouping	Accommodation
Chipmunk	House in family groups with neutered males	Similar set-up to an aviary preferable Deep litter floor with lots of vegetation, branches and climbing platforms within the cage as species is both arboreal and terrestrial Accessories include: tubes, branches, nest boxes, aerial rope walkways and wooden chewing blocks Must be located away from electrical radiation sources such as televisions, computers and strip lights as radiation waves highly stress chipmunks and will affect their behaviour. This occurs even when the appliance is off but still plugged in
Ferret	Ferrets are social and can be housed together in female (jill) pairs or small groups with neutered males (cobs)	Minimum of two ferret lengths in each direction Mesh sides (2.5 cm maximum) and mesh or solid base are recommended as ferrets can dig and squeeze through very small gaps Access or incorporated run recommended or at least regular walks on lead Accessories to include: large-diameter tubes, branches, nesting box, ropes, split levels and toys

- Dust baths should use non-toxic and non-irritant fine-grained sand
- Pure pumice sand is the usual constituent of commercially available sand and is sometimes mixed with Fuller's earth (a mineral that absorbs animal hair oils), conditioners and dietary supplements
- Some believe children's play sand is suitable if sterilised, whilst others state the grain size is too big. Using a proprietary mix is recommended.

Vivarium set-up

A vivarium usually accommodates a reptile, amphibian or invertebrate. The most important considerations for vivarium set-up are that it replicates the natural environment and allows the animal to self-regulate through the provision of microclimates that have temperature and humidity variations. It should also allow the animal to exhibit a range of its behavioural repertoire.

The major distinction between different vivaria is whether they accommodate temperate, tropical, desert or amphibious species that are either (semi- or totally) fossorial, terrestrial or arboreal.

Substrates

All substrates should be specific to exotic use so that they are hygienic and non-toxic. The choice depends on the species and its habitat along with personal preference and cost. However, substrates affect humidity, particularly in microclimates, and animals may rely on the substrate to assist self-regulation through burying. There-

fore, to be both structurally and temperature-stable as well as moisture-retentive, substrates may need to be mixed.

Common types of vivarium substrates include:

- Pea or aquarium gravel – suitable for amphibian vivaria
- Sand – aquarium, play or reptile sand (fine quartz sand): there are some concerns with impaction, abrasion and low humidity
- Calcium sand – a mineral-enriched, supposedly digestible substrate: there are some reports of impaction, and it can be dehydrating
- Sphagnum moss – highly absorbent, non-toxic
- Bark chippings – avoid cedar or pine as toxic if ingested; orchid or cypress is preferable
- Alfalfa pellets – edible, quite harsh but absorbent.

Proprietary products such as presterilised reptile bark, aspen bedding and vivarium carpets are also available. Risks of impaction can be reduced if the animal is removed from the enclosure for feeding.

Heating

The term 'cold-blooded' is inaccurate as no animal is truly cold-blooded. An animal's metabolic rate correlates directly with temperature. The distinction lies in the method through which they generate heat. Endothermic mammals generate their own heat within the body, whereas ectothermic animals obtain heat from their environment.

Two methods through which ectotherms obtain heat

- Thigmotherms obtain heat directly from contact with warm object, e.g. rocks that have absorbed heat from the sun are warm to the touch – snakes are commonly thigmotherms
- Heliotherms obtain heat indirectly by basking under heat sources (bright sunshine in the wild).

Equipment available to heat vivaria

- Thigmothermic: hot rocks – concealed heating element in replica rock (there have been some reports of burns if prolonged contact is allowed) and heat-mats – a slender heating element in a plasticised mat that emits low levels of heat
- Heliothermic: basking/spotlamps, infrared lights and ceramic bulbs/heaters (infrared and ceramic emit low or no light and are therefore good for night heating).

Amphibian enclosures often have one of the above but an aquarium heater will be required to heat the water itself, unless the body of water is small enough to remain at a suitable constant temperature through standard vivarium heating. Particular care must be taken when heating a damp environment.

Heating considerations

- Thermostatically controlled heating maintained at the optimum temperature for the individual is vital
- Temperature plays an important role in food metabolism and vitamin D synthesis
- Heating adds to the comfort and well-being of the occupant
- Temperature fluctuations, even within a few degrees, can cause stress and ill health in exotics. However, normal daily temperature changes between night and day should be allowed but must fall within the correct parameters for the species concerned
- Natural thigmothermic or heliothermic behaviour should be allowed
- A thermal gradient should be present to allow thermal regulation.

Lighting

The lighting regime needs to accommodate the natural behaviour of the species, be it nocturnal, diurnal or crepuscular, and supply a suitable ultraviolet (UV) spectrum for the correct time duration. Photoperiod and UV spectrum affect metabolic activity such as food metabolism and vitamin D synthesis and can influence biorhythms, stimulating hibernation or breeding behaviours.

Considerations of lighting

- Control photoperiod by timers to mimic species-specific natural day length
- Proprietary UV bulbs emit differing light spectrums and should be correct for species. Broad-spectrum bulbs replicate daylight and emit low levels of UVB
- Types of lighting include UV-emitting fluorescent tubes, halogen, metal halide and mercury vapour bulbs (the latter two can provide both heat and UV, but levels may be too high and pose a health risk to some)
- Both UVA and UVB light are required in differing quantities depending on species. UVA affects activity cycles and UVB aids in vitamin D_3 synthesis. Self-regulation should be permitted through a UV gradient or the provision of shades via hides and foliage where appropriate
- An incorrect lighting regime can lead to metabolic diseases.

Ventilation

Correct ventilation ensures that appropriate humidity and temperature levels are maintained. The movement prevents stale air accumulating and reduces the risk of damp spots that can harbour pathogens.

Considerations of ventilation

- Modern vivaria incorporate ventilation in their construction
- Most have a low covered vent where fresh air enters and a higher covered vent that allows stale air to pass out of the vivarium using convection
- Ventilation can be passive (convection) or active (mechanically powered)
- Choice depends on the size and type of set-up and the number of inhabitants
- Any mechanical parts must be beyond the animal's reach and any vents should be covered in a permeable membrane that is of a diameter not only small enough to prevent the escape of the occupants but also their prey if they are fed live foods such as fruitflies.

In desert vivaria active ventilation can cause too powerful an influx of air which cools the environment too much. Therefore passive ventilation such as the diametrically staggered vent system or simply a screened lid is usually sufficient.

Humidity

Correct levels of humidity appropriate for the species are important. Complications such as dysecdysis in reptiles and tail necrosis in rodents (ringtail) can occur if humid-

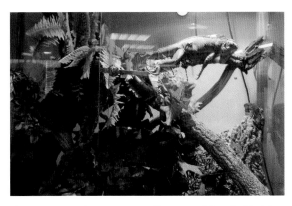

Figure 20.1 An iguana set-up. (Courtesy of Reptile World, Devon.)

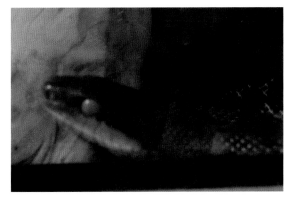

Figure 20.2 A snake about to enter ecdysis – note the cloudy eye. (Courtesy of Reptile World, Devon.)

ity is too low whilst damp conditions can lead to respiratory infections.

- Humidity should be measured using a hygrometer, particularly in vivaria as many reptiles and amphibians have little tolerance of fluctuations in humidity levels
- Humidity in vivaria can be controlled through specialist equipment such as foggers, filtered and aerated water features, regular misting/spraying and the addition of plants
- Ventilation affects humidity and is the predominant method of control in mammalian enclosures.

Furnishings

The type of furnishings that are included in a vivarium should be predominantly to benefit the animal. While it is acceptable to include aesthetic furnishing such as imitation vines and plastic plants to improve the overall appeal of a vivarium it is meeting the fifth freedom – the need to be protected from pain, suffering, injury and disease – that should be of most concern. Thus it is important to consider the following:

- Providing a complex environment that allows temperature, UV and humidity regulation as well as the expression of natural behaviours. This should include raised platforms, hides, rocks, plants (real or plastic) and branches (even terrestrial/fossorial species should be allowed access to low branches). These items should have a variety of surfaces and texture to aid ecdysis (Figure 20.1).
- Providing branches of differing diameter and texture for arboreal species as muscle fatigue could occur with uniform branches and access to rougher surfaces assists with ecdysis (Figure 20.2)

- Providing deep substrates for fossorial and semifossorial species
- Providing appropriate-sized hides that are accessible for both animal and handler
- Rocks are a useful addition, not only as platforms and for hide creation, but also as a heat source for thigmotherms, as they can be placed over a heatmat to absorb the heat so that any animal resting on it is warmed by a diffused and naturalistic heat supply.

Aquarium set-up

The basic principles of aquarium set-up are common to all types of tanks and also apply to vivaria housing amphibians. It is foolish to assume a fish tank is easy and, although cold freshwater tanks can be easier to maintain, they still take a lot of commitment. Care with positioning should be taken as bright light can encourage algal growth, radiators can affect the temperature and noise emitted from radios and televisions can cause stress.

Filtration

- The most important factor is water filtration – without meticulously clean, oxygenated water the inhabitants will quickly perish
- Several types of filtration system are on the market, all of which generally work very well when maintained regularly
- All use biological methods to break down fish waste from ammonia to nitrite, and finally into nitrate by providing a medium where bacteria flourish
- The differences arise in how they convert fish waste and whether, in addition, they mechanically remove particulate matter, chemically remove impurities or use UV light to sterilise the water.

Tank maintenance

Daily checks on the inhabitants, temperature and filtration operation should be carried out with weekly checks on water chemistry using appropriate testing kits. Depending on the effectiveness of the filtration system tank maintenance should be carried out approximately bimonthly, to include:

- Siphoning off approximately 10–20% of the water and replacing it with dechlorinated tapwater or reverse osmosis (RO) water (available from aquarists) that is heated to the same temperature as that within the tank
- Cleaning and/or replacing the filter medium
- Agitating any pebbles used as a substrate to loosen particles of dirt so they can be collected during siphoning
- Removing algae from sides of glass.

During maintenance care should be taken to add only dechlorinated water as the chlorine in tapwater can remove the protective mucous film fish have, leading to stress and possible infection. This can be achieved by adding a proprietary chemical dechlorinator or, if your water treatment company only uses chlorine in the treatment process as opposed to chloramines, by leaving tapwater out overnight to allow the chlorine gas to evaporate (Table 20.2).

Livestock

- Ensure correct stocking density – total length of fish per gallon (4.5 litres) of water (1 inch (2.5 cm) of fish per gallon, as a very rough guide). This varies with the type of aquarium set-up
- Consider the individual nature of each species
- A community tank should only house non-aggressive species

- Stressed 'peaceful' fish can be observed when inappropriately placed in an aquarium with territorial tank mates! Therefore territorial fish should be housed in tanks large enough to accommodate anti-social tendencies
- Special care needs to be taken with predatory fish
- A general rule of thumb is that any fish small enough to fit inside the mouth of another is fair game!
- Gradually introduce fish to avoid overloading the filtering system. It is imperative to wait until the filter has matured – meaning that bacterial colonies have grown in sufficient numbers to begin to remove waste – before any livestock is added
- When adding fish it can help to feed other inhabitants first to reduce their inquisitive nature and lessen the stress of the new addition
- Always allow the bag containing the fish to acclimatise to the same temperature as the tank water by leaving the sealed bag to float in the tank for approximately 10 minutes before release
- Some aquarists recommend removing the acclimatised fish from the bag and placing it in the aquarium rather than opening the bag and emptying the entire contents into the tank as the water may contain contaminants or parasites from the aquatic shop. However, if the shop is reputable this should not be the case and it is less stressful to allow the fish to swim gently from the bag than subjecting it to the trauma of capture once more.

Tank design

- Overall design of the tank should be suitable for the species and the type of set-up (Table 20.3)
- Avoid tanks that are built for aesthetic purposes rather than welfare as tanks that serve as a coffee table or those that are tall and narrow can have welfare implications: a cup placed on top of a glass tank can

Table 20.2 Types of filtration			
Biological	**Mechanical***	**Chemical***	**Ultraviolet***
Beneficial bacteria break down fish waste into ammonia, then nitrite, and finally into harmless nitrate. Basic models consist of a small canister with a pump and a sponge insert or an under-gravel system	Filters out debris and particulate matter through media such as sponges, gravel or varying sizes of sieve-like structures	Purifies water through chemical reactions. Sponge filters can be impregnated or separate containers are attached to the filtration system. Activated carbon can remove medications, tannins and other compounds whereas zeolite is used to remove excessive ammonia in freshwater tanks	Ultraviolet radiation is used to destroy harmful pathogens present in the water
*Although effective in aiding water purification, none of these filtration systems should be used without a biological component.			

Table 20.3 A basic guide to various aquarium set-ups

	Brief description	Heating	Lighting	Salinity	Substrate/accessories
Cold-water set-up	A cool freshwater tank to accommodate species such as goldfish and white cloud mountain minnow that recreates temperate riverine environments – rarely heated. May even need cooling in hot summers	Usually none	Broad-spectrum ultraviolet lighting controlled to mimic day length	None	Gravel, cold water or plastic plants, lava rocks, bogwood, hides, evaporation trays
Tropical set-up	A heated freshwater tank to accommodate species such as angel fish, neon tetras, clown loaches and Siamese fighting fish that recreates tropical riverine environments	Thermostatically controlled heating around 22–28°C	Broad-spectrum ultraviolet lighting controlled to mimic day length	None	Gravel or large-grain sand Tropical or plastic plants, lava rocks, bogwood, hides, evaporation trays
Marine set-up	A heated salt-water tank to accommodate species such as blennies and gobies. It often recreates open-sea environments and the more involved reef environments that accommodate clownfish, corals and invertebrates	Thermostatically controlled heating around 22–26°C	Specific ultraviolet lighting depending on the type of corals, controlled to mimic day length	Specific to species, approximately 1.020–1.025, measured by specific gravity – will require protein skimmer	Fine sand, live rock, corals hides, evaporation trays
Brackish set-up	A heated salt-water tank to accommodate species such as cichlids, gobies and puffer fish. It often recreates tidal environments	Thermostatically controlled heat source	Broad-spectrum ultraviolet lighting controlled to mimic day length	Specific to species Approximately 1.005–1.010 Measured by specific gravity Will require protein skimmer	

cause stressful noise vibration and as fish generally swim in a side-to-side motion across the tank; tall, narrow tanks can be restrictive
- Materials are usually either acrylic or glass
- Glass is generally more popular due to its clarity and scratch resistance; however, modern acrylic is lightweight, durable and stronger, without the discoloration problems of the past

- Any décor that is placed in the tank should be specific to aquaria as chemicals can leach into the water and affect its quality and stress the fish
- Factors to control depend on inhabitants and include temperature, light spectrum and water chemistry, including carbonate hardness, general hardness, pH, salinity/specific gravity, phosphorus, ammonia, nitrite and nitrate levels.

Furnishings should be specific to the set-up and species but might include:

- Hides
- Air stone, pump and one-way valve to aerate tank safely
- Plants (plastic or real).

Points to note

Any electrical cables from aquarium equipment should hang with a loop below the plug socket to prevent any drips entering the socket.

Items used for siphoning water such as buckets must not have been in contact with any detergents or other contaminants.

Aviary set-up

Aviary design

The overall design of an aviary should allow access to both external and internal environmental conditions and again meet the five freedoms. Therefore:

- The aviary should contain water and dust bathing facilities, hides, nest boxes, perches and a variety of toys that are regularly scrubbed and disinfected
- It should offer protection from inclement weather, particularly avoiding the prevailing wind
- It should allow access to rain, sunshine and fresh air
- Perches should be of varying sizes to inhibit foot deformities or conditions such as bumblefoot
- Ideally, perches should be fruit tree branches (non-toxic and allow bark stripping)
- Position perches in various locations to allow access to a range of conditions
- Ensure enough perches are in protected situations
- Avoid siting perches over food or water vessels to prevent contamination with excreta
- With doves or pigeons, perches should be placed side by side as dominant birds tend to prefer higher perches and proceed to defecate on subordinates.

Size and construction

- The aviary should allow short-duration full flight and accommodate the size of the species
- All timbers have to be treated and metal should be galvanised
- Some aviculturalists suggest weathering for up to a year to remove toxicity, particularly when housing hookbills, to avoid zinc toxicity complications
- Social species should be housed in appropriate numbers to avoid overcrowding and competition for resources

- Construction consists of two layers of mesh, approximately 5 cm apart
- The outer layer has a 1-cm diameter to prevent vermin entering and the inner layer has a diameter smaller than the head of the smallest species
- Wire must be thick enough to withstand powerful beaks
- Mesh should extend 20 cm below the surface to ensure the aviary is vermin- and predator-proof
- Entrance must incorporate a double-door system preventing direct access to the outside. This ensures that, as long as both doors are never left open at the same time, any escapees are contained
- Mesh suspended above the aviary prevents predators stressing the birds. Sparrowhawks can attempt to catch aviary birds, and during the flight response, injury or death can occur.

Plastic owls have limited success in deterring winged predators, and may actually be a stress factor.

Flooring

- Ideally, the floor should be raised so ground predators are not the same level as birds on the flight floor
- A 75-cm height difference is recommended
- Concrete is hard-wearing and easy to powerwash and disinfect
- Concrete floors should:
  - Incorporate slope to aid drainage
  - Be rough so not slippery underfoot
  - Be left uncovered or topped with a layer of clean gravel, sand or soil
- Alternatively put predator/vermin-proof mesh under a layer of turf at a depth of 25 cm to rise and overlap with the mesh of the aviary panels
- Substrates should be periodically replaced.

Some aviculturalists do not recommend wood chippings or sawdust as both can harbour the fungi *Aspergillosus fumigatus* that causes the respiratory condition aspergillosis. However, this is a naturally occurring fungus and is often carried by healthy birds. It only really causes a problem with immunosuppressed or malnourished birds and is kept at bay with good hygiene. Thus, as long as effective hygiene is maintained and no build-up of excreta is allowed, chippings could be used in some circumstances as they do allow larger birds such as parrots to forage for food.

Roofing

- Slanted or with an apex to facilitate drainage
- Guttering can be used to minimise water runoff into the aviary

- Have both open and covered areas
- Suitable roofing material such as felt, bitumen-covered wood or UV stable corrugated plastic is used
- Regular cleaning is needed to prevent algal and leaf litter build-up.

Accessories

- Provision of appropriate toys for Psittaciformes
- Extra stimulation (human interaction, puzzles) provided for intelligent species such as African grey parrots
- Passeriformes are generally not as interested in toys but enrichment can be provided in the presentation of novel food forms (pesticide-free dandelion leaves, watercress, pine cones)
- Some species, e.g. toucans, enjoy picking leaves of branches, thus non-toxic vegetation can be added periodically or the aviary can be planted if the floor type allows
- Large potted plants can be included, although hygiene considerations apply
- Advantages of plants include the provision of a visual barrier, wind break, perches and hiding places
- Plants can also increase humidity and provide a cool refuge during warm weather
- Natural hides such as hollow bark can offer additional enrichment.

Special considerations

Although the majority of the preceding considerations of aviary design apply to birds of prey there are further considerations to take into account. This is dependent on whether the birds are:

- Domestic and regularly flown by a falconer
- Rehabilitating wild birds
- Kept as though they were wild.

Rescued wild birds that are being rehabilitated for release back into the wild are kept in aviaries with the minimum of human interaction. Disturbance from external sources such as dogs barking and machinery should be prevented. Birds of prey that are being kept as though wild are not regularly flown and need to have an aviary that provides enough flight space to facilitate natural behaviours.

NUTRITION

An exotic's diet should meet all of its nutritional needs. Researching its wild diet and investigating captive diet recommendations is vital. Diet formulation will depend on the species' feeding strategy, lifestage and physiological requirements as well as preferred method of obtaining food. The palatability, presentation and frequency need to be correct for each species. Small mammals need to forage frequently to meet their fast metabolic rates whereas some snakes may only eat a few times a year.

Diet considerations

- Palatability and presentation: snakes have evolved to catch warm-blooded, fast-moving prey, yet are often offered a limp, damp, defrosted rodent!
- Lifestage – physiological differences during lifestages affect the nutritional requirement
- Interpreting behavioural cues can help. Increased alertness or aggression may indicate hunger but be aware of species such as Burmese pythons that will gorge themselves
- Avoid selective feeding in small mammals by leaving dried food until it is eaten before replacing. The pellets of proprietary feeds contain much of the vitamin and fibre content and are often left until the end as they are not as appealing as the nuts and seeds. By constantly topping up you are allowing the mammal to pick the more calorific morsels and leave the nutritionally superior pellets, thus contributing to an unbalanced diet and obesity
- Environmental conditions can affect appetite, particularly in reptiles, as temperature, humidity and lighting regimes can influence feeding. Specific needs must be met, particularly fibre and protein requirements and vitamin and mineral ratios. Snake and raptors must ingest whole animals to obtain the correct calcium: phosphorus levels. Raptors also need this to produce pellets
- Species-specific needs exist, such as intestine inoculation in hatchling iguanas. In order to obtain the correct gut flora for effective digestion, hatchlings eat soil and adult faeces. Without early access to these, nutritional complications may arise (Troyer 1984).

Correct levels of vitamins and minerals, appropriate to the species, need to be included in a captive diet. Nutritional complications such as hypervitaminosis (vitamin excess) and hypovitaminosis (vitamin deficiency) can arise if a nutritionally balanced diet is not provided. One particular consideration is the calcium:phosphorus ratio, as one is inversely affected by the other (as the level of one increases, the other decreases and vice versa). Absorption of calcium is hormonally controlled by, among others, vitamin D_3, the precursor of which is synthesised in the dermis of reptiles in the presence of UVB light. Many live foods are calcium-deficient and, without supplementation, resorption of calcium from the bones can occur, leading to metabolic bone disease. Some foods, such as spinach, kale, beetroot and chard, contain high levels of oxalic acid, a compound that binds calcium thus preventing its absorption, and should be limited in the diet.

Water must be provided in an accessible way to the species. Some animals such as birds of prey obtain all their water from their diet, whereas rodents need constant access to water that cannot be contaminated by their urine (e.g. provided in a bottle instead of a bowl). Many tropical species of lizards will only drink droplets of water off leaves, or indeed accumulated within their own coils (Cook's tree boa (*Corallus caninus*)), whereas amphibians can absorb it through their skin. Again, researching the species to ensure its hydration needs are met is a must. Many vivarium inhabitants will require regular misting of both themselves and the habitat in addition to the provision of a water bowl large enough for the species' needs, be that purely to drink from or to immerse itself fully in. Box 20.1 explores feeding exotics.

HEALTH AND WELFARE

General

Many exotics have very different needs to more typical pets. The use of correct environmental parameters cannot be overstated, especially in relation to fish, reptiles and amphibians. This is particularly the case as the use of incorrect parameters present from the start could lead to abnormal signs that are actually assumed to be normal as they have occurred since the animal's initial introduction to the set-up. Although not necessarily fatal, undue stress and discomfort resulting in long-term health issues may occur. Aside from environmental conditions, ill health can arise through inappropriate diets, genetic predisposition and opportunistic infection/parasitism. Therefore it is important to identify signs of ill health and abnormal behaviours to facilitate effective diagnosis and treatment. This is achieved by regular health checks.

Box 20.1

CONSIDERATIONS OF FEEDING EXOTICS

Examples of feeding strategy

Herbivores: vegetarian, varied and balanced food items usually with supplementation

Frugivores: fruit, varied and balanced food items usually with supplementation

Insectivores: few animals are strictly insectivores; in more cases it is the preferred food source; gut-loading of prey is paramount to ensure a nutritionally balanced diet

Nectarvores: nectar-varied and balanced food items, usually with supplementation

Carnivores: meat, usually whole bodies

Omnivores: combination of any of the strategies in varying proportions

Molluscivores: usually snails; may take slugs but not always exclusive of other food items; additional supplementation is usually required

Foliovores: almost strictly foliage eaters – varied and balanced food items, usually with supplementation

Grazers, foragers, stalking or ambush hunters

Lifestage and physiological considerations

Increased protein/calorific requirement: growth, pregnancy, lactating, egg laying

Lower protein/calorie requirement: geriatric

Aestivation, torpor and hibernation are states of lowered metabolism

Lifestyle: sedentary or active – affects calorie requirement

Snakes approaching ecdysis rarely feed until after shed is complete

Presentation to encourage feeding

Warm dead rodents to normal body temperature – keep their fur dry

Wiggle prey to stimulate live animals: squeeze the prey's nose for blood

Many insectivorous lizards require the movement of live food to stimulate feeding behaviour

Fast prey may need to be stunned or slowed by cooling (this is effective with crickets)

Avoid feeding too many live foods at once as crickets can attack predators and induce a fear response that may inhibit eating

Other considerations

Live food versus frozen or dried

Gut-loading live foods

Supplementation: vitamin and mineral needs can be species-specific and must be met

Correct calcium-to-phosphorus ratio is very important in exotics; dust live food and vegetables; ground-up cuttlefish may be fed to some species

Frequency: specific to species and lifestage

Timing: diurnal, nocturnal, crepuscular

Freshness: nutritional quality deteriorates over time

Remove predatory animals from enclosure before feeding to prevent them associating the keeper entering the enclosure with food (this can help prevent striking in snakes)

Use suitable equipment such as long-handled graspers to prevent injury to the handler

Rabbits and guinea pigs are caecotrophic and the soft caecotrophs are eaten directly from the anus regularly

Health checks may include:

- Visual observation of behaviour, gait and posture. General appearance, condition of coat and colour of mucous membranes
- Clinical measurements, e.g. respiration rate, heart rate, blood pressure and pulse
- Measuring intake of fluid and solids
- Weight monitoring
- Monitoring urine and faecal output, to include rate, frequency and consistency
- Assessment of teeth, claw and beak length/condition
- Checking eyes, ears, mouth and anogenital region for signs of infection or discharge.

An important note should be made about health and safety when dealing with any animal. Some animals pose a risk not only through injury, but also through the transmission of zoonotic diseases. Some common exotic diseases can be passed on to humans through both direct and indirect contact and it is paramount to adhere to strict hygiene controls.

In addition isolation and quarantine facilities should exist. Any sick or injured animal should be isolated to prevent the spread of disease, aid treatment and reduce the risk of cross-contamination. Regular screening of bloods and faecal matter can be carried out until no evidence of pathogens remains before reintroduction.

All new animals should be initially quarantined to allow any disease or health issues to become apparent before contact with any other animals has occurred. It also allows observation to assess temperament and individual needs.

Exercise

The provision of regular exercise opportunities should be available to all animals kept in captivity. This should:

- Be suitable for the species
- Be safe (e.g. on a lead or by the provision of solid exercise wheels, not wire rungs, as limbs and tails can become trapped)
- Be accessible
- Allow natural behaviour (e.g. scent marking, foraging, flying, jumping).

Grooming

Species-specific grooming requirements need to be met. Examples include:

- Regular grooming of long-haired mammals to avoid matting and fly strike

- The provision of dust baths, particularly for chinchillas, as fur will matt if allowed to get wet
- Nail clipping – small mammals, passerines and lizards
- Beak trimming (coping in birds of prey) – some psittacines and chelonians may require trimming by a trained expert if overgrowth occurs – this can indicate nutritional problem
- Teeth filing – rabbits often develop dental problems and may require their teeth to be regularly filed. Clipping with nail clippers is not recommended unless the operator is highly competent as the tooth can split, leading to infection within the root.

Fish

If ideal tank conditions are maintained and new introductions are quarantined, fish should not generally become ill. Most diseases develop as a result of a decline in immunity brought on by stress. Stress factors can include temperature fluctuations, changes in water chemistry and bullying by aggressive tank mates. Many of the pathogens occur naturally in the aquarium and it is only when the fish are weakened that they take hold.

Reptiles and amphibians

As reptiles and amphibians live in such controlled conditions captive-bred animals should rarely become ill. Unfortunately complications commonly arise because of inexperience, lack of knowledge and inappropriate care. Most health issues in reptiles and amphibians are due to either incorrect parameters and/or inappropriate feeding (Table 20.4).

Mammals

Generally these animals are healthy if cared for correctly and vaccinated appropriately. However some complications are common. For instance, due to years of inbreeding by laboratories and the fancy show trade, rats and mice can be prone to tumours and respiratory complaints. Rodents and lagomorphs have continually growing incisors and are prone to malocclusions as they do not wear down their teeth as much in captivity and traits such as reduced jaws are selected for in some breeds of rabbits (Table 20.5).

Birds

Many birds commonly kept in captivity can carry zoonotic respiratory diseases, as is currently well documented with the threat of avian flu. Captive-bred birds are fairly resilient if conditions are right but when

311

Table 20.4 Common health problems in reptiles and amphibians

Endoparasites

Endoparasites: nematodes, seven cestodes (tapeworms), pentastomids (arthropods) and protozoa	Symptoms can include vomiting, bloody mucoid diarrhoea, distended abdomen, septicaemia, weight loss and anorexia

Ectoparasites

Ticks, mites, blowfly and occasionally leeches	*Ophionyssus natricis* affect snakes, where they attach under scales. Cloacal mites (*Cloacarus* spp.) can affect aquatic turtles. Tortoises kept outdoors can be at risk of myiasis in unhygienic conditions or when suffering with diarrhoea as well as tick infestation. Some wild-caught species of reptiles can be imported with tick infestation, such as *Amblyomma* and *Aponomma* spp.

Bacterial infections

Blister disease/scale rot/vesicular dermatitis or necrotising dermatitis – watery blisters on ventral surface, septicaemia and secondary infection	Commonly caused by poor husbandry, particularly moist, dirty environments with low temperatures and poor ventilation. Also caused by contact with excessive build-up of excreta on vivarium floor. In severe cases, infection may pass into the body causing septicaemia (infection of the blood) and organ failure
Septicaemic cutaneous ulcerative disease (SCUD)	SCUD is a bacterial infection caused by *Citrobacter freundii* affecting aquatic chelonians. Once blood stream is infected, ulceration of the skin and loosening of the scales occur
Stomatitis (mouth rot): purulent discharge, excessive salivation, swelling/reddening around or in the mouth, inability to close the mouth, reduced or absent tongue flicking, necrosis	Stomatitis can be a bacterial, fungal or viral infection often caused by stress, inappropriate environmental conditions, overcrowding, internal or external parasites, trauma, poor nutrition and the stereotypic behaviour of nose rubbing against glass vivaria. It can also occur after hibernation in chelonians
Salmonellosis: all reptiles and amphibians – mild to severe intestinal upset, abscesses, septicaemia, skin slough	Nearly all species of reptiles and amphibians are carriers of salmonella but it is particularly common in snakes and chelonians. It is a potentially serious zoonotic disease that can be a danger to vulnerable people such as the elderly or very young. Perfectly healthy animals can be asymptomatic carriers
Red-leg disease – amphibians – inappetance, bloated and lethargic. Ulcerated lesions	Common bacterial (*Aeromonas* spp.) infection in amphibians causing red ulcerations of varying size on body but more commonly on legs. Poor environmental conditions such as overcrowding, spoiled food, faecal-contaminated water, trauma to the skin, low temperatures and exposure to toxins such as pesticides are thought to lead to the infection
Runny-nose syndrome: tortoises – clear watery nasal discharge, sneezing, laboured, audible breathing, lethargy, depression and anorexia	Serious condition with multifactorial aetiology that if left untreated can progress into pneumonia and may be fatal. Some individuals can be latent carriers

Other health issues

Dysecdysis: partial ecdysis with retained skin in patches on body or around digits, tail tip, nostrils and eyes	Necrosis and digit and tail tip loss can occur due to reduced blood supply as the dry skin constricts and acts as a tourniquet. Spectacles can remain attached to the eyes of snakes and become ulcerated. Condition is usually caused by inappropriate environmental conditions such as low humidity and temperature. The provision of rough bark, stones, clean damp vermiculite or sphagnum moss, water baths and microclimates that allow suitable humidity should prevent occurrence. Treatments include gently bathing toes or tail tips and placing snakes in snake bags or pillowcases with warm, wet towels. Retained spectacles can be left to next shed if environmental conditions are improved. If they still remain attached, gently swabbing with cottonwool buds and hypromellose (false-tear solution) can be effective

Continued

Table 20.4 *Continued*	
Dystocia (egg binding) or postovulatory stasis: difficulty laying, straining, distended abdomen, long gestation period, depression, anorexia, cloacal swelling/prolapse	Common in chelonians, lizards and, occasionally, snakes. Often caused by hypocalcaemia (low calcium levels) but also lack of laying sites, overcrowding, inappropriate environmental parameters, deformed eggs, pelvic fractures or malnutrition. Radiography and veterinary intervention indicated
Vomiting and regurgitation: usually snakes	Can occur if snake is handled roughly postfeeding. May also occur if snake has been force-fed, particularly if exposed to low temperatures afterwards. Can also indicate a worm infestation
Gout: accumulation of uric crystals: visceral (organs) or articular (joints)	Usually caused by dehydration, kidney damage or, more commonly, an inappropriately high-protein diet. Often a problem when herbivorous species such as iguanas are given proteins such as live foods or dog food
Overgrown beaks and claws: chelonians/lizards	Can occur due to lack of abrasive substrates in the vivarium
Metabolic bone disease (MBD): all species of reptiles	MBD covers a range of disorders caused by an imbalance of vitamin D_3, calcium and phosphorus. These nutrients are vital to bone growth and maintenance, muscle contractions and blood coagulation. In the case of calcium deficiency (hypocalcaemia), the body will obtain it from internal sources such as bone which can lead to often irreversible symptoms such as deformed growth, softening of the bones and shell (in chelonians) and increased susceptibility to fractures. Generally the calcium-to-phosphorus ratio should be around $2:1$ in growing reptiles and $1.5:1$ for adults. Vitamin D_3 should be provided by ultraviolet B light and within the captive diet. Lack of supplementation, incorrect calcium-to-phosphorus ratio, incorrect vivarium parameters or inappropriate food items are the usual causes of metabolic disease. It is important to note that some vegetation such as beet leaves, cabbage, peas, potatoes and rhubarb contains oxalates that can inhibit calcium absorption; however this is only a serious issue when access to minerals is low
Other nutritional disorders: thiamine deficiency, hypovitaminosis A, hypocalcaemia	Thiamine deficiency: usually seen in fish-eating species such as garter snakes fed thawed frozen fish that are deficient in thiamine – results in neurological disorders
	Hypovitaminosis A is usually caused by dietary deficiency and results in many symptoms, including skin complications, respiratory infections and renal and liver problems. Hypocalcaemia: see metabolic bone disease (above)
Tail autotomy	Spontaneous tail shedding is a defence mechanism in many species of lizard and can be caused by rough handling. Regrowth usually occurs but is often stunted and less colourful. Cleaning of wound is recommended to prevent infection
Obesity: gout, metabolic bone disease, fatty-liver syndrome	Caused by inappropriate diet or overfeeding. Can affect lizards, chelonia and some snakes (particularly if fed fat rodents). Change to correct diet postdiagnosis
Posthibernation anorexia (PHA): tortoises	Treatment requires fluid therapy, tubing with high-energy and protein food replacement mixture such as critical care formula and supportive care

stressed can be more susceptible to disease (Table 20.6).

HANDLING AND RESTRAINT

General handling considerations

Before handling an animal it is important to assess the situation. Draw on previous knowledge of the species and take into account its normal behaviour. Try to take the route of least resistance where possible when handling animals – if they are reluctant, and don't have to be moved immediately, then leave them! Be a little cunning – for instance, if it is an arboreal snake that is coiled around a branch and won't let go, then remove the branch. Before approaching, observe the animal and interpret its behaviour and consider the following:

- Does it look stressed, relaxed, in pain, aggressive or domineering?

Table 20.5 Common health problems in mammals

Endoparasites

Helminth worms: all small mammals	Small infestation may show no signs but severe infestation can lead to loss of condition, vomiting, diarrhoea and weight loss. Many are species-specific and almost all can be treated with anthelminthics
Coccidiosis: rabbits	Causes diarrhoea, staining or mucus present in faeces, anorexia and hepatic failure. Two forms exist – hepatic and intestinal. Both are contracted by ingesting oocysts, usually in contaminated feed or water or during grooming of the feet

Ectoparasites

Mites, ticks, fleas and lice: all small mammals	Many are species-specific and need to be correctly identified. Clinical signs: pruritus, hyperkeratosis, papular lesions, alopecia, scurf and anaemia (particularly in young animals with a heavy parasite burden)
Myiasis (flystrike): rabbits	Associated with diarrhoea arising from poor diet and husbandry. Clinical signs: matting and soiling of perineal fur, lesions, presence of eggs or maggots, loss of condition, depression and lethargy. Maggots must be removed and wound treated, and this process may require sedation

Viral

Myxomatosis: rabbits	Viral infection transmitted by biting insects; prevented through vaccination. Symptoms include periocular oedema, secondary respiratory infection, difficulty eating and drinking and disorientation
Distemper: ferrets	Serious, fatal paramyxovirus infection that is spread in the urine of infected dogs, foxes and mustelids; vaccination is available. Clinical signs: brown oculonasal discharge encrusting the lips, nose, chin and eyes, hardening (hyperkeratosis) of footpad, lethargy and coma
Aleutian disease: ferrets	A parvovirus infection caused by different strains of varying strength and varying immune response, transmitted by direct contact and not usually fatal
Influenza: ferrets	Ferrets are susceptible to most strains of influenza that infect humans, including both types, A and B
Viral haemorrhagic disease (VHD): rabbits	Calicivirus spread by contaminated faeces; often fatal. Clinical signs: inappetance, depression, collapse, breathing difficulties, fits, nasal discharge, high temperature and death

Bacterial

Wet tail/proliferative ileitis: hamsters (at weaning)	Clinical signs: lethargy, inappetance, fluid diarrhoea with wet, soiled and matted area around the anus and tail. Often fatal, sometimes within 24 hours. Supportive treatment and antibiotics can be administered
Salmonellosis can affect all animals: diarrhoea	Clinical signs: often watery and containing mucus or blood, vomiting, inappetance, weight loss and abortion in guinea pigs. Zoonotic
Pasteurellosis: rabbits	*Pasteurella* spp. infection associated with overcrowding, particularly breeding colonies, and poor housing. Clinical signs: sneezing, oculonasal discharges
Tyzzer's disease: affects most small mammals	Caused by *Clostridium piliformis*, leading to enteritic symptoms
Necobacillosis: rabbits – ulceration and necrosis of skin around lips, nose, face and neck	*Fusobacterium necrophorum* infection associated with poor hygiene, trauma/abrasion and malocclusion. Good results seen with improved hygiene and the administration of topical and oral antibiotics. Clinical signs: ulceration/necrosis of lips, nose and face
Pododermatitis: small mammals	Bacterial infection resulting from hock sores developing in overweight or immobile animals

Fungal

Dermatophytosis (ringworm): affects small mammals	Fungal infection caused by *Trichophyton mentagrophytes* or *Microsporum canis*

Continued

Table 20.5 *Continued*

Other health issues

Trichobezoar (hairballs)	Overgrooming can be caused by parasitic irritation, dental disease and intestinal complications often arising from inadequate fibre content in diet or boredom. Increasing fibre content of diet may be beneficial
Barbering: whiskers/fur chewed short	Often dominance aggression injury in rodents
Impacted cheeks: distended, swollen cheeks, difficulty eating	Caused by accumulation of food due to boredom, inappropriate diet or excessive access to food
Ringtail: necrosis of skin around tail	Circular constrictions around tail prevent blood supply causing sloughing of skin. Thought to result when relative humidity is too low
Malocclusion: overgrown incisors common in rodents and lagomorphs	May result in ulceration, inappetance, anorexia; veterinary treatment is required to resolve dentition then ensure appropriate diet with sufficient fibre/forage content

Table 20.6 Common health problems in birds

Ectoparasites

Mites	Scaly face mite, scaly leg mite, red mite, feather and feather follicle mite, air sac mite. Diagnosed by skin scrapings
Lice	(Usually) species-specific *Mallophaga* spp. that chew feathers. Treat with antiparasitic preparations
Flies: maggot infestations, presence of keds (wingless form of horsefly)	Can be found in passerines, raptors and pigeons. Treat with permethrin

Endoparasites

Tapeworms (cestodes), roundworms (nematodes)	Lethargy, emaciation and diarrhoea. Diagnosis is through screening droppings/crop tube for eggs. Treat with anthelminthics and remove intermediate host
Protozoan parasites: *Giardia* spp., *Hexamita* spp., *Trichomonas* spp., coccidiosis	Weight loss, diarrhoea, feather plucking. Diagnosis through faecal smears and treated with antiprotozoals
Bumblefoot: abscessation, swelling and tissue necrosis	Bacterial infection of foot categorised by severity. Usually caused by poor hygiene and prolonged use of uniform perches. Antibiotics and cleansing of lesions successful in early stages

Bacterial infections

Avian mycoplasmosis	Common in cramped, overcrowded conditions with poor ventilation
Salmonellosis	Zoonotic bacterial infection that causes enteric signs in humans
Enteritis	Infection of intestinal tract, usually with *Escherichia coli* or *Campylobactor* spp.
Chlamydophilosis/psitticosis/ornithosis: nasal discharge, sneezing, lack of condition	Zoonotic bacterial infection spread by faecal, oral and respiratory secretions as well as feather dander. Birds can be carriers with no symptoms or may exhibit classic 'sick-bird syndrome' (hunched and fluffed up) or even death. More common in imported and smuggled birds improperly quarantined. Zoonotic

Viral infections

Newcastle disease/paramyxovirus	Notifiable disease caused by paramyxoviruses commonly affecting pigeons but also found in other species. Dyspnoea, tachypnoea, oedema, torticollis, listessness, wing droop and sudden death
Psittacine beak and feather disease (PBFD)	Deformed feathers and abnormal beak. Usually found in psittacine species

Continued

Table 20.6 *Continued*

Fungal infections

Aspergillus	Airborne fungal spores infect respiratory tract of vulnerable birds and germinate. Affects stressed, immunosuppressed and sick birds. Zoonotic

Other health issues

Obesity, liver disease	Affects birds allowed to feed selectively on nuts and seeds
Gout	Often seen in older budgies, cockatiels and parrots fed an unbalanced diet
'Going light': loss of weight and condition	Symptom of stress and underlying infection seen in overcrowding and exhibition birds
Zinc poisoning	Poor-quality galvanised caging where zinc oxide powder forms and is ingested
Teflon and smoke/cooking fat inhalation	Odourless fumes are released when Teflon-coated pans and oil are overheated, resulting in respiratory failure and death
Cold or heat stress	Can be a contributory factor to illness due to immunosuppression
Broken feathers through trauma or disease – can prevent flight	Repair by imping if one or two primary feathers affected or wait until next moult. Some diseases cause deformed feather regrowth
Trauma	Most common causes of trauma are aggression or induced panic, usually from the presence of predators or other stimuli such as loud noise
Dystocia	Difficulty laying – multifactorial – diet, age, size of clutch/egg, nesting material, first clutch, environment, obesity through drug therapy. Eggs require removal
Crop impaction	Common in juveniles due to overeating and ingestion of substrate. Treated by flushing out contents of crop
Feather plucking	Often due to lack of stimulation but also stress, excessive preening during breeding season, poor husbandry and hormonal imbalance

- Can you hear any vocalisation, unusual or otherwise?
- What sort of animal is it – is it a predator or prey animal? Is it particularly flighty? Will it tend to exhibit a fight-or-flight response, fear aggression, or other defence mechanism?
- Is the animal toxic/poisonous/venomous?
- Is the animal a potential carrier of zoonotic diseases?
- Do any of the handlers have allergies to any animals?
- Is handling equipment necessary (Table 20.7)?
- Is the handler suitably dressed?
- Should you approach openly or covertly, down wind?
- What is the animal's physiological state – is it pregnant/gravid, lactating, exhibiting signs of entering breeding condition? Is it preparing to shed or in the process of shedding? Reptiles can be more irritable before and during ecdysis
- Is it a geriatric or juvenile animal? Young animals can be more unpredictable whereas older animals may have complications such as arthritic limbs

- What is your previous knowledge of the animal? Is there an owner or keeper you can consult?
- What is the size of the animal? How many people will you need to catch and restrain it (Figures 20.3–20.5)?
- How large is the enclosure? Do you need to partition some of it off to aid capture?
- Do you have a suitable transport container ready in advance?

ADMINISTRATION OF MEDICINE

The following routes of administration are applicable to most exotic species, except fish.

- Oral
- Intramuscular injection directly into muscle tissue
- Intraosseous injection directly into the bone cavity, appropriate when venous access is difficult
- Subcutaneous injection under the skin
- Intravenous injection directly into the vascular system through a vein

Table 20.7 Equipment that may be required for handling exotics

Fish	Birds	Reptiles and amphibians	Mammals
Two nets, one smaller than the other	Goggles (protect eyes from long beaks)	Goggles if dealing with species such as spitting cobras	Cat grabber possibly useful for aggressive ferrets
Long, narrow bag for transporting – two-thirds air and one-third water	Coveralls and sturdy footwear (no open-toed shoes)	Coveralls and sturdy footwear (no open-toed shoes)	Coveralls and sturdy footwear (no open-toed shoes)
Insulated box (polystyrene)	Gauntlets/gloves	At least two helpers for large species of snake	Gauntlets/gloves
Wet towel can be used to restrain larger species for short duration	Hook (long-necked species)	Snake hook used to lift coil near head in larger species whilst handler supports rest of body	Crush cage again possibly with aggressive ferret to administer medication
Insulated material to pack box during travel – helps maintain water temperature and buffers movement	Net: framed opening assists with capture in aviary	Snake fork: a wooden stick with V-shaped end can be placed behind head to restrain poisonous snakes	Harness may be used for exercising ferrets and rabbits
	Towels can be used to restrain wings of larger birds	Snake bag: similar to pillow case – darkness is calming and snake can coil	Pet pal/cat carrier or other suitable carrier
	Jessies: small leather straps tied in falconer's knot around ankles of bird held whilst on glove	Harness may be used for exercising large species of lizard	Towel can be used to wrap fractious animals
	Hood (falconry) used to keep bird calm before flying	Small pet pal can be placed over small lizards that shouldn't be handled and stiff card slipped under to prevent escape	Cat bag can be used to restrain rabbits

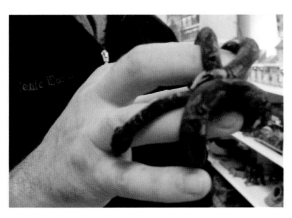

Figure 20.3 Handling small snakes. The snake is allowed to coil loosely around the hand. (Courtesy of Reptile World, Devon.)

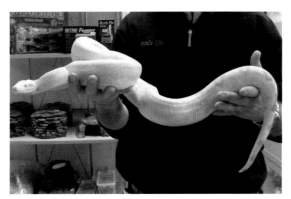

Figure 20.4 Handling medium-sized snakes. Note the handler supporting the tail and the relaxed posture of the snake. More agitated snakes could be restrained by gently gripping the snake directly behind its head with one hand. (Courtesy of Reptile World, Devon.)

- Intraperitoneal injection into the abdominal cavity. Allows larger amounts of fluids to be administered during fluid therapy – not used for medication.

Although some larger fish can be injected it takes expertise and significant experience as it involves removing the fish from water which can stress it considerably. It is far more common to add a suitable medication to the aquarium water. This is then removed after treatment through the use of activated carbon, as mentioned before. Absorption of drugs is also possible through the

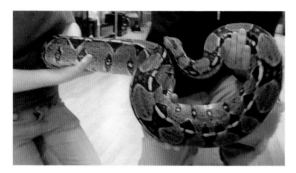

Figure 20.5 Handling large snakes. At least two people should assist with large snakes to support the weight of the animal and prevent coils sagging. This is a docile animal, but more agitated animals may require restraint directly behind the head. Handlers should remember to keep their backs straight and their knees bent when lifting heavy animals. Never place any snake, whatever its size, around the neck because of the risk of constriction and biting. (Courtesy of Reptile World, Devon.)

skin of amphibians and medication can be administered through bathing.

REPRODUCTION

General

Before embarking on any breeding programme, four questions must be asked:

1. Why are these animals being bred?
2. What will happen to the offspring?
3. Have the breeding requirements of the species been sufficiently researched?
4. Is all the required equipment/expertise available?

If all of the above can be answered and the reason for breeding is legitimate with reliable, informed and equipped keepers available to home all of the offspring, then breeding an animal can be considered.

Figures 20.6–20.10 illustrate how to determine the sex of lizards, snakes, tortoises and rodents.

Replacing stock through captive breeding is far preferable to wild-caught purchases and the scope of information available to breeders has vastly improved over the last few years. It is now possible to research accurately the breeding requirements of many common and not so common species of exotics. This expertise is invaluable as there are many factors that affect breeding success, including reproductive strategy of the species, their fecundity rate, whether the offspring are altricial or precocial and how to stimulate reproductive behaviour. See

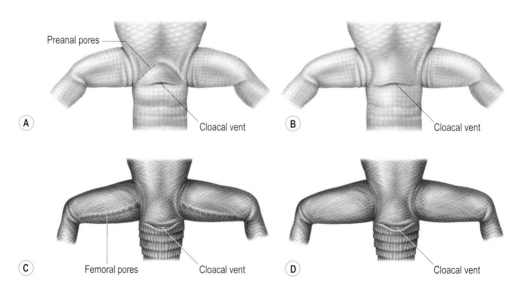

Figure 20.6 Sexual differentiation in lizards. (a) and (c) – male; (b) and (d) – female. (Reproduced from Aspinall V 2006 *The Complete Textbook of Veterinary Nursing*. Butterworth Heinemann, London, with permission.)

Table 20.8 for details of reproductive considerations and Table 20.9 for a guide to sexing exotic animals.

A separate breeding area or tank is often needed as slightly different parameters may be required to stimulate breeding. Nesting material may need to be provided. This might be in the traditional sense or, in the case of egg-depositing fish; vertical glass panels, artificial spawning mops or an upturned flowerpot. One or both of the parents may need to remain with the eggs or young or be removed as soon as the eggs or young have been laid or born or hatched. To prevent complications such as cannibalism or territorial conflicts young fish, reptiles and amphibians are usually reared separately.

Fecundity

An animal's fecundity is defined by its reproductive success and different breeding strategies have evolved as a result. Animals are usually either K-strategists or r-strategists. K-strategists usually live longer and invest more time in a few young, often providing parental care, whereas r-strategists will usually have a shorter lifespan and invest less time in several young, usually providing little parental care.

LEGISLATION AND TRADE

Moral issues

People want to keep exotics for a variety of reasons, usually because they find the animal fascinating and wish to have one to observe and care for.

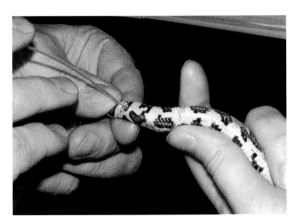

Figure 20.7 Use of a probe to determine the sex of a snake. (Reproduced from Aspinall V 2006 *The Complete Textbook of Veterinary Nursing*. Butterworth Heinemann, London, with permission.)

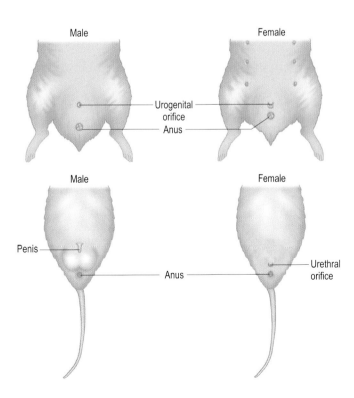

Figure 20.8 General method of sexing small rodents. (Reproduced from Aspinall V 2006 *The Complete Textbook of Veterinary Nursing*. Butterworth Heinemann, London, with permission.)

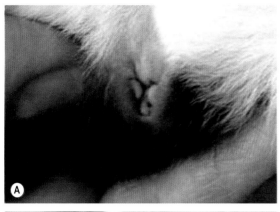

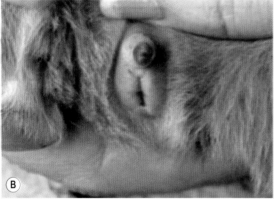

Figure 20.9 Sexing guinea pigs. (a) Female; (b) male.

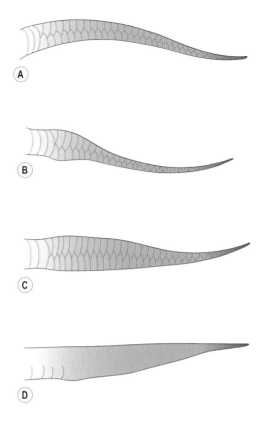

A and B – Female tail, ventral and lateral views. The tail base enlargement noticeable in some females (see B) appears to be male glands but note that the tail tapers rapidly.

C and D – Male tail, ventral and lateral views. Tail base is thick and this thickness extends for some distance beyond the vent.

Figure 20.10 Differentiation in male and female snake tails. (a, b) Female; (c, d) male.

Reasons exotics are kept

- Commercial trade
- Zoos and other animal attractions
- Educational purposes
- Research
- Breeding programmes.

However, some people are aesthetically attracted to exotics because of their danger factor and do not always consider the implications of owning an animal that can be dangerous, poisonous, reluctant to be handled, aggressive or prone to grow large. Too often, little consideration is given to the amount of care an exotic needs, which can include:

- Cost
- Specialist equipment
- Veterinary expertise
- Importance of environmental conditions
- Longevity of species (species such as tortoises and parrots can outlive their owners!)
- Space
- Care during holiday or periods of sickness.

Although extensive legislation exists to protect traded exotics, the problem lies with enforcement and the extent of illegal activity. Table 20.10 outlines legislation which has an impact on keeping exotic species.

The UK is one of the most proactive countries involved in combating wildlife crime and the illegal trade in exotics which relies on a multiagency approach. Experts from the police, government officials and customs and excise, along with the involvement of other organisations such as the Royal Society for Prevention of Cruelty to Animals (RSPCA), the Royal Society for Protection of Birds (RSPB) and Trade Records Analysis of Flora and Fauna in Commerce (TRAFFIC), work closely together.

Table 20.8 Reproductive considerations

	Fish	Birds	Reptiles and amphibians	Small mammals
Reproductive strategy	Live bearers Mouth brooders Nest builders Bubble nest builders Egg scatterers Egg depositors Substrate spawners Peat divers	Egg-laying reproduction with either precocial (waterfowl) or altricial (parrots) young	Viviparous Oviparous Oviviparous Parthenogenesis (whiptails and komodo dragons)	Live birth to either precocial (guinea pigs) or altricial young (rodents etc.)
Stimulating mating behaviour	Altering photoperiods Temperature changes Removing and reintroducing mates Conditioning – more live foods Provision of nesting material Mimicking rainy season	Altering photoperiod Availability of certain foodstuffs, particularly nuts and seeds in parrot species, as these are required by the young Provision of nesting material	Altering photoperiod Temperature changes Humidity changes Presence of mate Winter cooling Provision of nesting material	Many will breed throughout year if conditions and food supplies are favourable. Others are stimulated by photoperiod, temperature and food item changes Provision of nesting material

Table 20.9 Sexing exotics

Fish	Presence of gonopodium Tubercles on gill plates and/or pectoral fins Behaviour – males often harass females or become territorial Sexual dimorphism – size and shape differences Sexual chromatism – colour differences Vent differentiation
Birds	DNA – sexing Sexual dimorphism/chromatism – size, shape, plumage colour, e.g. peacock Laparoscopy
Reptiles and amphibians	Sexual dimorphism Males are often larger and possess greater ornamentation, e.g. horns (Jackson's chameleon) Size of dew flaps (male iguanas) Extendable dew flaps (male anoles) Larger nuchal crests (male plumed basilisks) Presence of spurs Presence of preanal pores/femoral pores Tail size/length (snake length after vent, tortoises wider in and longer in males) Presence of hemipenal bulge or a large vent Sexual dichromatism, e.g. male iguanas are usually greener DNA sexing Probing/laparoscopy Temperature-dependent sex selection in geckos and crocodiles
Small mammals	Sexual dimorphism Anogenital distance Presence of testes in males Teats absent in male gerbils, chipmunks, hamsters, mice and rats Note: female chinchillas have a large urinary papilla that can be mistaken for a penis which is larger and generally points towards the head in males. In rabbits the vulva is round with a small slit in the middle and generally points towards the head, whereas the penis is more cone-shaped and generally points towards the back of the animal. Pressure may need to be applied to both sides of the anal area to pop out the vulva or penis Male ferrets have an obvious fold of skin (prepuce) on the underside and evident testes

Table 20.10 Current legislation affecting exotics

Legislation affecting exotics	How it relates to exotics
The Animal Welfare Act 2006 came into force on 6 April 2007	Inroduced a welfare offence which places a duty of care on pet owners to provide for their animal's basic needs, such as adequate food and water, veterinary treatment and an appropriate environment in which to live. Previously the duty of care had only existed for farm animals Any person responsible for an animal has a legal duty to ensure that its needs are met as required by good practice. These include: • the need for a suitable environment • the need for a suitable diet • the need to exhibit normal behaviour patterns • the need to be housed with or apart from other animals • the need to be protected from pain, suffering, injury and disease Penalties for neglect and cruelty include fines of up to £20 000, a maximum jail term of 51 weeks and a lifetime ban on some owners keeping pets. Enforcers such as the Royal Society for Prevention of Cruelty to Animals (RSPCA) have more powers to intervene if they suspect a pet is being neglected The Act raised the minimum age for buying a pet, or winning one as a prize, from 12 to 16, without parental accompaniment
Wildlife and Countryside Act 1981	It is illegal to allow any animal which is not ordinarily resident in Great Britain, or is listed on Schedule 9 of the Wildlife and Countryside Act 1981, to escape into the wild, or to release it without a licence
Convention on International Trade in Endangered Species of wild flora and fauna (CITES)	CITES regulates international trade in over 33 000 species, of which approximately 28 000 are plants. CITES places endangered species in one of three different appendices: • Appendix I: species threatened with extinction and that are, or may be, affected by international trade. Trade is only permitted in exceptional circumstances • Appendix II: species that are not necessarily threatened with extinction but may become so unless trade is closely controlled by a permitting system. Appendix II also contains look-alike species, which are controlled because of their similarity to other regulated species. The majority of CITES species are listed in Appendix II • Appendix III: species which are protected in at least one country and for which the cooperation of other parties is needed to control international trade If the animal being imported is listed in Appendix A or B of CITES, a relevant export and import licence to bring it into the country (unless it is coming from within the European Union) will need to be obtained. These licences are passed on from the supplier to the retailer who must then pass them on to the new owner
Dangerous Wild Animals Act 1976	An animal listed in the Schedule to this Act will need a licence issued by the local authority
Welfare of Animals (Transport) Order 1997	This covers the transport of all vertebrate animals and also 'other cold-blooded animals'. It covers a wide range of principles, including protection of welfare during transport, space allowances, fitness to travel, treatment of sick animals, feed, water and rest periods, duties of transporters and documentation
Pet Animals Act 1951–1983	The Pet Animals Act requires pet shops to be run under local-authority licence. The Act requires that animals are at all times kept in suitable accommodation (in terms of size, temperature, cleanliness, lighting and ventilation), that animals are adequately supplied with suitable food and drink and are inspected at suitable intervals and that all reasonable precautions are taken to prevent the spread of infectious disease among animals
Control of Trade in Endangered Species Regulations 1997 (COTES)	COTES is the UK law that was brought in to enforce the rules agreed in the convention (CITES). The maximum penalty for offences under these regulations is 5 years' imprisonment

There are also concerns with the legal trade in terms of welfare. These include:

- The method of capturing wild-caught species
- Welfare of native-farmed species
- Welfare during transport
- Mental and physical implications of keeping exotics in captivity, particularly if wild-caught.

WILD-CAUGHT VERSUS CAPTIVE-BRED

Exotics are generally marked as captive-bred, farmed captive-bred or wild-caught. Wild-caught refers to an animal being taken from the wild whereas farm-bred refers to enclosed breeding farms within the native habitat of the animal where eggs or offspring are harvested. Obviously wild-caught animals will suffer considerable stress during capture and transport due to the unfamiliarity of human contact. They are also more likely to carry parasites and harbour diseases. Although slightly more used to contact, farm-bred reptiles are not always in much better condition than wild-caught reptiles due in some cases to poor husbandry and transportation. Captive-bred refers to animals that have been bred in captivity. They tend to be healthier animals with fewer parasites and can be more domesticated due to human proximity. They are usually considerably more expensive.

The parrot family has more globally threatened species than any other bird family, with many species listed on Convention on International Trade in Endangered Species of wild flora and fauna (CITES) Appendices I and II. The level of exportation of wild-caught birds is unsustainable. Only captive-bred and reared parrots should be bought as pets.

Most mammals are captive-bred and reared. However, the appeal of more unusual species and the willingness of people to pay can lead to trade in some wild-caught animals.

IMPORT AND EXPORT AND QUARANTINE

When importing any animal strict policies have to be adhered to in order to avoid contravening animal health and disease control legislation. Any legislation discussed in this chapter should only be used as guidance as policies and procedures can be updated at any time. It is therefore recommended that current versions of any legislation discussed here are referred to.

In order to import an animal into the UK several requirements will need to be met, including:

- The possession of all relevant documentation
- Fitness to travel
- The animal is not about to give birth, or has not recently given birth
- The animal is not a neonate – newborn animals and newly weaned animals are not accepted for carriage
- The use of a recognised animal freight carrier that is a member of the International Air Transport Association (IATA)
- The use of containers that conform to the IATA Live Animals Regulations
- The use of labels that conform to the IATA Live Animals Regulations.

Several different documentations may also be required. These might include:

- Export paperwork issued by the authorities of the exporting country
- Import paperwork issued by the Department for Environment, Food and Rural Affairs (DEFRA)
- Supplementary veterinary paperwork from a vet, treatment declarations, fitness-to-fly forms, acclimatisation certificates and blood test results
- Pet Travel Scheme (PETS) passport if applicable
- Declaration forms from the owner
- Airline customs and excise forms
- CITES licences.

Import from non-European Union countries

Generally most imports from outside the EU of non-CITES-listed exotic animals (that are not pets or mammals capable of carrying rabies) will require an import licence and a health certificate. The import licence will need to be applied for and granted before the animal arrives in the UK. Health certificates are issued by an official veterinarian stating that the animals, at the time of export, do not show any obvious signs of disease and that they do not come from a holding or an area covered by restrictions due to a disease outbreak. The animals will have to enter the UK via a border inspection post and, once inspected, will be issued with a border-crossing certificate by the State Veterinary Service of DEFRA. Additionally, they may require an export licence from the country of origin.

CITES

Any CITES-listed animal will require a permit to allow trade for commercial purposes. Animals listed on Appendix I are only licensed in exceptional circumstances. Any licences issued must pass along with the animal from the breeder to the supplier and on to the purchaser.

Rabies

Most mammals that are imported into the UK are subject to a 6-month quarantine period unless they fall under the PETS scheme.

Pets

As reptiles and amphibians do not transmit or carry rabies, there are no animal health import requirements for pet reptiles. These animals can be brought into the UK as long as they are accompanied by their owner and a self-certificate or a letter from a vet stating that the animals are fit and healthy to complete the journey and they are transported correctly. The certificate must state that the animals, at the time of dispatch, show no obvious signs of disease and that the holding of origin was not subject to any animal health restrictions. There are currently no limits on the number of pet reptiles and amphibians that an owner can bring into the UK.

PETS scheme

The pet scheme allows mammalian pets to travel between the EU and some non-EU countries without a quarantine period. Rabbits and other rodents travelling within the EU and some non-EU countries are not subject to any requirement with regard to rabies. Those travelling from other EU countries and from Andorra, Iceland, Liechtenstein, Monaco, Norway, San Marino, Switzerland and the Vatican are able to enter the UK on any route at any point of entry, subject to the agreement and conditions of carriage of the transport company. The maximum number of all types of pet animals (not only rabbits and rodents) each person may bring into the EU from most non-EU-listed countries is five. Ferrets may move between EU and some non-EU countries.

Birds

Due to the threat of bird flu, conditions for the import of birds other than poultry were changed in July 2007. As a result commercial importation of wild-caught birds is not permitted and captive-bred birds must come from approved establishments in a limited list of countries with a high avian health status and reliable veterinary services. Quarantine and testing procedures have been tightened and a list of approved quarantine establishments in the EU has been issued (there are currently none in the UK).

Psittacines

Each bird must be individually identified with either a leg ring or by microchip and be accompanied by a health certificate signed by an official veterinarian in the country of origin. Examination must be within 48 hours of export and certify that the birds do not come from, and have not been in contact with birds from, a holding on which psittacosis has been diagnosed in the past 2 months and that they do not come from a holding or an area covered by restrictions due to an outbreak of Newcastle disease or avian influenza or where avian influenza has been diagnosed in the last 30 days.

Non-psittacines

Imports of non-psittacines must be accompanied by a health statement signed by the seller or the exporter in the country of origin stating that the birds, at the time of export, do not show any obvious signs of disease and that they do not come from a holding or an area covered by restrictions due to an outbreak of Newcastle disease or avian influenza. Imports can only come from an approved list of countries.

Quarantine

Captive birds imported into the UK from approved countries must complete a minimum of 30 days' quarantine in an approved quarantine facility or centre. Imported birds shall be transported directly from the border inspection post of entry in England to an approved quarantine facility or centre. During the quarantine period an official veterinarian will inspect the quarantined birds at the beginning and end of the quarantine period and further inspections may be carried out if the official veterinarian feels it necessary due to the current disease situation. All quarantine and inspection costs will be met by the importer.

Bibliography

Aspinall V (ed.) 2006 The complete textbook of veterinary nursing. Elsevier, Spain

Cowdrey D 2002 Switching channels wildlife trade routes into Europe and the UK. WWF/Traffic International, Cambridge, UK

Girling S 2003 Veterinary nursing of exotic pets. Blackwell Publishing, Oxford

http://www.uvguide.co.uk

Pendry S, Inskipp C, Allan C 2006 Wildlife trade law: a UK enforcer's factfile. Traffic International, Cambridge, UK

Troyer K 1984 Behavioural acquisition of the hindgut fermentation system by hatchling *Iguana iguana*. Behavioural Ecology and Sociobiology 14:189–193

Further reading

Girling S 2003 Veterinary nursing of exotic pets. Blackwell Publishing, Oxford.
Indepth information on the treatment of exotics as well as husbandry and health issues.
Aspinall V (ed.) 2006 The complete textbook of veterinary nursing. Butterworth Heinemann, London.

Excellent chapters on comparative anatomy of exotics and restraint, handling and drug administration.
http://www.anapsid.org
http://www.degutopia.co.uk
http://www.reptileuvinfo.com
http://www.theparrotsocietyuk.org/husbandry.shtml

First aid

This chapter explores common first-aid scenarios that can occur in animals and describes how to approach them. The rules and aims of first aid are stated with transportation options and there is a discussion of how to monitor the first-aid casualty to prevent deterioration.

DEFINITION OF FIRST AID

First aid is the immediate treatment of injured animals or those suffering from sudden illness.

LEGISLATION THAT APPLIES TO THE FIRST-AID SCENARIO

First-aid scenarios are governed by the Veterinary Surgeons Act of 1966, which was amended to give veterinary nurses (qualified and listed) the power to do considerably more than a layperson if under the direction of a veterinary surgeon under schedule 3. Recently the schedule 3 amendments have been updated to include exotic pets, wildlife and large animals in addition to companion animals.

A layperson has the right to administer first aid, but only as an interim measure, designed to preserve life and alleviate suffering until a veterinary surgeon is able to attend the animal. Veterinary nurses have a greater knowledge of the situation than laypersons and so are able to assess the situation more accurately. For example, a veterinary nurse would have sufficient knowledge to pass a stomach tube in an animal suffering from a gastric dilation. However, giving medication or gastric lavage, in this case, would exceed the powers of schedule 3 and would not be acceptable (medication could be administered if directed by a veterinary surgeon).

RULES AND AIMS OF FIRST AID

First aid is based on three aims and four rules.

Aims

1. To preserve life
2. To prevent suffering
3. To prevent the situation deteriorating.

Rules

1. Do not panic – ensure your own safety first
2. Maintain the airway
3. Control haemorrhage
4. Contact the veterinary surgeon as soon as possible.

It is essential to be able to differentiate between:

- Life-threatening emergencies
- Emergencies requiring prompt attention
- Situations requiring only advice (Table 21.1).

TELEPHONE CALLS

The telephone call is often the first point of contact with the client or veterinary surgery in an emergency situation. Veterinary practices often establish protocols to encourage good practice when answering the telephone and to ensure that in the first-aid situation prompt action is initiated. This should include first-aid advice for the client, a synopsis of the emergency to be taken and recording the client's details.

It is often difficult for owners to be objective when assessing their pets and occasionally they will not want to deal with the nurse or receptionist. Although this can be frustrating you should always be sympathetic to the owners' wishes and deal with them in a calm, patient and sympathetic manner, whilst obtaining all the relevant information. Always try to sound professional and leave the client feeling reassured. Ideally try to speak to the owner on a first-hand basis. Second-hand conversations can often be inaccurate.

In the first-aid situation, several basic questions must always be asked:

- What are the owner's name, address and telephone number (and contact number if applicable)?
- What is the nature of the injury?
- What is the extent or degree of the injury?
- When did the accident happen or when was it first noticed?
- Has the condition improved or deteriorated? If so, how quickly?
- What are the animal's age, sex and breed?
- Is it on any present medication? If so, what?
- Where is the animal?
- In the case of poisoning, what poison has it consumed?

Always ask for a contact number in the first instance in the event of a disconnection. Clients should also be made aware that animals can bite when frightened or injured. If appropriate, instructions should be given on how to make a muzzle. Remember, if the animal is experiencing breathing difficulties a muzzle should not be applied.

History taking is very important because:

- The type of emergency can be determined
- Relevant instructions can be given to the owner
- It allows you to prepare the surgery for the arrival of the patient, e.g. setting up the oxygen, intravenous catheters and fluids.

Table 21.1 Classifications of first-aid emergencies		
Life-threatening emergency	Require immediate treatment/action by the owner at home or by the nurse in the surgery	**Examples** Road traffic accident Gastric dilation/torsion Respiratory failure Cardiac failure
Emergencies but not life-threatening	Require immediate attention – bring to the surgery	Fractures
Minor emergencies	Telephone advice could alleviate suffering until a veterinary surgery can attend the patient	

HANDLING AND TRANSPORTATION OF INJURED ANIMALS

Never try to remove an animal until it has had a preliminary examination, unless the situation is life-threatening, e.g. there is traffic or falling masonry. This will allow the injuries to be protected during transportation. The injured animal is often frightened and so might be aggressive if cornered or approached too quickly. Always reassure the patient, whilst making slow deliberate movements. Dogs are much more inclined to be aggressive than cats.

It is good practice to loop a lead or belt over the animal's head. If having difficulty, ask somebody to keep the animal's attention by standing in front of the dog and then approach quietly from behind to apply the lead. When on a lead dogs usually become more confident and biddable; however, on occasions the dog catcher may have to be employed. When the dog is under control a muzzle should be applied providing the animal is not dyspnoeic or has substantial face injuries.

When restrained a brief examination can be performed:

- Ensure there is a patent airway – extend the head and pull out the animal's tongue, removing any vomitus or foreign bodies
- Control haemorrhage
- Immobilise fractures
- Dress wounds.

Allow the patient to assume the most comfortable position until it can be transported or until the veterinary surgeon arrives. This generally tends to be wound-side down. Ask the owner to stay with the animal, to provide reassurance and comfort. Cats should be approached quietly and confidently. If possible stroke the cat's chin and then gently slide your hand around until you can scruff the cat. An examination can then be carried out. Sometimes it is necessary to lower an inverted box over the cat gently and then to slide a piece of hard cardboard underneath it so that the cat comes to lie on it. Alternatively a blanket or coat can be used to improvise.

Transportation

Ideally the animal should be moved with the minimum discomfort to the patient whilst not disturbing any bandages or dressings. Animals can be divided into one of two groups: ambulatory, i.e. those that can walk, and non-ambulatory, those that are unable to walk. Generally animals that are ambulatory are usually in less pain if they are allowed to walk themselves rather than being carried. Always give encouragement – use the voice.

Non-ambulatory casualties are unable to walk and therefore need to be transported either by hand or by some other means. Cases involving suspected spinal fractures should not be lifted in the arms but provision should be made to ensure the spine is kept straight and provided with support.

Small dogs and cats

- Slide one hand around the hindquarters and the other under the sternum, supporting the weight along the forearm
- Hold the animal firmly around the neck with one hand whilst holding the foreleg furthest away from the body with the other hand. Make sure the animal's neck remains extended.

Medium-sized dogs

- One arm should be placed around the front of the sternum
- The other should be placed around the pelvis, supporting the weight of the dog
- The animal is held close to the handler's chest
- Try to hold the injured side closest to your chest
- Lift the dog with a straight back and bent knees
- Always ask for help if the dog is too heavy (remember, if the dog is over 20 kg two people will be required to lift it).

Large heavy dogs

- Always lift with two or more people
- One person should stand at the animal's shoulder with an arm around its neck and the other around its thorax
- The other person should hold one arm under the abdomen and the other around the pelvis
- Keep your back straight and knees bent
- Beware of injuries to the animal's abdomen.

Boxes and baskets

These are suitable for cats and small dogs. They can be made from wicker, metal, wood or plastic. In an emergency washing baskets can be useful. Whichever is used there are three basic rules:

1. They must be escape-proof
2. They must have adequate ventilation
3. They must permit constant observation of the patient.

The animal must be lifted with minimal stress:

- Push a piece of hardboard under the animal and then, while holding the board, place the animal into the basket
- Gently scruff the animal with one hand whilst supporting the trunk with the palm of the other hand
- In the case of vicious animals, scruff with one hand and lift up bodily. Gently support the hindquarters with the other hand.

Stretchers

Always use a stretcher if the animal:

- Has suspected spinal fractures/injuries
- Has collapsed with despond
- Has collapsed with thoracic or abdominal injuries
- Has collapsed with unconsciousness
- Is severely injured.

There are several methods of stretching an animal but the same principles apply:

- Have a flat, rigid object which is strong enough to support the animal
- It must be able to fit into the vehicle!

Different types of stretcher include wood or hardboard sheets, wire mesh or plastic-coated fencing, sacks or coats mounted on poles and blankets.

To transfer the patient on to the stretcher:

1. Place the stretcher close to the patient's back
2. Apply a tape muzzle (if there is no respiratory distress)
3. Roll the patient on to its chest and push the stretcher underneath as far as possible. Allow the animal to collapse on to its side again and thus on to the stretcher. Avoid twisting the animal's spine.
4. Alternatively, grasp the skin along the back at several points and pull the patient (gently!) by the skin on to the stretcher. This requires several people, and the pulling must be done in unison to avoid spinal damage. This is the method of choice if a spinal fracture is suspected.

When in transit the patient needs to be observed and restrained constantly to ensure that the condition does not deteriorate, dressings are not disturbed, the animal does not escape or fall off a seat and it cannot interfere with the driver of the vehicle. There should always be a second person in the vehicle, preferably the owner, for several reasons. Having the owner in the vehicle will reduce the risk of causing a crash; the owner will be able to give a full case history to the veterinary surgeon and the animal will be able to be comforted. If, however, a second person is not possible then the animal must be restrained by securely fastening it to the door or ideally placing it in a transporting cage or carrier.

Small mammals

Small mammals such as hamsters, rabbits and guinea pigs should be transported in small containers, which will prevent them from rolling around in transit. This is especially true for suspected fracture cases as immobilisation of limbs can prove difficult. Remember that cardboard boxes can be chewed. Keep the animal quiet, warm and in the dark to reduce stress.

Exotics

Exotic animals, e.g. iguanas and tortoises, can be transported in containers, again ensuring that they cannot roll about. Snakes can be placed inside pillowcases for ease of movement. Birds may be transported in their own cages with all accessories removed to prevent further injury and covered with a towel to prevent further stress. Sealed cardboard boxes with air holes would be the method of choice: they must be of a suitable size so that the bird cannot open its wings and cause damage.

TRIAGE

Upon admission at the veterinary surgery the animal should be examined, a provisional diagnosis made and treatment given. Each animal should have an identity collar or band placed on it for identification. A full history should be obtained from the owner; it may be advantageous to do this away from the patient so that the owner can give full attention to the recorder.

All arrivals should be classified under the practice's system and patients prioritised according to their individual immediate needs (Box 21.1). A triage plan can be made up which categorises patients according to their need for treatment, often using class I–IV, where class I is near to death and class IV indicates that treatment is required within 24 hours. Unconscious animals should always be treated immediately as their condition can degenerate rapidly into an irreparable state.

Box 21.1

DEFINITION

Triage

Triage is the prioritisation of critically ill or injured patients into those requiring immediate treatment

Primary survey

Once triage has been carried out primary survey can commence. Primary survey addresses the ABCs of airway, breathing, bleeding, cardiovascular, circulation and level of consciousness.

Ask the following questions:

- Is the airway patent? Clear it if necessary
- Is the animal breathing? Give artificial respiration if necessary
- Does the patient have a pulse? Give cardiac massage if necessary.

At the primary survey stage the following treatment or actions may be undertaken:

- Supply oxygen if necessary to prevent hypoxia: possibly intubate
- Avoid placing leads around the neck of a patient with head, neck, ocular or respiratory injuries or difficulty
- Observe ventilatory pattern
- Place a fleece or pad on the table to prevent hypothermia
- Allocate an assistant to document procedures
- Commence a thorough examination
- Control severe haemorrhage
- Cover open wounds
- Take temperature, pulse and respiration
- Do an electrocardiograph
- Measure blood pressure
- Give fluid therapy if appropriate
- Perform diagnostic tests: an emergency blood profile, electrolyte assay and urine analysis can prove valuable
- Do a thoracentesis/abdocentesis
- Place a catheter
- Start drug therapy (particularly for seizures)
- Give analgesia – butorphanol would be the agent of choice due to its short duration.

Remember that oxygen is of the utmost importance. If time is wasted preventing blood loss, the dyspnoeic patient will be cyanotic and may have suffered irreparable loss of brain function. Alternatively an unattended main arterial bleed could leave the animal severely anaemic to the extent that there are insufficient circulating red blood cells to maintain oxygenation throughout the body.

Examination of the patient – secondary survey

Once the patient has had a primary survey then a secondary survey can be conducted. This stage involves making a full examination giving appropriate first aid.

Box 21.2

A CRASHPLAN MNEMONIC

A: Airway, breathing, bleeding
C: Circulation, cardiovascular system
R: Respiration
A: Abdomen, analgesia
S: Spine
H: Head
P: Pelvis, perineum, penis
L: Limbs
A: Arteries, veins
N: Nerves, neurology

The mnemonic 'A CRASHPLAN' can be used as an aid or individual practices may employ their own policy (Box 21.2).

Thorough clinical notes should be taken during the secondary survey; it is useful to have two people available at this stage as one can examine the animal while the other can make notes.

General examination

It is useful to obtain a body weight for the animal as losses can be dramatic in the critical care patient and it can aid in correct fluid restoration regimes. Always observe the animal visually prior to palpation.

State of consciousness

- How does the animal respond to stimuli, e.g. light, sound, touch?
- Is the animal alert?
- Does the animal have normal reflex responses?

If the answers to the above are no, then the patient is probably very seriously injured, ill or shocked.

Behaviour

- Is the animal acting normally? An owner may have to give this information as what is considered normal behaviour may differ between clients
- Abnormal behaviour may include excitability, depression, sluggishness or hyperaesthesia.

Respiration

- The character and rate should be taken into consideration
- Causes of alteration of respiratory pattern should be noted

- Laboured breathing is suggestive of alveolar damage or collapsed lungs, perhaps due to pneumothorax or a ruptured diaphragm
- Rapid, shallow breathing suggests pain first and foremost, but could also indicate shock, thoracic wall injury or abdominal crisis.

Cardiovascular assessment

The following should be considered:

- Heart rate and rhythm – ascertain if arrhythmia is present
- Pulse quality and rate – assess the pulse at different sites
- Blood pressure
- Possible central venous pressure

- Monitor the capillary refill time (CRT) and general mucous membrane colour
- Assess temperature at extremities
- Compare pulse to heart rate
- Check packed cell volume
- Assess jugular vein for distension
- Compare lung and heart sounds: this can help differentiate between cardiac conditions (auscultate with a stethoscope).

Temperature

- Assess body core temperature
- Assess extremities, e.g. tongue, paws, face, tail.

A general head-to-toe examination should then be performed to ascertain any other injuries; refer to Figure 21.1.

Nose	
Mouth	
Teeth	
Eyes	
Skull	
Ears	
Limbs	
Ribcage	
Thorax	
Abdomen	
Spine	
Pelvis	
Perineum	
Tail	
Body surface	
Reflexes	

Figure 21.1 General head-to-toe to toe-to-head examination form.

General rules to apply

- If everything is going well – worry! Question your methodology
- Record everything. What one person considers insignificant can be another person's inspiration to a diagnosis, a precursor to deterioration in the patient's condition or a reason to persevere in a hopeless case
- Even when the patient is considered stable constant monitoring for the initial 24 hours should be performed (or at least every 10 minutes)
- Patient monitoring/hospitalisation records should be attached to the kennel/cage and *must* include *all* medical and treatment details, i.e. the checklist plus urination, defecation and vomitus.

First-aid cases can be extremely stressful for all parties involved. Do not attempt procedures you are unhappy to perform and do not feel afraid to ask for help. Due diligence from the veterinary practice to formulate a first-aid action plan can help the staff, the client and, most importantly, the patient.

SHOCK

Shock is a clinical term used to describe a clinical syndrome characterised by a fall in cardiac output. This leads to inadequate oxygen and nutrients reaching the peripheral tissues and waste products from tissues not being transported away. The result is abnormal cell function and the body starts to undergo progressive changes, which can ultimately lead to death.

Signs of shock can include:

- Pallor of mucous membranes – blood supply is directed to the vital organs and vasoconstriction occurs in the peripheral blood vessels
- Increased CRT due to reduced blood volume taking longer to refill the capillary
- Increased respiratory rate to counteract the reduced blood volume to supply sufficient oxygen to the body
- Rapid, feeble pulse (which may not detectable)
- Coldness of extremities and mouth due to vasoconstriction of peripheral blood vessels
- Dull and depressed animal
- Convulsions and collapse (this happens if the brain becomes short of oxygen – hypoxia).

Hypovolaemic shock

This occurs when the circulating blood volume drops to a level which is inadequate to meet the body's requirements; it can be due to haemorrhage, loss of plasma or severe water and/or electrolyte losses (vomiting/diarrhoea).

Vasculogenic shock

Vasculogenic shock occurs when the circulating blood volume is normal but the capacity of the blood vessels (mainly veins) is increased. It may be drug-induced, e.g. by acepromazine, and is usually a result of overdosing. There are three types:

1. Neurogenic: nervous tissue trauma, e.g. in the central nervous system
2. Anaphylactic shock: allergic reaction, e.g. toad venom or bee sting will present with oedema around the sting/bite
3. Endotoxic shock or septic shock: due to release of endotoxins from bacteria invading the body.

Cardiogenic shock

This is not very common in animals. It is caused by reduced cardiac filling, e.g. pericarditis, or by reduced cardiac emptying, e.g. abnormalities such as cardiomyopathy.

First aid for the shocked patient

1. This will depend upon the cause of the shock – it may be necessary to treat other conditions first (remember ABC)
2. Prevent any further haemorrhage – this will stop the circulating blood volume from dropping any lower
3. Oxygen therapy may be given under vet's instructions
4. Do not apply direct heat or give drugs that will cause the veins or arteries in the skin to dilate (get bigger): this could lead to more blood loss or reduce the animal's temperature. It also diverts the blood away from the vital organs – heart, lungs and brain
5. Make the animal comfortable and prevent heat loss – make sure the animal is in a warm, quiet area. It may be advisable to dim the lighting as well. Use vetbeds and heat pads under and over the animal
6. It is likely that the vet or vet nurse will set up and administer intravenous fluids
7. You may offer oral fluids (little and often) at the veterinary surgeon's direction. Do not do this of your own accord as fluids are contraindicated in certain conditions, e.g. vomiting
8. Monitoring the patient – ideally this should be constant as shock patients can deteriorate rapidly. The patient should be monitored at least every 10 minutes, including:
   - Level of consciousness
   - Mucous membrane colour

○ CRT
○ Pupillary (light makes the pupil constrict) and palpebral reflexes (eyelids blink when touched)
○ Character and rate of pulse
○ Character and rate of respiration
○ Any other signs.

These should be written up on the patient's chart and the vet should be told immediately of any worries or changes in the animal's condition

9. Nursing care is vital in these cases. You can provide a lot of support for the shocked animal but remember that a shocked patient is often disoriented and in pain, so lots of cuddles may be too much! Move quietly and talk in a calm and soothing manner.

RESPIRATORY EMERGENCIES AND FIRST AID

There are many degrees of respiratory injury, ranging from shortness of breath to a cessation of breathing. Underlying disease processes, trauma or other cause such as poisoning may cause respiratory injuries.

Causes of respiratory failure include:

- Trauma, e.g. foreign body, pulmonary oedema, laryngeal paralysis
- Pulmonary embolism
- Neoplasia – primary or secondary metastasis
- Overdose of anaesthetic
- Pneumonia
- Pleural effusions – hydrothorax
- Paralysis to respiratory muscles – tetanus, botulism
- Laryngeal paralysis
- Poisoning, e.g. with Paraquat
- Pressure on diaphragm – gastric torsion
- Collapsed lungs
- Diaphragmatic rupture.

Clinical signs can vary but often include:

- Cyanosis
- Tachypnoea
- Orthopnoea
- Dyspnoea:
  - Laboured breathing:
    ○ Obstructed upper airway
    ○ Fluid in alveoli/asphyxiation
    ○ Collapsed lungs (pneumothorax, haemothorax, pyothorax, diaphragmatic rupture)
    ○ Decreased oxygenation of blood
  - Rapid, shallow breathing:
    ○ Shock
    ○ Paralysis of respiratory muscles
    ○ Pain
- Tachycardia, weak pulse

- Collapse
- Unconsciousness.

Rapid and effective treatment is essential if the patient is to survive.

Respiratory arrest

Acute respiratory failure represents a true emergency requiring urgent medical attention. The lungs cannot oxygenate the blood or excrete carbon dioxide. Causes include obstruction, anaesthetic overdose, toxins and pneumonia or some form of physical restriction to the thorax, e.g. ascites or a ruptured diaphragm. Clinical signs include hypoxia and cyanosis, tachypnoea, tachycardia and perhaps arrhythmias, open-mouth breathing (orthopnoea) and anxiety, which will become drowsiness and ultimately unconsciousness (Table 21.2).

Ruptured diaphragm

The main cause of a ruptured diaphragm is road traffic accidents. Clinical signs are dependent upon the location and severity of the damage caused to the diaphragm. They may include:

- Respiratory distress
- Dyspnoea

Table 21.2 First-aid actions for respiratory failure	
Establish and maintain a patent airway	Suction to remove mucus or other secretions Intubation, if required Tracheotomy if required
Provide oxygen via	Endotracheal tube Nasal tube Face mask Oxygen mask
Drug therapy	Diuretics to correct pulmonary oedema Bronchodilators to improve ventilation Respiratory centre stimulants if depressed
Thoracentesis	To relieve hydrothorax or pneumothorax
Nursing role	Ensure therapy is carried out Monitor vital signs Keep careful records of patient's condition Advise owner regarding patient's condition

- Cyanosis
- Mediastinal shift
- Bowel sounds in thorax on auscultation.

Mediastinal shift is the movement of the contents of the mediastinum which displaces the heart to the right-hand side; therefore auscultation will give louder heart sounds on the right-hand side of the thorax than on the left-hand side, as in the normal animal.

Acute pulmonary oedema

This is a condition caused by congestion of the lungs leading to the passage of serous fluid from the capillaries into the interstitial tissues/alveoli. It is caused by left ventricular heart failure, chest trauma, uraemia or the inhalation of chemical irritants. Clinical signs are similar to the previous condition but rales on breathing will also be seen.

Collapsed lungs

Collapsed lungs can be caused by:

- Open pneumothorax, where a wound penetrates the pleural cavity
- Closed pneumothorax, where there is no wound leading to the body surface, but lungs are injured internally, tearing the pleural membrane
- Haemothorax, where there is damage to a blood vessel and blood collects in pleural cavity: as a result, lungs float and can't expand
- Diaphragmatic rupture, where there is pressure of the abdominal contents on the lungs or pressure reduction in thoracic cavity
- Beware – infection and contamination are common with these injuries.

Thoracic wounds

- Causes include road traffic accident, bites and staking accidents
- Clinical signs include abnormal breathing patterns, open pneumothorax and subcutaneous emphysema
- Subcutaneous emphysema: there is crackly skin due to the accumulation of air under the subcutaneous layer of the skin.

Resuscitation

See Figure 21.2 for actions to be taken when cardiac pulmonary arrest occurs.
Remember:

- Ventilation must be performed simultaneously with cardiac massage – think of the ABC rule

- Two people can manage better than one
- If alone, apply cardiac massage for 5 seconds then inflate the chest three times, then repeat
- If the heart does not restart after 3 minutes of cardiac massage the patient can be declared dead.

ADVANCED CARDIAC LIFE SUPPORT

This is defined as any invasive procedure or administration of medication.

If resuscitation is unsuccessful after 5–10 minutes, advanced cardiac life support (ACLS) can be tried. Open-chest cardiopulmonary resuscitation must be considered, particularly in severely hypovolaemic patients, severe trauma patients or patients suffering from pleural effusion. The reliability of external chest compressions has to be questioned in larger breeds of dog.

Drugs

The agent will vary depending upon arrhythmia, electrolyte disorder, acid–base status and underlying disease factors. If there is no intravenous line, a urinary catheter can be placed in an endotracheal tube and adrenaline (epinephrine), lidocaine or atropine can be administered at double dose. The catheter is then flushed with sterile saline and ventilation is continued. Drugs can be administered via normal intravenous routes, including the lingual vein. Intracardiac injections should only be considered as a last resort as they can lead to further damage to the cardiac tissue.

Ventricular fibrillation

Electrical defibrillation can be administered after trying a precordial thump to the heart. For external defibrillation 7–10 Joules and for internal defibrillation 1/10th of this rate can be given, and repeated up to three times consecutively at the same dose. If unsuccessful, double the initial dose and administer adrenaline, then defibrillate twice more at twice the initial dose. In between defibrillation basic cardiac life support should be continued.

Heimlich manoeuvre

The Heimlich manoeuvre is used as an emergency measure to try and remove foreign bodies from the respiratory tract. The aim is to apply pressure to the diaphragm to cause a cough, which will dislodge the object.

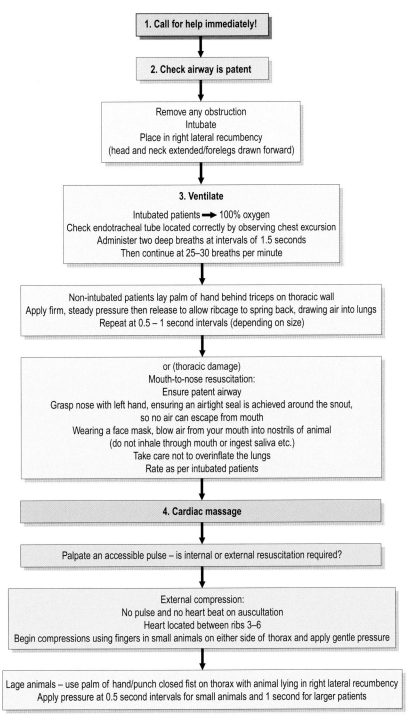

Figure 21.2 Actions to be taken when cardiac pulmonary arrest occurs.

Method

- Suspend the patient upside down by the hindlegs
- Remember to maintain health and safety at all times
- Punch the animal just below the xiphisternum
- If this does not work, use both hands on either side of the thoracic girdle and compress sharply
- Repeat up to four times.

Hanging the patient upside down aids in the evacuation of the foreign body. If after four attempts the object has not been removed, an emergency tracheotomy should be considered.

CLASSIFICATION OF HAEMORRHAGE

Haemorrhage can be classified according to:

- Type of blood vessel damaged
- Time at which bleeding occurs
- Destination of blood loss.

Type of blood vessel

Arterial haemorrhage is categorised by bright red blood; it pumps forcefully and has a definite bleeding point. Venous haemorrhage is categorised by darker red blood, with little or no spurting from the wound and a definite bleeding point. Capillary haemorrhage is bright red blood; it involves small volumes which slowly ooze from the wound and there is no definite bleeding point.

Time at which bleeding occurs

Primary haemorrhage is immediate bleeding, reactionary haemorrhage is bleeding that occurs within 24–48 hours of the original injury and secondary haemorrhage is bleeding that occurs 3–10 days posttrauma.

Destination of blood loss

External haemorrhage involves bleeding from the body surface and is clearly visible. Internal haemorrhage is bleeding into body cavities or the tissues and is hidden.

Control of haemorrhage

The body has four natural factors which act to stop initial bleeding:

1. Retraction of the cut ends of blood vessels: as the vessel is damaged the ends involved coil backwards on themselves, creating a jagged edge, reducing the lumen so the clot which forms has a smaller diameter to fill.
2. Falling blood pressure: the blood pressure will drop as blood is lost, which in turn will slow the remaining volume of blood circulating around the body, enabling the clot to lodge in the damaged area.
3. Back pressure: the haemorrhage at the damaged area, for example in dead space in the body, will create back pressure. Consider a gap in the tissues which the blood is filling: it can only contain a certain amount of blood and once full will exert its own pressure back on the blood that is entering, i.e. equilibrium will effectively be achieved, stopping the bleeding.
4. Blood clotting: the blood contains thrombocytes and numerous clotting factors which are activated when blood vessels are damaged to create strands of insoluble fibrin which form a net in the damaged area, trapping cells and debris to form a clot which acts as a plug for the hole created (Figure 21.3).

First aid for haemorrhage

There are five common methods which can be employed:

1. Direct digital pressure
2. Artery forceps
3. Pad and pressure bandage
4. Pressure points
5. Tourniquet.

Direct digital pressure

This involves the application of direct pressure with clean hands; the fingers can be applied directly to the skin on either side of the wound to push the ends together to help prevent further bacterial infection. If the wound is too large for this, place your whole hand or a piece of material, e.g. tea towel, over the wound.

Artery forceps

These tend only to be used in cases of severe haemorrhage and by veterinary professionals. The artery forceps are used to grab the ends of the cut blood vessel, stopping the bleeding, and then the ends are ligated with catgut.

Pad and pressure bandage

This method uses a pad of swabs or cotton wool placed on to the wound and then bandaged under pressure into place. The procedure may need to be repeated if the blood soaks through. It is not advisable to remove the

Clotting process:

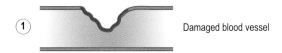

① Damaged blood vessel

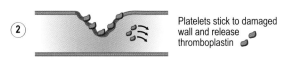

② Platelets stick to damaged wall and release thromboplastin

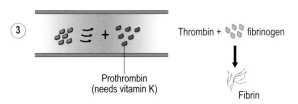

③ Thrombin + fibrinogen

Prothrombin (needs vitamin K)

Fibrin

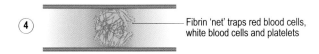

④ Fibrin 'net' traps red blood cells, white blood cells and platelets

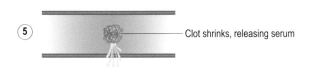

⑤ Clot shrinks, releasing serum

Figure 21.3 Clotting.

pad – keep adding layers on top until the blood does not come through. If the wound is on a limb, bandage the whole leg to avoid swelling.

Padding materials form a cushioning and supportive layer, they provide protection to bony prominences and are usually made from natural or synthetic fibres (Table 21.3).

Table 21.3 Padding materials	
Cotton wool	Natural fibre, cheap, good absorptive properties
Softban	Soft, natural padding, available in various sizes and thicknesses
Foam	Synthetic, comes on rolls, varies in size

Pressure points

There are certain points on the body where an artery can be compressed against a bone to reduce bleeding. There are sites which can be used on the dog and cat:

Brachial artery

- Runs along the inside of the humerus then behind the biceps
- Pulse can be felt in distal (farthest away from body) third of humerus
- Pressure applied here arrests haemorrhage below the elbow.

Femoral artery

- Runs over the proximal (closest to body) third of femur on the inner surface of the thigh
- Pressure here arrests haemorrhage below the stifle.

Coccygeal artery

- Underside of the tail
- Pressure at the root will arrest haemorrhage from the tail.

Tourniquet

A tourniquet restricts all the blood vessels to a wound and should only be used in severe cases. It should be fixed a few inches above the wound. The pressure is adjusted so it is tight enough to stop bleeding but it must not be left on for more than 10–15 minutes. If it needs to be in place for longer then release it to allow some blood to the tissues below to perfuse them and preserve their integrity, then reapply the tourniquet. Never leave a tourniquet in situ unattended.

Other first-aid methods for haemorrhage include electrocautery and diathermy which use direct heat or heat produced by electrical currents to coagulate blood vessels. Styptics have an astringent action on tissues and blood vessels, i.e. they cause constriction; they are used in nail clipping and examples include ferric chloride, potassium permanganate, silver nitrate and acetic acid. They are also available as commercial dressings, e.g. lysostat, and a swab soaked in adrenaline solution can be used to treat epistasis.

WOUNDS

A wound is a disruption in the normal integrity of the soft tissues or a forcible break in the continuity of the soft tissues. This can be caused by an insult, which can be on purpose, e.g. surgery, or incidental, e.g. trauma.

Wounds can be either acute (of sudden onset) or chronic (long-term) (Box 21.3).

Wound categories

Wounds can be classified by type or by the degree of contamination present.

Many wounds can fall into more than one category (Table 21.4).

Incised wounds

- Caused by sharp instruments, e.g. knives, glass, scalpel blades
- Their edges are clean-cut and easily defined

- Avulsed wounds are common on limbs where animals have stood on glass
- Simple incised wounds heal very quickly on their own
- They normally haemorrhage considerably due to lack of recoil of vessels
- They tend to heal very quickly if held together
- Generally incised wounds leave minimal scarring.

Box 21.3

DEFINITIONS

Acute

Wounds induced by surgery or trauma
Healing time is dependent on the depth and size of the lesion but generally heals normally

Chronic

Wounds resulting from different causes
Depending upon their pathology, they may take many months or years to repair, e.g. decubitus ulcers

Table 21.4 Wound types	
Open	Involves a break in the body surface, e.g. skin or mucous membranes Blood loss can be evaluated Main groups: incised, lacerated and puncture wounds
Closed	No break in body surface Includes bruising and ruptures
Abrasion	When epidermis has been eroded to expose the dermis, i.e. the full thickness of the skin has not been broken
Avulsed	Where a flap of skin is forced away from the body but still remains intact at some point
Contused	Any wound where bruising is present
Clean	Surgical wounds Elective wounds Highly vascular tissues not predisposed to infection
Clean contaminated	Minor contamination is evident Surgical wounds with minor break in aseptic technique Elective surgery in tissues with normal resident bacteria flora, e.g. gastrointestinal tract No spillage of organ contents
Contaminated	Moderate contamination is evident Fresh traumatic injuries, open fractures, penetrating wounds Surgery with gross spillage of organ contents Presence of bile or urine Surgical wounds with major break in asepsis
Dirty	Grossly contaminated or infected Contaminated traumatic wounds more than 4 hours old Perforated viscera, abscess, necrotic tissue, foreign bodies

Lacerated wounds

- Most common type of wound
- Usually caused by road traffic accidents, barbed wire, dog fights
- Wounds are irregular in shape with jagged edges
- Skin has been torn apart, sometimes completely
- Severity depends upon how deeply the wound penetrates
- Haemorrhage is surprisingly small and normally is due to ragged tearing of the blood vessels
- High risk of bacterial contamination
- Healing is normally slow
- Risk of scarring.

Puncture wounds

- Produced from blows by sharp instruments, e.g. nails, thorns, teeth and bullets
- The skin wound may be quite small, with a deep track running down into the underlying tissues
- High risk of bacterial infection because:
  - Bacteria can be carried into wound at the time of injury
  - Small wounds heal over very quickly, trapping bacteria inside
- Often overlooked by owners
- Can form a small abscess
- Sometimes contain a foreign body, e.g. thorn
- Sometimes object has gone straight through tissue, e.g. bullet
- Avulsed wounds can occur with puncture wounds:
  - Generally happen in dog fights
  - Animal is picked up by its scruff
  - Underlying tissues are ripped away
  - Only teeth puncture wounds show in the skin
- Very prone to infection.

Abrasion

- Name given to a graze or scrub wound
- Do not penetrate full thickness of the skin
- Usually caused by a glancing blow
- Superficial wound, therefore only capillary bleed
- Often contaminated
- Rarely serious; however very painful
- Healing takes place under a scab.

Categorisation of wounds by contamination

Depending upon the degree of contamination open wounds can be classified into the following groups (Table 21.4):

1. Clean
2. Clean contaminated
3. Contaminated
4. Dirty.

Management of these wounds varies according to the severity of the injury and the patient's condition. Generally, contaminated and dirty wounds are not good candidates for primary closure. Until contamination and infection are eliminated, open wound management is necessary. Dead and dying tissues need to be removed or debrided to minimise the potential for bacterial infection and create a viable wound bed.

Wound healing

Wound healing is a dynamic process, i.e. more than one stage of healing will be occurring at any given time (Table 21.5). Soft tissue heals as a result of epithelial regeneration and fibroplasias. This occurs when the wound undergoes the three phases of soft-tissue wound healing:

1. Exudative – inflammatory – debridement phase
2. Proliferative – collagen phase
3. Maturation phase.

Table 21.5 Wound healing	
Phase	**Characteristics**
Inflammatory	Begins immediately after injury Formation of blood clot Platelets stimulate release of growth factors
Debridement	Part of inflammatory phase Characterised by influx of white blood cells into wound Macrophages/monocytes Occurs approximately 6 hours posttrauma Wound healing is sustained by release of growth factors from variety of cell types
Repair (proliferative collagen/fibroblastic)	Begins 3–5 days posttrauma Invasion of fibroblasts and development of granulation tissue Wound strength is increasing exponentially
Maturation	Remodelling of collagen of the scar and slow gain in wound strength Begins approximately 3 weeks after injury and may take weeks to years to complete

There is minimal wound strength during the first 3–5 days of healing. Corticosteroids delay all types of wound healing. A wound never regains the strength of normal tissue.

First-intention healing

If the edges of the wound are not widely separated and held together by blood clots then new vessels grow into these clots from the side of the wound. Healing components are brought to this site to produce the fibrous scar tissue that will tie the wound edges together permanently. Epithelial cells quickly spread across the narrow scar and start producing a new skin layer. Provided there is no sepsis the healing will take place in 5–10 days. It can only take place in incised wounds where the edges are in opposition or can be achieved with stitching or bandaging.

Second-intention healing/granulation

This is usually how lacerated, avulsed and infected wounds heal. The repair may take several weeks because the wound edges are widely separated. Clusters of granulation tissue are produced on the wound and multiply to form an area of granulation tissue. This tissue is moist and bright red with an uneven surface and is very easily damaged and will haemorrhage profusely if disturbed. It grows upwards towards the skin surface and when it has reached the level of the skin, new epithelial cells spread across the top to complete the healing process.

Third-intention healing

This occurs when large or very contaminated wounds are allowed to heal initially by second-intention healing and then are closed by sutures. This allows granulation to take place after the infection has been removed.

Wound contamination and infection

There is a difference between wound contamination and infection. All wounds created under aseptic techniques are contaminated by microorganisms from the environment. Transient microbes do not normally invade the surrounding tissues; however, because there is no host immune response to these organisms they will multiply and cause infection. Infection is the process whereby organisms bind to tissue, multiply and invade tissue. This in turn will elicit an immune response – this means that the numbers of microorganisms have increased to a point at which the body is unable to control them. This is often characterised by erythema, oedema (Figure 21.4), pus, pyrexia, pain and change in colour of exu-

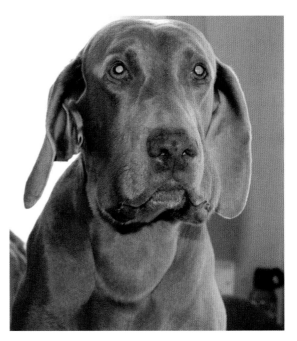

Figure 21.4 Excessive facial oedema due to pharyngeal trauma.

dates, unpleasant odour and an elevated neutrophil count.

Other factors that can create infection include:

- Foreign bodies
- Excessive necrotic tissue left in wound
- Excessive bleeding creating high levels of iron
- Compromised local defences, e.g. burn patient
- Immunosuppressive drugs, e.g. prednisolone, cyclophosphamide
- Obesity
- Length of time wound is open to environment
- Poor surgical technique
- Poor surgery management.

Factors that can affect rate of healing include:

- Type of wound
- Age of wound
- Infection
- Contamination
- Age of animal (an older animal will heal slower)
- Other health problems:
  - ○ Diabetes mellitus: slower healing and predisposition to wound infection
  - ○ Cushing: steroids: slower healing
  - ○ Liver disease: reduced amounts of clotting factors
- External drug factors
- Radiation therapy

- Movement – if edges of wound move against each other the tissues are continually being destroyed, e.g. on joints
- Disturbances in circulation – heavy contusions can impair local circulation, leading to necrosis of tissues which will need to be removed before healing occurs
- Self – trauma, e.g. licking: movement, infection and damage.

First-aid management of wounds

In the first-aid situation the wound must be protected to prevent further damage. This helps to control haemorrhage, prevent additional contamination and immobilise extremities. Remember, if there is a significant amount of blood loss you should treat the animal for shock.

Always follow this set course of action:

1. Treat for shock
2. Control haemorrhage
3. Remove the cause of the injury (remember that penetrating objects can be acting as a plug so remove them at your discretion)
4. Clip hair from around the wound
5. Cleanse the wound using lavage
6. Dress the wound (Table 21.6).

Lavage

- Removes debris and loose particles and tissue from the wound
- Reduces the number of bacteria
- If infection is suspected, can take a tissue biopsy prior to lavage
- Use large volumes of warmed, sterile, normal saline (dilute chlorhexidine solutions can irritate the tissues involved, although they are often employed for lavage).

Use of antibacterials

Systemic or topical use depends upon several factors:

- Patient's condition
- Immune status

Table 21.6 Dressing materials	
Dry dressing	Absorb fluid from wound (blood/exudate/pus)
Impregnated gauze dressing	Impregnated with materials depending on use (Vaseline/antibiotics) Keeps wounds moist

- Nature of surgery (elective versus emergency)
- Location of wound
- Duration of surgical procedure
- Surgeon's experience
- Environment.

Patients in good health, with adequate immune status, undergoing a relatively short (less than 90 minutes) elective orthopaedic or soft-tissue procedure (not abdominal) performed by an experienced surgeon in a clean surgical facility using aseptic technique should not require antibiotics. In clean surgical wounds preoperative antibiotics should be considered in cases of shock, severe trauma, long procedures, foreign bodies, poor blood supply, malnutrition, obesity or if disease is present. Broad-spectrum antibiotics should be used in chronic wounds. Applying topical preparations can be counterproductive. Although they have an antimicrobial action, they can have adverse effects on wound healing. Generally water-soluble products tend to impede wound healing more than ointments or creams. Solutions tend to evaporate. Ointments and creams remain in contact for too long, preventing drying of the wound. A clean wound in a healthy patient is best left to heal without using topical preparations. Aseptic technique and appropriate clean management of the wound are more appropriate.

FRACTURES

A fracture is a complete or incomplete break of bone continuity, with or without displacement of the resulting fragments. Figure 21.5 shows classification of fractures. Complete fractures are more common. A complete fracture is a break right the way through the bone and an incomplete fracture is only part of the way through the bone; with displacement the break is not in its normal anatomical position and if it has no displacement it is broken but remains in its normal position.

Fractures are classified according to the nature of the break (e.g. complete or incomplete) and the direction of the fracture line (Table 21.7). They can also be classified as uncomplicated or simple, or complicated or comminuted.

Simple fracture

- An uncomplicated fracture
- It has only one fracture line
- It can be with or without tearing and laceration of the soft tissue
- No wound leading from the fracture to the skin
- The direction of the fracture line may also be described

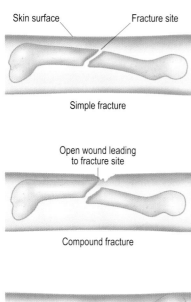

Simple fracture

Compound fracture

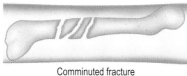

Comminuted fracture

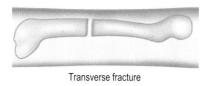

Transverse fracture

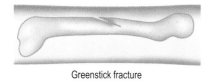

Greenstick fracture

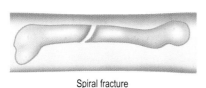

Spiral fracture

Figure 21.5 Classification of fractures. (Reproduced from Aspinall V 2006 *The Complete Textbook of Veterinary Nursing.* Butterworth Heinemann, London, with permission.)

Table 21.7 Classification of fracture sites	
Diaphyseal	Fracture in the diaphysis/midshaft Further divided into proximal, middle or distal
Physeal	Fracture through the growth plate of an immature animal; also known as Slater–Harris fracture Still open, cartilaginous, weaker than bone Proximal or distal
Epiphyseal	Articular fracture
Condylar	Fracture of epiphysis when the condyles are involved Distal humerus/distal femur Could be an avulsed fracture
Supracondylar	Fracture through shaft of humerus or femur just above condyles

- Transverse fracture: the line of the break is at 90° to the shaft of the bone
- Oblique fracture: the line of the break is at an oblique (/) angle to the shaft of the bone
- Spiral fracture: the line of the break spirals around the shaft of the bone.

Comminuted fracture

- Also known as a complex fracture
- It creates three or more fragments
- Sequestra or splinters of bone that become separated from the main bone are common with these fractures; the sequestra will eventually die as they have no blood supply.

Open fracture

This is a fracture which is exposed by an open wound, i.e. the fracture communicates with the external environment. This poses the potential for infiltration by pathogenic organisms. The wound can be gaping or a pinpoint, e.g. puncture wound from a canine tooth; the fracture is still classified as open.

During initial surveys it is advisable to check for skin penetration or look for gas shadows on radiographs to indicate an open fracture.

Closed fracture

This is a fracture which is not open, i.e. has no communication with the external environment. The skin barrier around the bone fragments is not breached and no communication with the environment occurs. It should be checked regularly as these can easily become open fractures.

Incomplete fracture

An incomplete fracture occurs when the bone is fissured (cracked) but the fragments are not separated by the fracture line or when the bone is only partially broken. The periosteum (covering of bone) is not torn. These fractures are common in juvenile animals where they are called greenstick fractures: the bone cracks and finer cracks run from it. They often heal with rest and casting.

Fissured fractures

These are mere cracks in the bone and are common in the bones of the face and skull; they are usually only serious if accompanied by haemorrhage (where it is the bleeding that is the primary issue).

Deferred fractures

Bone has been fractured but the fragments do not separate until or unless some extra force or strain is exerted upon the bone affected.

Pathological fracture

This is a fracture of a bone weakened by disease during normal use. It can be due to a generalised disease process, e.g. calcium deficiency, or a localised disease process, e.g. tumour in bone.

Avulsion fracture

In an avulsion fracture a bony prominence is torn away from the rest of the bone, usually by the pull of a muscle. These fractures are common in the condyles of femur and humerus, and are also known as distracted fractures.

Depression fracture

A fragment of bone is forced in below the level of the surrounding surface; they are common in the bones of the skull or in the vertebrae.

Complicated fractures

In complicated fractures some other serious injury is produced in addition to the fracture: for example, a dislocation of the hip in addition to a fractured femur or tearing a nerve.

Impacted fractures

One fragment of the bone is jammed inside another, usually at an angle; these often result from fall injuries where the upper part of the broken bone is forced into the lower portion.

Ununited fractures

In ununited fractures union has not occurred after the normal healing time. It may be due to delayed union because of illness, lack of rest or debilitation. Sometimes a piece of tissue, e.g. muscle, becomes placed in the fracture site, preventing healing.

Penetration fracture

These are caused by penetration of a foreign body such as a bullet and are usually incomplete fractures.

Definition of fracture sites

Most fractures occur in the long bones, e.g. femur, humerus. In veterinary medicine it is essential that as much information as possible can be recorded about the nature of a fracture, therefore a classification system exists to describe the location of the fracture site upon the long bone (Table 21.7).

Causes of fractures

Fractures may be pathological in nature, e.g. caused by disease, or as a result of excessive trauma. It is important to try and establish exactly how a fracture was caused as this will provide vital clues to what type of fracture is present.

Trauma can be classified as either indirect or direct. Indirect trauma can be where a limb is trapped in a hole or twists when falling and the bone is broken by the excessive leverage or indirect force applied to it. Direct trauma results in fracture from sheer physical force, e.g. a kick, gunshot or road traffic accident.

Fracture diagnosis

Fractured areas often present with:

- Uselessness of the affected site
- Crepitus of the fragments:
  - ○ Either felt or heard
  - ○ Can be due to arthritis
  - ○ Avoid excessive palpation: further soft-tissue damage

343

- Unnatural mobility:
  - Lameness
  - Masticatory problems
  - Smaller animals are more difficult to diagnose
- Deformity or distortion:
  - Visible or palpable
  - Compare to other limbs
- Inflammation:
  - Always present
  - May be due to another condition
  - Swelling present in early stages then replaced by a generalised oedema
- Localised heat
  - Due to inflammation
- Pain:
  - Related to inflammation
  - Tissue damage
  - Indirect tenderness can be more reliable than direct as this can be due to soft-tissue damage
  - Local tissue shock will exist for 20–30 minutes after incident and may reduce the sensation of the pain
- Contusions:
  - Discoloration of the affected area
- Radiographic signs:
  - Break in continuity of the bone
  - Radiolucency where fragments are distracted
  - Radiopacity where fragments are compressed or superimposed.

Fracture first aid

You should never try to reset or reduce the fracture in the first-aid situation. If you suspect a fractured spine it must always be supported.

The aim of first aid is to:

- Minimise movement
- Alleviate pain
- Prevent the condition deteriorating.

Always:

- Handle the broken limb as little as possible
- Control haemorrhage
- Support the fracture.

Remember the animal will be in pain and likely to bite. Always utilise restraining equipment, i.e. a muzzle, or consider stabilising the fracture postanalgesia.

Specific fracture first aid

- Cover any open wounds
- Immobilise fracture before moving animal
- Spinal fractures – keep straight

- Control haemorrhage
- Avoid drug therapy until the animal has had a full clinical examination.

Support dressings

1. Robert Jones bandage
2. Bandaging – the affected part can be bandaged to the unaffected parts so that the healthy part acts as a splint, e.g. scapula can be bound against the ribcage
3. Splints:
   - Zimmer splint:
     - Made of malleable aluminium backed with foam
     - Can be shaped to limb then bandaged to increase rigidity
   - Gutter splints:
     - Straight, non-malleable plastic with foam
     - Again, bandage to increase rigidity
     - Lack of movement limits use.

Fracture healing

1. A haematoma forms 6–8 hours posttrauma
2. Tissue and bone fragment necrosis initiates the inflammatory response
3. Haematoma is replaced by granulation tissue and stem cells to begin repair of fracture
4. Stem cells migrate from the periosteum and endosteum into fracture gap accompanied by new blood vessels derived from periosteal and medullary vessels
5. New tissue is synthesised, forming a callus
6. Callus consists of fibrous tissue, cartilage and bone
7. Callus envelopes bone ends, increasing stability as cartilage ossifies into new bone
8. Eventually the bone fragments are rigidly united by callus and clinical union takes place
9. Then follows a period of bone remodelling: initial callus is gradually removed and new bone is deposited
10. Accurate alignment of fracture fragments will lead to restoration of original bone shape. If more realignment occurs, then remodelling will shape bone to minimise pressure of exertive forces upon it, i.e. maximise its resistance.

The aim is to restore the functional anatomy of the fractured bone. This is achieved by restoring the continuity of bone, the length of bone and the functional shape of bone and maintaining soft-tissue function.

Reduction is the process of bringing fracture fragments back into correct anatomical alignment. This can be an open reduction, e.g. surgery, or closed reduction by manipulation. Fixation is where bone fragments are immobilised in correct alignment until clinical union occurs. The bone's blood supply must be preserved.

Rate of fracture healing

If no complications occur fractures then heal within 12–16 weeks in adult dogs and cats. Remodelling may continue for months or even years. Healing is usually assessed by patient progress in conjunction with radiographs, checking callus formation and mineralisation. Factors that affect healing include:

1. Age – immature animals heal quicker than adults, adults heal quicker than geriatrics
2. Osteomyelitis – inflammation and infection of bone marrow
3. Debilitation
4. Location of the fracture – cancellous bone heals quicker than compact bone
5. Blood supply – muscle coverage increases blood supply and therefore increases healing
6. Oblique fractures heal quicker than transverse fractures as there is an increased area for tissue regeneration
7. Success of reduction
8. Movement – immobilisation should occur.

Complications

These include:

- Non-union: complete failure of fractured ends of the bone to unite
- Delayed union: fracture healing progress is slower than expected
- Malunion: heals in poor alignment
- Osteomyelitis: infection delays healing
- Fracture disease: inability to flex the joints in a limb after fracture healing; one or more joints may be rigid in the affected limb due to scar formation
- Short limb: shortening occurs with inadequate reduction of overriding fracture fragments; limb function is often affected.

SPRAINS

The definition of a sprain is an injury which occurs when a synovial joint has been violently forced to move too far in one direction. It causes stretching and damage to the synovial membrane, ligaments and other soft tissue in the process, but the joint remains normal. Common sites of sprains are the shoulder, the stifle, the carpus and the tarsus. Clinical signs include swelling of the joint capsule, tenderness on palpation of the joint, especially

when moved in the direction of the stretched tissues, 50–90% lameness and no gross deformity of the limb. Treatment is to rest the joint to minimise swelling, perhaps apply a pressure bandage (Robert Jones) and use cold compresses to reduce inflammation.

STRAINS

The definition of a strain is the stretching or tearing of a muscle or tendon. Common sites are the muscles of the limbs. Clinical signs include 30–70% lameness, localised tenderness and swelling with no gross deformities. Treatment is rest, splinting the limb if necessary, application of a cold compress, a support bandage if applied immediately and hot fomentations, and the use of heat pads long-term relieves pain.

RUPTURED TENDONS

The definition of a ruptured tendon is a form of severe strain or injury in which the tendon is either partially or completely torn as a result of sudden violence.

Always check wounds to distal limbs for tendon damage. The tendons may also rupture due to indirect violence, e.g. twisting the leg awkwardly can rupture the Achilles tendon. Common sites include the tendons of the distal limbs and the gastrocnemius tendon (Achilles tendon). Clinical signs are: the animal's claws may stick upwards rather than down; if the Achilles tendon is affected the animal is unable to keep the hock straight and therefore, as it places its foot on the floor, the tarsus sinks to the ground; and the animal walks with the metatarsus on the ground like a kangaroo.

BANDAGING

An essential aspect of animal first aid is to be able to:

1. Carry out routine bandaging procedures
2. Advise clients on care and protection of bandages
3. Recognise problems with bandages.

Reasons for bandaging include:

- Support:
  - ○ Fractures, dislocations, sprains, strains, healing wounds
- Protection:
  - ○ From self-mutilation, infection, environment
- Pressure:
  - ○ Prevent oedema, haemorrhage

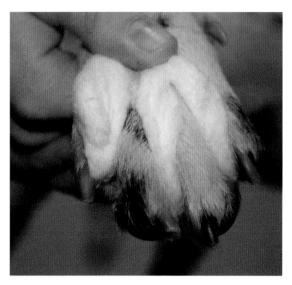

Figure 21.6 Bandaging technique in the dog: padding the toes.

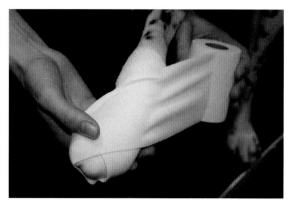

Figure 21.8 Application of adhesive bandage.

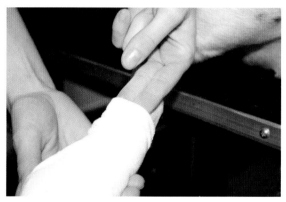

Figure 21.9 Checking the tension of the bandage. Two fingers should be able to fit inside the bandage comfortably.

How to apply a simple bandage

1. Select suitable materials (Table 21.8) and position the animal conveniently
2. Restrain the patient
3. Prepare the area to be bandaged – ensure it is clean, pathogen-free and dry
4. Apply a suitable dressing to the affected area
5. Apply a layer of padding to prevent sores, decubitus ulcers (with foot bandages, remember to pad between the toes)
6. Apply a layer of bandaging material (conforming)
7. Apply a layer of covering material (Table 21.9)
8. Check the fit of the bandage – tight/loose.

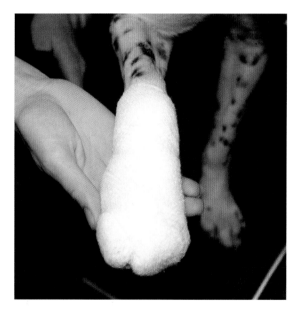

Figure 21.7 Application of conforming bandage.

- Immobilisation:
  - To restrict movement to promote healing or provide pain relief.

See Figures 21.6–21.9 for bandaging techniques and types of application.

Note that materials should overlap by one-half of the bandage width and should be applied at a constant pressure to ensure there are no pressure points on the bandage. For ear bandages it is advisable to draw an

Table 21.8 Bandaging materials

White open weave	Natural material Non-conforming Frays easily
Conforming bandage	Follows shape of area to be bandaged Strong, neat
Cohesive bandage	Self-adhering Does not stick to hair or skin Strong, flexible Conforming
Tubular bandage	Elasticated Made of cotton or nylon Apply using applicator Limbs/tails
Crêpe bandage	Used in human first aid – triangular bandage Washable/reusable Can use head/thorax

Table 21.9 Bandage covering materials

Zinc oxide tape	Adhesive Inelastic Non-conforming Frays
Elastoplast	Adhesive Elastic Varying size Conforming
Non-adhesive tape	Adheres only to itself, not the patient

arrow indicating the location of the pinna to prevent damage when the bandage is removed.

Care of a bandage

- Keep it dry
- Avoid self-mutilation
- Avoid soiling with excrement
- Watch for oedema
- Watch for discharge
- Watch for skin irritation
- Watch for odours

- Check bandage is neither too tight nor too loose (you should be able to fit two fingers snugly into the top of the bandage).

Problems and how to avoid them

Self-mutilation

- Elizabethan collars
- Muzzles
- Discipline
- Bitter sprays
- Sedation.

Soiling/wetness

- Only take the animal out when dry and when necessary
- Use a plastic bag
- Use an old intravenous fluid bag with the top chopped off: boot with bandage
- Avoid licking.

CASTING

- Casts can be used to immobilise a limb
- Use fibreglass, plaster of Paris or commercial casting preparations
- Casts must be monitored carefully and padding layers should be applied to avoid ulcers on the bony prominences.

FIRST AID FOR FITS AND CONVULSIONS

See Box 21.4 for useful definitions.

A partial seizure is one which is restricted to a focal area of the brain, therefore the corresponding area of the body is the only part affected, e.g. the animal goes blind or cannot use one limb. A grand mal is a seizure with no localising signs which has a brief period of restlessness followed by unconsciousness, generalised muscular activity, excessive salivation, nystagmus and often urination or defecation. A petit mal is a mild, very brief generalised seizure.

Seizures/epilepsy

- Epilepsy – a medical condition where seizures will recur; not due to a short-term problem or an underlying disease
- Seizure – manifestation of a fit: can usually be related to a short-term problem or underlying disease.

DEFINITIONS

Fit

An episode characterised by inappropriate and involuntary motor activity. The most common manifestation is a convulsion

Convulsion

A series of involuntary contractions of the voluntary muscles

Note: convulsions are a symptom of a neurological disease but not a disease themselves

Seizure

A convulsion or attack of epilepsy, subdivided into:

Audiogenic

Brought on by sound

Cerebral

Attack of epilepsy

Eleptiform

Resembling epilepsy or its manifestations

Focal

Partial seizure

Generalised

Grand mal

First-aid treatment of fits/convulsions

Signs of a convulsion include:

- Head shaking
- Facial twitching
- Spastic collapse
- Paddling
- Excessive salivation
- Nystagmus
- Increased respiratory rate
- Spontaneous urination/defecation
- Duration is on average 1–2 minutes
- May be continuous, and if so, is more severe.

The main first-aid consideration is to prevent the animal causing any further injury to itself.

Action

1. Make the animal secure – minimal external stimulation, place in a darkened area, pad around the animal
2. Take a history to try and establish the cause (this is important in case it is poisoning)
3. Contact veterinary surgeon
4. Monitor and record all vital signs
5. Make ready drug therapy.

Treatment

If the patient is found convulsing:

- If at surgery, intravenous catheterisation or intravenous diazepam is indicated (under the direction of the veterinary surgeon)
- Be aware that the patient will be dissociated, therefore likely to bite, so care should be taken
- Place blankets around the patient:
  - To protect the animal from injury whilst thrashing about
  - To act as a sponge for any urine passed
- Lower lights in room and quieten area if possible
- Constant observation.

After the convulsion

- Clean away excessive salivation
- Ensure airway is patent
- Avoid unnecessary stimulation via touching
- Move the patient to a cool, padded, darkened kennel if not already in such a location
- Observe frequently.

If the patient is a known epileptic animal that has been stabilised, all staff members should be notified. Again intravenous anticonvulsant therapy is administered and the patient must receive its normal routine of anticonvulsant, as these agents are often time-specific.

GERIATRIC FIRST-AID EMERGENCIES

Elderly animals suffer from many generalised malaises due to the degeneration of their anatomical and physiological systems.

The main first-aid scenarios which may present in the geriatric patient are:

- Heart attacks
- Fits/convulsions
- Metabolic failure
- Cerebrovascular accident.

Heart attacks

Heart attack is a cardiopulmonary arrest; cardiopulmonary arrest is a sudden cessation of functional ventilation and effective circulation. It is often precipitated by:

- Hypovolaemia
- Metabolic acidosis

- Respiratory failure
- Underlying cardiac disease, e.g. cardiomyopathy, congestive heart failure.

Successful recovery depends on the patient's history, health status, previous drug therapy, precipitating event and the skill of the veterinary team. Only 1–10% patients are successfully revived. Clinical signs include:

- In the conscious patient, loss of consciousness and cessation of respiration – gasping may occur just after cardiac arrest
- Pupils become fixed and dilated within 30–45 seconds
- CRT can remain normal for several minutes after cardiac arrest if the cardiovascular system was normal prior to the incident
- Mucous membranes may be cyanotic, grey, dusty pink, pale or normal – beware anaesthetised animals on 100% oxygen
- No palpable pulse is present
- Diagnostic electrocardiogram will show asystole and absence of an audible heart beat.

First-aid actions

1. Assess patient – what is the patient's previous health status?
2. Call for help! For successful resuscitation 2–3 people are required with most animals
3. Begin basic cardiac support – if indicated, begin advanced cardiac life support.

Metabolic failure

Aged animals can suffer from numerous metabolic disorders, including dehydration, hypokalaemia leading to metabolic acidosis, hyperkalaemia leading to metabolic alkalosis and other electrolyte disorders. Hypokalaemia can occur in patients suffering from polyuria and polydipsia (chronic renal failure) which are both common in the elderly animal. Clinical signs include muscle weakness, ventroflexion of the neck in cats, gastrointestinal weakness, poor renal water conservation, poor cardiovascular function and cardiac arrhythmias. Treatment is to obtain a thorough history, correct the underlying disease and/or dietary problems and to restore the acid base balance via specialised fluid therapy.

Hyperkalaemia can be life-threatening and should be treated promptly and the underlying cause must be treated. Hyperkalaemia can be caused by oliguric or anuric renal failure, urethral obstruction, Addison's disease, diabetes mellitus, tissue breakdown or renal insufficiency. In severe cases the patient may present in a moribund state, be suffering from circulatory collapse and be exhibiting muscle weakness or periodic paralysis.

Treatment is to discontinue all medication, intravenous catheterisation, indicated fluid therapy, indicated drug therapy and possibly peritoneal dialysis.

Cerebrovascular accident

This is a disorder of the blood vessels serving the cerebrum, resulting from an impaired blood supply to the brain. It would be called a stroke in human medicine. Clinical signs are akin to a 'funny turn' and should not be confused with vestibular syndrome, which is much more common in elderly canine patients.

Hyperthermia: heat stroke

Clinical signs include:

- Pyrexia
- Tachypnoea/orthopnoea
- Restless
- Cyanosis
- Profuse salivation
- Collapse, which may lead to coma and subsequent death.

Treatment

- Oxygen
- Intubate
- Cool – cold-water baths, hose pipe, ice packs
- Check rectal temperature at least every 15 minutes until it reaches 39°C
- At this point, put the animal into a cool kennel and offer copious water – keep checking the patient's temperature every 30 minutes
- Chilled intravenous fluids.

Hypothermia: frostbite

- Usually affects young, small, drowned, small animals and animals under general anaesthetic.

Clinical signs

- Sleepy/lethargic
- Lack of appetite
- Weakness which may lead to coma
- Subnormal temperature.

Treatment

- Massage with warm towels
- Warmed intravenous fluids
- Bedding, heat pads/lamps, hot-water bottles, hair dryer.

349

POISONING

A poison can be defined as a toxin or toxic agent. An animal is said to be poisoned when the poisonous agent produces clinical effects in the animal.

An antidote is a substance which neutralises a poison by rendering it harmless or establishing a body reaction.

It is essential to have knowledge of common poisons and their effects if you work with animals. A general poisoning protocol would be to:

- Obtain a comprehensive history
- Give first-aid advice over the telephone
- Examine the patient and perform first aid/supportive therapy
- Obtain samples of any body fluids, e.g. vomit, faeces, urine and agent for forensic examination or in case litigation is undertaken
- Samples must be clearly labelled with:
  ○ Name and address of owner
  ○ Animal's name and description
  ○ Time and date of collection
  ○ Signature of collector
- Be professional – remain impartial in cases where a third party may be suspected of involvement
- Ensure access to a poison information unit is available.

Veterinary Poisons Information Service (VPIS)

This is an organisation that provides a 24-hour service to subscribing veterinary surgeons. It can supply data on the clinical effects of a number and range of poisonous compounds, advise on the treatment of specific poisons and advise on antidote therapies if applicable.

Action in a suspected poisoning case

See Figure 21.10 for action to take in a suspected case of poisoning.

Poisoning is not common and in most cases can be attributable to an animal eating something it shouldn't have access to and not maliciousness.

General considerations

Species of patient

Pups chew most things and eat them, e.g. plants, rat bait. Cats are cautious but will ingest toxins on their coat via grooming or eat poisoned prey, and they are more susceptible to liver damage from drug overdose as they have a poor liver enzyme system. Birds are susceptible to inhalant toxins. Horses and large-animal species may inadvertently graze on poisonous plants in their

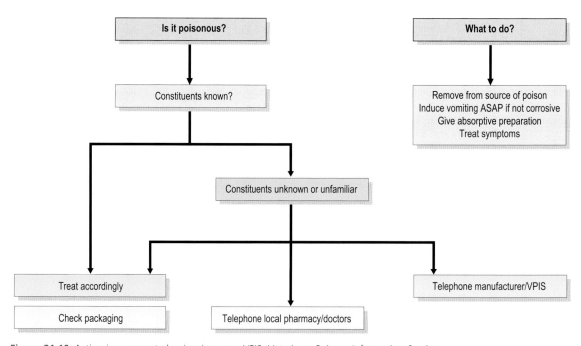

Figure 21.10 Action in a suspected poisoning case. VPIS, Veterinary Poisons Information Service.

pastures. Reptiles and amphibians are susceptible to toxins in water to which they may become exposed.

Common poisons

There are three main groups of poisons:

1. Those classed as available substances because they are toxic. These are generally palatable and often ingested in large quantities, e.g. rat and mouse bait, molluscicides, insecticides and pesticides
2. Those which are substances not intended for consumption but that have toxic effects, e.g. antifreeze, bleach, oil, creosote and paint stripper
3. Naturally occurring substances such as bee and wasp stings, snake venom and poisonous plants.

Poisons can also be grouped according to their effects on the animal. This helps when determining the treatment, as most poison cases cannot be specifically diagnosed primarily. Due to the rapid actions of poisons, treatment must be initiated immediately. If the general type of action of the poison is determined then a general treatment can be begun.

Possible treatment regimes

One regime is to increase the metabolic rate and thus excrete the poisonous agent. Most poisons are metabolised by the liver then excreted by the kidney, so in poisoning cases these organs must be operating at their maximum capabilities. This can be helped to be achieved by:

- Intravenous fluids, diuretics, oral fluids
- Manipulation of urine pH can increase the rate of excretion of poisons, e.g. aspirin is acidic, therefore if urine is made alkaline then there will be rapid excretion of the aspirin
- Increasing liver function by the administration of anabolic steroids and water-soluble vitamins.

If the patient has central nervous system depression:

- Increase consciousness/maintain by oxygen therapy and respiratory stimulants, e.g. Dopram-V.

Maintain body temperature:

- In hypothermic poisons: increase body temperature
- In hyperthermic poisons: decrease body temperature
- Monitor the rectal temperature periodically.

Anticonvulsant therapy

- Some poisons cause convulsions which can be treated with diazepam

- Beware – some agents cause fits, then central nervous system depression, and treatment for convulsions can worsen this effect, leading to a quicker death.

Groups of poisons

Irritant/corrosive

- These directly damage the tissues they contact
- Skin and mucous membranes are most affected
- An example is bleach.

Narcotic/sedative

- Similar effects to sedative drugs and anaesthetic agents
- Cause sleepiness, depression, collapse, unconsciousness, coma and death
- Examples include alpha-chloralose, anticonvulsants, antidepressants and sedatives.

Convulsants

- Cause central nervous system to become hyperactive
- Result in twitching, shaking, overactivity, convulsions and death
- Rapid onset of action
- Examples include metaldehyde, strychnine, nicotine, lead and phenols.

Anticoagulants

- Reduce coagulation in cardiovascular system, leading to haemorrhage
- Examples include warfarin and salicylates (aspirin).

Summary of route of access to poisons

- Baits against pests
- Eating baited prey
- Licking contaminated hair
- Drug overdose
- Poisonous plants
- Absorption through skin/mucous membranes
- Inhalation
- Malicious administration.

General methods of treatment

Successful treatment depends upon:

- Prevention of further absorption of poison
- Identification of poison
- Treating the symptoms
- Giving an antidote if available.

351

Inhaled poisons

- Carbon monoxide
- Acrolein (overheated fat)
- Lead (paint fumes)
- Nicotine
- Actions:
  - Improve ventilation
  - Give oxygen therapy
  - Keep animal quiet
  - Intermittent positive-pressure ventilation if necessary.

Ingested poisons

The aim is to remove as much of the poison from the gastrointestinal tract as possible and prevent as much as possible from being absorbed into the blood stream. Methods to facilitate this include inducing vomiting by administering emetics, use of absorbents such as charcoal to neutralise the poison in the stomach and fluid therapy to dilute the poison. The use of emetics needs to be carefully considered, especially if the poison is unknown, as if it is an irritant substance it could cause more damage as it comes back out of the digestive system.

Emetics

There are two classes: direct and indirect. Direct emetics are taken orally and cause irritation to the stomach, thereby inducing vomiting.

Examples

- Mustard solution – 2 teaspoons/cup warm water – ineffective
- Salt solution – 2 teaspoons/cup water – ineffective/ electrolyte imbalance
- Washing soda crystals – 1/2 pea-sized orally – effective
- Fingers down throat – you will get bitten!
- Hydrogen peroxide – dilute or corrosive
- Syrup of ipecac.

Indirect emetics are injected into the blood stream and act via the brain nerve centre to induce vomiting.

Examples

- Apomorphine – do not give to cats
- Xylazine.

These can only be used under guidance from a veterinary surgeon and somebody should always stay with the animal whilst it is vomiting to monitor it.

Emetics must not be given if:

- Poison is corrosive/irritant
- Animal is convulsing
- Animal is unconscious
- It is 4 hours or more since ingestion.

Gastric lavage

It is recommended that this procedure is performed under sedation or anaesthetic. The animal is intubated using the largest endotracheal tube available. The cuff is inflated to prevent water entering the respiratory tract. The end should be at least 4 cm from the animal's mouth. The method is as follows:

- Measure a wide-bore stomach tube and insert to the mark
- Tilt the body so the stomach is higher than the mouth
- Add plain water into the (warmed) stomach tube, allow it to drain or use a syringe and add little and often rather than one large amount
- Continue flushing until water returning is clear
- Keep sample of poison and measure pH
- Add a small amount of crushed inactivated charcoal to stomach to absorb any remaining toxins.

Surface poisons

These are often corrosive or irritant. They may be ingested, causing damage to the digestive tract and may be licked off or absorbed through the mucous membranes.

Non-oily compounds

- Examples include disinfectants
- If unknown, wash with copious amounts of water
- If known, take appropriate action.

Liquid oily compounds

- Clean with Swarfega or equivalent (detergent)
- Rinse well until smell of contaminant has disappeared.

Solid oily compounds

- Example includes tar
- Clip fur if the compound will not wash off
- If contamination is close to the skin, apply liquid paraffin, margarine or butter to the area or try to remove it with solvents such as acetone
- Put on a buster collar to prevent ingestion/skin damage.

Note that some chemicals will be corrosive to humans too, so wear protective clothing.

Acids/alkalis

Examples include:

- Battery acid – sulphuric acid
- Sodium hydroxide
- Formic acid (in disinfectants)
- Acetic acid
- Paint strippers.

Their effects are as follows:

- Cause contamination of the skin/gastrointestinal tract
- Signs include stomatitis, ulceration, enteritis, dermatitis, salivation, vomiting and diarrhoea
- Treatment – with an acid, give alkali and vice versa
- Do not use emetics but attempt gastric lavage
- Use absorbents/protectants.

Ethylene glycol

- Antifreeze
- Palatable due to its sweetness (dogs)
- Signs:
  - Central nervous system depressant
  - Depression
  - Weakness
  - Ataxia
  - Metabolised to oxalic crystals which are deposited within body tissues
- Causes acute renal failure: convulsions, uraemia, acidosis, coma, leading to death (within 24 hours if a large amount is ingested)
- Treatment:
  - Ethanol within 4 hours of ingestion
  - 20% alcohol + 5% sodium bicarbonate to correct acidosis 55 ml/kg intraperitoneally
  - Charcoal
  - Anticonvulsants
  - Intravenous fluid, diuretics (monitor urine output)
  - Peritoneal dialysis.

Lead

- Source: old pipes/paint/batteries/golf balls/lino/putty/solder/fishing weights
- Usually affects dogs
- Accumulative poison
- Signs:
  - Anorexia
  - Vomiting
  - Diarrhoea/constipation
  - Abdominal pain
  - Acute irritation
  - Mucus discharge
  - Depression, aggression, excitement – central nervous system effect
  - Hyperaesthesia
  - Muscle spasms
  - Convulsions
  - Paralysis
  - Blindness
  - Death
- Treatment:
  - Gastric lavage, not emetics
  - Bathe skin with olive oil/water
  - Intravenous fluids
  - Possible glucosaline if dehydrated
- Insecticides:
  - Surface toxins usually ingested by cats via grooming
  - Signs include salivation, hyperactivity, ataxia
  - Treatment: emetics, anticonvulsants, bathing, fatty foods and drinks, e.g. milk is not to be given as it increases absorption in the gastrointestinal tract.

Organophosphates

- Dichlorvos (e.g. sheep dip)
- Signs: vomiting, salivation, constricted pupils, muscle twitching, sweating, dyspnoea, bradycardia, paralysis, convulsions, coma and death
- Treatment : atropine sulphate injection.

Borax

- Nippon/ant killers
- Honey-based, therefore attractive to dogs and cats
- Signs: vomiting and diarrhoea, collapse, convulsions, paralysis, death
- Treatment: symptomatic.

Molluscicides

Metaldehyde – slug pellets

- Signs: excitement, anxiety
- Tremors
- Tachycardia/ tachypnoea
- Hyperaesthesia
- Nystagmus
- Ataxia
- Hyperthermia
- Salivation
- Convulsions, coma, death
- Treatment: barbiturates (in fits), emetics and oxygen.

353

Methocarbamol – slug bait

- Signs: hypersalivation, vomiting, colic, dyspnoea, ataxia
- Treatment: atropine sulphate every 3–6 hours.

Rodenticides

Alphachoralose – green

- Bait/poisoned prey
- Signs: hypothermia, depression, incoordination, coma
- Cats become excited and aggressive, twitch ears and convulse
- Treatment: warmth, emetics, avoid sedatives, stimulant drugs.

Warfarin – blue

- Bait/poisoned prey
- Anticoagulant poison: the animal may bleed to death
- Signs: haemorrhage, shock
- Pale mucous membranes, anaemia, haematomas
- Tachypnoea/tachycardia
- Lameness
- Vomiting and diarrhoea
- Collapse and death
- Diagnosis – measure stage 1 clotting time
- Treatment: care when handling, vitamin K, blood transfusions, oxygen, avoid blood-thinning drugs.

Strychnine

- Used for moles/birds
- Very rapid onset of action
- Signs: sudden death, hyperexcitability, tremors, convulsions, vomiting, salivation, acid–base disturbances
- Treatment: anticonvulsants, gastric lavage with 1/1000 potassium permanganate
- Calciferol (excess vitamin D)
- Signs: anorexia, depression, diarrhoea, arching of back, polyuria, polydipsia and kidney failure
- Treatment: emetics, high fluid intake, low-calcium diet, avoid sunlight.

Poisonous plants

Laburnum

- All plant is poisonous
- Common in puppies

- Central nervous system stimulants, therefore signs include vomiting, excitement, convulsions, respiratory failure, leading to death
- Treatment: emetics, symptomatic.

Nicotine

- Ingestion of plant, cigarettes, cigars
- Affects parasympathetic nervous system
- Signs: salivation, abdominal pain, vomiting and diarrhoea, convulsions, paralysis, tachypnoea, tachycardia, coma, leading to death
- Treatment: gastric lavage.

Other common poisonous plants include:

- Fungi
- Horsetails
- Bracken
- Yew
- Monkshood
- Rape
- White mustard
- Hemlock
- Deadly nightshade
- Acorns
- Ragwort.

Drugs with toxic effects

All drugs have the potential to be toxic but some have greater safety margins than others. Absolute overdose is when an animal is given an incorrect dose. A relative overdose is a normal dose given but the animal cannot metabolise or excrete it perhaps due to age (young or old) or liver or kidney disease.

Use in inappropriate species, i.e. given to an animal it was not intended for (often human drugs), can result in overdose. Drugs used in inappropriate combinations can result in the combining agents rendering them potentially toxic.

An example is aspirin which acts as a cumulative poison; small dogs and cats are susceptible. Clinical signs include:

- Vomiting
- Inappetite
- Ataxia
- Depression
- Acid–base disturbances
- Hypoglycaemia
- Convulsions
- Reduced clotting time
- Gastrointestinal tract irritation
- Hyperthermia.

Treatment includes gastric lavage, emetics, charcoal and purgatives.

Paracetamol is another common drug that can be toxic to cats. In cats it converts haemoglobin to methaemoglobin and 'muddy' mucous membranes are seen. It causes liver damage and haemolysis with clinical signs including cyanosis, icterus, haemoglobinuria, anaemia, anorexia, vomiting, toxaemia, facial oedema, tachypnoea and tachycardia. Treatment is ascorbate (which converts methaemoglobin back to oxyhaemoglobin), drugs to protect the liver, oxygen and blood transfusions.

Diagnosis/sample taking

Samples which may prove useful include:

- Food that has been ingested
- Samples of vomit
- Postmortem samples (stomach, liver, kidneys, urine).

Some poisons leave a distinctive odour on the body:

- Carbolic soap: phenols
- Almonds: cyanide
- Formaldehyde: metaldehyde.

Samples

- All samples should be placed in glass containers as plastics can react with some chemicals
- May require specific fixing agents (usually 70% alcohol) – consult the lab
- Refrigerate until posted
- Label the sample accurately with the identity of animal, owner and sample taker; in legal cases seal and sign bottles
- Lab must be provided with complete clinical history, i.e. drug therapy
- Labs only search for specific poisons – list ideas
- Ensure the client is aware of the cost involved before undertaking forensic examinations.

FIRST AID FOR INJURIES TO THE HEAD

Ophthalmic emergencies

A true ophthalmic emergency is a situation where a delay in treatment would jeopardise the function of the eye. However the eye is a very sensitive structure and any injury to it should be dealt with as soon as possible.

Examination should occur in a darkened room to assess pupillary and palpebral reflexes and to assess pupil size (anisocoria can indicate brain damage). An ophthalmoscope should be used to examine the extra-

---

Box 21.5

DEFINITIONS

Blepharospasm

Swollen eyelids, screwed up against the light

Chemosis

Oedematous conjunctiva bulging up over eyelid margin

Epiphora

Excessive tear production

Photophobia

Dislike of bright light

---

ocular structures for damage such as lacerations of head and periocular tissues, fractures, position and size of the globe, movement of the eye, discharge and blepharospasm. Examine the intraocular tissues for damage but avoid touching as it is very easy to damage them. Look for lacerations, foreign bodies, haemorrhage, abrasions, oedema, opacities, abnormal positions and any evidence of self-trauma (Box 21.5).

Proptosis

- Acute forward displacement of the eye beyond the boundaries of the bony orbit and the eyelids, leading to prolapsed eyeball
- Common in brachiocephalic breeds
- Often caused by blunt trauma or can be due to excessive restraint.

Clinical signs

- Worst-case scenario – eye is completely out of its socket – this is exophthalmos
- Haemorrhage
- Eyelids contracted and turn inwards
- Medial rectal muscle is often damaged, causing the eye to be displaced laterally.

Lid injuries

- These can be due to foreign bodies
- Commonly due to scratches, bites and lacerations.

Clinical signs

- Swelling
- Oedema
- Haemorrhage
- Possible tissue loss.

Conjunctival injuries

- Vary from superficial damage to full-thickness lacerations
- Due to trauma or foreign bodies
- Superficial ulcer
- Deep ulcer
- Complicated ulcers
- Penetrating corneal wounds
- Penetrating foreign bodies
- Chemical keratitis.

Clinical signs

- Blepharospasm
- Epiphora, blood
- Subconjunctival haemorrhage
- Total eyelid closure
- Wrinkled cornea.

Anterior uveitis

- Inflammation of the uvea can be due to trauma, neoplasia, inflammation or infection
- Red and painful appearance to the eye
- Miotic pupil, corneal oedema (cloudy)
- Diagnosed using ophthalmoscope.

Hyphema

- Haemorrhage within the anterior chamber of the eye can be due to trauma, neoplasia, bleeding disorders
- Presents as a red eye due to anterior chamber being filled with fresh red blood
- This can darken as and when the blood clots.

Glaucoma

- Glaucoma is an increase in intraocular pressure
- If not treated within 12–24 hours it can result in permanent damage to the optic nerve and retina, leading to blindness
- Normal intraocular pressure is 15–30 mmHg
- Measure using a tonometer: 50 mmHg will cause permanent damage
- Inherited in Basset Hounds, American Cocker Spaniels and Bouviers amongst others
- Can be a secondary complication of uveitis or due to neoplasia or anterior lens luxation.

Clinical signs

- Eye presents very painful and red
- Corneal oedema can be seen
- Mydriatic pupil
- Abnormal papillary light reflexes
- Vision impairment may or may not be present.

Retinal detachment

- Presents with all or virtually all vision loss
- Can be due to trauma or neoplasia or of medical cause.

Foreign bodies

- These easily lodge under the eyelids or beneath the third eyelid
- If present for a long time they will present with a purulent discharge
- Cleanse eye but do not use antiseptic solutions, as they will sting
- Use ice packs and cold compresses to reduce inflammation
- If non-penetrating, remove if possible
- Topical anaesthetic agents will help
- Be careful not to leave any behind
- Small debris, e.g. grit, can be removed by lavage
- If a foreign body does not move during lavage, assume it has penetrated the eye and do not attempt to remove it.

Fractured skull

- Fractures of the orbital bones can cause trauma to the eye
- Usually there is only bruising – seen as a red blob on sclera
- Eye globe may present bulging out due to haemorrhage behind it
- Papillary reflexes may be impaired
- Animal may be concussed
- Apply cold compresses and treat shock.

Direct trauma

- Direct trauma is caused by blows and kicks
- Can cause haemorrhage
- Treat shock.

Chemical damage

- Flush eye and cover with dressing and await veterinary surgeon
- Alkaline solutions: can use vinegar solutions
- Acidic solutions: can use a bicarbonate solution
- Hot fat: use liquid paraffin
- If in doubt, use sterile saline and flush thoroughly.

Stings and allergic reactions

- Animals often stick their head in areas where they shouldn't, resulting in bites, stings or allergic reactions

- Treat with cold compresses to reduce inflammatory response
- Will present with oedema of the conjunctiva.

Ear injuries

These can be classified into damage to the pinna, foreign bodies and vestibular syndrome.

Pinna injuries

- Can be due to trauma, particularly dog bites, insect stings, snake bites
- Aural haematomas.

Clinical signs

- Head shaking
- Oedema
- Haemorrhage
- Discharge
- Closed wounds due to bites will incite an inflammatory response and therefore will be hot and painful
- An aural haematoma will be swollen but cool to the touch
- Haemorrhage from the pinna should be treated using pressure and bandaged
- Be careful if clipping wounds here as it is very easy to tear the ear flap
- Aural haematomas can be drained but often require surgical intervention
- Self-trauma is to be expected so be prepared!

Foreign bodies

- Often grass seeds but can be virtually anything small enough to fit in the ear.

Clinical signs

- Head shaking
- Pawing at ears or rubbing along the floor
- Purulent discharge
- Pain, especially on palpation externally
- Often lodge at base of ear canal.

Treatment

- If you can see the foreign body and the patient is amenable, try and remove it
- Can use lubricant agents to soothe, e.g. olive oil, liquid paraffin
- Surgical intervention may be required.

Vestibular syndrome

- Owners will often think their pet has suffered a stroke, as the symptoms are remarkably similar to human strokes
- Caused by an injury to the vestibular system in the inner ear and not by a cerebrovascular accident as in humans
- Very hard to determine what has caused injury but may be due to inner-ear inflammation or encephalitis.

Clinical signs

- Sudden onset
- Tends to affect older patients
- Nystagmus
- Head tilt, uncoordination
- Some present in collapsed state
- Pedal reflexes are often dulled but eye reflexes are usually unaffected.

Treatment

- Very little you can do except tender loving care to patient and owner
- Confine the animal in a warm, darkened kennel to restrict movement and prevent any further damage
- The veterinary surgeon may try steroid therapy but patients often do not recover fully.

Other head injuries

- Fractures due to trauma or pathological causes
- Common in mandible, maxilla and mandibular symphysis
- Fractured or missing teeth (Figures 21.11 and 21.12) will need treatment to remove
- Wounds: treat as for wound first aid, remembering ABC (see above).

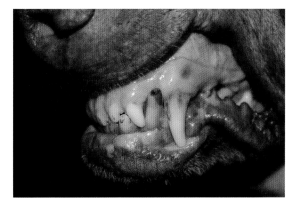

Figure 21.11 Broken canine tooth: note the accumulation of tartar on the intact canine tooth.

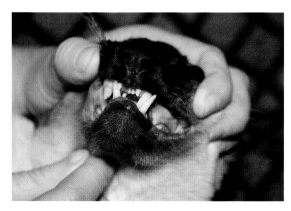

Figure 21.12 Cat dentition after a road traffic accident. Note the broken and missing teeth, and misalignment of the jaw.

STINGS AND BITES

Snakes and other reptiles

- The only native UK venomous snake is the adder (it has a distinctive V on its head)
- Current fashion is for people to keep more exotic and potentially poisonous pets
- Clinical signs of bite are the bite wound, inflammation, oedema, reddening and heat
- Treatment:
  - Identify poison/reptile
  - Prevent further absorption by applying a tourniquet (watch constantly and remove the tourniquet after 15 minutes and reapply it)
  - Flush wound
  - Administer antivenom
  - Treat shock and symptoms.

Toad poisoning

- Toad skin is coated with a toxic slime to prevent ingestion

- Cats and dogs will often pick toads up and ingest a dose of poison
- Clinical signs: profuse salivation, pawing at head/mouth
- No specific treatment: flush with water and wipe away saliva
- Possibly use atropine/corticosteroids.

Insect stings

- Rarely severe unless animal undergoes anaphylactic reaction, leading to asphyxia
- Clinical signs characterised by inflammatory response
- Bee stings: remove sting (it has a backward barb), grasp as close to the skin as possible to prevent squeezing the poison sacs, bathe with alkaline bicarbonate solution: 1 teaspoon bicarbonate to 0.25 litre of water
- Wasp stings: bathe with acidic vinegar solution: 50:50 vinegar:water
- In some cases treatment with antihistamines/corticosteroids is indicated.

Bibliography

Aspinall V 2006 The complete textbook of veterinary nursing. Butterworth Heinemann, London

Dallas S 2006 Animal biology and care. 2nd edn. Wiley/Blackwell, Oxford

Lane D R, Cooper B, Turner L 2007 Textbook of veterinary nursing, 3rd edn. Butterworth-Heinemann/BSAVA, Oxford

McIntyre D, Drobatz K, Haskins S et al. 2003 Manual of small animal emergency and critical care. Wiley/Blackwell, Oxford

Moore M 2000 Manual of veterinary nursing. BSAVA, Oxford

Pratt P W 1998 Principles and practice of veterinary technology. Mosby, Philadelphia

Simpson G 1994 Practical veterinary nursing, 3rd edn. BSAVA, Oxford

Warren D M 1995 Small animal care and management. Delmar, New York

Chapter | **22** | *Jane Williams*

Nutrition

This chapter identifies the essential nutrients that animals require in their diet and the functions for which these are needed. Life stage and clinical nutrition principles are explored with reference to specific animal species.

Nutrients are substances present in food that are required by organisms for:

- Growth and repair of body
- Metabolic processes
- Energy source.

Obtaining nutrients is so important that many organisms have undergone specific adaptations in response to their nutritional needs and the means by which they obtain and process food. An organism's body plan and lifestyle are adapted to its individual method of obtaining food. Heterotrophs are organisms that must obtain their energy and nourishment from the organic molecules manufactured by other organisms. They include all animal species; macromolecules are eaten, broken down and then assimilated to meet the animal's own needs. For example, when you eat a fillet steak it is broken down into amino acids via the digestive system and then these amino acids are rebuilt into muscle tissue in your body.

Ingestion is the process of food being taken into the digestive system. Digestion is the breakdown of food inside the organism to its basal nutrients to enable them to be utilised, e.g. lipids are digested to their basic components, fatty acids and glycerol. Absorption describes the passage of nutrients through the cells lining the digestive tract and into body fluids or blood. Elimination is the final stage of the process when undigested and unabsorbed food is ejected from the body.

MODES OF NUTRITION

Animals ultimately depend upon plants for their food, energy and oxygen.

They can be divided into one of three main categories: herbivores, which are classed as primary consumers and eat exclusively or mainly plant material; carnivores, which are flesh eaters, classified as secondary consumers and consume herbivores or each other; and omnivores, which are animal species that eat both plants and animals. An obligate carnivore is an animal that requires meat in its diet, e.g. cat.

Adaptations of herbivores include:

- They eat only algae or plants
- Their diet may be restricted to certain parts of a plant, e.g. roots, leaves or a specific plant or plants
- Many aquatic herbivores are filter feeders, e.g. whale, which filters plankton
- Plant cells contain a large quantity of cellulose and are difficult to digest. Herbivores have various adaptations to overcome these problems
- Insects have tough, piercing mouthparts to enable them to pierce cellulose cell wall and suck sap or nectar from the tonoplast
- Other herbivores eat vast quantities of food, e.g. cows, grasshoppers, locusts, elephants, and usually excrete lots of waste, almost unchanged
- Some possess specialised teeth and jaws with wide molars for grinding plant material; some species of rhinoceros use their lips to break open seeds
- Others have specialised digestive systems which are longer and more elaborate than those of carnivores
- There is a symbiotic relationship with microorganisms in their digestive tracts; microorganisms break down the cellulose cell walls, allowing access to cell nutrients, e.g. cow, horse, termites.

Adaptations of carnivores include:

- Carnivores eat meat and possibly bones
- They need to find and capture prey and possess adaptations for this purpose
- Hydra have long tentacles with stinging cells to paralyse their prey
- Vertebrate carnivores have a multitude of adaptations
- Frogs have a fast-moving tongue
- Lions have sharp teeth, muscular legs and claws
- All have well-developed canine teeth for stabbing during combat and developed molars for tearing or shredding meat into easily swallowed chunks
- They possess a specialised digestive tract and digestive juices designed to break down proteins
- Their digestive tracts are shorter than those of herbivores because meat is easier to digest.

Adaptations of omnivores include:

- Omnivores include both plant and animal material in their diet
- These are obtained via a variety of mechanisms
- Aquatic filter feeders tend to ingest both plant and animal material
- Earthworms ingest plant and animal material in soil and utilise organic material before egesting the remainder
- They are generally equipped with highly developed senses (especially smell and taste) to distinguish between foods

- Their dentition displays a mixture of carnivore and herbivore adaptations, as do their digestive systems.

SYMBIONTS

A symbiotic organism lives in intimate association with a member of another species. One or both of the organisms usually derives nutritional benefit from the association. There are three types: parasites, commensalists and mutualistic organisms.

Parasites

These live on or in the body of another living organism (the host) from which they obtain their nourishment. Ectoparasites such as fleas and ticks live on the outer surface of the host's body; endoparasites, e.g. tapeworms and roundworms, live inside the host. Parasites nourish themselves either from food ingested by the host or from sucking the host's blood. An effective parasite will not kill its host before it provides passage to a suitable replacement.

Commensal organisms

This is an organism that derives benefit from its host without either doing harm to the host or benefiting its host. Commensalisms are common in the ocean, e.g. hermit crab shells and worm burrows contain uninvited guests obtaining shelter and food from the host.

Mutualistic partners

This is a relationship between two species of organism that live together for their mutual benefit. They may be unable to survive independently of each other, e.g. the flagellate protozoan that lives in the intestine of the termite. Termites eat wood but cannot produce enzymes to digest it. The flagellate cannot chew wood and cannot survive outside the termite's intestine but does produce the enzymes necessary to digest cellulose. Therefore termites cannot survive without the flagellate. Newly hatched termites lick the anus of other termites to obtain their own essential supply of flagellates.

FEEDING MECHANISMS

Three general feeding mechanisms are recognised:

1. Mechanisms for dealing with small particles
2. Mechanisms for dealing with large particles
3. Mechanisms for dealing with fluids and soft tissues.

There are many adaptations to facilitate effective feeding, including:

- Suspension feeders: these filter small particles out of the water
- Substrate feeders: these live on or in their food and eat their way through it
- Fluid feeders: these ingest nutrient-rich fluids from a living host
- Nectivores: these ingest nectar
- Parasites: these gain food from a host source
- Bulk feeders: mostly animal species which eat relatively large pieces of food.

Animals that feed on food masses are often heavily adapted for this task. The animal must be able to locate, hold (and sometimes capture) and swallow the food mass. Some animals employ toxins to immobilise prey. Invertebrates lack true teeth, but may have beaks or tooth-like structures to seize or break up food. Fish, amphibians and reptiles use teeth to grip their prey until it is swallowed and they do not actually chew the food item. True mastication (chewing) is only found among mammals. Mammals have four types of teeth: incisors for biting, cutting and stripping; canines that seize, pierce and tear; and premolars and molars for grinding and crushing food. Teeth may be modified or eliminated to reflect the feeding habits of the animal. Herbivores often have suppressed or absent canines and well-developed molars, with many species possessing open-rooted (continually growing) teeth due to the extent they grind food and wear down their teeth. Carnivores have well-developed canines for seizing prey, with premolars and molars that are adapted for slicing through meat.

Animals that feed on fluids also have specific adaptations. This method of feeding is common in parasites, but many free-living forms also feed on fluids. Some internal parasites do not have a gut and simply absorb nutrients from the surrounding fluids. Some bite or rasp the tissues of the host to suck blood or obtain fluids.

NUTRIENTS

Nutrients are the elements or components of food. An essential nutrient is a substance which is required by an organism for normal life but cannot be synthesised by its own body. Therefore essential nutrients must be obtained from the diet.

There are six essential nutrients:

1. Water
2. Protein
3. Fat
4. Carbohydrates

Table 22.1 Classification of nutrients

Macronutrients	Protein
	Fat
	Carbohydrates
Micronutrients	Vitamins
	Minerals

5. Vitamins
6. Minerals.

These can be divided into macronutrients, those that are needed in large quantities, and micronutrients, those that are required in relatively small amounts (Table 22.1).

Water

Water is essential for life. It is required for metabolism, cell integrity, transportation and excretion. Water balance is tightly monitored as part of the homeostatic control of the body. A daily intake is required to replace the insensible or obligatory water losses from urine, faeces, sweat, respiratory tract water vapour and secretions such as milk. Water is sourced from foodstuffs or drunk directly but in other species it may be absorbed via the skin from the environment. Fresh drinking water should always be available for all animals.

Protein

Proteins are large complex molecules. They are made up of long chains of amino acids called peptide bonds. There are 20 amino acids which are arranged in different sequences to give all the different types of protein within the bodies of animals. Protein is essential within the diet to provide animals with the amino acids that they cannot synthesise within their own bodies, i.e. the essential amino acids. Proteins are required within the body for the following functions:

- To regulate metabolism – enzymes and hormones are types of protein
- In growth and repair – tissues are made up of proteins
- For structural support – within the cell membrane and in connective tissues
- As a source of energy from the diet.

Non-essential amino acids are still required to produce proteins within the body but can be synthesised within the cells using other amino acids or nitrogen compounds. Animals have increased needs for protein when they are:

- Pregnant
- Lactating
- Growing
- Undergoing repair of damaged tissue.

Animals can become deficient in certain amino acids or generally not ingest sufficient protein within their diet, which will lead to physical problems. Protein deficiencies result in:

- Poor growth
- Weight loss
- Poor hair quality
- Anorexia
- Compromised immune status
- Muscle wasting, which may lead to emaciation or cachexia
- Eventually death.

Because they are obligate carnivores, cats require an extra essential amino acid from their diet (taurine) and a higher percentage of protein content in their diet. Taurine insufficiency can lead to eye and heart problems, e.g. feline retinal degeneration and dilated cardiac myopathy, reproductive failure, growth abnormalities in kittens and reduced immunity. Protein is not the richest source of energy that can be obtained from the diet but will be used as an energy source if an animal undergoes a period of inappetance due to starvation or prolonged disease.

Fats/lipids

Fats consist of one glycerol molecule which has attached to it three chains of fatty acids. A molecule of glycerol and its three associated chains of fatty acids comprise one triglyceride. The combinations of the fatty acids give the different types of fats available within the diet. Fatty acids can be saturated or unsaturated. Each chain of fatty acids consists of the individual fatty acids joined together by carbon bonds. The carbon bonds can be singular or double between the fatty acid molecules. If the carbon bond is a single bond then no more fatty acids can join on to that portion of the chain and it is said to be saturated. If the carbon bond between the fatty acids is a double bond then another fatty acid could join if the double bond was broken into two single bonds. Chains of fatty acids containing double carbon bonds are said to be unsaturated. Fats/lipids are required to:

- Provide energy: lipids are the most concentrated form of energy available from the diet
- Increase palatability of food
- Provide essential fatty acids
- Act as a transport medium for the fat-soluble vitamins A, D, E and K

There are three essential fatty acids, all of which are polyunsaturated:

1. Linoleic acid
2. Alpha-linoleic acid
3. Arachidonic acid.

Again, since cats are obligate carnivores, they require an animal dietary source of arachidonic acid as they are unable to synthesise or ingest sufficient quantities from other sources. Essential fatty acids have a role in kidney function and reproduction, form part of the cell membrane and are needed for the production of prostaglandins. Deficiency results in:

- Dull coat
- Hair loss
- Fatty liver
- Anaemia
- Reduced fertility.

Diets that have a high fat content are more prone to putrification as the fat component becomes rancid, and this can lead to the destruction of other nutrients, particularly vitamin E. Fats are solid and lipids are a fluid consistency at room temperature.

Carbohydrates

Carbohydrates are made up of simple and complex sugar molecules. Simple sugars, e.g. glucose and fructose, consist of two sugar molecules with a single bond, a monosaccharide. Sugars containing two bonds are known as disaccharides, e.g. lactose and sucrose, and are harder for the body to digest.

Complex sugars consist of chains of sugar molecules with numerous bonds joining them, e.g. starches, which are even harder to digest, thus providing a slow-release source of energy. Cooking sugars, both simple and complex, increases their digestibility. Carbohydrates provide the body with useable energy and a stored source of energy, either as fat deposits or as glycogen in the liver. Animals can synthesise enough glucose to meet their metabolic needs without an external dietary source provided that there is sufficient glycerol and amino acids within the body. Indigestible complex sugars are also known as dietary fibre. Dietary fibre or roughage, e.g. cellulose, pectin and lignin, is usually sourced from plants within the diet. Dietary fibre helps to bulk the faeces and slow down the rate of passage of food through the digestive system, which can prove valuable in the management of some medical cases.

Vitamins

Vitamins are organic compounds which help to regulate the body's processes. Vitamins cannot be synthesised in the body and must therefore be obtained via the diet. Vitamins are either fat-soluble or water-soluble. The fat-soluble vitamins are A, D, E and K whereas the water-soluble vitamins are B-complex and vitamin C. Water-soluble vitamins are required in higher amounts than the fat-soluble ones since they are constantly being excreted (via urine) from the body. Oversupplementation of vitamins is known as hypervitaminosis and undersupplementation of vitamins is called hypovitaminosis. Fat-soluble vitamins can be toxic because they are stored in the body and can achieve much higher concentrations than the levels required for health.

Minerals

Minerals are also known as ash. Minerals are inorganic nutrients which are divided into macrominerals and microminerals (Tables 22.2 and 22.3). Macrominerals are required in relatively large quantities and microminerals are only required in trace amounts. Calcium and phosphorus are the most important minerals in terms of lifestage nutrition. The ratio between these two minerals should be maintained at 1:1 or a maximum of 2:1 and should be monitored, especially during growth periods. An imbalance in the ratio of calcium to phosphorus ratio can occur due to a deficiency in vitamin D, which can

lead to rickets. Trace or microminerals are mostly toxic if there is oversupplementation or excessive amounts are administered in the diet.

TYPES OF FOOD

Complete diets provide balanced nutrition for specific animal species and often lifestage or clinical condition. A balanced diet can be defined as a diet which provides all the necessary nutrients for the optimal maintenance of the physiological function of an animal, whatever its lifestage. They can be meat, dry or semimoist or a calculated combination of foodstuffs (Table 22.4). A complete diet provides all the animal's nutritional needs if matched to weight and lifestage and fed alone. Complementary diets provide part of an animal's dietary needs; again they may be meat, dry or semimoist. If complementary diets are mixed together they can form a balanced diet but care should be taken not to have too much of any one essential nutrient. Supplementary foods are extra to the normal, such as treats and titbits, or they could be vitamins or mineral supplements. Again, care should be taken not to overfeed as this may lead to dietary problems.

Table 22.2 Macrominerals		
Mineral	**Function**	**Deficiency**
Calcium (Ca)	Structure of skeleton/bones and teeth Required during growth, late pregnancy and lactation Blood clotting Nerve and muscle function	Nutritional secondary hyperparathyrodism Skeletal abnormalities, e.g. rubber jaw, lameness High levels of calcium: hip dysplasia
Phosphorus (P)	Bone and teeth development (in proportion with calcium) Metabolic processes	Skeletal abnormalities
Chloride (Cl)	Osmotic pressure Acid–base balance Water balance	Fatigue, exhaustion, decreased water intake, retarded growth, dry skin, hair loss
Magnesium (Mg)	Bone and teeth development Energy metabolism	Muscular weakness, convulsions High levels of magnesium: fluid
Potassium (K)	Osmotic pressure Acid–base balance Water balance Nerve and muscle function	Muscular weakness, poor growth, lesions of heart and kidneys
Sodium (Na)	Osmotic pressure Acid–base balance Water balance Nerve and muscle function	Fatigue, exhaustion, decreased water intake, retarded growth, dry skin, hair loss

Table 22.3 Microminerals

Mineral	Function	Deficiency
Arsenic	Growth Red blood cell formation	Unlikely
Chromium	Carbohydrate metabolism	Unlikely
Cobalt	Component of vitamin B_{12}	Unlikely if sufficient B_{12}
Copper	Haemoglobin synthesis Structure of bones and blood vessels Melanin production Enzymes	Impairs absorption and transport of haemoglobin Can cause anaemia (but so can excess)
Fluoride	Bone and teeth development	Unlikely
Iodine	Thyroid hormone production	Hypothyroidism Excess – hyperthyroidism
Iron	Haemoglobin and myoglobin Utilisation of oxygen	Anaemia, weakness, fatigue Excess is toxic
Manganese	Chondroitin sulphate and cholesterol synthesis Enzymes associated with fat and carbohydrates	Defective growth, reproduction and problems with lipid metabolism
Molybdenum	Enzymes	Unlikely
Nickel	Membrane function Nucleic acid metabolism	Unlikely
Selenium	Glutathione peroxidase	Dogs – degeneration of skeletal and cardiac muscles Other species – reproductive problems
Silicon	Bone and connective tissue development	Unlikely
Vanadium	Growth, reproduction and fat metabolism	Unlikely
Zinc	Enzymes Epidermal integrity Immunological homeostasis	Poor growth, anorexia, testicular atrophy, emaciation and skin lesions

FOOD ADDITIVES

Food additives are chemical substances which are added to the diet to perform an additional function. Additives are used to:

- Preserve foodstuffs
- Enhance palatability
- Provide flavour
- Provide vitamins or minerals
- Conserve moisture
- Preserve texture
- Provide colour.

Little research has been undertaken in animal diets into the cumulative long-term effects of chemical food additive substances.

FEEDING REQUIREMENTS OF DOGS AND CATS

The animal care industry has a strong influence on what people feed their pets. Many commercial companies provide veterinary nurses and pet store staff with access to further qualifications within the field of nutrition, e.g. Nutritional Advisor Programme (Hills) and Pet Health Counsellor (Pedigree). Body condition scoring is a way of evaluating body fat stores and confirms whether the energy intake is suitable (Figure 22.1).

Feeding requirements of dogs and cats vary with lifestage, mental, physical and environmental stresses and disease status. Hunger is a craving for food stimulated by a decrease in blood glucose, a decrease in circulating amino acids and an increase in gastric motility. Lifestage

Table 22.4 Forms of feed

Forms of feed	Factors to consider
Fresh meat/fish	Bulk for storage Is it fresh? What is its age? Is there any contamination? Used for cats, dogs, snakes, lizards
Frozen meat/fish	Ensure it is properly defrosted Bulky Needs good storage Used for cats, dogs, snakes, lizards
Dairy products, e.g. milk	Freshness Contamination Storage Used for cats, dogs
Vegetables	Storage Contamination by microorganisms Freshness Vitamin and mineral content Used for rabbits, guinea pigs, chelonia, lizards, birds
Canned food	Storage Cross-contamination (in a fridge) Contamination (when opened) Bulk Long shelf-life Used for cats, dogs
Dry food	Storage/bulk Contamination by water, microorganisms, vermin Vitamin and mineral use-by date Mixers, complete or complementary feed (biscuits) Store in airtight container Used for cats, dogs, rabbits, birds
Semimoist	Airtight container Use-by dates Contamination Used for cats, dogs, lizards
Prepacked, powdered, pelleted grain, cereals, seed, fish food	Airtight containers Cross-contamination Vitamin/mineral use-by dates: this is important for small mammals and birds Contamination, e.g. by microorganisms Must be correctly stored

feeding is providing a balanced diet that is suitable for the animal according to its stage of life; common lifestage diets include puppy/kitten or growth, adult maintenance, adult light, geriatric and working dog.

Dogs are omnivores; they have different energy and nutrient requirements depending upon their age and their environment. Breed and activity level must be considered; for example, indoor or outdoor dog, age, and lifestyle and neutered or entire. Cats are obligate carnivores; they have an essential need for taurine and arachidonic acid to be provided by their diet. Age and lifestyle, i.e. indoor or outdoor cat, should be considered when choosing diets. All-meat diets can lead to potential skel-

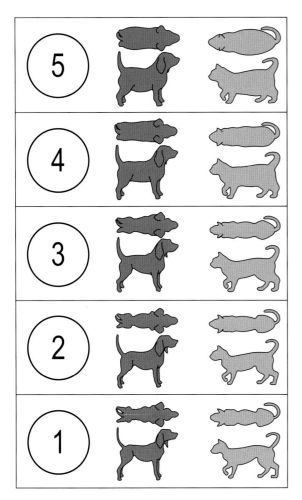

Figure 22.1 Body condition scoring. (Reproduced from Aspinall V 2006 *The Complete Textbook of Veterinary Nursing*. Butterworth Heinemann, London, with permission.)

etal problems in young dogs and vegetarian feline diets can lead to heart and ocular problems in cats, due to inadequate taurine levels.

Malnutrition is a condition that has resulted from inadequate nutrition. Care should be taken when reintroducing food as the animal's metabolic and digestive system may not cope with large quantities of food. Free access to food can result in diarrhoea or vomiting. A diet that is easily assimilated containing high-quality protein is indicated to rebuild tissues. Obesity is commonplace in modern pets. If they lose weight too quickly, cats can die as a result of metabolic acidosis. Animals can yo-yo like people: it is better for them to lose weight slowly and maintain their weight loss. Feeding reduced-calorie, high-fibre diets which satisfy hunger by slow release of glucose due to slow digestion is indicated.

Growth diets are indicated for young animals and pregnant or lactating adult animals. In dogs breed is important during the growth phase as giant breeds such as Great Danes require a slower growth rate than small breeds such as Yorkshire Terriers and commercial diets are available to satisfy these needs. Growth, pregnancy and lactation require additional protein, calcium and phosphorus levels to adult diets. Pregnant animals do not have increased nutritional requirements until the third trimester of the gestation period. Adult foods are calculated to provide optimum nutrition for an adult animal; a light or reduced-calorie version is usually available in most commercial brands for animals that are good doers or who have reduced energy requirements, e.g. indoor cats or neutered animals. Working diets are another version of an adult diet but have a higher calorific content to satisfy animals which expend more energy due to the nature of their role in society, e.g. sheep dogs or gundogs. Geriatric or senior diets tend to have reduced calorific content and have a high-quality biological protein source, making them easier to digest, and additional vitamins and minerals to compensate for the reduced efficiency of the older pet's digestive system.

Prescription or clinical diets

These are specially formulated diets designed to provide optimal nutritional requirements for the aid or prevention of disease. The nutrient content and quality are adapted to meet the clinical requirements of the animal. For example, postoperative diets have a high biological source of protein and they are often partially predigested to facilitate absorption. Renal diets contain a high biological protein source at a reduced amount, increased calories from non-protein sources, low salt content to prevent hypertension, reduced phosphorus to deter progression of renal disease and increased fibre and fatty acids. The aim of clinical diets is to preserve or improve the function of organs and body systems affected by disease. Proprietary examples are available for:

- Renal disease
- Postoperative care
- Diarrhoea
- Diabetes mellitus
- Cardiac disease
- Constipation/colitis
- Liver disease
- Cardiac disease
- Dietary sensitivity
- Skin disease
- Uroliths
- Neoplasia
- Senility.

FEEDING REQUIREMENTS OF HERPTILES AND BIRDS

Reptiles have a lower metabolic rate than endotherms, therefore they require a lower calorific intake to maintain their body weight. Environmental influences should be considered: temperature, humidity, light quantity and quality all affect feeding and intake. Dietary requirements are dependent on age, size, breeding status, season and nutritional status. Generally the smaller the reptile, the less it eats. Diets should have an overall ratio of calcium to phosphorus of 1.5 : 1; in captivity vitamin D supplementation is often required.

Food type and presentation are important and food should be consumed within 30–40 minutes of being offered but allow longer for ill, nervous or new animals to feed. Feed in a designated area with water should always be available. Often reptiles will not drink directly from a bowl but can take water from foliage, off the walls or roof of the cage and therefore the cage should be regularly sprayed with a fine mist of water throughout the day.

Captive birds can be subdivided into caged birds, hard bills and soft bills, and raptors. Hard bills, e.g. parrots, extract the kernel of seeds and nuts by cracking the hard husk using specially adapted beaks. Soft bills feed on fleshy fruits and/or invertebrates. There is some overlap between the two categories, particularly when birds are breeding. Hard bills need seed appropriate to their size, i.e. for budgies and canaries canary seed, rape seed, millet and sunflower, and for larger psittacines peanuts and pine nuts. Food containers must be checked to ensure they are not just full of empty husks.

Generally birds only eat food they recognise or have become imprinted upon. Unfamiliar food or a new feeding dish may even frighten a bird. Abrupt changes in diet should be avoided as they can result in starvation and death.

Introduce changes very, very slowly over weeks. Birds need at least six different food items in their basic diet to avoid malnutrition. It is advised to feed a commercially produced balanced diet. Supplementation is a good idea to offer a broad-spectrum supplementary ration. This ration could consist of:

- Green food – lettuce, watercress, chickweed, parsley, dandelion
- Sprouted seeds
- Vegetables – carrots, turnips, beetroot
- Fruit – oranges, apples, grapes.

Certain items can be puréed into a mash with a little animal protein, e.g. boiled egg, cheese or milk, to provide a source of vitmain A, D_3 and B_{12}. Insectivores will require live food such as crickets or mealworms. Frugivores will require syrupy foods but not molasses.

Raptors require a staple diet which will probably consist of 1-day-old male chicks, which can be obtained from local hatcheries, falconers and pet food suppliers. These are stored frozen and defrosted daily as required. Care should be taken to ensure they are fully defrosted and at body temperature before feeding. The entire chick is fed, including skin and feathers as these are required for roughage and to ensure good calcium levels. Do not offer more food if there is still food present in the bird's crop.

Wild birds tend to feed mostly at first light and again in late afternoon. Therefore it would be advisable to feed caged birds at regular intervals, not ad libitum. If a bird is ill or kept in low temperatures, offer food fairly frequently, i.e. six times daily. High-energy foods such as hemp, rape and niger seeds should be reduced in summer (it is warmer, therefore birds do not burn as many calories). Very small birds should have low-level lighting in winter to enable them to feed overnight as 12 hours is too long a period without food. Grit is required by most seed-eating birds for proper function of the gizzard. The grit must be of an appropriate size, changed regularly and should consist of both soluble (oyster shell/egg shell) and insoluble (quartz/igneous stone) types.

FEEDING REQUIREMENTS OF HORSES AND LIVESTOCK

The same principles apply to large animals as to small animals. Different species, breeds and lifestages will require suitable balanced complete diets. Ruminant species such as the cow will require access to large quantities of forage provided by grass, straw or silage depending upon management systems for long periods of time. In beef breeds supplementation by commercial concentrates to facilitate quick gains of muscle mass may be used. Pigs that are raised indoors will be fed a commercial concentrate and outdoor husbandry systems may have this supplemented by the opportunity for natural foraging. Sheep have access to grass pasture which may be supplemented by forage or concentrates. Horses should have access to grazing or forage and depending on the workload this is often supplemented by a wide variety of concentrates. Pregnant, lactating and growing animals will have increased protein and calcium requirements; in livestock young animals are often reared away from the dam using milk and concentrates but using artificial teat systems. Body scoring systems are routinely employed to monitor nutrition and management in livestock species. Table 22.5 shows feeding methods used in animals.

Table 22.5 Feeding methods used in animals

Automatic feeding systems	Time and quantity can be set Often used in livestock husbandry Useful if the owner is out for long periods of time or on holiday Some systems can be started by the animal pressing a lever or button
Scatter feeding	Scatter food around the animal's enclosure Makes animals work for their food: • They exercise • They burn energy • It mentally stimulates them • It keeps the animal's weight down • It can be a problem if there are lots of animals in an enclosure as it is difficult to monitor the amount each animal is eating Food can go off if it isn't eaten
Container feeding	Food contained in one place Containers are available in different sizes, shapes and designs to meet all species needs Can be moved around enclosure and could use more than one Can get damaged and spilt and bullying can occur Again, it is difficult to monitor which animal is eating what if more than one are housed together
Demand feeding	Animals are fed on demand Can be an automated system which the animal stimulates when it is hungry by pressing a lever/button Is also seen in young animals when they are suckling and during the weaning process Can be used in zoos as part of a feeding regime linked to training/public displays Used in exotic species which may only eat at variable times Can offer food but it must be removed if it isn't eaten after a set time
Hiding food – enrichment	Used to make animals work for their food Physical and mental exercise
Mimicry of hunting	Mental and physical exercise To encourage eating
Food as a reward	During training programmes Emotional guilt, e.g. if out for a long time

Bibliography

Ackerman N 2008 Companion animal nutrition: a manual for veterinary nurses and technicians. Butterworth Heinemann, Oxford

Agar S 2001 Small animal nutrition. Butterworth Heinemann, Oxford

Aspinall V 2006 The complete textbook of veterinary nursing. Butterworth Heinemann, London

Dallas S 2006 Animal biology and care, 2nd edn. Wiley/Blackwell, Oxford

Lane D R, Cooper B, Turner L 2007 Textbook of veterinary nursing, 3rd edn. Butterworth-Heinemann/BSAVA, Oxford

McDonald P, Greenhalgh J, Edwards R et al. 1995 Animal nutrition. Longman, London

Moore M 2000 Manual of veterinary nursing. BSAVA, Philadelphia

Pratt P W 1998 Principles and practice of veterinary technology. Mosby, Philadelphia

Simpson G 1994 Practical veterinary nursing, 3rd edn. BSAVA, Philadelphia

Warren D M 1995 Small animal care and management. Delmar, New York

Chapter | **23** | *Lucy Dumbell and Donna de Haan*

Animal welfare and the law

This chapter will consider the importance of an animal's welfare requirements, discuss how we could measure an animal's welfare status, review key pieces of legislation aimed at improving animal welfare and how that legislation is produced and enforced, and look at the future of animal welfare.

DEFINITION OF ANIMAL WELFARE

Everyone has a different opinion on what constitutes a good state of welfare for an animal and this is a question for which there is no one standard answer. Unfortunately, because of this the whole topic of animal welfare is highly controversial. Many definitions exist for animal welfare. Some authors suggest that an animal has a high level of welfare if it is free from injury and pain, whilst other authors believe that an animal should be emotionally content, as well as physically healthy and fit. One definition of animal welfare that is widely used is that of Broom (1986), who wrote that welfare is 'the state of an individual as regards its attempts to cope with its environment'. It is important to note that welfare status can vary between very poor and very good, and we should always state whether an animal has good or poor welfare.

Now we have considered what animal welfare is, we should question why it is important. Historically people did not always believe that an animal had feelings, and therefore if an animal had no feelings it did not matter how it was treated. Throughout the 17th and 18th centuries many writers discussed whether animals could feel emotions and whether this mattered. As animals cannot talk it is hard to prove conclusively that they have feelings and therefore suffer. Jeremy Bentham, an 18th-century social reformer, said: 'the question is not Can they reason? nor Can they talk? But, Can they suffer?' With this in mind it is now felt by the majority of people today that if an animal shows the ability to suffer then we should care how we treat it.

Today, it is written into American and European Union (EU) law that animals have feelings (are sentient). As well as this ethical argument there are other well-recognised consequences of poor welfare in animals. These include reduced growth rates, reduced fecundity (the ability to produce offspring), reduced immune competence, abnormal behaviour, reduced longevity (length of life), increased social aggression, reduced self-maintenance behaviour and decreased efficiency of digestion. These are undesirable characteristics for any carer of a domestic or captive animal as they result in reduced productivity, greater expense to maintain health and expression of undesirable (and sometimes socially unacceptable) behaviours.

The EU recognises that animals contribute to human quality of life and their welfare status affects their ability to do this. It is well recognised that upbringing has a large effect on people's attitudes towards animals and their welfare. As it is extremely difficult to get agreement on a clear definition of animal welfare, even between two individuals, when people come from different backgrounds their opinions on the topic tend to differ even further. The EU believes that improving animal welfare requires a coordinated approach, recognising that different countries have different attitudes and approaches to animal welfare for legal, socioeconomic, political, ethical and cultural reasons.

All of these factors mean that, although the majority of people agree that if we influence an animal's life we should care about its welfare, there is still debate and disagreement as to what constitutes an acceptable level of welfare for an animal.

MEASURING ANIMAL WELFARE

As there are so many opinions on what animal welfare is, assessing welfare status is challenging. Many authors have tried to describe and classify factors that improve an animal's welfare status. One suggestion has been that you can divide factors into life-sustaining needs, e.g. water, health-sustaining needs and comfort-sustaining needs (Hurnik and Lehman 1988) (Figure 23.1).

According to Broom (1986), an animal's welfare status will result from its interaction with its environment and therefore it can only be observed accurately when it is within its usual environment. When assessing an animal's welfare status, therefore, it is important to view the animal within its environment. When undertaking an assessment it is widely recognised that there is not a single measure of welfare that is accurate and therefore it is currently recommended to use a combination of different measures. This combination should include methods from at least two of the three categories of welfare measures:

1. Behavioural measures
2. Physiological measures
3. Neurological measures.

Probably the most common combination of these is to use a physiological measure, e.g. heart rate or hormone concentration, and a behavioural measure, e.g. a time budget or the presence of undesirable behaviours. Neurological measures are increasingly being used in research; however currently they are relatively poorly understood and therefore seldom used in real-life situations.

One method of assessing an animal's welfare is to consider the five animal freedoms. These key concepts were initially written by the Brambell Committee (1965), which was reviewing the welfare aspects of factory farming in the UK in the 1960s. From their initial recommendations the five freedoms were developed into their present form by a member of the British Farm Animal Welfare Council (FAWC). The five animal freedoms are:

1. Freedom from thirst, hunger and malnutrition
2. Freedom from discomfort
3. Freedom from pain, injury and disease
4. Freedom to express most normal behaviour
5. Freedom from fear and distress.

The five freedoms have been adopted as the key principles underpinning animal welfare in the UK and the USA. Although they were initially developed for farm animals they have been interpreted to provide guidance for all animals.

For any measure used to assess animal welfare we should be able to describe clearly what it entails, and assess whether the animal has poor or good welfare when considering the method. When the five animal freedoms are assessed in this way it becomes clear that they are not always a useful scale to assess animal welfare against.

Freedom from thirst, hunger and malnutrition

The freedom from hunger and thirst is often considered to be fairly easy to measure in many species, as a veterinary surgeon would be able to measure the consequences of hunger and thirst – malnutrition and dehydration – fairly easily and accurately. Hunger and thirst are, however, feelings, sensations, and as such, measuring them, rather than their consequences, can be difficult in animals as they cannot talk. Despite this our knowledge about what, and in what quantity, an animal eats and drinks is quite comprehensive for many species and so this is one of the easier freedoms to measure.

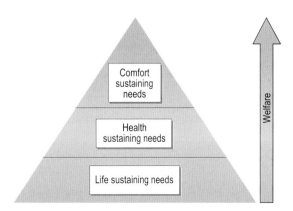

Figure 23.1 Welfare measurement via provision of factor.

Freedom from discomfort

Assessing to what extent an animal feels discomfort is difficult. There are many definitions of discomfort but they all agree that discomfort can be mental or physical. As such this is a challenging area to measure. The majority of measures of this freedom revolve around assessing aspects of the animal's environment that are presumed to give comfort, e.g. the provision of suitable housing and bedding as required, rather than actually assessing the individual animal's levels of discomfort. Therefore the accuracy to which one can interpret this freedom is probably low.

Freedom from pain, injury and disease

A veterinary surgeon could, for many commonly domesticated species, assess whether an animal is injured or diseased with a high degree of confidence and accuracy. For more unusual animals this, although seemingly simple, can pose a challenge to the most experienced veterinarian. The assessment of an animal's pain level is a lot more difficult. The International Association for the Study of Pain (IASP) defines pain as 'an unpleasant sensory and emotional experience associated with actual or potential tissue damage or described in terms of such damage'. It is widely agreed that pain is undesirable as it causes delayed healing, prolonged recovery time and changes in an animal's physiology and observable behaviour. There is a growing amount of interest in how we can assess an animal's pain levels, both the private conscious experience of pain and the observable behaviour associated with this feeling. Different people are known to demonstrate a large amount of variability in 'the greatest level of pain of which a subject is prepared to tolerate' – their pain threshold (defined by the IASP). It is also known that the pain threshold demonstrates interspecific variation (i.e. differs between species) and yet only pain levels larger than an animal's pain threshold are likely to be detectable through observing behaviour, currently the most common way of diagnosing pain. Therefore this third freedom is also difficult to use as a measure of animal welfare if considered in its entirety.

Freedom to express most normal behaviour

The freedom to express most normal behaviour is widely considered the most difficult freedom both to assess and to satisfy. If this freedom is to be met several factors have to be considered, including the current state of scientific knowledge about the normal behaviour of the species, the degree to which that individual animal conforms to the values known for that species, the knowledge of the carer and assessor, and the degree to which the carer is prepared to take behaviour into account when designing management methods. Often how an animal is managed is determined by a historical course of events. Although the reasons why those management methods were originally designed may no longer be valid, the traditions that have arisen surrounding them make difficult a truly objective assessment of the necessity for the management method. This is particularly true for companion animals, which are often expected to fit into their owner's lifestyle, sometimes with little consideration for the impact their owner's lifestyle decisions have on them.

Freedom from fear and distress

Fear is an emotion experienced when anticipating an unpleasant event and is therefore extremely difficult to assess in humans, and even more difficult to assess in animals. It is known that within humans fear is a very personal emotion, depending heavily on previous experiences and upbringing. There is no reason to think that this is not true for animals as well, if indeed we accept that they are capable of experiencing emotions. Distress is a term that has many different implications, but certainly has both physical and mental causes. It is often used when an animal is unable to cope with a factor, and as such is an extreme condition and is incompatible with high levels of animal welfare. Overall it can be seen that this freedom is difficult to assess, although by the extreme nature of the concepts it entails it is likely to be easier to assess than, for example, discomfort.

The five freedoms therefore set out an ideal scenario for an animal experiencing a high level of welfare; however they are of little practical use when it comes to assessing an animal's welfare, except in the most general and idealised scenarios. Nevertheless they do represent a unified vision of optimal animal welfare that presents a powerful image to aim for.

LEGISLATION

Legislation is the action of upholding and creating rules (laws) that have authority as they are supported by an official body. Legislation is a term that can also be used to refer to a group of laws. When considering legislation it is worth knowing who created the laws, who is governed by them and who upholds them. The UK, USA and EU all have legislative bodies composed of two legislative chambers (bicameral). The Parliament of the United Kingdom of Great Britain and Northern Ireland, the

United States Congress and the legislative body of the EU are the official bodies that create the laws for these nations. The laws that these bodies create are then enforced by a judicial system, which is a system of courts of law for the administration of justice to the people (and lands) that are governed by these laws, in the name of the state (or sovereign). The judiciary is also the branch of government responsible for interpreting the law. The executive branch of government manages the smooth running of the state, leads a lot of policy and heavily influences which legislation is proposed or revised.

USA

US Congress

In the USA citizens are subject to three levels of government:

1. Federal level
2. State level. All states have to have a written constitution and follow a republican form of government. Every state has a bicameral legislative body (except Nebraska, which is unicameral with 'The Legislature'); these are called a range of terms, including The Legislature, General Assembly and Legislative Assembly. Although the US Congress has powers over all states for issues that affect commerce and allocates funds, laws can vary hugely between states. In Massachusetts and New York, agents of animal welfare organisations can be appointed special officers to enforce legislation relating to animal cruelty. The laws on tail-docking in dogs also vary hugely between different states. The state judiciary is typically headed by a state supreme court (although the name can vary), which hears appeals of legal issues, while lower state courts conduct trials
3. Local level. All the states are divided into counties (called boroughs in Alaska and parishes in Louisiana). The structure of local government varies between states but local governments can be grouped into five classes which all differ in the powers they possess and the geographical areas they control. Local governments only have the powers that their state gives to them and therefore these also vary between states.

Due to this complex and tiered system legislation in the USA can seem confusing and even contradictory at times.

Animal welfare legislation in the USA

In the USA the US Department of Agriculture (USDA) monitors animal welfare and has an Animal and Plant Health Inspection Service (APHIS) which leads the way in setting standards for the humane care and treatment of animals. The USA has had an Animal Welfare Act since 1966, has passed amendments in 1970, 1976, 1985 and 1990 and compliance with this law is monitored by APHIS. The US Animal Welfare Act 1966 is applied to warm-blooded animals, except pets owned by private citizens and those used for food, fibre or other agricultural purposes. The US Animal Welfare Act 1966 states that minimum standards of care and treatment should be provided for animals, including appropriate housing, handling, sanitation, nutrition, water, veterinary care and protection from extreme weather and temperatures. These are all minimum standards and people are encouraged to exceed them.

Animals used in research are also protected by the US Animal Welfare Act, which requires that researchers minimise the pain or distress experienced by an animal and forbids unnecessary duplication of a specific experiment. Research establishments can set up their own ethics committee that must submit evidence to APHIS of complying with the Animal Welfare Act 1966. APHIS inspectors can make unannounced inspections at least once annually to businesses, and can issue Official Notices of Warning or civil penalties or submit evidence to USDA for further action.

Some species also have specific acts protecting them, e.g. The Horse Protection Act (1970, amended in 1976), which aims to protect horses participating in shows, sales, exhibitions and auctions from soring. Soring is where the horse's forelegs are irritated by injecting or applying chemicals or mechanical irritants and often this is so painful that the horse develops permanent scars. The aim is to accentuate the gait, as usually a horse in pain will lift its limbs higher and more quickly off the ground, which is considered as being desirable behaviour in some breeds.

The EU

Governance of the EU

The EU is a political and economic community that has, as of 2008, 27 member states: Austria, Belgium, Bulgaria, Cyprus, Czech Republic, Denmark, Estonia, Finland, France, Germany, Greece, Hungary, Ireland, Italy, Latvia, Lithuania, Luxembourg, Malta, Netherlands, Poland, Portugal, Romania, Slovakia, Slovenia, Spain, Sweden and the UK. Only the European Commission can formally propose legislation, although the Council of Europe and the European Parliament form the legislature. For a law to be passed these two legislative bodies do not have to agree (codecision); however, this is usually the case. EU legislation comes in two forms:

1. Regulations, the strongest act of law that the European Parliament recognises

2. Directives, which require member states to achieve a stated result, but it is up to them how they achieve this.

Animal welfare legislation in the EU

The EU first passed legislation concerning farm animal welfare in 1974 and at that time this gave guidance on slaughtering farm animals. The Treaty of Amsterdam, which has been in force since 1 May 1999, states the position of the EU on issues connected with animal welfare. It specifically states that animals are capable of experiencing feelings (sentience), including pain, and requires member states to consider the animals' welfare requirements.

The EU believes that it should legislate to improve animal welfare and prevent cruelty, although it says that some specific issues should be the responsibility of member states (e.g. the use of animals in sporting events such as bullfighting). An EU action plan on animal welfare was developed in 2006 with the 'aim of developing and guaranteeing animal welfare and protection within the EU and in other parts of the world' by 2010. It identified five areas of action necessary to achieve this:

1. Upgrading minimum standards
2. Promoting research and substitute methods for animal testing
3. Introducing welfare indicators
4. Ensuring that professionals and the general public are better informed
5. Supporting international initiatives for animal protection.

The EU also provides guidance on specific groups of animals, e.g. the European Convention for the Protection of Pet Animals, which is aimed at promoting the welfare of pet animals. It gives details of the minimum standards required when keeping pets and discusses stray animals and also humane education programmes. Not every EU member state is participating in this convention and notable absences include the UK.

The United Kingdom of Great Britain and Northern Ireland

The Parliament of the UK

The executive body in the UK consists of the Prime Minister, who is the head of the largest political party in the legislature, and the Cabinet. The Parliament of the United Kingdom of Great Britain and Northern Ireland is the supreme assembly with law-making powers over all other government institutions for England, Scotland, Wales, Northern Ireland and their associated colonies. It

has an upper house, the House of Lords, whose members are not elected by the population, and a lower house, the House of Commons, whose members are democratically elected. Laws usually begin as either a green paper, which is a document on which there has been consultation with interested parties (stakeholders), or a white paper, which is a statement of policy. When a bill is proposed both houses have to agree on it before it can be passed to the sovereign, currently Queen Elizabeth II, for royal assent, when it becomes an Act. Laws can apply to the whole of the UK or specific parts of it.

The judicial system in the UK differs depending in which country you reside. Scotland (led by the Scottish Parliament) has a separate system with the highest court for criminal cases being the High Court of Judiciary, and in civil cases the House of Lords. Matters surrounding the Scottish, Welsh or Northern Ireland Assembly are considered by the Judicial Committee of the Privy Council.

Animal welfare legislation in the UK

The first piece of legislation concerning animal welfare passed in Great Britain was the Protection of Animals Act 1822 (amended in 1835 and 1849). In 1900 the Wild Animals in Captivity Protection Act was passed and these two were subsequently amalgamated in 1911 to the Protection of Animal Act, which has only recently been superceded by the Animal Welfare Act 2006.

The aim of the Animal Welfare Act 2006 is: 'To reduce animal suffering by consolidating and bringing up to date legislation that exists to promote and improve the welfare to farmed, domestic and captive animals'. The development of the Act began with the UK government's Department for the Environment, Food and Rural Affairs (DEFRA) launching a public consultation in January 2002, which led to the draft Animal Welfare Bill being published in July 2004. This was then amended and introduced to the UK Parliament on 13 October 2005 and finally gained royal assent on 8 November 2006, when it became the Animal Welfare Act 2006. The Act came into effect on 6 April 2007. This is an example of the lengthy process that frequently occurs before any Act comes into effect.

The Animal Welfare Act 2006 applies to vertebrates (other than humans) that are commonly domesticated in the UK and are under the control of humans (whether temporarily or permanently). It aims to:

• Protect animals from harm
• Promote welfare, license or register activities involving animals
• Support the development of codes of practice
• Extend powers to help animals in distress

- Grant enforcement powers to investigate allegations of cruelty (including animal fights)
- Allow local authorities to prosecute people who break the Act
- Set out postconviction powers.

The Animal Welfare Act 2006 only applies to England and Wales as Scotland has its own legislation, the Animal Health and Welfare (Scotland) Act 2006, which came into force on 6 October 2006. The Animal Health and Welfare (Scotland) Act 2006 has many similarities with the Animal Welfare Act 2006, including placing a duty of care on those caring for animals, raising the animal ownership age to 16 and banning the use of animals as prizes. It also supports the response to serious outbreaks of animal disease, allowing biosecurity codes to be established and extending slaughter powers in the event of exotic animal disease.

There are many different individual pieces of legislation to promote and safeguard the welfare of animals in the UK. These are outlined in Table 23.1. There are also international agreements that influence, and are often coded for within, national legislation. One such agreement is the Convention on International Trade in Endangered Species of wild fauna and flora (CITES) 1979. The aim of this agreement is to ensure that trade of wild plants and animals does not threaten their survival. This is a voluntary agreement, with each government that joins being termed a 'party'. The UK is one of the 172 parties (as of November 2007) which, once they have joined, are legally bound to uphold its ideals.

ANIMAL WELFARE ORGANISATIONS

There are many organisations that promote animal welfare. Some of them focus on one particular issue, e.g. the League Against Cruel Sports (UK), or group of animals, e.g. British Horse Society (UK), but some organisations are more general:

- The Royal Society for the Prevention of Cruelty to Animals (RSPCA) evolved from the Society for the Prevention of Cruelty to Animals, which was established in 1823. The RSPCA is a UK-based charity and states that it 'will, by all lawful means, prevent cruelty, promote kindness to, and alleviate suffering of animals'
- The People's Dispensary for Sick Animals (PDSA) cares 'for the pets of needy people by providing free veterinary services to their sick and injured animals and promoting responsible pet ownership'. It was founded in 1917 and is now Europe's largest private employer of fully qualified veterinary surgeons and nurses and is based in the UK

- The Humane Society of the United States (HSUS) was established in 1954 and aims to celebrate animals whilst confronting cruelty. It deals with wide-ranging issues, e.g. animal fighting, trading in seal fur, and also provides advice and campaigns for improvements in animal welfare
- The World Society for the Protection of Animals (WSPA) aims to promote animal welfare in areas of the world where animals are not protected. It identifies four priority areas: improving conditions for companion animals, promoting sustainable exploitation of wildlife, improving welfare of farm animals and providing disaster relief for animals.

These are just a few of the many organisations worldwide that are involved in animal welfare.

THE FUTURE OF ANIMAL WELFARE

During the last few years, attention has focused on not only passing legislation to promote animal welfare but also planning how to encourage and support carers in improving and prioritising an animal's welfare. The Animal Health and Welfare Strategy for Great Britain covering Wales, Scotland and England was written in 2004, showing where DEFRA wanted to be in 2014, and aims to:

> develop a new partnership in which we can make a lasting and continuous improvement in the health and welfare of kept animals while protecting society, the economy, and the environment from the effect of animal disease.

The Animal Welfare Delivery Strategy 2007 was published in October 2007 by DEFRA with the goal that 'all those who are responsible for animals must ensure good standards of welfare for them and those who have contact with, or benefit from, animals must pay due regard to their welfare'. The delivery strategy was to plan and monitor how the Animal Health and Welfare Strategy for Great Britain and the Animal Welfare Act 2006 were implemented in England. It applies to animals kept for pleasure or profit, including companion animals, agricultural animals, game and wildlife, and has five key themes.

1. Everyone involved in animal health and welfare should work together in partnership
2. All those with an interest in animal health and welfare must have a good understanding of their responsibilities, including animal owners
3. To ensure that animals are cared for appropriately and in accordance with existing welfare standards and are therefore more likely to be healthy, and less likely to contract or spread disease

Table 23.1 Some of the animal welfare legislation in the UK

Act	Scope of application	Main points
Abandonment of Animals Act 1960	Any animals in England, Wales and Scotland	It is an offence under this act to abandon any animal without reasonable excuse in circumstances likely to cause it unnecessary suffering
Protection of Animals Act 1911 amendments, most recently in 2000	Any domestic or captive animal in the UK	It is illegal to cause unnecessary suffering to an animal (or permit this to happen) by overt acts or omission of care. Prohibits animal fighting and baiting, poisoning and inhumane operations
Animal Boarding Establishments Act 1963	England, Wales and Scotland	Requires establishments where boarding of cats and dogs is a business to be registered with the local authority. The local authority has to be satisfied with standard of care and welfare of the animals
Welfare of Animals during Transport Order 1997	All vertebrates and cold-blooded animals in England, Scotland and Wales. Version for Northern Ireland, 1997. Scottish revision in 2006	It is an offence to cause undue injury or suffering. Gives space allowances, treatment for sick animals, feed, water and rest periods, duties on transporters for all animals. Specific arrangements for certain species, farm livestock, horses and poultry, also domestic and wild animals. Some exemptions for journeys less than 50 km. (Supersedes Transit of Animals (Road and Rail) Order 1975 in the main)
Veterinary Surgeons Act 1966	Lists people qualified to practise veterinary surgery in UK	Veterinary surgery is defined as 'the art and science of veterinary surgery and medicine' and incorporates diagnosis, advice based on diagnosis and medical or surgical treatment of (or operations on) animals. Controls the addition to and removal of names from the register depending on education and conduct. This Act is administered by the Royal College of Veterinary Surgeons (RCVS) and safeguards animals from incorrect diagnosis and potentially harmful treatments
Veterinary Medicines Regulations 2005	England, Wales and Scotland	Regulates who can dispense and provide appropriate advice on the medicines that an animal should receive
Animal Health Act 2002	England and Wales	Gives specific provision to deal with disease control and biosecurity guidance, strengthening the Animal Health Act 1981

4. To spread the message that preventing animal diseases has obvious benefits and is also cost-effective
5. To clarify the role of the government in providing leadership and helping to raise animal health and welfare standards.

The EU believes that there needs to be clearer guidance on scientific research, the implementation of animal welfare guidelines, awareness-raising, education and promotion of best practices. The European Commission published a new Animal Health Strategy for the EU for

2007–2013, noting that 'prevention is better than cure' and aims to provide 'the best possible framework for animal disease control in Europe' (Kyprianou 2007). This strategy has four goals:

1. To ensure a high level of public health and food safety by minimising the incidence of risks from animal diseases, food-borne diseases and biotoxins and chemical risks to humans
2. To promote animal health by preventing or reducing the incidence of animal diseases, and in this way to support farming and the rural economy
3. To improve economic growth/cohesion/competitiveness, assuring free circulation of goods and proportionate animal movements
4. To promote farming practices and animal welfare which prevent animal health-related threats and minimise environmental impacts (in support of the EU Sustainable Development Strategy).

There are also some species that have specific provision, e.g. donkeys, mules and horses are covered by the Equine Health and Welfare Strategy for Great Britain (www. equinehealthandwelfarestrategy.co.uk), launched in March 2007, which sets out a 10-year vision where:

1. All horses are healthy and are treated humanely
2. Everyone responsible for horse health and welfare fulfils their duty of care.

In order to achieve these goals everyone involved with horses must understand their responsibilities, know how to meet them and ensure that:

- Health and welfare standards, and other information necessary to support each individual's duty of care, are appropriate, up to date and accessible
- The risks of infectious diseases, including those entering the UK from abroad, are addressed and managed effectively
- The health and welfare status of the horse population is adequately monitored
- Significant health and welfare problems are identified and addressed.

Animal welfare is an area which has had increased legislative attention. As such it is currently at the forefront of both the political and social consciousness. It is to be hoped that it remains there to ensure animals can benefit whilst continuing to contribute to our quality of life. Never before have humans been so influential over the welfare, and even the existence, of other species of animals. In a time when it is suggested that we are altering the climate of our planet, our collective responsibility towards those we share this planet with has never been stronger.

Bibliography

Bentham J 1789 An introduction to the principles of morals and legislation. Latest edition 2005 Adamant Media Corporation, Boston

Brambell F W R 1965 Report of the technical committee to enquire into the welfare of animals kept under intensive livestock husbandry systems. HMSO, London

Broom D M 1986 Indicators of poor welfare. British Veterinary Journal 142:524–526

DEFRA 2004 The animal health and welfare strategy for Great Britain. Defra Publications, London

Hurnik J F, Lehman H 1988 Ethics and farm animal welfare. Journal of Agricultural Ethics 1:305–318

Kyprianou M 2007 A new animal health strategy for the European Union (2007–2013) where 'prevention is better than cure'. Office for Official Publications of the European Communities, Belgium

Further reading

Animal and Plant Health Inspection Service. Available online at: www.aphis.usda.gov/

British Horse Society. Available online at: www.bhs.org.uk/

Department of Environment, Food and Rural Affairs. Available online at: www.defra.gov.uk/

European Union. Available online at: europa.eu/

Farm Animal Welfare Council. Available online at: www.fawc.org.uk/

Humane Society of the United States. Available online at: www.hsus.org/

International Association for the Study of Pain. Available online at: www.iasp-pain.org//AM/Template.cfm?Section=Home

League against Cruel Sports. Available online at: www.league.org.uk/

People's Dispensary for Sick Animals. Available online at: www.pdsa.org.uk/

Royal Society for the Prevention of Cruelty to Animals. Available online at: www.rspca.org.uk/

United States Department of Agriculture. Available online at: www.usda.gov/

World Society for the Protection of Animals. Available online at: www.wspa.org.uk/

Management of zoological collections

This chapter explores the history of zoological collections and describes how management, identification and husbandry techniques have evolved in recent times. It discusses the role of the modern zoo keeper and the importance of modern captive animal collections to conservation.

THE ROLE OF ZOOLOGICAL COLLECTIONS

Over the years the word 'zoo' has come to describe a collection of animals that people are allowed to view and, although safari parks, sanctuaries and rescue centres would all argue this point, as far as the general public are concerned, this is the case. Indeed, in the UK any collection of animals that is open to the public, either paying or non-paying, for 7 days in a year has to have a zoo licence to allow it to operate. However there are differences between animal collections. This chapter is a personal description of the different types of collection but it is by no means definitive and you must make up your own mind as to your own definitions.

In reverse order, rescue centres tend to concentrate on either a very specific, native species or family of animals (such as swans or pinnipeds) or on domestic species. In the case of native species, they will usually take in sick or injured animals in the hope that they can nurse them back to health and potentially release them into the wild. Failing this they will either humanely destroy them or house them in captivity for the rest of their natural lives. When they work with domestic species they are often dealing with abused or abandoned pets which they will care for until a new owner can hopefully be found.

Sanctuaries and rescue centres do cross over but sanctuaries tend to care for a wider range of species, such as primates or felids, and they are generally set up either to save animals from abuse (for example, dancing bears or photographers' chimps), habitat destruction or poaching. They are more likely, though not always, to be set up in the animals' natural range, and if this is the case they are often supported by money from abroad, either raised from the general public or from other animal collections. For example, several orang utan sanctuaries are funded in this way. Some people are of the opinion that rescue centres and sanctuaries should be places designed simply to hold the animals and not to breed them, but it seems that many of them find it hard to resist the temptation of breeding the animals once they have them in captivity. Unfortunately, this can sometimes exacerbate the very problem they were hoping to solve.

When safari parks came into existence the whole idea behind them was to have the animals in huge paddocks through which the public could drive. However due to public demand safari parks are changing and most now have a central area that is far more 'zoo-like' where visitors can leave their cars and stroll around looking at the animals in enclosures. Indeed, a few zoos have gone the other way and have open-plan paddocks through which the public can either drive or be driven in large trucks to give the safari experience.

Most zoos tend to be in or close to a town and because of this they are generally quite small. The enclosures are therefore smaller too but the variety of animals kept is far larger than any of the other types of collections. Modern, responsible zoos are realising the restrictions of space and are choosing species to match. Generally far fewer zoos now keep elephants, for example, leaving the keeping and breeding of these huge animals to the collections that have the space and facilities to look after them correctly. The problem is that these animals are very long-lived, and as most breeding collections are not willing to take on animals that are past breeding age, numerous zoos will have ageing elephants in their collections for many years to come.

The changing role of zoos

When the first animal collections were created they were purely for the entertainment of a chosen few, usually royalty or the wealthy. As time passed zoos slowly became more common and accessible to the masses but their role stayed basically unchanged. It was not until well into the 20th century, as the plight of many species was becoming obvious, that it was realised that there was a reservoir of endangered species in captivity and that we had the capability to breed these animals to increase the world's populations. Although this has worked in a few cases, unfortunately it has had very limited success.

As time progressed it became painfully obvious that zoos alone would never be able to save many – if any – species from extinction. Rather than just trying to increase numbers they had to make sure that there was still somewhere for the animals to live that was safe and protected. This meant that another way had to be found and the focus of zoos had to change accordingly. Many zoos now concentrate on working with the animals and habitats in situ. To do this the home zoo, which is hopefully able to make a profit, uses the funds raised to support both research and conservation in the animals' habitat country, wherever that might be. Sometimes the organisation may purchase areas of land and conserve the habitat or it may pay for an education or research programme in the country to encourage indigenous people to conserve wildlife for future generations. To do this they may implement ecotourism projects where tourists will come to the area to observe the living wildlife. This aims to encourage people to conserve the animals for

business and long-term profits rather than simply view them as a dwindling food source. Zoos, both large and small, also offer financial support to other conservation organisations or may work in cooperation with them.

To complement this most zoos will have both education and research departments. These will work both within the animal collections and in the habitat countries. Few other organisations cover as wide an age range and academic levels in their education programme as a zoo. Almost all zoos will have some programme for preschool children and the best ones will continue right the way through to PhD level. This results in numerous opportunities for research projects both within the zoos and wherever else the zoo is involved (see below). In addition we must take into account all the passive education that takes place as the zoo visitors tour the zoo grounds reading labels or listening to organised talks as well as any organised events that take place, such as evening talks or educational promotions.

The position and duty of a modern zoo in society

So where does a zoo fit in today's world? They are undoubtedly a place of entertainment for the public: this is still the main reason why people pay to come in and we must remember this. If visitors do not enjoy their time at the zoo they will not come back and without visitors zoos cannot survive to continue the work they do in other areas. The World Association of Zoos and Aquaria calculates that over 600 million people visit animal collections each year (www.waza.org).

As mentioned above, zoos are also a major force in the education system of many countries. In the UK alone, 740 000 pupils use the education services of zoos with over 400 000 receiving formal education (www.biaza.org.uk). Don't forget that it isn't just animals that you can learn about in zoos: zoos can also be used to teach about human behaviour, building design, tourism and media and are also often used as a source of inspiration for art students. This is now one of the main strengths of zoos – they are a great reservoir of knowledge and information.

As mentioned previously, zoos now conduct much of their conservation in a different way to a few decades ago and we are yet to see if this will be truly effective. It should be mentioned that the more traditional methods of conservation (i.e. breed and release) do still take place but they are relatively rare and are far more carefully planned than previously.

It is pleasing to see how many communities have taken their local zoo to their hearts and are interested in everything that the zoo does. This can also have its drawbacks as occasionally something may happen to a popular animal and there will be a major backlash of bad publicity against the zoo for a while, but generally people are very supportive. However, this could be a short-lived situation: it was only two or three decades ago that zoos were being attacked by the press and various anti-zoo organisations on a regular basis and many closed as a result.

One of the main catalysts for the change in public perception was the advent of the 'fly on the wall' documentaries that became popular in the 1990s. This allowed viewers to see what was happening behind the scenes, to appreciate the problems that zoos face and to see the passion of the staff who work there. In a recent survey being a zookeeper was the most desired job in the UK (if the pay was better), compared to the situation in the 1990s, when staff were told to check beneath their cars for explosive devices. To capitalise on this many zoos now run a Keeper for the Day programme where members of the public pay to work with the keepers. Not only does this scheme generate revenue but it also demonstrates the new openness of animal collections, which can only be a good thing.

Without zoos most people would never see some animals in the flesh and without this, how can we expect them to have the desire to help conserve them? Whenever zoo visitors stop and think about the status of an animal in the wild and feel that they want to do something to help them, then the zoo has done a good job.

ZOO LEGISLATION

The modern zoo has to comply with many forms of legislation, both legal requirements that are set by the relevant governments and those that are self-imposed by the governing body of the region in which the collection is located. A discussion of relevant types of legislation follows but readers are advised to check on the regional zoo association's website, government or ministry websites and the health and safety body's website. In the UK these are www.biaza.org.uk, www.defra.gov.uk and www.hse.gov.uk.

Animal collections have to comply with the following guidelines. The names and exact details vary depending on the country in which the zoo is based, but most apply to some extent.

Zoo licence

This is the licence that allows the zoo to operate. As noted above, a zoo is defined as an establishment that allows the public access to view its animals on 7 days in any 12-month period. Whether the public are charged

an admission fee or not is irrelevant. A team of inspectors will tour the establishment and if it meets the requirement it will be given an operating licence for 4 years. Subsequent licences last for 6 years. The UK guidelines are set out in the Secretary of State's Standards for Modern Zoo Practice, details of which can be found on the Department for Environment, Food and Rural Affairs (DEFRA) website (www.defra.gov.uk).

Health and safety

As society in general becomes more likely to sue an establishment for any injury, whether physical or psychological, it is prudent to ensure that you are fully up to date with the correct health and safety legislation for your country. Once again these should be easily found on the relevant government website. Most zoo managers have to complete some form of risk assessment on all jobs within the zoo that staff are involved in as well as any activities that are organised for the public. These forms will highlight any potential problems or dangers, and ask for a date for the safety measures to be implemented. It is also important to ensure that all staff are made fully aware of any risks involved with their job and are issued with all the appropriate protection equipment such as masks, gloves and goggles.

All the appropriate paperwork and posters should be on display and easily accessible. UK zoos are subject to regular health and safety checks by their local authority.

Hazardous substances are also covered by their own legislation to ensure correct usage and disposal. This affects not just cleaning materials but also many of the chemicals that the veterinary department will be using.

Accidents

All accidents should be reported to the zoo management and recorded, no matter how small. The possibility of a serious infection from a relatively small cut is very high in the conditions in which zoo staff work. More serious injuries, to both staff and public, usually have to be reported to the local authorities and in some cases an investigation will take place. Zoos often ask for near-miss incidents to be reported in the hope that future accidents will be averted.

Firearms

Almost all zoos will be required to have at least one person with a firearms permit or licence to dispatch an animal if a dangerous situation such as an escape occurs. As vets often have to have a firearms licence to use their dart guns, they may often have a licence for other weapons as well. Ideally several people should be able to use the guns and there should be a selection of weapons to choose from.

Anyone on the firearms team should also have regular training from a recognised body such as the police force to ensure that they are competent and confident with the weapons.

Animal transportation

This is one of the most complicated and time-consuming regular procedures in the zoo world. The biggest problem is that lots of organisations require various tasks and paperwork to be completed before an animal can be moved. The ministry that controls farming and animals in both the exporting and importing countries will require several tests to be done on most animals to help prevent the spread of disease. If a disease is currently prevalent in the country of export then the move may be halted indefinitely.

The Convention on International Trade in Endangered Species of Wild Fauna and Flora (CITES) certificates will have to be gained before some animals can be moved. For more details on this, see www.cites.org. There are numerous laws on the movement of animals, regarding the amount of time an animal remains in a crate or transporter as well as the size of that transporter. Many of these laws are based on farm and domestic animals but sometimes concessions are made for the movement of exotic animals. Obviously you cannot transport a fully grown giraffe by plane and it would have to take the slower route by land and sea.

ISO 14001

As many animal collections now style themselves as environmental parks and wish to set an example, they often try to reach the ISO 14001 Environment Management Standard, which is an internationally accepted standard to show that a company is reaching set criteria regarding the environment. It affects all parts of the business and is constantly monitored to ensure that standards do not slip.

Buildings

Wherever you are in the world the chances are that buildings have to conform with certain standards. To ensure this, planning permission often has to be sought before a project can be started and the plans have to show that the building will reach certain standards of safety as well as meet any environmental criteria that may be in force.

Other legislation that will need to be considered includes laws covering subjects such as food hygiene in catering outlets, fire precautions, including regular drills for the staff and regular checks of all equipment and safe disposal of animal waste, including the disposal of animal bodies. The list is almost endless and as a general rule, the more diverse a collection, the more legislation that will be involved.

THE ROLE OF THE ANIMAL KEEPER

How the role has changed

The role of zoo keepers in most collections has probably changed faster in the last few decades than in most other professions that do not rely heavily on information technology. For a long time keepers were farm workers who just happened to look after different species of animals. They would be expected to come into work early, clean the animals out and have the zoo looking tidy before it opened, usually at 10 a.m., after which they would either have to be on show to the public to answer questions or be hidden out of sight so that they didn't spoil the look of the place. They weren't expected to know about the natural history of their animals; rather the public were far more interested in the personalities of the animals they were looking at, how dangerous they were and how cute were the babies.

This has slowly changed, sometimes for the better and sometimes for the worse. Interactions with the animals began to be expected and the rise of the chimp's tea party and the circus-like elephant shows took place. Although this lasted for quite some time, things did change when conservation started to come to the forefront. The more enlightened zoos began to consider breeding their animals rather than continually taking from the wild – sometimes this was out of necessity as supplies from the wild started to dry up. To do this they needed staff who knew what was needed to breed the animals successfully, so the role of the keeper changed to that of a true animal carer.

With the passage of time it became apparent that a well-trained committed group of keepers was one of the mainstays of all zoos (although by no means the only one). Managers began to invest in their staff by enrolling them on nationally recognised courses for exotic animal management, by paying for them to attend conferences to further their education and by trying to ensure they had the time to study and learn about their charges. This soon came to the attention of other bodies such as the media and education, who realised that there was a resource here to be used.

Modern keepers no longer just have to know how to use a broom and shovel to clean and a knife to cut up the vegetables (although that is still a major part of the job). They now have to be ready to appear on live or recorded national television or radio at a moment's notice, to answer numerous requests from students about their animals, to know about the natural history of a species as well as the individual (television documentaries have made the public far more knowledgeable and demanding in their questions), to give informed public talks, to continue to attend conferences although now they give the presentations, to have a working knowledge of veterinary procedures so that they can assist when necessary, to assist or carry out research on their animals and also to consider continuing their education beyond the zoo-provided courses.

When managers used to look for staff they would choose ones who looked strong enough to work all day and had good 'stock sense'. Now it is realised that brains are just as important as brawn. Keepers are the public face of the zoo and as such have to be presentable, knowledgeable and polite. They are the ambassadors for their zoo around the world.

Daily routines

The title of this section is a misnomer. There is no such thing as a routine day in a zoo and that is one of the main attractions for the people who work there. At the end of almost every day you should be able to ask yourself 'what did I do that was new today?' or 'what did I learn today?' Probably the easiest way to show what a normal day should be like is to break the day up into bite-sized pieces for both a keeper and a animal manager at a typical UK zoo (Table 24.1) and then show what can happen on a day when things don't go quite to plan (Table 24.2).

As can be seen, it does not take much to change the daily routine completely – just one special visitor and one sick animal. All staff have to be flexible and although Table 24.2 showed how such problems affected the keeper and manager, they would have had a knock-on effect for several other departments as well:

- Any planned procedures that the vet had arranged would have been cancelled or rescheduled
- If the animal was well known by the public the press office would have had to prepare a press release
- Any planned repairs in the building needing the keeper's presence would have been postponed
- If the animal was due to be moved the curator would now need to cancel or organise a replacement
- Staff at the front entrance would need to tell visitors that the animal was off display.

This shows how zoos work as a community. Something that happens in one department has a knock-on effect all around the institution and possibly even further afield.

All other departments have their daily routines. Ground staff keep the grounds clean and the gardens tidy, the press office checks to see if they are likely to be asked about an international story that has hit the press, vets monitor for any diseases such as foot and mouth in the region as well as deal with the animals on site and maintenance deals with repairs in the public areas as early as possible. The list is endless and ever-changing but is targeted at providing a good product, continually improving the animals' welfare and reaching the goals of the collection.

Qualifications

As zoos include such a wide variety of professions within the same organisation it is impossible to list all the qualifications that are needed. Stop and think of some of the different jobs involved in running even a medium-sized zoo (Box 24.1).

This box by no means gives a complete list but for most of these jobs the zoo will be looking for either the relevant qualification or a fair amount of experience. Although working in zoos is never well paid, there is no shortage of competition for jobs as zoos are generally considered good places to work. Most of the qualifications that are needed will be similar to the general

---

Box 24.1

JOBS IN A ZOO

Accountant	Librarian
Adoption coordinator	Marketing manager
Animal curator	Play area supervisor
Artist	Press officer
Bar staff	Receptionist
Carpenter	Researcher
Catering manager	Research student
Cleaner	Sales person
Director	Secretary/personal assistant
Driver	Storeman
Education officer	Teacher
Environment officer	Toilet attendant
Events coordinator	Tree surgeon
Functions manager	Vet
Gardener	Vet nurse
Gate keeper	Volunteer
Grounds keeper	Volunteer coordinator
Horticulturist	Waiting staff
Human resources	Website supervisor
IT officer	Welder
Keeper	Works supervisor
Labourer	

Table 24.1 A routine day at the zoo

Time	Keeper	Manager
7.45	Arrive at work and get changed	Arrive at work and get changed
8.00	Visual check of all the animals keeper is responsible for	Check that all the staff are in and inform them of the day's events
8.15	Go to the zebra house to assist with animal training	Fill in the daily report sheet
8.30	Service the nocturnal house	Walk the entire section
9.30		Report to the curator for the day's instructions
10.00	Go to the mess room for tea break	Go to office for tea break
10.30	Clean and feed the bongo	In office answering e-mails and bringing records up to date
11.30	Clean and feed the kangaroos	
12.00	Assist with the cleaning of the bison	Attend meeting with the science department
12.30	Lunch	
13.15		Lunch
13.30	Work on enrichment for the section	
14.15		Meet vet to discuss upcoming procedure
14.30	Collect browse for the section and feed to the animals	
14.45		Give a talk to MSc students
15.00		
15.15	Public talk	
15.45	Stock up the section with hay, straw and feedstuff	In office answering e-mail, post and phone queries. Working on studbook and staff matters
16.15	Prepare the evening feeds	
16.30	Feed and shut in animals for the night	
17.00	Complete the day's record keeping	Check that all staff have finished safely
17.15	Finish work	
17.30		Finish work

workplace, the exception once again being the keeping staff.

Most of the regional organisations such as British and Irish Association of Zoos and Aquariums (BIAZA: UK), the Association of Zoos and Aquariums (AZA: USA) and ARAZPA (Australasia) recommend a course for the keepers to go on. This ensures that there is continuity between the region's zoos to ensure that everyone understands the level attained. In the UK we have the Advanced National Certificate in the Management of Zoo Animals (ANCMZA), which is a 2-year correspondence course (for more details go to www.sparsholt.ac.uk). Each zoo

has a zoo tutor who will mentor the students who are marked on both their course work and exams. Each region will have its own preference as to the style of the course and the amount of work involved. In addition there are numerous degree and MSc courses, details of which can be found on the internet.

Once you work for a zoo there are plenty of opportunities to further your education. Most staff dealing with the public will go on some form of training to finetune their skills and many staff may also be given media training. Practical courses are common too, from chain sawing to forklift truck driving, not to mention first aid.

Time	Keeper	Manager
Table 24.2 A not-so-routine day at the zoo		
7.45	Arrive at work and get changed	Arrive at work and get changed
8.00	Visual check of all the animals keeper is responsible for	Check that all the staff are in and inform them of the day's events. One member of staff is off sick
8.15	Go to the zebra house to assist with animal training	Fill in the daily report sheet
8.30	Service the nocturnal house	Walk the entire section
9.00		Meet member of the public who is paying to work on the section for the day
9.15	Find sick animal in nocturnal house	Get a report of a sick animal
9.30	Assist with the catch-up of the sick animal	Assist with the catch-up of the sick animal
9.45	Assist the vet with the sedation	Assist the vet with the sedation
11.15	Clean and feed the bongo	Help out on the section that is short-staffed
11.30	Clean and feed the kangaroos	Attend meeting with the science department
12.00	Assist with the cleaning of the bison	
13.00	Lunch	
13.15		Do most important paperwork
13.30	Finish off the nocturnal house work	Lunch with a VIP visitor
14.15	Collect browse	
14.30	See vet to check on sick animal	See vet to check on sick animal
14.45	Return animal to the enclosure and monitor	Give a talk to MSc students
15.00		
15.15	Public talk	
15.45	Stock up the section with hay, straw and feedstuff	Report to curator on day's events. Assist on section that is short-staffed
16.15	Prepare the evening feeds	
16.30	Feed and shut in animals for the night	
17.00	Complete the day's record keeping	Check that all staff have finished safely
17.15	Finish work	
17.30		In office replying to e-mails, post and phone calls
?		Finish work

ANIMAL IDENTIFICATION AND ANIMAL RECORDS

Reasons for identification

As discussed in the next section there are numerous methods of individually identifying an animal but the first question we need to address is: why is this necessary?

The primary reason for being able to identify each animal is to aid record keeping. The quantity of information kept on each animal is always increasing and it is often recorded and kept by several different people (keepers, vets, curators and studbook holders), so it is vital that they all know which animal they are referring to in their records.

It had long been held that it was enough for the keeper simply to be able to tell the animals apart but as soon as that keeper leaves or the animals are moved to another part of the collection, then all that knowledge is lost. I have lost count of the number of times that keepers (including myself) have been 100% certain of the identity of an animal, only for the records to prove beyond a shadow of a doubt that they were wrong. Too many things can change on an animal as it grows older, or even as the seasons change, for this to be a reliable method of identification.

It is no use to a breeding programme if the animal recorded as number 376 is paired with animal 454 and no one can tell you which animal is which! Equally the vet will need to be certain that he or she is indeed giving the right animal the right treatment. This is particularly relevant in the case of vaccinations, which are usually spaced a year apart. Returning to the breeding situation, it is also worth bearing in mind that several species of animal look alike to the naked eye and without accurate records going back generations, hybrids could soon occur. This is even more likely in the case of subspecies which are far more likely to be able to interbreed. Also, imagine being unable to confirm the identity of one of your animals that is being transferred to another zoo and 6 months later it transpires that you sent away your only breeding female!

With the current tiger population, for example, it has been possible to go back in time through the generations via the records and find out when possible cross-breeding of subspecies has occurred. The offspring of these animals can be traced back through the generations to the modern day and prevented from any further breeding to ensure the pureness of the subspecies. The same has been done with the captive orang utan population to remove all offspring from Bornean and Sumatran hybrids from the breeding plan, usually by various contraceptive methods.

If you have a large number of animals of one species you need to be able to identify the animals as they are moved from one cage to another, or if you have to remove one particular individual. This is a common problem with many smaller and more easily transported animals such as birds and rodents.

The permanent identification of animals has also proved to be useful when animals have been released back into the wild. As the animals can be monitored it is possible to study both dispersal and survival rates. The discovery of non-marked animals also indicates that they are successfully breeding in their new situation.

Even in the larger groups of animals where the identification methods may not be easily seen on a day-to-day basis (herds of ungulates or large troops of primates), it is at least possible, when an animal dies or is removed for treatment, to tell which one it is.

Finally some of the methods of identification are only temporary and these are generally used to allow animals to be studied easily for a short period of time by people who do not have the time to identify the animals by any other method.

Methods of identification

There are many different methods of identification used in modern zoos (Table 24.3). Several of them are now becoming outdated, as new methods are developed and people's perceptions change, and are only found on older animals. It is not uncommon for an individual animal to have more than one method of identification – one that is visible to the naked eye for daily observations and one that cannot be lost but can only be read by the animal being restrained or having died:

- Certain species are required to have tags by law, e.g. cattle and sheep in the UK
- Tattoos on the knuckle or around the eyes are allocated certain numbers. The animals are tattooed with dots in these places and the value of the dots is added up to find out the animal's number. Tattoos around one eye or hand have the value of units and on the other of tens (Figure 24.1).
- Branding is very rarely, if ever, carried out in modern zoos
- With freeze branding the hair usually grows back completely but is white in colour
- Horn branding is where marks are carved into the animal's horn or cut with a hacksaw
- Notching consists of taking a small notch out of an animal's extremity such as ears, webbed feet, ridge scales on reptiles or tortoise shells. Toe clipping is also a form of notching. The areas notched have similar values to the tattoos above

Table 24.3 Identification methods

Method	Positives	Negatives
Natural markings, e.g. feather patterns, coat patterns, deformities, size	Non-invasive, can often be seen from a distance, no cost	Can change either over a long time or quickly, e.g. during a moult; information may be lost if an animal or keeper is transferred off a section. Size will also change over time
Dyes and coloured sprays	Easy to apply without harming the animal. Easily seen from a distance. Only short-term, ideal for research studies. Good for seeing breeding in some species, i.e. ram pads	Only short-term: dyes can transfer from one animal to the other causing confusion. In extreme cases new colours may potentially affect animal behaviour
Ear tags	Come in a large range of colours and can be numbered to ease individual identification. Easily applied to young animals	Small tags are not easily seen from a distance and large ones can be obtrusive. Tags can be caught in fences and pulled out, injuring the animal. Adult animals may require sedation to have an ear tag put in
Tattoo	Permanent. If done carefully, can be fairly unobtrusive	Can only be done on areas of bare skin. If numbers are used, can be disfiguring
Branding	Permanent	Can be disfiguring. Considered barbaric by general public. Painful to the animal for some time. Difficult to see with long-haired species. Sedation may be necessary
Freeze branding	Permanent. Does not destroy the hair follicles as branding does. Reported to be less painful than traditional branding	Brands have to be large. Would not work with light-coloured species
Horn branding	Fairly permanent. Easily seen	Can only be done with certain species. Has to be done on an adult animal so sedation is often required. Occasionally animals may lose their horn or horn sheath. Can only be done with straight lines so Roman numerals are usually used: not everyone can read these
Notching	Easily seen	Also may be considered barbaric. A simple injury to an animal can change the number of that animal, causing confusion
Transponding	Easy procedure with young animals. Low failure or loss rate of transponders. Every animal can have an individual identification number	Slightly painful. Animals need to be restrained or sedated. Currently several companies produce transponders and not all readers are compatible with all readers. A fairly expensive method of identification
Necklaces	Easy to read. Unlimited number of combinations. Can be temporary or permanent	Very obvious. Potential of strangulation

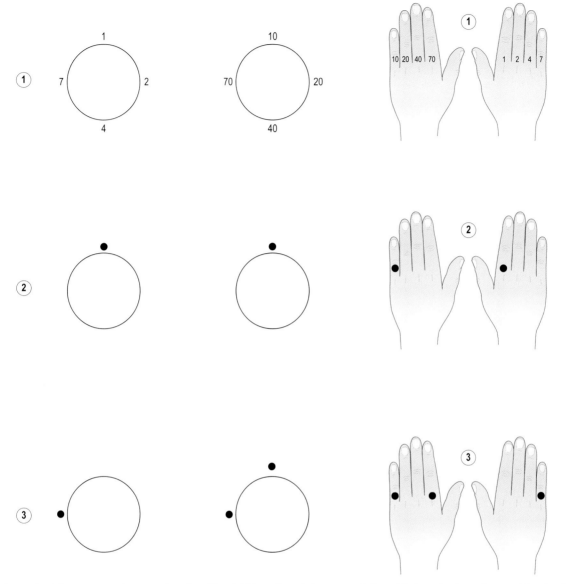

Figure 24.1 Tattoos around eyes and on knuckles. (1) The value of the tattooed dots; (2) the animal number 11; (3) animal number 87.

- Transponders may need to be implanted by a vet; at the very least training is needed. Some countries require that imported animals are transponded as this is a fairly secure method of identification
- Necklaces are often used during observation by students to ease the problems of identification.

Methods of recording

Table 24.4 outlines the different methods of recording information about animals. Remember that this is not the only information that is recorded at zoos. Various items, from the seemingly mundane numbers of visitors and the weather to the parasite burdens of the stock at different times of the year, will all be saved for future reference.

The last three rows of Table 24.4 are due to be replaced by a new system called Zoo Information Monitoring Network System (ZIMS), to improve the transfer of knowledge as there have been problems with the non-compatibility of some of the programs in the past.

Table 24.4 Recording methods

Method	Description
Keeper diaries	Kept by the keepers on a daily basis, recording anything relevant that happened on the section or that may prove relevant in the future, e.g. animal behaviour, breeding behaviour, jobs done, changes in diet, types of browse fed. These are how the day's events are passed on to any keepers who were not working on that day. They are often copied into a more permanent format at a later stage
Record cards	One of the first methods of official record keeping in zoos. Each collection has its own style. Many zoos still use this method, particularly if not all staff have easy access to computers. With long-lived species it is important to redo the cards every few years before the information becomes illegible
Daily return	An official record kept by senior staff on a department including such things as animal moves, deaths, births, sicknesses and transfers. Also records staff who are on duty or on leave
Animal Record Keeping System (ARKS)	A computerised system that records all the relevant information for an individual as well as allowing the user to display all the animals currently in a group or that have been in the past. It is possible to select as much or as little information as desired and it is the easiest way to send information about an animal from one institution to another
Medical Record Keeping System (MEDARKS)	A similar system to ARKS that is aimed primarily at the veterinary aspect of the animals in the collection
Studbooks (Single Population Analysis and Records Keeping System: SPARKS)	Another similar system that concentrates on assisting the user to decide on the best pairing within a species and the numbers of that species in captivity. This is usually used for monitoring populations from more than one collection

Studbooks

In their simplest form, studbooks are a list of all the animals of a given species that are alive in a country, region or even globally. It is what the studbook holder can do with this information in the studbook that makes them an indispensable tool in the modern zoo world. With the program Single Population Analysis and Records Keeping System (SPARKS) and the correct training, the user can trace the lineage of any given animal as far back as the records go and also, more importantly, work out the animal's relationship to any or all currently living animals. This is known as the mean kinship of an animal.

Having this information means that the animal can be ranked in importance. For example, a male that has no siblings or offspring is probably going to be quite high in the rankings whereas one that has six siblings and has sired 20 offspring will be close to the bottom. The studbook holder will now make recommendations as to which animal should breed with which. Generally like is paired with like – the most important male should

breed with the most important female and so on down the rankings to the level where the recommendation is that these animals should not be allowed to breed any more. Any animal that comes from the wild is known as a founder and these are the most important animals in any studbook. Although zoos rarely take animals from the wild these days, odd ones do still turn up from sources such as customs confiscations or injured animals from sanctuaries.

This is a very time-consuming job that requires a lot of training and data inputting, particularly if you are setting up a new studbook. It also relies on the cooperation of all the zoos involved. Everyone in the zoo world should know that the recommendations are for the best of the species but sometimes a zoo may be unwilling to part with an animal. Maybe it is a favourite of the staff, it is a good breeder providing the zoo with plenty of babies for the public to see or maybe the zoo simply can't afford to pay for the transfer. Until all zoos accept that the studbook holder's recommendations are the best for the animals and should be carried out, there will slowly be a degradation in the genetic material of the

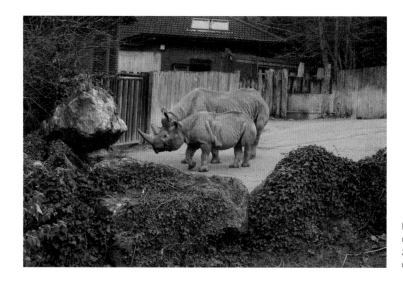

Figure 24.2 Reproductive achievement can be a viable measure of success for zoological collections and an important contribution to conservation.

animals in captivity. The target for most studbooks is to retain 98% of the genetic purity of a species over a period of 100 years.

Surprisingly, one of the easiest methods of helping to achieve this target is to slow down the breeding of a species. Every generation bred is going to cause new problems for the studbook, such as:

- Individuals unable to breed for one reason or another
- Unplanned matings: maybe an animal was not taken away from a group soon enough and was allowed to breed
- Overcrowding caused by the population growing combined with the increasing number of animals that are not wanted for breeding.

If the animals are allowed to breed unchecked you could have a new round of youngsters each and every year. However if you prevent them from breeding on alternate years then the number of youngsters is immediately halved and you have time to catch your breath. The most practical, but controversial, option is for zoos to cull the surplus unimportant animals to allow the more important ones to breed (Figure 24.2).

ZOO RESEARCH

This is one of the major growth areas in zoos and it covers almost all levels of research. If you have a look at the e-mail inbox of any zoo you will see that there are a very high number of queries from students from all over the world. These may be answered by one of several departments within the zoo from the animal and veterinary departments to the education and research depart-

ments. Queries will come from many levels of education, from school projects right up to PhD students. These are just the tip of the iceberg as they represent only those students who are making the most of a facility to aid their research.

Most zoos have a research department of their own and indeed in several countries it is a requirement of a zoo to conduct research of some description. It has only been in recent years that zoo research has been accepted as a worthwhile discipline; previously it had been frowned upon by scientists who did the 'real' research on the animals in the wild. However, with the passage of time, academics are starting to appreciate that there is a whole wealth of information that can be gained only from these captive animals.

One of the major areas of research is in the field of nutrition, with two main directions being taken. One is to see how much of any food that is eaten is actually absorbed and used by the animal; this can help us to understand what the animal requires in the wild. This is vital information if a release is planned. The other is to research the types of food that we feed to our animals to see how they compare with any known wild diets, thus helping us to improve our captive diets. One thing to bear in mind at this point is the problems involved with sourcing the correct foodstuffs for our animals. Fruit is the main problem for two reasons: the fruit that humans eat has far more sugar in it and it is usually fully ripe. Wild fruits have far lower levels of sugar and rarely have the opportunity to ripen fully before being eaten. Not surprisingly, very few fruit suppliers have large supplies of unripe, sour fruit. The other problem is that most animal feeds are made with domestic or farm animals in mind and people require far different things from these animals than we do from the ones in zoos. Farm animals have to grow quickly or produce large amounts of produce such as eggs or milk and as a result need a diet that will give them the energy to do this. Zoo animals are still basically wild animals; certainly their body's requirements will not have changed much and they will be very efficient at surviving on poor-quality or low amounts of food. Feedstuff produced for domestic animals is too good and will cause obesity, hoof overgrowth and numerous other problems. Fortunately continuing studies by zoo researchers and food-producing companies mean that a wider range of species-appropriate feeds are now more readily available.

Another type of research that can be carried out very successfully in the captive situation is into the behaviour of the animals. It is believed to be important that captive animals' behaviour mimics that of the wild counterparts as much as possible and the only way that we can find this out for sure is to study the animals. This research often goes hand in hand with studies involving environmental enrichment and as such will usually involve the animal departments as well as the students.

Another form of research that often requires cooperation with another department, this time the veterinary department, is reproductive research. Once again this is research that is of vital importance to the future survival of many species in captivity.

One point worth making is the fact that zoos are quite reticent about the type of research they do. If they wish to do anything that is considered to be invasive they may well have to apply for a licence. As this is often public knowledge, many will shy away from this as it opens them up to criticism from animal rights organisations. It is usually perfectly acceptable to collect samples from an animal during a veterinary procedure or sometimes if it is part of a regular health check but as each region has its own rules this must be checked.

HOUSING AND HUSBANDRY

What are the animals' needs?

By now you will have realised that there are several different versions of the five freedoms (Chapter 9) and although the wording may change slightly, the general concept remains the same. These are the mainstay of deciding what the animals in your care need and deserve. They can be supplied in many different ways: correct housing is a necessity and there is no excuse for keeping an animal in poor conditions except for the shortest of times. Such occasions will be beyond the zoo's control, such as a building or enclosure being damaged and the animals having to be temporarily rehomed while repairs are effected or animals having to be kept inside due to an infectious outbreak in the vicinity.

Adequate space is always a problem with animals in captivity and we will never be able to provide most species with as much as they have in the wild. However, many animals only have such large home ranges to ensure that they can meet all their needs. If you can provide them with food, water, breeding opportunities, seclusion, shelter, stimulation and exercise within their enclosure they will have less of a desire to go further afield to look for it.

A correctly designed building should provide all the animal needs in terms of shelter, heating and nesting places but it is important that enough are provided for the whole group. When the enclosure is correctly designed it will also allow the animal to express its natural behaviours. Keeping a burrowing animal on a solid floor will soon result in a very stressed animal that could well have injuries to its front feet.

Always try to keep the animals in the correct social group. One animal on its own may not look much of an exhibit but if that is how it lives in the wild then that is how it should be kept. Some naturally solitary animals will share an enclosure with another if it is big enough but you have to ask yourself which is the most important – a single animal that the public might not be able to see very well or several animals in the same enclosure that are continually pacing? In my experience if the reason why an animal is on its own is explained to the public they understand.

With a little thought most enclosures can be made to suit the animal they are intended for and to meet all their requirements while also being attractive to the public.

Enclosure design

This is a subject that almost any animal professional can wax lyrical on indefinitely. It is a very subjective topic and as soon as any design is built everyone comes up with ideas that they think would have improved it in some way. Almost all the suggestions are valid and almost all will have been discussed at some point by the design team and rejected for one reason or another.

The design team should consist of a variety of people from different disciplines and should meet regularly during any new build to ensure that all problems are dealt with as they occur.

Zoo design is a very specialised subject and few architects have much experience with it. They have to be prepared to turn many of their preconceived ideas on their heads and be flexible with their design. Many designs begin with the management of the zoo locating a site in the grounds for development and providing the architect with a rough drawing or plan of what they require. The architect will now draw up the first set of plans for the design team to look at.

The design team should consist of senior staff from the zoo, staff who will be using the building on a regular basis, representatives from the maintenance department and the architect. This team will be supplemented by specialists both from outside and within the zoo as the need arises. There should be as many meetings as necessary to get the plans exactly right before building starts. Many more concepts have to be considered than in normal human housing:

- Everything has to be easily cleaned and therefore all electrics have to be waterproof
- Fixings for perching and enrichment have to be provided
- There has to be easy access for long lengths of wood for perching
- There has to be the ability to separate and catch up animals
- Drainage has to be good and easily serviced
- In cold climates back-up heating systems should be provided
- There should be several entrances for the animals to go into the house from the paddock so that one animal cannot monopolise the only entrance
- Everything has to be 'animal-proof'; most non-animal people cannot appreciate the strength or dexterity of animals
- Double-door systems will often be required for added security.

This is just a short list to start you thinking. If you are ever lucky enough to be involved in designing an enclosure you will soon realise that altering just one small feature has a knock-on effect to many others. Also this is only for the fabrication of the building: it now needs to be made to look pleasing to the public so you have to start involving aspects of landscape design such as rockwork (real or artificial), substrates and planting. After this you have the outside paddocks to consider as well.

Compromises sometimes have to be made for both animals and public. It is natural for animals to want to hide away from the public sometimes and it is natural for the paying public to feel cheated when this happens. There are things that can be done to help this situation. If you have a ground-living species that likes to lie alongside a log or in an area of undergrowth then make sure that the logs point towards the viewing area and don't run parallel to it. Equally with clever planting animal runs and tracks that go through vegetation can be viewed by the public while still giving the animals a sense of security. Don't forget other tricks such as mirrors and cameras to see into sleeping and nesting areas as well as one-way glass so that the animals cannot see the visitors at all.

Zoo design does not stop with the enclosure alone. Think where that enclosure fits into the layout of the zoo. When it is built is it going to affect the flow of visitors around the grounds? Are you going to need extra food outlets, toilets and the like? In extreme cases, will it boost your visitor numbers to the extent where parking needs to be increased? Do you need new roads so that the building can be serviced? Will you need to lay new pipes and cables to deal with the increased waste and power use?

The most obvious change over the years has been from the small barred cages that were once so common to the large, airy enclosure of today. Sometimes these changes can be surprisingly small but can make a world of difference. Look at an old enclosure and imagine it with the concrete floor dug up and plants put in. Now change the old bars with glass and what was once a terrible enclosure is now perfectly suited for its resident.

Some useful further reading is the proceedings of the zoo design conferences, which can be obtained from the secretary of the Whitley Wildlife Conservation Trust (trustsecretary@wwct.org.uk), and the Zoolex website (www.zoolex.org).

Mixed exhibits

More and more collections have mixed exhibits. This is where two or more different species are kept together in the same enclosure. A typical example is the average tropical house which can house mammals on the floor as well as birds and reptiles in the trees; occasionally mammals will get in on the arboreal act with the introduction of bats into the enclosure. There are many advantages and disadvantages to mixed exhibits, as can be seen in Table 24.5. The advantages and disadvantages balance out and most problems can be overcome if they are thought through carefully and the staff are willing to adapt and put in a little effort.

Environmental enrichment and its aims

So what is environmental enrichment? Frankly, it is nothing new. The first time that people threw a stick for a dog, let a kitten play with a ball of wool or spread the cattle food out around the paddock rather than leave it in a pile, they were carrying out enrichment. Anyone that owns or works with animals will deal with animal enrichment on an almost daily basis. As a result there are lots of different definitions for environmental enrichment, but here we will describe it simply as when an animal keeper, pet owner, lab technician, hobby farmer or smallholder does something to improve the welfare of animals.

Table 24.5 The advantages and disadvantages of mixed exhibits

Advantages	Disadvantages
The public find them very enjoyable. They are usually planted out well or at least themed to mimic a habitat and there is a high density of animals so there is plenty to see	Very difficult to feed an animal or species individually as most will have access to all the feeding stations
It allows the zoo to hold more animals than usual in a given area. Where perhaps 30 animals of one species would fight, 15 of one and 15 of another may not	For the reason given above it can be difficult to administer medication
A good educational tool, showing how animals live together or sometimes how animals from different parts of the world have evolved to fill the same niche	Very difficult to catch an individual of any species if it needs treatment or is to be moved to another collection. Traps have to be employed
Animals often breed well in these types of enclosure because of the 'natural' environment and stimulation	Breeding is very difficult to control: because of the 'natural' environment there are plenty of places for the animals to nest
Interaction between species can help with keeping the animals occupied, therefore reducing the necessity for environmental enrichment	Occasionally mistakes can be made with the species that are mixed, resulting in one species preying on another
A good environment for studying animal behaviour	A particularly aggressive individual may dominate an area of the enclosure, excluding all other animals. This can be a particular problem if it dominates a resource such as food or water

In zoos we want to keep our animals active at the times when they should be active, we want to keep them fit and healthy and we want them to show similar behaviours to their wild counterparts. Animal collections are constantly under a microscope: we invite the public in to view our work, the press is often waiting for us to make a mistake and in the UK we have to reach the Secretary of State's Standards for Modern Zoo Practice. All of this means that we have to provide a good product, which means that we have to maintain suitable enclosures, provide a wide variety of animals for the public to see and ensure these animals are in the best possible health both mentally and physically and it is with this final point that enrichment can help (Figures 24.3 and 24.4).

One of the big problems encountered with all types of captive animals is that of stereotyping. This is when behaviour (often part of the animal's natural repertoire) is repeated excessively for no apparent gain. People often think that this is just a problem with zoo animals. We have all seen animals pacing in a zoo; often it is the big cats that show this behaviour, or at least they are the ones that do it the most noticeably because of their tendency to pace the perimeter of their cage, often near the public barriers. However a lot of other animals will also pace. Sometimes the repetition is so complicated that it will take a considerable length of time before it becomes

clear exactly what they are doing. It doesn't just involve pacing, it might be any other odd behaviour that animals do. It could be overgrooming, where the animal may develop bald or even sore patches; feather plucking in birds may also be a result of overpreening and is usually considered to be the result of boredom; R&R (regurgitation and reingestion) is when an animal, often a primate, will force itself to be sick and will then promptly eat its own vomit – the list of aberrant behaviour is almost endless. It is not just zoo animals that are affected either: farm animals will constantly lick the sides of their stalls or may be seen throwing their head back repeatedly. We have all seen and probably laughed at (although we may not admit to it) the home videos sent in to television programmes of the dog or cat walking a repeated route and doing a neat back flip at the end. It might be funny but in truth it is probably a seriously disturbed animal. In labs too, mice and rats stuck in small cages for all of their lives will often develop strange rituals, and in extreme cases animals in any location or situation will start to harm themselves to relieve the boredom. We call this self-mutilation or self-injurious behaviour.

One of the main aims of enrichment is to try and improve the health or at least the fitness of an animal (Figure 24.5). In the wild there is no such thing as a free meal; every animal has to work for its food. It may look as if the wildebeest wandering across the plain eating the

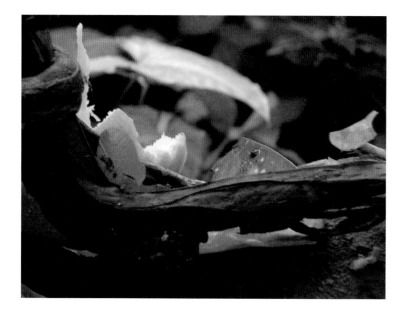

Figure 24.3 Mimicry of natural environment as enrichment in tree ants.

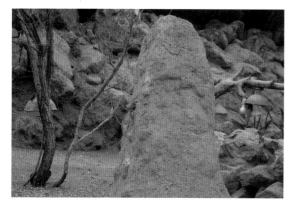

Figure 24.4 Food enrichment: false termite mound with hidden food compartments.

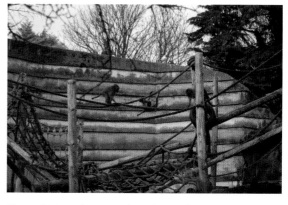

Figure 24.5 Environmental enrichment for baboons.

grass under its feet has a life of leisure, but the fact is it never stops wandering – it will clock up thousands of miles each year of its life. Compare that to its counterpart in the zoo. Even in the most expansive of paddocks we can't even dream of equalling that sort of mileage. The problem will be aggravated if all food (which is often more nutritious than the wild diet) is just placed in a pile in front of the animal. Why should the animal exercise? Why not just eat the food and then sit down and ruminate for the rest of the day. If the food is put in small piles in various parts of the paddock, or if the hay is placed under a pile of branches it will take a lot longer to eat for a start and you will probably find that animals will spend a far greater time moving around exploring the paddock in case you have put a pile down that they haven't managed to find yet. Enrichment is also useful

to encourage animals to make full use of their environment.

Enrichment has often been used to aid people with the management of their animals. One of the main times that we might use it is when we are mixing animals for the first time, and it is used simply as a distraction to help alleviate any aggression that may occur. Also problems sometimes occur when one of the animals in a group dominates the others at feeding time. Enrichment will often increase the number of feeding stations or increase the time that the food is available so that one animal simply can't commandeer it for the whole day. Figure 24.6 shows examples of enrichment.

It is vitally important to study the animals before, during and after the enrichment is given to them. It is no use thinking that you have put the enrichment in and

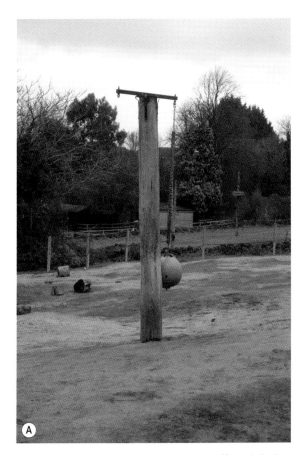
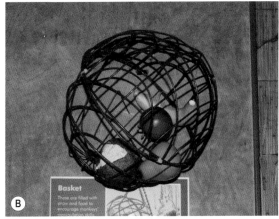
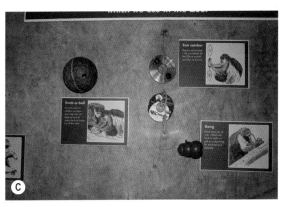

Figure 24.6 Examples of enrichment. (a) Giraffe and elephant enclosure; (b) basket and fruit; (c) sensory enrichment.

all problems are now solved. As an example, a small troop of baboons was given a large termite mound-style feeder to make them spend more time feeding as they would not know when the food was going to appear. When the feeder was first given to them the mealworms could come out of several points around the feeder. This seemed to be the sensible option as it was assumed that this would decrease aggression. What actually happened was the aggression in the group increased as the dominant animals kept moving from feeding point to feeding point, checking for mealworms. It was decided to reduce the number of feeding points to just one to see what would happen. The result was the dominant animal would wait at the feeding hole until he had eaten his fill or became bored and would then move on, allowing the next in line to take its turn and this went on all the way down the line: each animal knew its place and the aggression was reduced. An interesting byproduct of this enrichment was that the amount of social grooming in the group increased dramatically as they spent a lot more time grooming each other whilst waiting their turn.

Environmental enrichment also has the advantage of bringing the animals out on to public display without forcing them. They choose to come out and hunt for mealworms and probably will show no interest in the watching public.

Environmental enrichment can be subdivided into different types, as follows.

Manipulatory enrichment

This is an enrichment that is designed to be moved around or 'played with' by an animal. Examples are balls for big cats to knock about and carry, suspended logs for horned animals such as bison to butt and cardboard boxes to be destroyed by a variety of animals.

Sensory enrichment

This aims to stimulate animals' senses in an unaccustomed way. Herbs and spices can be used to make the animals investigate parts of the enclosure, sealed tubes with stones inside become rattles and icecubes are always enjoyed on a hot day.

Feeding enrichment

This is the easiest of all enrichments as it can be as simple as scattering food all over the enclosure, giving it to them whole instead of cut up or maybe hiding it in a device so that they have to work out how to access it.

One important principle is not to repeat an enrichment too soon as the animals will become bored and interact with it less.

For more information go to www.enrichment.org or www.reec.info. The latter website has several papers from regional conferences on environmental enrichment. Many zoos also include enrichment as part of their website.

THE ROUTINE CARE OF EXOTIC ZOO ANIMALS

This is not the place to go into detail about the daily care of the many types of animal you find in zoos. More than enough books and websites do that. What is more important is to point out that it is imperative to make sure that everyone involved in the care of the animals uses all the facilities that are available to them.

These facilities are manifold and could include such resources as:

- Approaching the other staff in the collection: often their total experience can add up to hundreds of years and that is a great deal of knowledge to call upon
- Staff from other collections are always willing to share their knowledge and there are several e-mail groups dedicated to this
- Don't be afraid to use books. As well as the ones dedicated to the captive management of animals there are many that have information on the animal in the wild rather than in captivity. This is useful information too: the habitat of the animal will tell you whether you need to provide heat, what sort of humidity is needed and how to fit out the enclosure plus what sort of food the animal is likely to need.

The main point of the routine care of zoo animals is that, along with the daily routine of the keepers, it should ensure that the five freedoms are met for all the animals (Chapter 9).

HEALTH AND WELFARE

Animal welfare

It can be difficult to explain to the general public why it is sometimes necessary to euthanase a seemingly healthy animal and even if there are legitimate reasons some of the more passionate visitors may become very vocal. Such situations include where a zoo perhaps has several males (some of which are castrated) but no females of a species. This species is critically endangered and we are crying out for more collections to hold breeding groups. The only way that this zoo will be able to take any females is to put down the castrated males to make space. These males are never going to be able to contribute to the breeding programme and in fact their very presence is having a negative effect on it. So what do you do? Do you wait another 10 years for these males to die of natural causes, by which time the other males may not be fit enough to breed, or do you put them down, put up with the bad publicity and do what you feel is best for the species? Although zoos do not face these questions on a daily basis they do still occur occasionally.

It must be emphasised that no zoo would take this as a first option; they will always try to rehome surplus animals, or preferably control breeding to prevent a surplus in the first place, but occasionally such a situation will happen. Usually it will occur with species that live in single male groups: as there are an equal number of males and females born there will always be spare males. With some species, such as the Western Lowland gorilla, it has been discovered that zoos are able to maintain bachelor populations, which does relieve the pressure somewhat, but you do still have the problem of these groups taking up space that could be used by breeding groups.

To make sure that a zoo does not overstep the mark and is doing everything correctly with as high a standard of animal welfare as possible, most will 'self-police' by setting up some form of welfare committee. This committee should have representatives from several departments of the zoo as well as outside experts and some lay people who have an interest in zoos or animals but are not professionally involved. These people will meet on a regular basis to discus any events that may have happened or problems that seem likely to occur in the future. Senior management should also be involved so that any decisions made can be enforced there and then.

Many of the studies carried out in zoos by their own students concentrate on the welfare of the animals in their care and we are always looking at ways to improve it. With some species we have just about got it right but with others we still have a little way to go and sometimes outside intervention is necessary. For example, recently the Royal Society for Prevention of Cruelty to Animals produced a report on the welfare of elephants in captivity in the UK (*Live Hard, Die Young*: www.rspca.org.uk/ elephants) and this forced the zoo industry to take a good look at itself. A report was produced by BIAZA (available online at www.wildlifeinformation.org) which countered many of the arguments but the benefit of the initial report was that the elephant-keeping community drew closer together, communicated with each other more and made real efforts to improve their animals' welfare. Only a few collections decided to stop keeping elephants as a result but everybody made changes to their management techniques, and as a result these elephants have some of the best facilities in the world and are the best-cared-for animals too.

Veterinary care

The veterinary care of animals in a zoo is of the utmost importance and many zoos have their own well-equipped veterinary departments. The bigger the zoo, the more likely it is to have such a department. There comes a point where it is economically more sensible to have your own vet team than it is to be continually calling in an outside veterinary practice. There are several degrees of veterinary cover in zoos, from the one mentioned above, to having a veterinary facility but calling in a vet to carry out the procedures, to having no facilities and fully relying on an outside practice.

Whatever system the collection has chosen to adopt, the roles of the veterinary officer will be broadly the same. The first and foremost will be to provide treatment to any animal in the collection that requires it but the vet will also be expected to provide a schedule of prophylactic treatment, including worming and vaccinations. In addition the vet will be expected to monitor all the treatments and the general health of the animals and probably be actively involved in some of the research projects that are taking place.

As with many departments within an animal collection, a veterinary department is one that can only cost money with no chance of any financial return and indeed setting up a full-size department is an extremely expensive venture. Apart from the wages of at least one vet and one vet nurse, it costs a small fortune to build and equip a facility that will be suitable for the wide range of animals found in most collections. The average veterinary practice only has to cope with a small number of species, although that number is increasing as more and more exotic pets are kept, whereas a zoo vet could be dealing with several different species a day all week and must have the equipment to deal with this variety.

This variety also means that specialist training is required and there are numerous additional courses in exotic animal medicine that can be taken either during initial training or at a later date. Most zoo vets will also need to call in specialists from other disciplines, both human and animal, as the need arises. An organisation called the International Vet Group will travel anywhere

in the world to assist in animal treatments and countless human doctors are willing to donate their time and expertise for the chance to work with something different.

THE MANAGEMENT OF COLLECTIONS

The management hierarchy of a typical zoo

There is no set formula in the management hierarchy of zoos. Each zoo will use whatever system suits it best for the size of the organisation.

There are numerous departments within a zoo and their individual roles will be described briefly in the next section. In Figure 24.7, the job titles edged in red show a direct hierarchy, i.e. they are junior to the person above but senior to the one below. The other job titles are all different roles in the same department and answerable to the first job title in black above them. In some instances (particularly in smaller collections) one person may fulfil several of these roles.

The departments of a typical zoo and their roles

A representative selection of the departments in a typical zoo is listed in Figure 24.7 and a brief description of their duties follows.

Animal departments

These are usually led by a curator or manager and will have several grades of keeper down to trainee. The department is responsible for all aspects of animal management as well as public relations and helping to keep the park respectable.

Veterinary department

The veterinary department is responsible for the health of the animals in the zoo, both reacting to problems as they occur and trying to be proactive to prevent them. The department will work closely with the animal departments and possibly the research department.

Catering department

This is one of the few parts of the zoo that will make money so it is important that it works well. It will probably be subdivided into several departments such as the main restaurant, outlets around the zoo and special

395

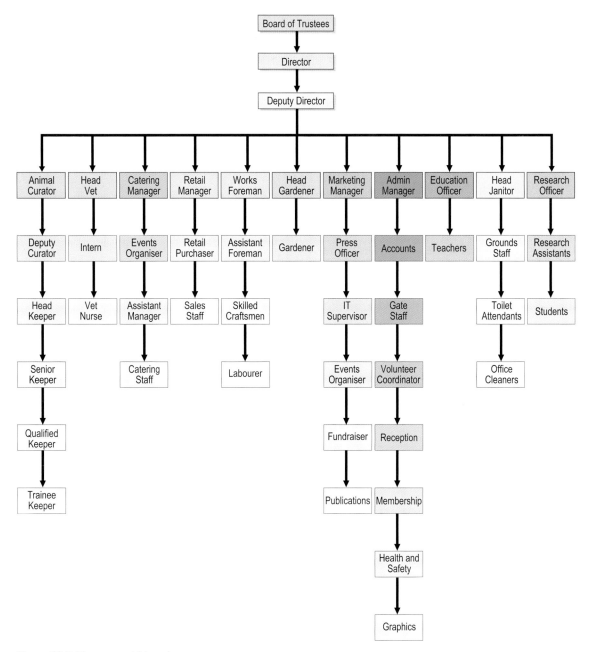

Figure 24.7 Management hierarchy.

functions. These functions will often take place out of hours and will sometimes require help from other departments.

Retail department

Again this is another money-maker for the zoo. There will be several outlets around most parks, with the main one near the main entrance. Some collections are now expanding this area with sales on the internet or by mail order.

Works department

The works department is a vital part of the zoo. Without it the place would literally fall apart. As well as regular maintenance these departments are often involved in any new builds that are taking place.

Gardens

The gardens are an often unsung part of the zoo but would soon be missed if they weren't there. As more exhibits are themed in zoos their role increases in both the design of the exhibits and then the maintenance.

Marketing

This department has several sections, most of which are related in advertising and publicising the zoo, from press releases about events such as interesting births to evening functions. The zoo website and publications will also be organised by this department.

Zoo administration

This is a 'catch-all' department that has a wide variety of functions, all of which are important in the smooth running of any business.

Education

Originally thought of as an 'add-on' that zoos ought to have, this department has now become one of the most important in the zoo with thousands of students passing through the department each year.

Janitorial

Janitorial is another of the unnoticed departments – until the job isn't done properly. Keeping an area of over 100 acres clean, not to mention the public conveniences that have been used by up to 10 000 visitors a day, is not an easy task.

Research department

This is another department that is rapidly growing in importance in the modern zoo. The research department continues further education where the education department leaves off, extending as far as PhD level. They will supervise all the students using the zoo as well as conduct research of their own. The research will often take place in situ as well as in the zoo and the department often works closely with the local university. The zoos conservation section is often part of this department.

Collection planning

In this section everything that animal collections have to think about in advance will be discussed. It must be remembered that many zoos have to be run as a business. In some countries they are fortunate enough to receive state support but this is not the case worldwide, and even these zoos still need to have a plan to show that they will use the money that they are given wisely.

There are two main types of plan: short-term and long-term. The long-term ones usually set out the aims of the collection for the next 10 years and these will be revised or rewritten every 5 years or so. It is impossible to make a 10-year plan last the full 10 years as the market changes far too quickly and it would be a big mistake to tie yourself down for that long. Equally it is important not to use this as a method of continuously postponing unpopular but necessary projects. What will be included in this plan are the larger projects that the zoo wishes to do; for example, 'use the site of the old elephant house for new tropical house' or 'develop relations with a production company to promote the idea of a new television series'. For many of these projects there is a great deal of work to be done before they come to fruition so a deadline is needed to make sure that people do not become complacent. Each department within the zoo will have its own aims, from a new outlet for retail to a new conservation area in Africa for science, and it is up to the board of directors (or their equivalent) to prioritise each of these and decide which ones the business should be investing in.

As time goes on these projects will move either in part or wholly to the short-term plan. For example, the new tropical house mentioned above may well be included in two such plans – the first year would be to plan and build the house, followed in the second year by fitting the house out and sourcing the stock for it. The short-term plan will also include many of the more mundane projects that happen in the collection such as maintenance schedules, replacement or disposal of stock according to breeding programmes and staff training.

From these initial plans a schedule for the whole zoo and budgets can be drawn up to make sure that everyone in the management team knows what is to happen that year and can plan accordingly. This is important in a business that relies on people visiting to make its money: it is important that the centre of the zoo is not a building site at the peak time of year and that retail have had time to stock their new outlet ready for those busy days. The animal departments will also need to know when any build is likely to be finished as it takes considerable time to import an animal from a zoo abroad, not to mention that the animal may have to be in quarantine for up to 6 months before it can go on show.

This involves a lot of meetings, coordination and good leadership to ensure that a zoo runs smoothly and is focused on its future and not, as has happened far too often, still living in the glory days of the past.

International cooperation

One of the biggest steps forward that zoos have made over the last few decades is in the way that they now cooperate for the good of the animals. There used to be considerable competition between collections, which is understandable as they are all trying to get a share of the same corner of the market, but they have learnt that there is more to be gained than lost by working together.

The obvious benefit of this cooperation is the improved welfare of the species in their care. No longer does every zoo in the world have to learn on their own how to manage each type of animal by trial and error. They can contact any zoo in the world and ask them for their diet or management technique and they will be happy to provide it. It would be easy to suppose that it is the new world of computers and communication that has allowed this to happen but in fact it started long before this came into existence.

As a young keeper I can remember an older member of staff complaining about the fact that he had been asked to show a visiting keeper from another zoo around and explain how our penguins did so well. His main complaint was that if he did that then they would know how to breed them as well! Fortunately this sort of opinion is no longer prevalent and we are all only too pleased that other people may want to know how we are managing our animals. Now, when two keepers from different collections have a conversation each of them will learn something from the other.

There are so many meetings, both international and national, held on all aspects of work in zoos each year that it is impossible for any one zoo to send representatives to them all. At least all the proceedings are published and these are well worth hunting down if you want to study a particular aspect of zoos. Once again, your regional organisation would be a good place to start. With the advent of the computer the ability to transfer information in vast amounts instantly to many people has made things so much easier, not just for the gathering and dispersing of knowledge but also for planning the survival strategies of many species.

Bibliography

Clubb R, Mason G A review of the welfare of zoo elephants in Europe. University of Oxford, Oxford

Management guidelines for the welfare of zoo animals – elephants, 2nd edn. BIAZA, London

Chapter | 25 | Jane Williams

Laboratory skills and microbiology

This chapter considers laboratory practice and common tests used as an aid to the diagnosis and treatment of animal disease. The essential skill of microscopy is explained thoroughly to enable students to perform microscopic evaluation of samples. Pathogenic microorganisms are classified into species and their individual characteristics considered in relation to how they cause disease and prevention of their effects.

HEALTH AND SAFETY IN THE LABORATORY

There are many potential hazards in the laboratory and it is important to be aware of the risks so that accidents and cross-contamination can be avoided.

There are a number of laws and regulations that govern the health and safety of workers in the veterinary laboratory.

Health and Safety at Work act 1974

- Governs both employee's and employer's responsibilities in the workplace
- Protects against risk
- Controls storage and use of dangerous substances
- Governs provision of personal protection equipment (PPE)
- Governs schedules of work and practice protocols.

Control of Substances Hazardous to Health 2002

- Controls the risk to the workforce from using/exposure to harmful substances at work
- Aim is to reduce occupational illness
- Examples include cleaning products, waste products, pathogens
- Control of Substances Hazardous to Health (COSHH) regulations include risk assessment, monitoring, training, information and supervision.

Reporting of Injuries, Diseases and Dangerous Occurrences Regulations 1995 (RIDDOR)

- These regulations describe procedures which must take place if death, serious injury or a work-related disease or injury occurs in the workplace
- Incidents are reported to the Health and Safety Executive (HSE)
- Injuries that must be reported include:
  ○ Injury which causes 3 or more days off work to the affected person
  ○ When reportable, work-related disease is diagnosed, e.g. tetanus
  ○ When a dangerous occurrence takes place, e.g. explosion, chemical leak.

First aid in the laboratory

- Standard first-aid procedures should be available in the lab
- All first-aid equipment and boxes should be checked regularly
- All should be easily accessible
- The first-aid box should be green with a white cross
- The names of first aiders and their location should be specified.

Safe working practice in the laboratory

- No food or drink at any time
- Protective clothing should be worn
- Long hair should be tied back
- Lab should be kept free from obstructions and clean
- No unauthorised personnel should be allowed to enter without supervision
- Waste should be disposed of correctly:
  ○ Clinical waste is disposed of by specialist company/incineration
  ○ Cadavers are disposed of by certified collector/incineration
  ○ Commercial waste is included with office waste, which is disposed of by council
  ○ Sharps are collected in a sharps bin, which is disposed of by specialist company/incineration
- Wash hands before and after working in the laboratory and in between tasks where appropriate
- Follow hazard symbols and manufacturer's instructions
- Standard operating procedures/protocols and schedules of work should be in place.

Waste disposal

In the laboratory you will often be given specific instructions on where to dispose of waste. Animal tissue may be kept separate from normal clinical waste; additionally potential hazardous waste, e.g. bacterial cultures, is normally autoclaved before disposal.

MICROSCOPY

To look at the detailed structure of cells it is necessary to look at the means available to examine them, i.e. microscopes. Refer to Table 25.1 for a comparison of light and electron microscopes.

Light microscopes

Single-lens type

- Simplest form of microscope
- Limited powers of magnification.

Compound light microscope

- Two lenses are used
- Light from the object passes through the first lens and is magnified
- This magnified image then acts as the object for the second lens, which magnifies it further
- For example, if the eyepiece lens has ×10 magnification and the objective lens has ×40 magnification, total magnification of the object would be ×400

Table 25.2 shows the magnifications commonly used for animal samples.

The degree of detail that can be seen with a microscope is called the resolving power or resolution. This measures its ability to distinguish two objects which are close together. A microscope with high resolution can distinguish two objects which are very close together whereas a microscope with low resolution will show the two objects as one. The resolving power of a microscope is inversely proportional to the wavelength of light used, i.e. the shorter the wavelength, the greater the resolution. This means that the resolving power of any light microscope is limited because the wavelength of light has a fixed range. Improvements can be made to a certain extent by the use of staining specimens, focusing techniques and methods of illumination.

Electron microscope

These were developed by scientists exploring the possibilities of utilising shorter wavelengths for magnification. The first electron microscope was developed in

Table 25.1 Comparison of light microscope and electron microscope

	Advantages	Disadvantages
Light microscope	Cheap to buy Cheap to operate – uses a small amount of electricity for a light source Small and portable Unaffected by magnetic fields Preparation of material quick and simple Requires little expertise Material rarely distorted by preparation Living and dead material can be observed Natural colour of material can be observed	Lower magnification – 1500 times Low resolving power – 200 nm Restricted depth of field
Electron microscope	Much greater magnification – over 500 000 times Much greater resolving power – approximately 1 nm Depth of field can be much greater	Expensive to buy – costs millions of pounds Expensive to operate – requires up to 100 000 volts to produce electron beam Very large and immobile – needs special rooms Affected by magnetic fields Preparation of material long and complex Preparation of material may cause distortion Only living material can be viewed – high vacuum kills material All images in black and white

Table 25.2 Magnifications commonly used for animal samples

Power of magnification	Magnification factor	Samples exampled
Low power	×10	Parasites Skin Urine deposits Faeces
Medium power	×40	As above, but in more detail Total red and white blood cell counts
High power	×100 (oil immersion)	Bacteria Blood cells Dry prep urine

1933. They use the same principles as the light microscope but swap beams of electrons for rays of light. The image produced cannot be seen by the naked eye: it is projected on to a screen from which black and white pictures or electron micrographs are produced. There are two types: transmission and scanning electron microscopes.

Light microscope

There are two types of light microscope: monocular (one eyepiece) and binocular (two eyepieces).

Parts of the microscope

Figure 25.1 shows parts of the microscope.

(a) Eyepiece – this has a lens in it with a magnification, usually of ×10
(b) Eyepiece tube – this houses the eyepiece and is removable to allow cleaning of eyepiece lens
(c) Head – the movable top of the microscope which can be rotated for comfort
(d) Coarse focus – larger of the focus knobs, used to focus initially

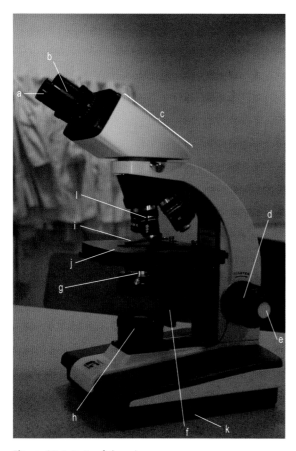

Figure 25.1 Parts of the microscope.

(e) Fine focus – smaller focus knob, used to focus for fine detail (should never need to be turned more than a quarter-turn to achieve clarity)

(f) Coaxial stage mechanisms – these manoeuvre the stage and therefore the slide, allowing thorough examination

(g) Substage condenser – ensure this is racked up before focusing; it plays a role in focusing for parasites. It controls the light on to the specimen

(h) Iris diaphragm – controls quantity of light from bulb to the slide (like the pupil in the eye)

(i) Spring arm – holds the slide securely upon the stage

(j) Mechanical stage – where the slide is placed

(k) Brightness control – controls amount of light flooding the slide

(l) Objective lens – various magnifications are available; it can be removed for cleaning.

Remember that the magnification of your sample will be the eyepiece lens multiplied by the objective lens, not just the objective lens! Always use a lens tissue to clean

the lens as normal tissue paper will scratch and damage the lens. Air puffers are available to blow off dust and if greasy spirit may be used to clean the lens (after oil immersion). When carrying the microscope support the limb and the base to prevent damage. After use place the lowest objective lens in position, rack up the condenser and set the light to its lowest setting and turn it off to prevent it blowing when the microscope is turned on. Replace the dust cover. If you have used the oil immersion lens then clean it before the oil dries.

How to use the microscope

Place the microscope on a secure, level area away from vibrating objects, heat, light or water supplies.

1. Set the binocular eyepieces for your interpupillary distance (the measurement between your two pupils) so only one field of vision can be seen

2. Place the slide uppermost on the stage in the slide clips (cover slip side up or, if there is no cover slip, you can usually scratch a bit of stain to see which side it is on)

3. Click the lowest-power objective lens into place

4. Rack the lens to just above the slide (watching it at all times), then slowly rack away from the slide using the coarse focus knob whilst viewing the slide (use both hands on both coarse focus knobs as the focus system is balanced and always using one knob will damage the microscope)

5. When the object comes into focus, transfer to the fine focus knob and finetune for clarity

6. Adjust the substage position for the best lighting; it is best to begin with the substage condenser raised and it can be lowered if required, e.g. for parasites

7. Use the mechanical stage travelling knobs to move the slide around to view the entire sample

8. Providing the focus is sharp, swing in the ×40 lens and adjust the focus.

Hint – the more powerful the objective lens, the closer the lens will be to the slide when in focus; if glasses are normally worn, remove them.

Troubleshooting

No image or very dark image or image dark and illuminated irregularly

- Microscope not switched on (check plug and base)
- Illumination control at low setting or off
- Objective nosepiece not clicked into place over lens
- Diaphragm closed down too much or off-centre
- Light failure.

Image visible and focused but pale and indistinct

- Diaphragm needs to be closed down further
- Condenser requires adjustment.

Image blurred and cannot be focused

- Dirty objective
- Dirty slide
- Slide in upside down
- Slide not completely flat on stage
- Eyepiece lens not set for user's eyes
- Fine focus at end of travel.

Dust and dirt in field of view

- Eyepiece lens dirty
- Slide dirty
- Dirt on lamp glass or upper condenser lens.

Oil immersion technique

1. Rotate the ×40 lens away from the slide
2. Take the oil and place a drop on top of the slide (enough to make a concave meniscus)
3. Click ×100 lens into place and carefully lower it into the oil; the oil should 'splat' but still be between the lens and the slide
4. Adjust the focus.

Vernier scales

Vernier scales are located on the mechanical stage. They are arranged at right angles to each other so that the readings on these two scales can be recorded for any particular point, providing coordinates which can be used to relocate an item on the slide. Each scale is divided into a main scale in millimetres and a Vernier plate, bearing 10 divisions each of 0.9 mm.

To read a Vernier scale:

1. Move the slide and observe which number the zero on the Vernier plate is opposite,
2. If the zero is between numbers, then record the lower one,
3. Observe the Vernier plate and record the increment which exactly matches the main scale, which will give a whole-number increment.

The centrifuge

The centrifuge is used to centrifuge or spin down samples for analysis or examination. It operates on a balance principle, therefore any samples being centrifuged should be balanced using an equivalent sample. This could be the same-size tube filled with a placebo substance, e.g. water. The sample tube and the balance should be on the same plane, i.e. opposite each other. The centrifuge should be kept clean and free from contamination. Contamination commonly occurs when the safety plate is not securely fastened over the samples, resulting in movement, breakage and spillage. Spillages should be cleaned up when they occur as samples like blood can be difficult to remove once dry.

Automatic analysers

Commercial analysers offer a reliable, accurate method of obtaining results which is less time-consuming than manual methodologies and offers a wider range of tests. Chemistry analysers produce clinical chemistry data to diagnose disease and monitor therapy. They are sensitive machines which require careful maintenance and the manufacturer's instructions for operating should be closely followed.

Most makes require a warm-up period to allow the light source, photodetector and incubator (if present) to reach the equilibrium (or factory setting) before use; it is usual practice to turn the machine on first thing in the morning and leave it ready for use. There are two types of analyser: wet or photometric colorimetry and dry analysers. Quality control is required to ensure accuracy. This can be achieved by analysing a known sample or doubling up a sample and sending one to an external laboratory and performing the other in house, then comparing the results.

COLLECTION AND PRESERVATION OF PATHOLOGICAL SAMPLES

All samples must be:

- Labelled with details of the owner and animal, date, type of sample and the practice details
- Collected aseptically to prevent contamination and inaccurate results
- Collected wearing appropriate PPE, e.g. gloves
- Collected into a suitable container which is secure to prevent leakage and contamination (Figure 25.2 and Table 25.3)
- Collected into appropriate preservatives and stored correctly to prevent inaccurate results.

Records required for pathological samples

- Detailed information about the patient's condition for the pathologist

Table 25.3 Blood collection tube colour and preservative

Anticoagulant	Vacutainer colour	Plastic tube colour	Use
Ethylenediamine tetra-acetic acid (EDTA)	Purple	Pink	Haematology Cerebrospinal fluid
Heparin	Green	Orange	Biochemistry Lead
Potassium oxalate with sodium fluoride	Grey	Yellow	Glucose
Sodium citrate	Light blue	Purple	Coagulation tests
Plain – no anticoagulant	Red	White	Serum is used for biochemistry
Citrate dextrose	Yellow		Cross-matching/blood typing

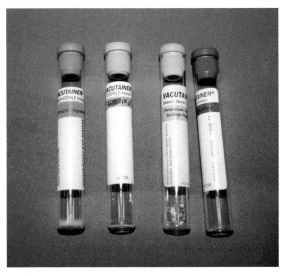

Figure 25.2 Vacutainers for blood collection.

Table 25.4 Toxicology sample collection methods

Sample	Container
Whole blood	Ethylenediamine tetra-acetic acid/heparin
Plasma or serum	Clotted tube
Brain, kidney and liver postmortem samples	Freeze, then send to laboratory as soon as possible
Stomach contents	Waterproof bag/vial
Foodstuffs	Watertight container
Environmental sample, e.g. soil	Sealable container

- Completed pathology request form
- Details of owner
- Details of patient: species, breed, age, neutered status
- Date of sampling
- Clinical history, including recent pathology results and treatment
- Site of sampling for tissue samples and whether whole tissue has been submitted
- Test or tests required.

Tissue samples and body organs

Tissue samples are often used to identify a particular lesion or mass. Histopathology is the microscopic exam-

ination of tissue. Tissues can be sampled by biopsy (live animal) and postmortem (dead animal). Biopsies can be incisional, whereby a sample area of a lesion or organ is removed for examination, or excisional, where the whole lesion or organ is removed. Once removed, samples should be stored in appropriate preservative to prevent deterioration (Table 25.4). Preservative should penetrate the whole sample and the sample size should be restricted to 2–3 cm thick. A slice of a lesion or an organ is preferable; this will encompass the outer edge and the inner core. It should include the border between healthy and diseased tissue. Bodily fluids can be preserved by making a fixed smear.

Blood

It is vital to use the container which has the right type of preservative substance within it and a good-quality

Table 25.5 Faults in blood smears

Fault	Cause of fault
Too thick	Too much blood
Too thin	Too small a drop of blood Spread too slowly
Alternate thick and thin bands	Spreading done with jerky motion
Streaks throughout the smear	Irregular edge to spreader Dried blood on edge of spreader Dust on slide or in blood
Spots where blood is absent	Grease on slide
Very narrow, thick smear	Smear made before the blood has run along the edge of the spreader or one side of the spreader was lifted during spreading
Unequal distribution of white blood cells	Could be normal or sample not mixed

sample should be obtained to ensure accurate results. Sample collection can be from the jugular vein, saphenous vein, cephalic vein or transverse facial vein (horse). Ideally tests should take place as soon as possible after collection but whole blood may be stored at room temperature for up to 2 hours and in the fridge for 2–3 hours; serum and plasma can be frozen once it has been separated from blood cells. Remember, before starting any test, the sample should be at room temperature. Table 25.5 shows faults in blood smears.

Hair/skin

Samples to be collected should not be from a cleaned area as this may remove bacteria. Hair plucks using Sellotape or fingers can be mounted on to a clean microscope slide for examination. Skin scrapes can be collected using a blunt scalpel blade, raising the area to be sampled between thumb and finger then scraping until it bleeds. The sample is placed on to a clean, labelled microscope slide and potassium hydroxide can be added to the sample to improve viewing of mites. Skin is examined under the microscope at ×10 and ×40 magnification.

Urine

Urine collection can be by catheterization, which collects a sterile sample using aseptic technique; cystocentesis, which also results in a sterile sample, and uses aseptic technique; or a free-flow sample from midstream flow: this has the potential for cross-contamination as the beginning of the urine flow often has mucus, skin bacteria and epithelial cells from the urethra within it.

If urine is not tested within 1 hour it should be refrigerated; if it is required for longer than 24 hours a preservative should be used. Toluene can be added: just enough is used to get a thin film floating on the surface of the sample and the sample is suitable for biochemistry. Thymol can be used but it interferes with glucose testing and biochemistry. Boric acid is the preservative of choice: it often comes in commercially made-up pots, used to preserve bacteria. It prevents bacterial multiplication for up to 4 days and preserves the sediment.

Faeces

Fresh samples should be used and ideally direct collection from the animal used to ensure freshness but there is a risk of rectal mucosa damage. Avoid contamination with bedding and collect as little air as possible in the sample as this will promote bacterial replication. Some faecal samples need to avoid the presence of air; for example, in the horse, strongyle eggs will hatch into larvae if air is present. Faeces can be stored in the fridge from 24 hours to 4 days but in a warm environment parasite eggs will hatch into larvae.

Body fluid samples

Numerous body fluids are used for diagnostic sampling. These include synovial fluid, peritoneal fluid, thoracic fluid, tracheal wash, fine-needle aspirates and cerebrospinal fluid. Most require skilled knowledge and aseptic technique to facilitate collection and the fluid should be stored in sterile containers. A tracheal wash is performed using an endoscope passed into the trachea. A small quantity of sterile saline is introduced then aspirated to examine for the presence of pathogens. Fine-needle aspirates are commonly performed to evaluate the cytology of lumps, cysts and other abnormalities. A needle and syringe are inserted into a cyst and then the plunger is depressed a number of times, leading to cells being collected within the syringe. These cells are then transferred to a microscope slide, stained and examined for neoplastic changes.

Virology

This is usually performed at an external laboratory. Samples that may be examined include:

- Blood: equine influenza
- Tissues: fetal tissues for equine herpesvirus

- Swabs: nasopharyngeal swabs for influenza, conjunctival swabs for ocular discharge, pus samples for culture
- Bodily fluids: semen for equine viral arteritis.

Samples are tested to diagnose disease, ascertain vaccine efficacy (with antibody titres) and ensure the disease is eradicated.

Packaging and posting samples

Pathological samples are potentially hazardous materials and could cross-contaminate the postal staff. Careful packing is required to protect staff and to prevent deterioration or spillage of the sample. Fluid samples, e.g. faeces, fluid, blood, serum, urine and tissue samples should be placed in an appropriate-sized sample tube, sealed and wrapped in absorbent material (cotton wool) – enough to soak up all of the sample if it spills – placed in a leak-proof plastic bag and then inserted into a padded envelope for posting (these are often provided by commercial labs). Dry samples such as hair plucks and smears should be placed in a suitable sealed container in a clean dispensing bag with a sealable top and then into a suitable container for posting. All pathological samples should be labelled with Pathological specimen, Biohazard (with symbol) and Fragile: handle with care.

When posting samples other factors need to be considered, including:

- Transit time: how long will the sample await collection?
- Public holidays: avoid weekends and holidays due to reduced postal service
- Sample durability: some sample types will deteriorate quickly
- Post versus courier: some labs will offer a courier service.

Delays may result in deterioration of samples or prevent the instigation of treatment regimes, which could be detrimental to the patient.

Biochemistry

Biochemistry is the analysis of plasma (or serum); plasma or serum is generally analysed to ascertain raised levels of enzymes which can indicate tissue damage. A number of different profiles are available depending on the depth of analysis required, e.g. preanaesthetic profiles tend to evaluate liver and kidney function whereas an animal with an unknown condition may be tested using a full-body profile testing all physiological systems.

Muscle enzymes, e.g. creatinine phosphokinase and aspartate aminotransferase, are tested for. Raised levels are seen in animals suffering from muscle and often liver disease.

Analysis of liver enzymes is used in the diagnostic evaluation of liver function. In the healthy animal the liver enzymes, e.g. alkaline phosphatase and aspartate aminotransferase, are present in hepatocytes but are released when liver damage is present. Liver function can also be determined by bile acid analysis as hepatic disease results in elevated bile acids in the blood.

Bilirubin is a pigment produced as a byproduct of red blood cell destruction; high levels can occur if biliary or liver disease is present.

Urea and creatinine are products of protein metabolism and are normally excreted by the kidneys through urine. In renal disease kidney function is reduced and therefore urea and creatinine remain within the blood. Azotaemia is a description of raised levels of urea and creatinine in the blood. Be aware that other factors can affect the animal, mimicking renal disease, e.g. dehydration, increased protein intake.

Blood glucose can be measured by biochemistry or a glucometer; a transient increase may be seen in animals that are pregnant or obese or who have been receiving certain drug treatments, e.g. corticosteroids.

- Hyperglycaemia: diabetes mellitus, postfeeding sample, stress, Cushing's, corticosteroids, pancreatitis, certain drugs, e.g. morphine
- Hypoglycaemia: neoplasia, hepatic insufficiency, hypoadrenocorticism, malabsorption, starvation, insulin (overdose/no eating).

Total plasma proteins (albumin and globulin) can be measured by refractometer or biochemical analysis; these show elevated levels in dehydrated animals and decreases with liver disease and immune dysfunction, respectively.

HAEMATOLOGY

Haematology is the study of the cellular components of the blood and associated clotting factors. Blood contains many different types of cell. These can be divided into three categories: erythrocytes or red blood cells; leukocytes or white blood cells and thrombocytes or platelets. Anaemia is an abnormally low erythrocyte count and may be acute or chronic.

Anaemia is classified according to aetiology into blood loss, excessive destruction of red blood cells or inadequate production of red blood cells. Haemolytic anaemia is a form of anaemia that results from the destruction of erythrocytes, often due to pathogens, genetic factors or toxaemia. Leukocytes can be divided into two groups: granular leukocytes (granulocytes) and agranular leukocytes (agranulocytes). White blood cell counts indicate animals' suffering from infection or inflammation.

Common laboratory investigations performed for erythrocytes include:

- Packed cell volume (PCV: microhaematocrit)
- Mean corpuscular volume (MCV)
- Mean corpuscular haemoglobin concentration (MCHC)
- Blood smears, which are a general evaluation of cell morphology.

Packed cell volume

- This is a percentage of the volume of whole unclotted blood occupied by erythrocytes
- Microhaematocrit is a method used to determine PCV, using high-speed centrifugation of blood in capillary tubes
- PCV values are increased in athletic fit animals and in high altitudes
  - ○ Increased PCV can indicate dehydration
  - ○ Decreased PCV can indicate anaemia
- The capillary tube containing the blood sample (preserved in ethylenediamine tetra-acetic acid (EDTA)) is centrifuged for 5 minutes at 10 000 revolutions per minute, then examined in a microhaematocrit reader
- You can record plasma colour, buffy coat height and height of red blood cell column
- Plasma colour may be pink (in haemolysis), yellow (in jaundice) or milky (in lipaemia)
- The buffy coat (the white blood cells and platelets which comprise a small layer in between the red blood cells and plasma) is normally 0.5–1.2% of the sample; a higher level indicates a possible rise in the leukocyte count.

Blood smears

Blood smears provide a general examination of the blood; they can be used to examine cell morphology, identify parasites and perform manual red and white blood cell counts.

You will need a spreader slide (in which one edge has been removed), a clean microscope slide, tissue, capillary tube and an EDTA blood sample. Place a drop of blood on the right-hand side of the microscope slide. The spreader is positioned at an angle of 45° to the blood, then inserted into the drop, allowing the blood to flow along its edge. The spreader is then pushed in one smooth continuous motion towards the left-hand side of the slide to produce a thin layer of the blood which in an ideal world would be one cell thick! The smear should have a head, body and tail and be thin enough to allow diagnostic examination. Air-dry the slide by shaking it rapidly and it should dry within 5 seconds if it is the correct thickness. It should then be stained straight away or, if this is not possible, fix the smear with absolute methanol for 5 minutes. The smear is stained to make examination easier using a differential stain (Diff-Quik), Leishman stain or Giemsa stain.

Examination of blood smears

Blood smears should be examined using the ×100 objective lens under oil immersion. Total red and white blood cell counts may be performed using a haematology analyser or a counting chamber. A differential leukocyte count provides an indication of the different types of white blood cell that comprise the total figure of leukocytes in the animal. Increases and decreases in white blood cell type can be indicative for diagnosis. Identify the type of white blood cell present, whether polymorphonuclear cells (neutrophils, basophils, eosinophils), lymphocytes or monocytes. It is important to identify correctly the different cells to ensure accurate diagnoses. The following criteria should be applied: cytoplasm colour, colour of granules if present, nucleus size and shape and the size of the cell. Once 100 cells have been counted, the figures obtained can be expressed as a percentage or as an absolute number.

Total white blood cell count equals the number of all types of white blood cell in 1 cubic millimetre of blood. The differential white blood cell count provides an indication of the proportions of the different types of white blood cell. The two tests are complementary and should always be performed in unison for accuracy.

URINE ANALYSIS

The collected urine sample should undergo macroscopic examination, microscopic examination and specific gravity. Many things can be ascertained from the general character of the sample: perform this first as other tests may change the results.

Macroscopic examination
Amount

- Try and measure – this is not always easy!
- More important in neonatal cases
- Polyuria: excessive urine
- Oliguria: little urine
- Anuria: no urine.

407

Colour

- Yellow is normal but intensity may indicate concentration
- Brown/yellow: bile pigments are present – may be caused by shock, renal problems, dehydration
- Red/brown: red blood cells and haemoglobin are present – may be caused by oestrus, foodstuffs, e.g. beetroot; the sample may be stale
- Bright red: urinary tract exit trauma
- Brown/black: azoturia, excess exercise.

Turbidity

- Normal urine will appear clear; abnormal urine will be cloudy
- Cloudiness may be due to:
  - Red or white blood cells
  - Crystals
  - Casts
  - Epithelial cells
  - Mucous strands
  - Sperm
  - Fungi/yeasts
- Centrifuge and examination of sediment are usually required to ascertain.

Odour

- Does it smell normal?
- Strong smell: concentrated
- Ammonia/stale smell: bacteria are present
- Sweet smell (pear drops): ketosis (diabetes)
- Poisoning cases may alter smell of urine.

Next invert and remix the sample before beginning the other tests.

SPECIFIC GRAVITY

Specific gravity is the weight of a substance compared with the weight of an equal amount of something that is taken as standard; it can be thought of as a measure of concentration. The specific gravity of water is 1.000. Specific gravity of urine determines how many undissolved substances or items are present in the sample. Increased specific gravity can indicate dehydration, shock, infection or diabetes mellitus. Decreased specific gravity can indicate renal failure (polyuria), liver failure, Cushing's or diabetes insipidus. It is tested using a refractometer.

Chemical tests

These are usually performed using commercially impregnated sticks that provide a quick and accurate result.

Care and storage of urine reagent sticks

- Keep away from direct sunlight
- Store in a cool, dry place
- Replace cap after use
- Do not handle reagent areas
- Always use fresh urine.

Method

- Invert urine sample to mix
- Dip all of the reagent areas into the urine (have a watch with a second hand ready)
- Tap the edge of the strip against container or on a piece of tissue to remove excess
- Leave for the allocated time and record results – be careful, as many of the individual tests are completed at different intervals.

pH is a measure of the acidity or alkalinity of urine:

- $< pH\ 7$ = acidic
- $> pH\ 7$ = alkaline
- 7 = neutral.

Microscopic examination

A well-mixed urine sample is centrifuged to separate the liquid and solid components of the sample. The liquid is discarded and a stain can be added to enhance viewing (Sedistain), then a drop of the sediment is placed on to a microscope slide, a cover slip is added and it is examined systematically on the ×10 and ×40 objective lens for crystals, cast and cells.

MICROBIOLOGY

Microbes are microorganisms (Table 25.6). Microbiology is the study of microorganisms.

Types of microorganisms

- Bacteria – mostly unicellular
- Fungi – multicellular
- Viruses – no cellular structure.

Microorganisms are named using a generic name (genus: capital letter) followed by scientific name (species: lower-case letter). For example, *Escherichia coli*.

Viruses are usually identified by the disease they cause, e.g. feline leukaemia virus. Microorganisms are very small and are measured in units known as microns or micrometres: 1 micrometre = 1/1000th of a millimetre. Viruses are even smaller and can only be seen using an electron microscope; they are measured in nanometres (nm); 1 nm = 1/1 000 000 mm.

Table 25.6 Comparison of microorganisms

Type	Size	Structure	Nutrition	Motility
Bacteria	0.5–5 μm	Prokaryotic (no membrane-bound nucleus), unicellular, cell wall	Mainly heterotrophic, saprophytic or parasitic	Some are motile
Virus	20–300 nm	Central core of DNA or RNA, protein coat, often has lipoprotein membrane	Heterotrophic, obligate parasites (require host)	Some are motile
Fungi	Variable	Uni- or multicellular chitinous cell wall, membrane-bound nucleus	Heterotrophic, saprophytic or parasitic	Non-motile except for some spores
Protozoa	10–200 μm	Unicellular, eukaryotic, no cell wall	Heterotrophic, saprophytic or parasitic	All motile
Algae	0.5–20 μm	Uni- or multicellular, cellulose cell wall, eukaryotic	Autotrophic	Some motile

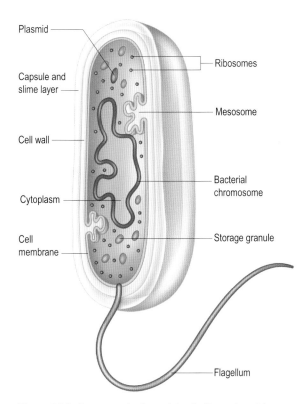

Figure 25.3 Structure of a bacterial cell. (Reproduced from Aspinall V 2006 *The Complete Textbook of Veterinary Nursing*. Butterworth Heinemann, London, with permission.)

Plasmid
Capsule and slime layer
Cell wall
Cytoplasm
Cell membrane
Ribosomes
Mesosome
Bacterial chromosome
Storage granule
Flagellum

Table 25.7 Classification of bacterial shape

Name of bacteria (classification)	Shape
Bacillus (bacilli)	Rods
Vibrios (curved bacilli)	Curved rods
Cocci Diplococci (remain in pairs after cell division)	Spherical
Streptococci	Chains of spheres
Staphylococci	Clusters – divide randomly in clusters
Spirillum (*Spirilla*) – rigid cell wall Spirochaetes – flexible cell wall	Spiral or helical cells

Viruses are not cellular and do not fit into the five kingdoms. They are classified as:

- Animal viruses
- Plant viruses
- Bacterial viruses.

BACTERIA ANATOMY

Figure 25.3 illustrates the structure of a bacterial cell and Table 25.7 gives the classification of bacterial shape.

Slime capsule

- Made of ectoplasm
- Protects cell

- Acts like glue to stick bacterium to host cells
- Prevents phagocytosis
- Increases virulence
- Acts as a food reserve.

Cell wall

- Unique shape (this allows treatment by drugs as specific drugs will target specific cell wall shapes)
- Protection – for example, it can prevent water entering the cell
- Varying thickness
- Made from a substance called murein.

Cell membrane

- Plasma membrane
- Inside cell wall
- Has selective permeability
- Has many folds, called mesosomes
- Mesosomes give an increased surface area for cell respiration and cell division to occur.

Cytoplasm

- Inside cell membrane
- Thick viscous fluid containing dissolved nutrients and waste products
- Within it are inclusion granules which store nutrients.

Ribosomes

- Inside cytoplasm
- Contain ribonucleic acid (RNA)
- Site of protein synthesis.

Bacterial chromosome

- Within cytoplasm
- No membrane around nucleus (like in animal cells)
- Small, with one circular or folded chromosome of deoxyribonucleic acid (DNA).

Plasmids

- One plasmid or more are usually present
- Small pieces of additional DNA.

Flagellae

- Appendages outside the cell wall
- Flagellae: movement

- Pili: hair-like; different types have roles in sex or attachment to cells
- Fimbriae: attachment.

Inactivation of bacteria

There are four main methods used to inactivate bacteria: oxidation, coagulation of protein, chemical combinations and osmosis.

Oxidation

- Add oxygen from the atmosphere to the bacteria
- This changes the chemical nature and destroys the bacteria.

Coagulation of protein

- High temperatures, e.g. boiling
- Coagulation or sticking together of proteins in the bacteria destroys the cell.

Chemical combinations

- Chemicals damage the structure of bacteria and destroy them
- For example, some disinfectants destroy the lipid envelope and allow excess fluid into the cell.

Osmosis

- Changing the concentration of fluid outside the bacteria causes water to be drawn out (placing it into hypertonic solution) and this desiccates or dries out the cell within
- This is achieved by placing the sample into saturated salt or sugar solutions.

Bacteria consist of approximately 80% water plus some fat and mineral content.

Conditions required for bacterial growth

- Suitable nutrients
- Correct temperature (ideal = $37\,^{\circ}C$)
- Correct pH
- Water
- Correct gaseous environment.

Replication methods

Bacteria reproduce by:

- Binary fission
- Spore formulation
- Conjugation.

Binary fission

- Most common method of replication
- Cell grows or elongates and the chromosome is replicated
- This gives a long cell with two identical chromosomes
- The chromosomes separate and the cell membrane begins to form a wall or septum in the middle of the cell
- The cell then divides into two daughter cells.

Sporulation/spore formation

- The bacterial cell becomes deprived of nutrients or a nutrient that it requires
- The bacterial chromosome replicates
- The cell then divides into two unequal parts
- The bigger portion is the forespore and the smaller portion is the endospore
- The cell membrane then surrounds the forespore
- Additional layers or spore coats are made and layered around the additional chromosome in the endospore
- When sufficient layers are made the cell self-destructs (lysis); the copied chromosome in the endospore is protected by the numerous layers surrounding it
- The endospore survives and can survive in a kind of suspended state until the right environmental conditions return, when it will regrow
- Examples include *Clostridium botulinum* (botulism), *Bacillus anthracis* (anthrax) and *C. tetani* (tetanus).

Conjugation

- This is a form of sexual reproduction
- It involves the passage of hereditary material from one bacterium to another
- The DNA is transferred by an appendage or pili
- Plasmids and additional genes are also passed over during the transfer
- Conjugation is common in Gram-negative bacteria.

Artificial culturing of bacteria

Bacteria can also be grown outside the body or the normal environment in laboratory conditions using culture media. Media are artificial nutrient substances upon which microorganisms may be grown in the lab. Culture media are available in a variety of types, including solid media (agar) and liquid media (broth). These are usually a nutrient broth or agar with additional substances added to them. Cultures are used to grow bacteria and to aid in their identification. Solid media allow individual bacterial colonies to be seen and their shape, size and colour to be recorded.

Toxin production

Toxins are poisons which damage cells of the host. Bacteria can produce endotoxins or exotoxins. In the body an exotoxin will stimulate the production of an antibody called an antitoxin. Endotoxins are part of the cell wall of some Gram-negative bacteria which are released when the cell dies; they are normally exceptionally heat-resistant, e.g. salmonella. Exotoxins are mainly produced by Gram-positive bacteria: these are extremely potent poisons but are normally easily destroyed by heat as they are proteins, e.g. *Staphylococcus aureus*.

Classification of bacteria – chemical reactions/staining

Table 25.8 Environmental classification of bacteria	
Aerobic bacteria	Need oxygen to survive
Anaerobic bacteria	Need carbon dioxide levels to be high to survive
Obligate aerobes	Bacteria that need oxygen to be able to reproduce
Obligate anaerobes	Bacteria that require carbon dioxide to replicate
Facultative anaerobes	Bacteria that grow in oxygen but can live without it
Microaerophiles	Bacteria that grow best when the oxygen concentration is lower than that of atmospheric air (less than 22%)

There are two types of stain: simple and differential.

Gram stains (differential stain)

- Gram-positive stain: purple
- Gram-negative stain: red

Ziel Neelsen stain/acid-fast staining

- Mordant: chemical is added to stain or dye to give greater penetration.

These are used to help identify which antibiotic to use:

- Penicillins – effective against Gram-positive organisms
- Streptomycin – effective against Gram-negative organisms
- Tetramycin – effective against a range (broad-spectrum).

411

Swabbing for bacteria

The aim is to isolate the organism to enable it to be cultured so that it can be identified and antibacterial sensitivity testing can take place. With nasal swab samples, pass the swab as far as possible into the nasopharynx and collect nasal secretions. Then send these to an external lab for diagnosis, which can take several days to weeks. Reproductive swabs can also be taken from the clitoral fossa or vagina. Serological testing is taken as soon as possible after the onset of clinical signs, followed by a convalescent sample approximately 2 weeks later. The serum sample is sent to an external lab where antibody titre levels are compared; a substantial increase in antibodies indicates infection. Remember that animals which have been vaccinated in the face of infection may display raised antibody levels due to vaccination or because of the infection.

VIRUSES

Figure 25.4 shows virus structure. Viruses are the smallest of the pathogenic microorganisms. They can only be seen under an electron microscope. They are identified by their shape and their cell inclusion bodies. Cell inclusion bodies are round, oval or irregular-shaped structures that are found in the cytoplasm or nuclei of viruses. They consist of genetic material, either RNA or DNA, and a protein coat called a capsid.

Virus

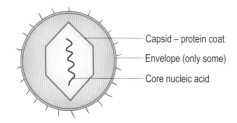

Shapes

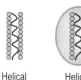 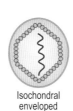

| Helical | Helical enveloped | Isochondral | Isochondral enveloped |

Figure 25.4 Virus structure.

Viruses can enter the body by a variety of routes:

- Bite, e.g. rabies
- Inhalation, e.g. cat flu
- Ingestion, e.g. parvovirus.

Most viruses are labile in the environment; this means they are easily destroyed by heat. All viruses require living tissue or somatic cells (normal dividing cells) to survive and reproduce. Viruses tend to concentrate on particular areas and this affinity is known as tropism, e.g. neurotrophic concentrates on nervous tissue. Virus shape can be described as helical, icosahedral or complex.

Virus structure

There are two parts to a virus, the genome or central core and the capsid, a protein coat which gives protection and shape. Many viruses are surrounded by a lipid layer or envelope for further protection.

Virus reproduction

Viruses reproduce by replication. Viruses require living cells to replicate. The virion, an infectious version of the virus, invades a host cell and takes control of the cell's nucleus. The virion then manipulates the nucleus to produce replicated versions of the virus. Once these are manufactured the virion releases toxins which break down the host cell membrane, releasing the 'new' virions to infect more host cells.

PROTOZOAL PARASITES

Protozoa are the lowest form of animal life. They are unicellular organisms which reproduce by binary fission.

Common protozoal infections seen in animals include:

- Coccidiosis – birds, rabbits
- *Toxoplasma gondi* – cats (zoonotic)
- *Hammondia* – cats
- *Giardia* – all domestic animals (zoonotic)
- *Sarcocystis neurona* (equine protozoal myeloencephalitis).

FUNGI

Pathogenic fungi are classified into two types: yeasts and moulds. Yeasts are unicellular and reproduce asexually by budding. An example is *Candida albicans* (thrush), which is found in the intestinal tract of healthy animals and other areas on unhealthy ones! Moulds are multicellular – they reproduce sexually and asexually to produce spores; examples include *Dermatophytes* (ringworm) and aspergillosis.

PRIONS

A prion is an infectious protein that causes disease. Scrapie in sheep and bovine spongiform encephalopathy (BSE) in cattle are examples of prions. The prions do not appear to contain any nuclei material and are often called spongiform encephalopathies due to the postmortem changes that occur within the brain tissue of infected animals. Prion diseases are fatal.

Bibliography

Aspinall V 2006 The complete textbook of veterinary nursing. Butterworth Heinemann, London

Bacha W J Jr, Wood L M 1990 Color atlas of veterinary histology. Lea & Febiger, Philadelphia

Blood D C, Studdart V P 1988 Baillière's comprehensive veterinary dictionary. Baillière Tindall, Philadelphia

Lane D R, Cooper B, Turner L 2007 Textbook of veterinary nursing, 3rd edn. Butterworth-Heinemann/BSAVA, Philadelphia

McCurnin D M, Bassert J M 2005 Clinical textbook for veterinary technicians, 6th edn. W B Saunders, Philadelphia

Meyer D J, Harvey J W 1998 Veterinary laboratory medicine; interpretation and diagnosis, 2nd edn. W B Saunders, Philadelphia

Moore M 2000 Manual of veterinary nursing. BSAVA, Philadelphia

Moore A H, Simpson G 1999 Manual of advanced veterinary nursing. BSAVA, Philadelphia

Pratt P W 1998 Principles and practice of veterinary technology. Mosby, Philadelphia

Simpson G 1994 Practical veterinary nursing, 3rd edn. BSAVA, Philadelphia

Torrance A G, Mooney C T 1998 Manual of small animal endocrinology, 2nd edn. BSAVA, Philadelphia

Chapter | 26 | Jane Williams

The veterinary profession, pharmacology and theatre practice

This chapter begins to explore the complexity of therapeutic care of animal species. It includes a brief introduction to organisations involved with the veterinary profession and the impact they have on animal welfare.

The basic principles of pharmacology are stated and related to administration routes and techniques used for delivering medication to a range of animal species. The role of the veterinary nurse in the operating theatre with respect to preparation of the patient and staff is considered and a basic introduction to surgical instrumentation is provided.

ORGANISATIONS INVOLVED WITH THE VETERINARY PROFESSION

There are a number of organisations within the veterinary profession and allied industries, e.g. animal health and welfare, that have an important effect on animal health and welfare practices. These include:

- Royal College of Veterinary Surgeons (RCVS)
- British Small Animal Veterinary Association (BSAVA)
- Veterinary Defence Society (VDS)
- British Veterinary Nursing Association (BVNA)
- British Equine Veterinary Association (BEVA)
- British Veterinary Association (BVA).

Royal college of veterinary surgeons

The RCVS is a regulatory body for veterinary surgeons and veterinary nurses in the UK. Its role is to safeguard the health and welfare of animals. It is committed to veterinary care through the regulation of the educational, ethical and clinical standards of the veterinary profession, thereby protecting the interests of those dependent on animals and ensuring public health.

British Small Animal Veterinary Association

The BSAVA exists to promote high educational and scientific standards in small-animal practice; it organises an annual congress for veterinary surgeons and veterinary nurses. It also publishes books, manuals, CD-Roms and videos on small-animal topics and the *Journal of Small Animal Practice*. It has its own charity, Petsavers, which funds clinical investigations into diseases of companion animals.

Veterinary Defence Society

This is an organisation that provides legal advice and support for veterinary surgeons by subscription.

British Veterinary Nursing Association

This organisation promotes veterinary nursing as a profession and is run by veterinary nurses for veterinary nurses. The BVNA implemented and governs the Animal Nursing Assistant course in conjunction with ABC Awards. It is involved with decision-making processes that affect the veterinary nursing profession, organises an annual congress for the veterinary nursing profession and publishes the *Veterinary Nursing Journal*.

British Equine Veterinary Association

BEVA aims to promote veterinary and allied sciences related to the welfare of the horse. It organises an annual congress for equine veterinarians and nurses and publishes the *Equine Veterinary Journal* and *Equine Veterinary Education*.

PRACTICE STRUCTURE

Figure 26.1 shows the typical structure of a veterinary practice. Box 26.1 shows the roles and responsibilities of veterinary practice personnel.

Patient records

Taking and recording case histories

When will a nurse need to do this?

1. Before examination by the veterinary surgeon or in his or her unavoidable absence
2. If the owner phones with a query which is to be related to a veterinary surgeon, or following which you must decide the urgency of the case

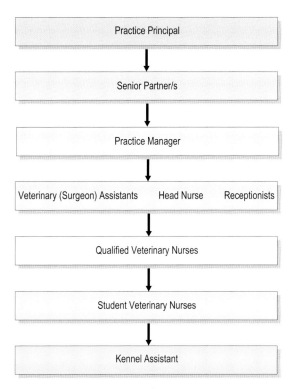

Figure 26.1 Typical structure of a veterinary practice.

3. If the owner has to leave the patient with you and cannot wait to speak to the veterinary surgeon.

Guidelines for history-taking

- Record everything you are told in written form – it is easy to forget information that you have memorised, and the smallest detail may turn out to be the most important
- It helps to use a standard case history form
- Following the same order of questioning also helps avoid omission
- Avoid leading questions: it may save time but can lead to inaccurate answers
- Use effective questioning – you will need to learn to obtain information quickly
- Taking a case history is as much about the ability to communicate as it is about medical knowledge!

What to ask and record

Owner details

- Is the person the owner or an agent acting on behalf of the owner?
- Name and address

Box 26.1

ROLES AND RESPONSIBILITIES OF VETERINARY PRACTICE PERSONNEL

Practice principal

Usually senior partner
Contact for Royal College of Veterinary Surgeons
Contact for insurance company
May be the radiation protection advisor

Senior partner

Responsible for staff in conjunction with practice principal
Formulates practice policy
Handles contracts, dismissals and grievances

Practice manager

Role varies within practices
Responsible for staff under the guidance of practice partners/principal
Responsible for holiday rotas and work rotas
Reception
Accounting/invoices
May or may not be responsible for nursing staff

Veterinary surgeon assistants

Consultations
Visits
Operations

Head nurse

Responsible for nursing team
May report to practice principal or practice manager

Nurse rota, holidays, on call
Nurse training, nurse clinics, general nursing duties, schedule 3

Qualified veterinary nurse

Responsible to head nurse
Nurse training
Schedule 3
Nurse clinics
General duties

Student veterinary nurse

Responsible to head veterinary nurse, then to qualified veterinary nurse
General duties under the guidance of a qualified, listed veterinary nurse or veterinary surgeon

Kennel assistant

Responsible for kennels, i.e. cleaning
Nursing should be left to the nurses
Practice may or may not have any kennel assistants
Reports to practice manager or head nurse

Receptionist

Responsible to practice manager (or head nurse if nursing staff)
First point of call
Very important person!

- Contact phone numbers, including mobiles and when the owner will be available on these numbers.

Animal signalment

- Name, age and whether age is accurate
- Species and breed
- Sex and neuter status (and if this is accurate)
- Value: commercial value, sentimental value and purpose, e.g. pet or breeding or racing or child's pony.

Been in owner's possession (BIOP)

- How long has the animal been in the owner's possession?

Animal temperament

- General/with people/with animals.

Present problem/major presenting complaint

- Why has the owner brought the animal in?
- Onset – sudden or insidious

- Order of signs – which came first?
- Duration
- Progression – improving, deteriorating or stable?
- Treatment – if any and what effect has it had?
- Any other animals or humans, i.e. contacts affected.

Past medical and surgical history

- Past illnesses, accidents, their treatment and outcome
- Vaccination status
- Parasiticide status
- Breeding history – last oestrus, any matings, their success
- Any known allergies?
- On any medication – home remedies or alternative?

Diet

- Type of food/amount of food
- Frequency of feeding
- Any change in diet
- Any access to other food sources.

Environment

- Housing/bedding
- Household products/detergents used
- Exercise
- Other animals
- Other people
- Any changes recently?
- Turnout.

System review

- This is not an examination of the animal but questioning the owner about the animal
- General demeanour and attitude – bright, alert, responsive, depressed, changed temperament
- Appetite and thirst:
  - Anorexia
  - Polyphagia
  - Pica
  - Coprophagia
  - Polydipsia
- Weight gain or loss
- Vomiting or regurgitation:
  - Food/bile/water/blood
  - How frequently?
  - How soon after eating/even if fasted or not eating?
- Diarrhoea:
  - Frequency
  - Urgency
  - Consistency
  - Blood/mucus
  - Tenesmus/constipation
- Eye/ear/oral:
  - Discharges (serous/mucoid/mucopurulent/purulent/serosanguineous)
  - Head tilt
  - Pain
  - Ability to eat/drink
  - Pruritus
  - Halitosis
  - Odour
  - Blepharospasm
  - Swellings
  - Perceived changes in vision or hearing
- Skin/hair:
  - Pruritus
  - Alopecia
  - Wheals/pustules/papules
  - Seborrhoea
  - Odour
- Respiratory/cardiovascular:
  - Change in breathing pattern
  - Abnormal noises, e.g. wheezing, snoring, roaring, whistling
  - Sneezing/coughing
  - Type of cough, e.g. dry, harsh or moist
  - Frequency of cough
  - Exercise tolerance
- Urogenital:
  - Discharges (serous/mucoid/mucopurulent/purulent/serosanguineous)
  - Dysuria
  - Pain on urination
  - Stranguria (straining)
  - Change in frequency (pollakuria = increase in urine)
  - Change in volume (polyuria, oliguria, anuria)
  - Blood in urine – haematuria
  - Change in odour/colour/turbidity
- Neurological:
  - Behaviour
  - Seizures
  - Ataxia
  - Head tilt
- Locomotion:
  - Lameness/pain – describe and which leg
  - Exercise tolerance
  - Muscle wastage
  - Generalised weakness
  - Joint swelling or heat or pain
- Anything else relevant to the case.

Preparing a summary case history

For both new and hospitalised cases you may be required to deliver a case summary for another staff member. Try and keep information concise. Using a list of headings can help ensure all relevant information is included:

- Brief history – animal signalment and chief complaint
- Previous history where relevant
- Present physical condition and demeanour/attitude
- Physical parameters recorded, e.g. temperature, pulse, respiration
- Results of diagnostic tests
- Fluid and nutrition status
- Medical and surgical treatments
- Progress
- Discharge information for owner (if appropriate).

Financial recording

It is important to record treatment, hospitalisation, surgery and drugs on the client's record. Many surgeries allocate charging for inpatients to specific staff members or a designated member of staff. Modern practices often have a computerised system which details set pricing schedules for veterinary products and services.

417

Preoperative consent forms

These constitute a legal document between the client and the vet. They should include:

- Owner signalment, including contact number and times
- Animal signalment
- Detailed description of procedures to be undertaken
- Estimate of cost
- Risk warning with regard to general anaesthetic, surgery, diagnostic testing or medical procedures
- Permission to undertake further treatment as required
- Client signature or that of the client's representative (must be over 16 years)
- Date
- Preanaesthetic blood test consent
- Microchip consent if neutering form.

Postoperative information forms

These act as client information sheets which provide instructions and reassurance after surgical or medical procedures. They usually inform the client on:

- Animal's dietary requirements
- Exercise requirements
- What to expect after the procedure
- Follow-up appointments
- Emergency contact details
- Medication instructions
- Care instructions.

Nurse clinics

Nurse clinics allow members of the nursing team the opportunity to enhance the veterinary–client bond. They are often organised as a complementary consultation event and cover a range of prophylactic health care issues, e.g. puppy or kitten clinics covering vaccination, worming and general training and obesity or weight control clinics. The nursing staff often has more time allocated to be able to discuss issues in depth with the client which can highlight problems and feed into veterinary consultations. They are fun and rewarding for the nurses taking part.

PHARMACOLOGY

Pharmacology is the science of the study of drugs (Box 26.2). When drugs are classified, the following information is required:

- How do they achieve their effect on the body?
- Which body system (or infective agent) do they act upon?

Box 26.2

PHARMACOLOGY DEFINITIONS

Therapeutics
The use of drugs in the management of a disease – manipulation of physiological functions

Therapeutic index
The ratio between the dose of drug that will cause toxic effects and the dose required to produce the desired effect
The lower the therapeutic index, the more dangerous the drug is

---

Box 26.3

PHARMACEUTICAL NOMENCLATURE

Generic name
The approved name of the agent, e.g. carprofen

Trade name
The brand name of the agent, e.g. Rimadyl

Pharmacological agents are usually organised into a pharmacy or designated dispensary.

Pharmaceutical nomenclature and terminology

Pharmaceuticals have a generic name and a trade name (Box 26.3). Box 26.4 lists common terminology used in reference to drugs.

Remember that some agents will contain more than one ingredient in their generic name and should be listed accurately.

Drug preparations

Drugs can act in different ways:

- Systemic action: throughout the body via the circulation: the route of administration is oral or parenteral
- Direct action: on a specific site: the route of administration is topical or local.

The information discussed so far provides useful underpinning knowledge for the veterinary nurse – but how do we decide which product is right for the job?

Box 26.4

DRUG TERMINOLOGY

Adverse reaction

Undesirable response
Varies from mild to fatal

Agonist

A drug has specific action by binding with an appropriate receptor

Antagonist

A drug that inhibits a specific action by binding with a particular receptor

Efficacy

The extent to which a drug causes the intended effects in the patient

Half-life

Time taken for 50% in quantity of the drug to dissipate from the body

Metabolism

The biochemical process that alters a drug from an active form to an inactive form or elimination from the body

Parenteral

The route of administration of injectable drugs

Residue

The amount of drug present in the tissues/products, e.g. milk/meat at a particular time

What to use?

The agent chosen will depend upon a number of factors:

- Type of drug required
- Speed of action required
- Where it acts upon
- Convenience of administration
- Contraindications and side-effects
- Cost
- Patient: species/age/temperament.

Speed of uptake

How fast a drug acts upon the patient can be directly correlated to the route of administration for the majority of agents. Remember that speeds do vary between drugs.

Detoxification

Drugs are detoxified by the body in the liver and kidneys. Waste metabolic products are excreted via the bile and urine collectively.

PHARMACOKINETICS

Pharmacokinetics is the study of the complex sequence of reactions that occur within the body after the drug is administered.

Therefore, there is a time lapse or limit from administration for the required percentage of drug to occur since detoxification begins immediately. This effect is counteracted by:

- Repeat dosing
- A high or loading dose followed by a reduction
- Continuous dosing
- Underdosing will have no or little effect
- Overdosing will lead to toxicity.

Primary factors that influence blood concentration levels of a drug and the patient's response are:

- Rate of absorption
- Amount absorbed
- Distribution throughout the body
- Drug metabolism
- Rate and route of excretion.

Bioavailability is the degree to which a drug is absorbed and reaches the general circulation. Factors that affect the rate of absorption include:

- Mechanism of absorption
- pH and ionisation status
- Absorptive surface area
- Blood supply to target area
- Solubility of drug
- Dosage form
- Status of gastrointestinal tract
- Interactions with other medication.

Systemic pharmaceutical compounds reach their target areas via the circulation where they pass or cross the cell membranes by one of the following transportation methods:

- Passive absorption, e.g. diffusion
- Active transport
- Pinocytosis.

How an individual agent is transferred from the systemic circulation into the cell will depend upon a number of variables, including:

IONISATION OF DRUGS

Acidic drugs only pass in an acidic environment
Alkaline drugs only pass in an alkaline environment
Acidic drugs in an alkaline environment will ionise
Alkaline drugs in an acidic environment will ionise

- Is the drug fat- or water-soluble?
- The size and shape of the drug molecule
- Is the drug ionised?

THE IMPORTANCE OF IONISATION

Compounds usually divide into ions when in solution, e.g. sodium chloride ionises into Na^+ and Cl^-. The chemical nature of compounds will affect their capability to pass through the cell membrane, which is constructed from a phospholipid bilayer, with hydrophilic and hydrophobic sections (these will relate to the charges upon the ion content in the lipid layers and cause the drug molecules to bind within the membrane). Only non-ionised, i.e. no overall negative or positive charge, drugs can pass through cell membranes with their absorption rate unaltered by their environment (Box 26.5).

General rules of thumb

Increasing the surface area of the target area will increase the rate of absorption. Increasing the blood supply will increase the rate of absorption. An intramuscular injection usually instigates a quicker reaction than a subcutaneous injection as muscle has a better blood supply. Poor circulation means a reduced blood supply, therefore a reduced rate of absorption. In fight or flight situations blood is diverted to muscles and away from the gastrointestinal tract. Therefore the rate of absorption is reduced. Inflammation results in an increased blood supply to the area and therefore the rate of absorption will increase.

Distribution

Figure 26.2 illustrates the absorption of drugs.

A concentration gradient exists between the drug in the interstitial fluid and the plasma within the cells. This should sound familiar – the metabolic process, which will occur when a concentration gradient is present with solutes in solutions and a semipermeable membrane, is osmosis. Therefore, the higher or steeper the gradient, then the quicker the rate of absorption. Drugs can bind

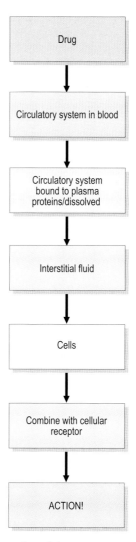

Figure 26.2 Absorption of drugs.

with plasma proteins which will render the agent inactive. Because the drug cannot be metabolised it will remain in stasis within the tissues until it is mobilised and a reaction will occur. When mobilisation occurs the drug is released into the blood stream and often gives an exaggerated or prolonged response. Barbiturates and a lot of anaesthetic agents behave in this manner.

PHARMACODYNAMICS

Pharmacodynamics is the study of the mechanisms by which drugs produce physiological changes within the body. Drugs can enhance or depress the physiological activity of a cell or tissue. Pharmacodynamics explores the sequence of events within the body that leads to the action of the drug by tracking the physiological sequence. Drug molecules combine with receptors within the cell, resulting in action. The efficacy of a drug, i.e. the measure of how it achieves its full potential, is relative to how well the drug molecule fits the receptor site it is intended for. The better the fit, the more efficient the drug.

Agonist

- High level of affinity
- High efficacy
- Specific action.

Partial agonist

- Less affinity
- Less efficacy.

Antagonist

- Blocks the action of another drug
- This is achieved by covering the receptor site
- Therefore no action occurs.

Figure 26.3 shows receptor and drug affinity models. Note that no drug produces a single effect.

Example: narcotic drugs

- Low dose: treatment for diarrhoea
- Higher dose: analgesic
- Higher dose: treatment for respiratory disease.

The potency of the drug will be the amount of the drug required to produce the desired effect; this will vary depending upon the condition being treated.

THERAPEUTIC INDEX

The therapeutic index is the relationship between the desired effect or action of a drug and its potential for toxicity, i.e. how much it takes to become dangerous. The therapeutic index is expressed as a ratio of lethal dose to effective dose ($LD_{50} : ED_{50}$). This ratio quantifies the drug's safety margin.

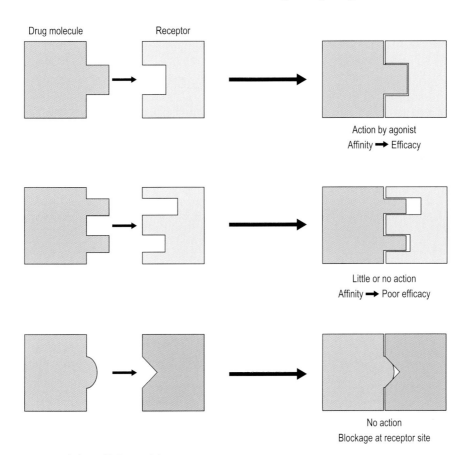

Figure 26.3 Receptor and drug affinity models.

Generally, larger numbers equate to safety. Therefore, a high therapeutic index is considered safe and a low therapeutic index dangerous.

Other possible problems

An adverse reaction is an undesirable response; this could be life-threatening or it could be just a rash. Idiosyncratic drug reaction is an unusual or unexpected reaction; again, this can be detrimental or advantageous. All of these reactions should be reported to the manufacturer.

SOURCES OF INFORMATION ON PHARMACEUTICAL AGENTS

There are many sources that can be utilised to research the pharmacodynamics, phamacokinetics and general information on the pharmaceutical agents used in animals.

- All drugs should have a datasheet available
- The NOAH compendium of datasheets provides useful information
- The pharmaceutical industry, i.e. the drug manufacturers
- The veterinary vade mecum
- The wholesaler/supplier
- The pharmacist
- The professional bodies, e.g. RCVS
- The vet.

DRUG CATEGORISATION

Drugs are classified according to their effect on the body and which area of the body they act upon. Most drugs in use in veterinary medicine may have more than one therapeutic use depending upon the dose prescribed.

The prefix 'anti' is often used in conjunction with the name of the organism the drug is designed to act against, e.g. antimicrobial (microbes) and antibacterial (bacteria). The suffix 'static' translates to a drug that causes pathogens it acts on to stop multiplying, allowing the body's own defences to counteract the attack; the suffix 'cidal' means that a drug will kill the pathogen it is active for.

EXCRETION/ELIMINATION

Drugs are eliminated either unchanged or as metabolites (biotransformation). Most drugs and metabolites are eliminated via the kidney, some are eliminated via the

gastrointestinal tract (not absorbed) and other metabolites are excreted via bile. Pulmonary excretion occurs for anaesthetic gases via pulmonary secretions. Drugs can also be excreted in milk, sweat, saliva or tears. In lactating animals transmammary elimination via milk may be significant and affect suckling young.

ADMINISTRATION OF MEDICINES

Medication may be administered via multiple routes (Table 26.1):

- Per os or orally
- Direct instillation or topically to the:
  - Skin
  - Pulmonary membranes
  - Per rectum
  - Intra-articular (on to joint surface)
- Parenterally via injections:
  - Intravenous
  - Subcutaneous
  - Intramuscular
  - Intraosseus
  - Intraperitoneum.

The route chosen will be determined by:

- The patient: temperament, condition
- The medication available: tablet, injection
- Pharmacological properties: some drugs will not work via certain routes and their efficacy may be reduced
- Convenience for administrator: home/vets
- Rate of absorption: certain routes are faster-acting for certain drugs.

Drugs need to enter their target cells or reach the cell membrane receptor sites to be effective.

$$\text{Absorption} \rightarrow \text{distribution} \rightarrow$$
$$\text{biotransformation} \rightarrow \text{elimination}$$

- Absorption, the rate and extent to which a drug leaves its site of administration, is dependent upon solubility:
  - Aqueous solutions have more rapid absorption than lipid solutions
  - Solid drugs need to dissolve first
- Bioavailability is the extent to which the drug enters the systemic circulation
- Factors that affect absorbability can change bioavailability.

Example

An oral preparation needs to be absorbed from the gastrointestinal tract, enter portal circulation then pass

Table 26.1 Comparison of administration routes

Route	Absorption	Use	Precautions
Oral	Rate and extent are highly variable and dependent upon many factors	Maximise compliance Convenient Economic Usually safe	Absorption (bioavailability) may be erratic and incomplete
Subcutaneous	Rapid if an aqueous solution; less rapid if depot formulations	Some less soluble suspensions and implantation of solid pellets or depot forms	Not suitable for large volumes Irritant substances cause pain and/or necrosis
Intramuscular	Rapid if an aqueous solution; less rapid if depot formulations	Moderate volumes Lipid vehicles Irritant drugs	Inadvertent intravenous injection Pain or necrosis at injection site
Intravenous	None (directly into circulation) Potentially immediate effects	Emergency use or large volumes Absorption bypassed	Increased risk of adverse effects Inject solutions slowly Not suitable for lipid solutions or insoluble substances
Pulmonary	Rapid, local administration for pulmonary disease	Usually for treatment of pulmonary disease	Irritant substances must be avoided Rapid absorption may induce high plasma concentrations and adverse effects

through the liver before it enters the systemic circulation.

Oral medication

- Tablets, capsules, liquids, pastes, powders, granules
- These have a long shelf-life
- They are manufactured uniformly with regard to drug content
- They are easily administered, and therefore there is good owner compliance
- They could be considered the least painful route
- There is a reduced risk of introducing infection (iatrogenic infection)
- There is a possibility of choking
- They may cause irritation
- There is a variable rate of absorption, depending on:
  ○ Age
  ○ Health status
  ○ Metabolic rate
  ○ Food in digestive tract
  ○ Physical state of drug (unionised/lipophilic form/acids (weak) are preferred and can be absorbed from stomach and alkalis (weak) from the ileum)
- Patients may not cooperate
- Oral medication may be mixed in feed: using tempting tasty bits such as cheese in dogs and cats or chopped carrots in horses may increase palatability

- The medication may be force-fed via a syringe – check with the vet: paste medication can be mixed with water
- It can be difficult to ensure correct dosages if the medication is spat out or inaccurate splitting occurs.

Method of oral administration to cats and dogs

1. Ask assistant to restrain animal
2. Check the patient's mouth is empty
3. Insert syringe tip at the side of the mouth underneath lip, pointing upwards towards back of tongue
4. Apply medication on to tongue
5. If administering a tablet or capsule, place it on the back of the tongue
6. Hold the animal's head up, trying to keep its mouth shut and massage the throat to encourage swallowing
7. A pill popper may be used as an aid.

Method of oral administration to large animals, including horses

1. Get assistant to restrain the horse: the horse may be tied up or may twitch
2. Check the animal's mouth is empty
3. Insert syringe tip at the side of the mouth pointing upwards towards the back of the tongue

4. Apply medication on to the tongue
5. Hold the horse's head up, trying to keep its mouth shut!

Remember health and safety: wear gloves and masks.
   Figure 26.4 shows oral administration of an anthelminthic to a horse.

Possible problems

- Accuracy: spilt dose, accessed by others, the animal may dislike the taste
- Aspiration of medication: aspiration pneumonia
- Injury to animal or handler.

Topical administration

- Topical administration may reduce the amount of drugs required systemically
- It may be the only effective method available
- It includes creams, ointments, powders, sprays and drops
- Also liniments: rub these on to the skin and they act as counterirritant or analgesic
- A lotic is a liquid suspension or solution that soothes
- Topical agents are applied to external surfaces of the body

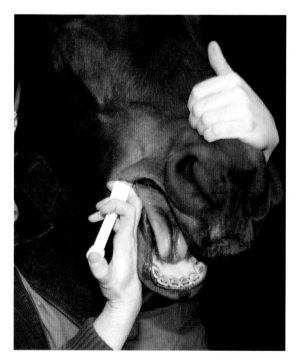

Figure 26.4 Oral administration of an anthelminthic.

- They may also be applied via an indwelling lavage system or nebuliser
- They can be applied to the skin, eyes, ears, lungs, rectum, vagina, uterus and joints.

Skin

- Shampoos – bathing
- Ointment – drug in base of oil/wax in water – semi-solid ointments work by water evaporating, leaving a thin layer of drug on the surface
- Cream: a drug in semisolid emulsion
- Dusting mixtures – adsorbent (cornstarch) or lubricant (talcum)
- Aerosols: drugs packed under pressure for ease of administration, e.g. ectoparasiticides.

Eye

- Tilt the patient's head back and use the fingers to open the eye
- Never touch the eye surface with a finger/nozzle/tube
- Drops – drop liquid on to the centre of the eyeball
- Ointment: apply by squeezing a line from inner canthus across eye surface; approach from the side
- Subconjunctival injections can be used.

Ear

- Drops/ointment
- Clean ear primarily to remove wax
- Restrain patient and extend pinna
- Introduce the nozzle into the ear canal, apply contents
- Keep hold of the pinna and massage the external auditory meatus: spread the contents over the ear.

Rectal/vaginal administration

- Via rectal passage or vagina and uterus
- Enemas, suppositories.

Intra-articular injections

- Can be used to apply medication to joint surfaces
- Must be done aseptically: clip and surgical scrub.

Parenteral routes

- Parenteral routes are more rapid and provide predictable levels of administration
- They are often the route of choice: often the intravenous route is used initially as this produces the quickest clinical response

- Animals are often uncomfortable at injection sites for 24–48 hours so location of repeat injections should be rotated
- Localised inflammation and infection may occur at the injection site.

Subcutaneous route

- Prepare injection (use an appropriate-sized needle gauge)
- Restrain patient (Figure 26.5)
- Site of choice:
  - ○ Scruff – small animals
  - ○ Side of neck cranial to scapula – large animals
- Area with poor blood/nerve supply
- Only use for non-irritant drugs
- Infection can be introduced via contaminated equipment
- Implants – hard concentrated drug, inserted under skin which release drug over a period of time, e.g. hormones in cattle.

Method of subcutaneous injection

1. Prepare injection (use an appropriate-sized needle such as 21G)
2. Restrain patient
3. Raise fold of skin
4. Moisten with surgical spirit (except for vaccinations and insulin, as spirit inactivates these)
5. Insert needle under skin and draw back
6. If there is no blood, slowly administer the injection
7. Massage the site gently
8. Record details
9. Dispose of equipment – clinical waste/sharps.

Intramuscular route

- Into muscle
- Common sites in small animals:
  - ○ Quadriceps femoris (hindlimb)
  - ○ Lumbar muscles
  - ○ Cervical muscles

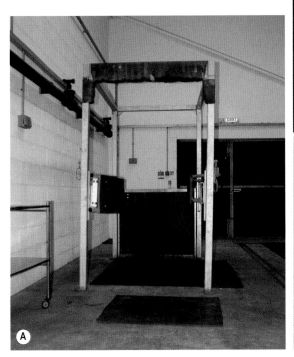
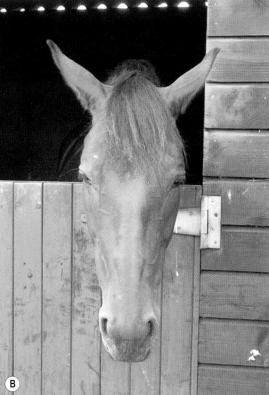

Figure 26.5 (a) Equine stocks can be used as extra restraint for examination or administration of medication.(b) A sedated horse.

- Common sites in large animals
  - Gluteals (rump): halfway between point of hip and tail base
  - Pectorals (brisket): either side
  - Neck: cranial shoulder blade, midway between dorsal and ventral surface
- Because muscle is dense large amounts cannot be injected at any one time
- These injections can be relatively painful for the animal so the patient may attempt to kick or bite.

Intramuscular administration routes

Large animal – neck

- This allows the handler to remain in a relatively safe area by the horse's shoulder
- There is a triangle defined by the nuchal ligaments along the crest of the horse's neck, the cervical vertebrae, which form a backward S-shaped curve from the horse's poll toward the point of the shoulder, and the scapula
- To locate it put the heel of your hand on the base of the horse's neck where it joins the shoulder, about midway between the crest and the bottom of the neck. The area covered by your palm is the injection site.

Large animal – pectorals

- Increased risk of being bitten, stuck with a front foot or run over by the horse
- The pectoral muscles tend to become sore easily and generally are only used when the horse is receiving prolonged treatment and is sore in other injection sites.

Large animal – gluteals

- Large, frequently used muscle mass which allows the handler to stand in a relatively safe area while giving the injection
- The disadvantage to this site is that it has very poor drainage if a needle abscess develops at the injection site. An infection at this site tends to spread up the loin and back and cannot be treated easily
- The proper location of this injection site is the intersection of a line between the tail head and point of hip and a line between the top of the croup and the point of the buttocks.

Small animal – quadriceps femoris

- The dog is restrained by an assistant
- The area to be injected is swabbed with alcohol to remove transient bacteria from the site

- The quadriceps muscle is located anteriorly to the femur; grasping the muscle mass in this area can help with visualisation
- The needle is inserted at right angles to the muscle belly, drawn back and if no blood is present the substance is injected
- The needle is withdrawn and the area is massaged.

Small animal – cervical and lumbar muscles

- These muscle groups are useful for fractious animals
- The patient is adequately restrained and the muscle group is isolated (cervical – neck; lumbar – just before the pelvis)
- Swab the site with alcohol
- Insert the needle on either side of the vertebrae into the muscle mass
- Again draw back to ensure there is no blood before injecting.

Method of intramuscular administration

1. Prepare injection
2. Restrain patient (using an assistant)
3. Prepare site – swab
4. Insert needle:
   - 21G (for solutions): inserted at right angles – often there is little response
   - Larger gauges, such as 18/19G (for suspensions), often elicit a response in large animals. Thump the site once or twice, then introduce the needle rapidly perpendicular to skin right up to the hub or pinch skin and slide needle in
5. Attach syringe and draw back
6. If there is no blood inject slowly
7. Massage site
8. Record details
9. Dispose of needle/syringe.

Possible problems

- Injury to animal and/or handler
- Self-injection
- Inadvertent damage to the structures, e.g. nuchal ligament (neck), vertebral column (neck), sciatic nerve (hindlimb)
- Pain, oedema, abscess, anaphylaxis.

Intravenous administration

- Quick-acting
- Most have an effect within 2 minutes
- Common sites:
  - Jugular vein – right or left
  - Cephalic vein
  - Saphenous vein

○ Lateral thoracic vein (horses)
○ Sublingual during general anaesthetic
- Used for drug therapy/fluid administration
- Can be via needle or via a catheter.

Method of intravenous administration – jugular vein

1. Prepare injection
2. Have assistant restrain patient
3. Operator clips, prepares surgically – scrubs vein with Hibiscrub swab then spirit swab
4. Operator stabilises vein (not where the operator has sterilised) by occluding it close to the thoracic inlet
5. Operator inserts needle into vein at 45° angle to skin, pointing upwards – blood should flow into needle/syringe if plunger is pulled
6. Assistant releases pressure and drug is slowly administered. Intermittently withdraw plunger to check location of needle
7. Remove needle and apply pressure for approximately 30 seconds to prevent haematoma.

Care should be taken to avoid the carotid artery. If the carotid artery is pierced, bright red frothy blood is seen spurting out of the hub. Remove the needle immediately and apply pressure for at least 5 minutes and seek veterinary attention.

Method of intravenous administration – cephalic vein

1. Prepare injection
2. Have assistant restrain patient
3. Operator clips and prepares surgically, scrubbing the vein with Hibiscrub swab then spirit swab
4. Assistant restrains the appropriate leg using fingers around the elbow joint to maintain stillness and occludes vein by applying pressure
5. Operator stabilises vein (not where the operator has sterilised)
6. Operator inserts needle into the vein at a 45° angle to skin pointing upwards – blood should flow into the needle/syringe if the plunger is pulled
7. Assistant releases pressure and the drug is slowly administered
8. Remove needle and apply pressure for approximately 30 seconds to prevent haematoma.

Possible problems with intravenous route

- Injury to animal/handler
- Self-injection

- Inadvertent puncture of arteries (if needle is placed too deep)
- Extravascular injection: tissue sloughs, oedema, pain, infection
- Anaphylaxis.

OBSERVATION OF ANIMALS AFTER ADMINISTRATION OF MEDICATION

The veterinary nurse or handler can be placed in an optimum situation to monitor patients after medication has been administered.

Why should patients be monitored after medication?

- Part of the job is to provide care for patients
- Compliance – to ensure the full amount of medication is taken/administered
- Accuracy – to observe injections have not gone into the wrong location
- Monitor for adverse reactions
- Record information.

Important factors to monitor

- Behaviour
- Clinical symptoms
- Clinical parameters – temperature, pulse, respiration, mucous membrane colour
- General health
- Abnormal signs
- Improvement
- Food/water
- Urine/faeces
- Signs particular to specific drugs.

How often should the patient be monitored?

- Immediately after administration
- Hourly
- Continuously
- The actual time period will often depend on the health status and condition of the animal.

Drug reactions

Adverse drug reactions produce a harmful effect but this is not the same as a side-effect. Patients at a greater risk of adverse drug reactions include those which are underweight due to less adipose tissue, hypoproteinaemic animals and individuals whose previous history is

Table 26.2 Classification of adverse drug reactions

Reaction type	Description	Details
A	Augmented – enhanced drug effect	Predictable Dose-dependent Common Low mortality
B	Bizarre – allergic reaction	Unpredictable Not dose-related High mortality
C	Chronic – due to continuous therapy	e.g. Iatrogenic, Cushing's disease from long-term use of steroids
D	Delayed – occurring a long time after treatment	Carcinomas from some teratogenic drugs
E	End of treatment – occurring on withdrawal of therapy	e.g. Cortisol insufficiency with steroid withdrawal

Box 26.6

DRUG INTERACTIONS

Giving drugs with food to aid absorption

Synergism: two drugs administered together to improve effect

Summation: two drugs given together but response is the same as if both given independently

Potentiation: two drugs given as one: one enhances the effect of the other

Antagonism: one drug inhibits the effect of the other

unknown or who have a known reaction to certain products. Refer to Table 26.2 for classification of adverse drug reactions.

Drug interactions are when products or substances are used cumulatively to treat a patient (Box 26.6). Unwanted interactions include:

- One drug affecting another
- Interactions can occur mixing drugs – outside as well as inside the body
- Food interactions
- Drugs administered via different routes can still interact.

Drug interactions and reactions can be reduced by:

- Familiarity with interaction and reactions for commonly used drugs
- Carrying out appropriate monitoring
- Reporting any reactions immediately to the veterinarian
- Storing drugs correctly

- Varying administration sites
- Considering staggering of oral medication
- Reporting any suspected drug reactions to Veterinary Medicines Directorate
- Not preparing drugs in advance
- Not mixing drugs in the same syringe
- Ensuring any previous drug reactions are clearly noted on case records
- Advising owners to keep a record.

SIDE-EFFECTS, CONTRAINDICATIONS AND DRUG REACTIONS

Side-effects of drugs

A side-effect occurs when a drug produces effects which are not desirable or are not part of a therapeutic effect other than those intended.

Common side-effects include:

- Urticaria
- Oedema
- Allergies
- Less commonly, anaphylactic shock.

Contraindications

Contraindications are datasheet warnings of the potential harmful effects of drugs or physiological interactions that may occur on administration of a product, often linked to the animal's physiological status. These can be avoided by reading the product datasheet and obtaining clear, detailed histories to make informed decisions regarding dispensing treatment.

Common contraindications

- Do not use in pregnant, lactating animals
- Do not use in animals with respiratory disease
- Do not use in animals intended for human consumption
- Do not use in animals undergoing steroid therapy.

SURGICAL NURSING AND THEATRE PRACTICE

Care of the patient

Preoperative care

The role of the veterinary nurse will probably include admitting the patient and possibly performing or assisting with preoperative diagnostic tests.

Admitting animals

- Make an appointment as this allows time to discuss the animal
- Use a separate room
- Be reassuring and professional
- Ask relevant questions about the animal:
  - Has there been any change since the last time the animal was seen by the veterinary surgeon?
  - When did the animal last eat and drink?
  - When did the animal last have any medication? What was the medication?
  - Does the animal have any known allergies?
  - When did the animal last urinate and defecate?
  - What sex is the animal?
  - Is it neutered? If not, when was it last in season?
- Vaccination status
- Temperament
- Any abnormalities
- Possibly identify any lumps or bumps with the owner present
- Ensure all animals are suitably restrained
- Note any items brought in with patient
- The owners may be allowed to see the operating/ hospital room for reassurance
- Ask the owner to leave before the animal is taken away
- Ask the owner to sign the consent form
- Ensure the owner knows the procedure for collection of animal
- Apply identification to the animal
- Isolate contagious/infectious animals
- Consider the animal's normal routine
- Weigh the animal

- Once an initial examination has been performed to establish health, premedicative agents that sedate and provide analgesia are often administered to the patient.

The consent form is an important legal contract between the surgery and the animal's owner. It is important to state clearly the full procedure that is to be performed and always confirm details of the pet and the procedure verbally with the owner. Do not use abbreviations. The signatory authority must be received from a person aged 18 years or over. The next stage will be to admit the animal into the hospital.

Perioperative care

Perioperative care occurs during the operation or the procedure. The role of the veterinary nurse will be to monitor the patient, perhaps monitor the anaesthetic or to assist the surgeon with the procedure.

Postoperative care

Postoperatively the veterinary nurse's duties may include cleaning the animal to remove blood stains from the coat, monitoring the animal, cleaning the animal's accommodation, contacting the owner, dispensing medication, printing advice forms, charging the client and/or pricing the operation, taking the patient to urinate and defecate, feeding and giving water to the patient, administration of medication and keeping the veterinary team informed of progress. When discharging the animal the nurse may be responsible for giving the owner discharge instructions, preferably before the owner receives the patient to ensure full compliance, booking follow-up appointments to check the animal or for suture removal and completing the cash/cheque/credit transaction.

Discharging

This should preferably be performed by a veterinary surgeon or a nurse who can fully explain the details to the owner and answer any questions. It should occur in a separate room and a confident approach with the owner should hopefully instil confidence in the owner that he or she will be able to cope. Explain thoroughly details of the procedure and tests performed and give clear aftercare instructions. It may be necessary to use non-veterinary terminology and ideally the owner should repeat important aspects of the animal's aftercare to the discharger to show he or she has understood. Medication regimes, exercise regimes and diet should be covered and appointments for follow-up checks should be made. Postoperative diets are usually bland and there are commercial formulations available which are partially digested to reduce the strain on the digestive system. Reunite the owner with the animal last to ensure that the owner listens to the instructions and not just fusses over the pet!

Theatre design and asepsis

The operating theatre should aim to be an aseptic environment, as even healthy animals undergoing a procedure will be compromised due to the surgery and the breach of the skin as their first line of defence (Box 26.7). Patient preparation should occur in the preparation area; then the animal should be brought to the theatre for a second and final scrub before being draped and undergoing the procedure. The theatre should contain the minimal equipment to function effectively to reduce the areas for potential pathogenic colonisation: theatre furniture includes the operating table, anaesthetic machine, monitoring equipment and an instrument trolley. The doors to the theatre should be swing action and should remain shut to reduce air flow and bacterial contamination and staff members should be restricted to the surgical team. Bacterial contamination can occur from transient bacterial populations on the patient and staff members' skin, bacteria from infectious patients and environmental bacteria. Nosocomial infections are infections that animals have acquired during hospitalisation and surgery.

Cleaning and hygiene of the theatre

This should be performed before surgery and between operations when instruments, waste and unneeded equipment should be removed. The operating table and any remaining equipment should be disinfected thoroughly. The operating schedule should also encourage hygiene by listing clean operations first, then clean contaminated operations, then contaminated operations

---

---

and finally dirty operations to reduce the number of pathogens in the environment. At the end of the day the theatre should be vacuumed and mopped with disinfectant, all designated equipment should be disinfected and restocked, and walls should be wiped down. Once a week all equipment should be removed to allow a deep clean to occur, which should involve scrubbing all areas of the theatre. Adequate sterilisation of equipment and instruments should also occur.

Theatre suite design should incorporate designated clean and dirty areas, allow sufficient room to manoeuvre and contain minimal equipment. Materials utilised should be impervious, washable, non-toxic and curved to avoid corners where bacteria can accumulate. Swing doors and knee- or elbow-operated scrub sinks are preferable. The ambient temperature should be approximately 21°C with 50% humidity and a minimum of 16 air changes per hour. Neonates and exotic species will require a higher ambient temperature of up to 28°C. The surgical team should all wear appropriate sterile clothing, i.e. scrub suits/gowns, clogs, masks, hair nets and sterile gloves, and these should be changed between operations. All members of the surgical team should undergo a full surgical scrub. During surgery there should be minimal movement and conversation, staff should show an awareness of surgical fields and all should know the theatre rules and protocols.

Preparation of the patient

Figures 26.6–26.8 show preparation areas and equipment.

Once the animal has been anaesthetised in the preparation area, the following steps should be taken:

1. Express or catheterise the bladder; animals should be encouraged to urinate before the operation. Catheterisation deflates the bladder, giving more space in the abdomen, and prevents strikethrough if the animal urinates during the procedure, which could potentially contaminate the surgical site
2. Clip the surgical field; a number 40 blade is used and the area around where the incision is to be made is clipped with a significant border to prevent contamination to the wound once open from the animal's coat. Vacuum or remove the hair from the site
3. Initial scrub of the surgical site is undertaken. A dilute solution of chlorhexidine or povidine-iodine is often used. Gauze swabs are soaked in the solution and used to clean the site. Once the initial dirt is removed, sterile gauze swabs are used to scrub the skin in a circular motion, working from the site of the incision to the outside edges of the clipped area. Once the peripheral hair has been touched discard the swab as it is now contaminated

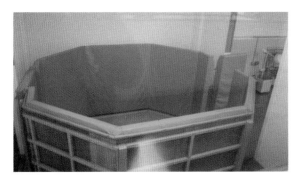

Figure 26.6 Overhead view of equine knockdown box.

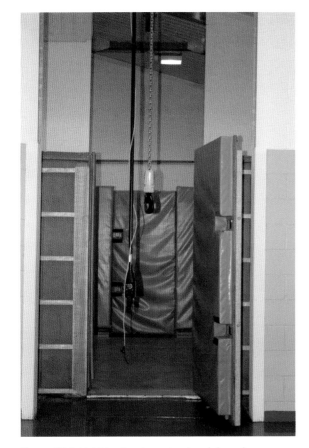

Figure 26.7 Hoist leading to equine knockdown box.

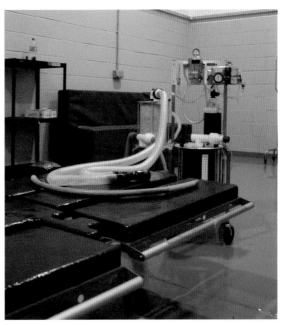

Figure 26.8 Equine anaesthetic machine and operating table.

allowed to dry but in some cases a more thorough repetition of the above is required.

Positioning the patient

The choice of position is usually made by the surgeon and will depend on personal preference, the size of the patient and the procedure being undertaken. When moving the patient respiratory patency must be continually checked as it is easy for the endotracheal tube to occlude. Animals are often placed in the supine or dorsal position (flat on their back) for thoracic and abdominal procedures; this may be associated with raising the table for head or rectal operations. The animal's legs will be secured with ties and cradles or wedges may be used to keep the body upright, although some operating tables have independent sides which are capable of tilting to hold the animal in position. The sternal position (lying on the abdomen) is used for spinal procedures and a lateral position (lying on one side) is often used for operations involving ears or limbs and for ovariohysterectomy in the cat.

Draping

The purpose of draping the patient is to create a sterile area around the surgical site. Two types of drapes are employed: fenestrated drapes have holes or windows cut into them and plain drapes do not. Both types are

4. A dry sterile swab dries the area using the same motion, then a germicidal agent such as isopropyl alcohol is applied in a sterile manner
5. The animal is taken to theatre, taking care not to touch the scrubbed site
6. The sterile scrub nurse performs the second scrub: often this is another application of alcohol which is

431

secured in place using towel clips. Drapes can be purchased in linen, disposable paper and plastic. The first drape is placed between the draper and the patient, the second is placed between the surgeon and the patient, the third is placed over the animal's head and the fourth is placed over the tail region. Care should be taken not to contaminate the wound. The drapes should cover the entire patient and the operating table, allowing only the surgical site to be exposed. The placement of drapes should be performed using cheatle forceps; another sterile drape is used for the instrument trolley.

Preparation of the surgical team

The surgical team also need to prepare for theatre. The resident and transient microbe populations need to be reduced on staff members and a methodical approach is employed. The preparation procedure involves scrubbing up, gowning and gloving.

Surgical scrub

1. For this you need a scrub sink, nail brush, cleaning agent in a dispenser (chlorhexidine or iodine), a sterile scrub brush and a sterile towel
2. Fingernails should be short and clean; water should be of a comfortable temperature with the taps ideally controlled using the elbows or feet
3. Thoroughly wash the hands and arms to the elbows with chlorhexidine
4. Holding the fingers under the stream of water, use a nail file to clean under the nails then discard the file and rinse the hands
5. Moisten the sterile scrub brush and place the cleaning agent directly on to it; using the sterile brush scrub the hand and arms from fingertips to elbow at least twice, rinsing between scrubs. The four sides of each finger should be scrubbed
6. After scrubbing, wash and rinse the hands only and allow water to drain down the arm before towel drying
7. The towel should be folded to open when you pick it up in the corner and shake it; never use the same piece of towel on different parts of the hands and forearms.

Gowning

1. Gowning should be performed directly after drying the hands following a surgical scrub
2. Gowns should be folded so the inner surface is exposed and the neck band is uppermost
3. Grasp the gown by the inside of the neck and allow the gown to unfold at arm's length
4. Place the hand and arms into each sleeve, then an unscrubbed assistant will fasten the ties; if the gown

has waist ties, lean forward to allow these to drop so the assistant can grab and tie them.

Surgical gloving

There are two methods employed: open and closed gloving. Surgical gloves should fit snugly and are available in powdered and non-powdered versions.

Open gloving

1. Open the inner wrap (sterile) of the glove packaging
2. The digits should be pointing upwards: check your left hand is opposite the left-hand glove
3. Pick up the everted cuff of the left glove with the thumb and forefinger of the opposite hand, touching only the inner folded-back cuff
4. Hold the glove open with the left hand, slide the right hand into the glove and push the fingers in
5. Do not push in the thumb but hook it under the rim of the right glove
6. Slide the gloved fingers of the right hand under the everted cuff of the left hand
7. Slide the fingers and thumb of the left hand into the glove and, using the right hand to help, ensure the glove is pulled over the cuff of the gown
8. With the gloved left hand, unhook the everted cuff from the right thumb, taking care only to touch the outer surface of the glove and pull the right glove completely over the thumb and cuff
9. Stand with the arms folded and the hands/forearms held aloft in a praying position to prevent contamination.

Closed gloving

1. The fingers and hand must remain covered by the gown at all times
2. Turn the opened gloves to face with the digits downwards
3. Use the left hand to pick up the left glove (on the right-hand side of the table), lining the thumb of the cuff and your own thumb up
4. The right hand picks up the right glove and, once the thumbs are lined, the left hand pulls the glove on to the right hand, making sure the cuffs of the gown are covered.

The scrub nurse

It is the role of the scrub nurse to prepare the instrument trolley, count swabs before, during and after surgery, aid the surgeon, pass instruments to the surgeon, swab (using a blotting action) any haemorrhage site, perform lavage as required and to dispose of relevant items in clinical waste.

The circulating nurse

It is the role of the circulating nurse to help prepare the surgical environment, instruments and team, to aid in positioning the patient, assist the anaesthetist, prepare the postoperative environment and any dressings that may be required, obtain any additional supplies, drugs or instruments required by the surgical team and to clear and clean the theatre at the end of the procedure.

Sterilisation

Sterilisation is defined as the destruction of microorganisms, including bacterial spores. Objects can be considered sterile or not sterile. Disinfectants do not provide sterility. Sterilisation can be achieved by either a chemical method or a physical method. Chemical sterilisation methods are said to be cold sterilisation methods, e.g. ethylene oxide, whereas physical sterilisation involves either dry heat, e.g. hot-air oven, or wet heat, e.g. autoclave and pressure. Boiling an item (in water at $100°C$) does not kill spore-producing bacteria or certain strains of virus and is therefore not considered to be a method of sterilisation.

Monitoring sterility

Time steam temperature strips

- The colour changes after the correct time, temperature and pressure have been achieved
- The strips turn from yellow to blue
- They should be put into the centre of the load to ensure sterilisation has occurred deep in the load.

Browne's tubes

- These are liquid-filled gas tubes
- Their colour change indicates sterility
- They change from red to orange to green (remember the traffic light system)
- They are dependent on the correct time and temperature.

Bowie–Dick tape

- This is a type of autoclave tape
- It is used to seal packs of instruments
- It has beige impregnated diagonal stripes which turn brown when they reach a certain temperature
- As with ethylene oxide, indicator tape does not guarantee sterility as it has no measure of time but it does indicate a certain temperature has been achieved.

Spore tests

- These are strips of paper impregnated with dry *Bacillus* species

- They are included in the load
- On completion they are removed and cultured to ascertain bacterial growth
- If there is no growth after 72 hours sterility is guaranteed
- The time delay involved makes this method impractical for daily monitoring but it is good practice to employ it as a checking mechanism.

Thermocouples

- These are leads which have heat-sensitive strips
- They are placed in various parts of the chamber
- The leads are passed through an aperture to a recording device
- They are usually used by service engineers to check heat is being achieved.

Packaging materials

Nylon film

- This is designed for autoclave use
- It is reusable (but brittle, so it may break)
- It comes in a variety of sizes
- It can be difficult to remove items and maintain sterility
- It is usually sealed with Bowie–Dick tape
- It can be double-folded and air contained within it should be expelled before sterilisation.

Autoseal pouches

- Disposable packaging which has a paper back and a transparent front
- Instruments are visible, which can prove useful
- It comes in a variety of sizes
- It is suitable for ethylene oxide or autoclave
- It is easy to open
- Care needs to be taken as the paper can become contaminated if it gets wet
- For single use only.

Paper wraps

- Like crêpe, they are flexible, conforming and disposable
- Good for use as an outer-layer wrap
- They should be sealed with indicator tape
- They are resistant to tearing and moisture-resistant.

Textile wraps

- Reusable
- They make good outer-layer wraps
- They are permeable to moisture and should be covered by a water-repellent wrap
- They possess good memory, i.e. they will lie flat on the instrument trolley.

Instrumentation

Early instruments were fashioned from butcher's, carpenter's and blacksmith's tools. Numerous different instruments have been designed specifically to fulfil a niche within surgical procedures. Instruments are made of martensitic or austenitic stainless steel, tungsten carbide or chromium-plated carbon steel.

Cleaning instruments

Instruments should be cleaned after use. Remove any sharps from the trolley immediately after the procedure has been finished. Separate delicate instruments from the heavier ones to prevent damage: immediately rinse them off with saline solution and remove organic matter as soon as possible. Blood will coagulate on instruments if they are placed in hot water, and is very difficult to remove.

Basic points to check

- Surgical instruments will rust and discolour if not maintained correctly and stored dry
- All instruments should be cleaned and decontaminated as soon as possible after use
- Do not allow dirty and soiled instruments to dry out: soak them in cold water if washing is delayed
- When using ultrasonic cleaners, use the correct concentration of cleaning agent and do not mix metals as it leads to electrolysis
- Do not use abrasive agents; use recommended cleaners only
- Do not soak for prolonged periods of time
- Rinse thoroughly after cleaning
- Dry thoroughly and check for damage
- Lubricate moving parts with water-soluble instrument lubricant
- Beware of using hard water in an autoclave as it will leave a residue on instruments – distilled water should be used.

Chemical solutions

A number of commercial instrument cleaning solutions are available. Gloves should be worn and manufacturer's instructions followed.

Ultrasonic descalers

These use ultrasound waves to clean instruments, often in conjunction with cleaning solutions. It is required to remove as much organic matter as possible from instruments primarily, then dilute an approved cleaning solution, place the instruments in the descaler and start the cycle. The descaler removes minute traces of blood.

Instrument classification

Scalpels

- Size 3 handle – small animal/10, 11, 12, 15 blade
- Size 4 handle – large animal/20, 21, 22 blade.

Dissecting forceps

- Consist of a handle with serration for grip
- Tips may be rat-toothed or serrated
- Used for intermittent, temporary grasping of tissue, skin, soft tissue or viscera
- Types include fine-tooth, heavy-tooth and plain dressing
- Plain are indicated for viscera and toothed for dense tissue.

Scissors

- Two blades: can be sharp or blunt
- Used for soft-tissue dissection (not skin) and suture cutting
- Types include Mayo for routine surgery, Metzenbaum, which have fine and long handles, Cartess, which are suture scissors, and Paynes scissors for removing sutures.

Figure 26.9 shows the types of surgical scissors.

Haemostats

- Artery forceps having a ratchet to maintain a closed position
- They have serrated blades and clamp tightly shut with a ring grip for fingers
- Used for occlusion of blood vessels
- Types include Spencer wells, Dunhill, Crile, Cairns, Kelly, mosquito and Kocher forceps.

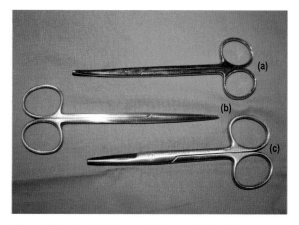

Figure 26.9 Surgical scissors. (a) Curved blade; (b) Metzenbaum; (c) straight blade.

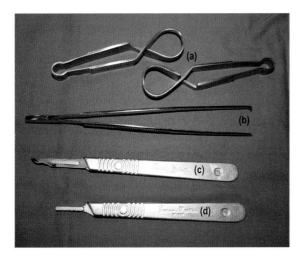

Figure 26.10 Surgical instruments. (a) Backhaus towel clips; (b) rat-toothed forceps; (c) scalpel with blade attached; (d) scalpel handle.

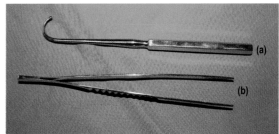

Figure 26.11 Gillies needle holders.

Figure 26.12 (a) Cat spay hook; (b) dissecting forceps.

Tissue forceps

- Have a ring grip for the fingers and a ratchet maintains a closed position
- The tip has a fine area of contact
- Used for prolonged grasping of soft tissue or viscera
- Types include Allis, Babcock and Duvalls.

See Figure 26.10 for examples of surgical instruments.

Towel clips/clamps

- Possess sharp curved tips which cross over
- Used for anchoring drapes to the patient
- Types include Backhaus and Mayo (curved) and Grays (straight).

Needle holders

- These have flat tips on the blades with a stippled surface
- They often have ring-shaped fingers and a ratchet to maintain closure
- They may be combined with scissor blades
- Uses include holding needles, suturing and knotting
- Types include:
  - Gillies: the disadvantage is that there is no ratchet, so you need to grip tightly: they also have a scissor action (Figure 26.11)
  - Olsen–Hegar: cutting edge and a ratchet; their disadvantage is that the cutting edge may cut thread

  - Mayo Hegar: they look like long artery forceps, and have a ratchet but no scissor action
  - McPhails: copper inserts in tips, handles on spring ratchet, squeeze to open and release needle.

Retractors

- Hand-held or self-retracting.

Hand-held retractors

- Have a grooved handle
- Hook-like end which may be flattened
- Used for retraction of soft tissue, viscera and bone
- Types include Langenbeck, Hohmann, Volkmann, Senn and Czerny.

Self-retaining retractors

- Ratchet which maintains open position
- Used for prolonged retraction of soft tissue, viscera and bone
- In muscle, use Gelpi, Wests and Travers
- For the abdominal wall, use Gossett and Balfour
- In the thoracic cavity, use Finichietto.

Figure 26.12 shows a cat spay hook and dissecting forceps and Figure 26.13 shows a selection of artery forceps.

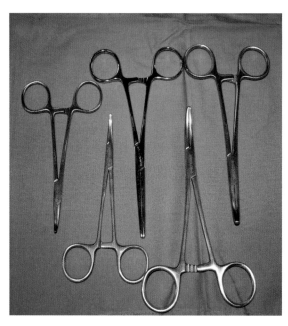

Figure 26.13 Selection of artery forceps.

Orthopaedic instruments
Curettes
- Oval-shaped cup
- Used to scoop out necrotic tissue
- One side has a sharp cutting edge
- If both ends have a scoop then it is called a Volkmann's spoon.

Osteotomes, chisels, gauges
- Cut and shape cartilage and bone.

Periosteal elevators
- Lift the periosteum and soft tissue from the bone surface.

Bone-holding forceps
- Grip bone fragments in fractures to allow fixation.

Bone cutters
- Rongeurs are used to nibble or cut small bits of bone/cartilage
- Cutters are employed for larger sections.

Rasps
- File and remove sharp edges of bone.

Retractors
- Hohmann retractors, which are hand-held, are used to hold muscle and tendons back.

Drills, saws, burrs
- These can be hand-held, battery- or air-operated.

Wire forceps
- Used for cutting or twisting wire.

Gigli wire/saw
- This is like cheese wire and is used for sawing through bone.

Bibliography
Aspinall V 2006 The complete textbook of veterinary nursing. Butterworth Heinemann, London
Bacha W J Jr, Wood L M 1990 Color atlas of veterinary histology. Lea & Febiger, Philadelphia
Blood D C, Studdart V P 1988 Baillière's comprehensive veterinary dictionary. Baillière Tindall, Philadelphia
Gorman N 1998 Canine medicine and therapeutics, 4th edn. Blackwell Sciences/BSAVA, Oxford
Lane D R, Cooper B, Turner L 2007 Textbook of veterinary nursing, 3rd edn. Butterworth Heinemann/BSAVA, Oxford
McCurnin D, Bassett J 2005 Clinical textbook for veterinary technicians, 6th edn. W B Saunders, Philadelphia
Moore M 2000 Manual of veterinary nursing. BSAVA
Moore A H, Simpson G 1999 Manual of advanced veterinary nursing. BSAVA, Oxford
Pratt P W 1998 Principles and practice of veterinary technology. Mosby, Philadelphia
Simpson G 1994 Practical veterinary nursing, 3rd edn. BSAVA, Oxford
Tracy D L 1994 Small animal surgical nursing, 2nd edn. Mosby-Year Book, Philadelphia
Wanamaker B P, Pettes C L 1996 Applied pharmacology for the veterinary technician. W B Saunders, Philadelphia

Chapter | **27** | *Jane Williams*

Fluid therapy and diseases

This chapter introduces the concept of fluid therapy and provides indications for its use in companion animal species. A range of common medical diseases exhibited in companion animal species are discussed with consideration of their management by the pet owner.

FLUID THERAPY

Fluid therapy is the management of fluid and electrolyte abnormalities in the animal body and is a fundamental aspect of clinical medicine. In the healthy animal fluid balance is maintained by oral intake combined with renal, gastrointestinal and insensible losses. The aim of clinical fluid therapy is to restore the normal fluid and electrolyte balance to the critically ill animal.

Fluid administration is an important therapeutic measure in the critically ill patient.

Fluid therapy objectives

1. In order to manage the administration of fluid therapy to the critically ill patient successfully it is vital that the patient is evaluated initially to identify the disease process involved (Table 27.1)
2. Identification of the disease involved will aid in the formulation of a successful fluid therapy plan.

Indications for fluid administration

A complete history in conjunction with a full physical examination of the patient will help to give the veterinary surgeon clues on whether or not fluids are indicated in the case. Blood profiling is an extremely useful tool to aid diagnosis of fluid and electrolyte imbalances.

The veterinary surgeon should question:

- Is the patient dehydrated?
- Are significant electrolyte disturbances present?
- Are there serious acid–base changes present?
- Are there ongoing fluid losses to be accounted for (vomiting/diarrhoea/haemorrhage)?

The answers should lead to the decision to use or not to use fluids. The next stage is to decide on a therapeutic fluid plan for that individual patient.

What route should the fluids be given by?

- Per os (PO)
- Subcutaneous (SC)
- Intramuscular (IM)
- Intravenous (IV)
- Intraperitoneal (IP)
- Intraosseus (IO).

Refer to Table 27.2 for a comparison of fluid administration routes.

What volume of fluids should be administered?

The volume to be delivered should be calculated to consider the levels of dehydration, previous fluid deficits

Table 27.1 Initial database for patients requiring fluid therapy

History	Water/food intake Gastrointestinal losses Urinary losses Heat exposure Trauma Haemorrhage Excess panting Pyrexia Diuretic use

Dehydration	<5%: not detectable
	5–6%: subtle loss of skin turgor
	7–8%: delay in skin elasticity, > CRT, tacky mucous membranes, sunken
	    eyes
	10–12%: tented skin, prolonged CRT, tachycardia, weak peripheral pulses +
	    collapse of veins
	12–15%: death imminent, moribund

Body weight	Acute decrease may be due to fluid loss Approximately 1 kg = 1000 ml fluid
Urinary losses	Catheterise + monitor
Circulatory losses	Place jugular catheter and measure central venous pressure
Laboratory findings Increased PCV and TPP	Utilise PCV and TPP Intravascular dehydration
Increased PCV and normal or reduced TPP	Dehydration with proteinaemia: splenic contraction
Normal PCV and increased TPP	Anaemia with dehydration, normal hydration and hyperproteinaemia
Reduced PCV and normal TPP	Anaemia with dehydration Anaemia with hyperproteinaemia
Normal PCV and TPP	Acute blood loss Normal hydration Dehydration with anaemia and hypoproteinaemia
Reduced PCV and reduced TPP	Blood loss Anaemia and hypoproteinaemia, overhydration
Urinalysis	If renal function is normal, reduced output with dehydration
Specific gravity	Elevated: normal response from healthy kidney Reduced: kidney problems may be underlying cause of dehydration
Biochemistry	K, Na: levels will indicate type of losses and fluid to use Elevated BUN + high specific gravity: non-renal cause Elevated BUN + low specific gravity: kidney possible source
Bicarbonate (total CO_2)	Help evaluate metabolic status and determine type fluid used

CRT, capillary refill time; PCV, packed cell volume; TPP, total plasma protein; BUN, blood urea nitrogen.

Table 27.2 Comparison of fluid administration routes

Route	Clinical name	Indications
Oral	Per os (PO)	Fluids must be hypotonic Need not be sterile Inexpensive Feeding tubes can be used to facilitate if prehension is limited or impossible Water and electrolytes are absorbed in bowel Contraindicated in cases with chronic vomiting, foreign bodies, postoperatively after abdominal surgery or if performing a water deprivation test (diabetes inspidus)
Subcutaneous	Sub-cut (SC/SQ)	Useful for small mammals, puppies, animals that are difficult to restrain Limited to small amounts of fluid 10–20 ml at each site depending on size of animal Common sites include dorsal aspect of back, lateral thorax and scruff Massage areas to encourage absorption Warm to body temperature Hypotonic saline or glucosaline is contraindicated and may cause diffusion of electrolytes into the tissues Not recommended if there is severe peripheral vasoconstriction
Intraperitoneal	IP	Fluids are injected directly into abdominal cavity Restrain animal in dorsal recumbency, clip area around umbilicus and scrub Useful for large volumes Risks include peritonitis, punctured viscera Can use hypertonic, isotonic, plasma expanders or blood via this route
Intravenous	IV	Most direct route straight into the blood stream Routes include cephalic vein, jugular vein, saphenous vein and sublingual vein (anaesthetised) Best route to restore circulation volume rapidly Risks include septicaemia, bacteraemia, phlebitis and thrombophlebitis
Rectal		Care must be taken as high risk of causing shock to patient Often used as a last resort Fluids at body temperature administered via a Higginson's syringe
Intramuscular	IM	Not really used for fluids Used for injecting small quantities, e.g. antibiotics
Intraosseus	IO	Useful route for exotics, small mammals and neonates Directly into medullary cavity of bone Quick route

and ongoing losses. The time period the fluids are to be delivered over should also be determined at this stage. Remember that overhydration is as potentially dangerous to the animal as dehydration.

What type of fluid should be used?

Administration of contraindicated fluids can compound the problems present with the electrolyte balance or precipitate unwanted fluid movement within the animal's circulatory system.

How fast should the fluids be given?

It is often a fine line between killing and saving an animal's life which can depend upon the fluid therapy plan.

What supplements should be added to the standard fluid?

Vitamins, antibiotics and other drugs can be added to fluids.

How will hydration be monitored?

Monitoring will directly contribute to other factors such as the rate of administration and volume of fluid to be given. A number of factors will be monitored, including:

- Skin tenting
- Mucous membrane colour
- Capillary refill time
- Body weight.

Body water recap

Body water makes up 60% of an adult animal's body weight. Intracellular fluid comprises two-thirds of total body water, and the remaining third is the volume of extracellular fluid in the animal. Extracellular fluid is then subdivided into interstitial fluid (75%) and intravascular fluid (25%).

Electrolytes

The principal intracellular cations are potassium and magnesium, which maintain intracellular fluid volume by osmotic movement. The principal extracellular ions are sodium, chloride and bicarbonate. The sodium-potasssium pump within cells maintains sodium and potassium. This system uses active transport on the cellular membrane to transport sodium and potassium against their concentration gradients for utilisation within the cell.

Because of this mechanism extracellular sodium levels can dramatically affect hydration on a cellular level. For example, in cases of severe water deprivation, an increase in sodium levels will precipitate water movement from the cell into the extracellular space, resulting in cell dehydration.

Regulation of fluid balance

Normal regulation of extracellular fluid is undertaken by the kidneys, which are also responsible for control of osmotic balance (renal tubules). Antidiuretic hormone (ADH) is released in response to changes in plasma osmolality, which increase water reabsorption from the renal tubules.

Baroreceptors in the cardiopulmonary circulation detect increasing levels whereas ones in the kidneys detect decreasing levels of circulating volume of extracellular fluid, stimulating the activation of renin–angiotensin. Renin–angiotensin stimulates the release of aldosterone and increased renal sodium absorption and potassium loss.

Maintenance of fluid requirements

Maintenance requirements are equal to the volume of fluid and electrolytes that is required on a daily basis to maintain normal total body water and electrolyte content. In a healthy animal water input should equal water loss.

Daily water losses occur from:

- Evaporation from respiration
- Faeces
- Urine.

Insensible losses, those which are unavoidable due to physiological processes, are estimated at a rate of 22 ml/kg per day. Sensible losses, those which can be manipulated by physiological processes, are estimated at a rate of 22–44 ml/kg per day. Maintenance fluid volume is considered to be the animal's sensible water losses and insensible water losses. If IV fluids are given for over 24 hours then electrolyte balances must also be addressed. The maintenance fluid volumes required are as follows:

- Cats: 66 ml/kg per day
- Dogs: 44 ml/kg per day
- Horses: 60 ml/kg per day in adults, 70–80 ml/kg per day in foals

Assessing the fluid patient

History

1. The first step is to access the degree of dehydration and electrolyte imbalance
2. Then identify the animal's disease
3. Identify the route of fluid loss to help identify electrolyte losses and acid–base balance
4. Discover the length of time of fluid loss
5. Estimate the quantity of fluid lost
6. Gather information on water and food consumption.

Increased fluid loss can result from:

- Polyuria – excessive urination
- Vomiting and diarrhoea
- Pyrexia, raised temperature, and associated panting
- Large burn wounds which would result in loss of fluid through exudates
- Excessive salivation
- Haemorrhage.

Physical examination

The physical examination aims to detect the degree of dehydration, although this can be difficult to assess accurately. The following are examined:

- Skin turgor: tenting. If it takes more than a few seconds for pinched skin to return to its normal position this suggests dehydration
- Moistness of the mucous membranes: dehydrated animals tend to have tacky mucous membranes
- Position of eyes: in dehydrated animals the eyeball is slightly sunken into its socket
- Heart rate: the heart rate increases as there is less circulating blood volume so the heart must work harder to compensate for this
- Peripheral pulses: these can be weak due to the lower circulating blood volume
- Capillary refill time: this will be longer in dehydrated animals as it will take longer for blood to refill the capillaries due to reduced blood volume in the animal
- Jugular distension: the reduced blood volume can cause the jugular to sag or distend as it is not as full of blood as normal.

Packed cell volume

Packed cell volume or PCV is an important diagnostic tool for the veterinarian to establish the condition of the circulatory system. It is a measure of the percentage of cells and by default the fluid component of blood. Therefore in dehydrated animals the PCV would increase as the ratio of fluid to cells is altered by a loss of fluid. Normal ranges for different species are known, but in some animals, e.g. the horse, breed and fitness can also influence the normal PCV, as can pre-existing clinical conditions and in an ideal world the individual animal's PCV would be established before it falls ill. The PCV reading can be used to calculate fluid deficits by subtracting the normal value from that taken and performing a simple calculation.

Total plasma proteins (TPP)

These are measured using the right-hand scale of a refractometer; dehydration causes elevated levels of plasma proteins for the same reason as the PCV increases, i.e. blood has effectively become more concentrated. PCV and TPP should always be assessed simultaneously as it is very unlikely that pre-existing disease will elevate both measurements.

Plasma electrolytes

Low concentrations of sodium, potassium and chloride always indicate a large fluid deficit but normal concentrations do not rule out a deficit. Hypokalaemia (marked reduction of potassium) causes severe muscle weakness and cardiac disturbances which can be caused by pro-longed diarrhoea or vomiting. The resulting cardiac dysrhythmias can be fatal.

Acid–base estimations

These need to be maintained within strict parameters. Acid–base balance is a measure of hydrogen ion (H^+) concentration and it is measured on the pH scale. Blood is slightly alkaline at a pH value of 7.35–7.45; if blood pH is below 7.35 the animal has acidaemia and if the pH is above 7.45 the animal has alkalaemia. Metabolic alkalosis and metabolic acidosis can influence the choice of fluid administered.

Urine output

Dehydrated animals normally present with oliguria, little or scanty urination, or anuria, absence of urination. The rate of urine production is directly proportional to the glomerular filtration rate, therefore to the renal perfusion rate, which reflects arterial blood pressure. A reduced urine output indicates severe hypotension (low blood pressure) so a return to normal urine production is a good prognostic sign.

Pulse

Changes in pulse rate, volume and rhythm are always present in the dehydrated animal and they should be assessed regularly. Palpation of peripheral pulses via femoral artery, sublingual artery and brachial artery will indicate the state of the circulation.

Respiration

Animals suffering a severe metabolic acidosis, as in chronic renal failure or diabetes mellitus, often hyperventilate. A return to a normal respiratory pattern is good news. The respiratory system should be monitored for rate and depth of respiration, by thoracic auscultation and monitoring arterial blood pressure.

Temperature

Differences between skin temperature between the toes, the oesophagus and rectal temperature can be useful in assessing the peripheral circulation. The normal temperature gradient is less than 3–4° but widens to 10° in hypovolaemic shock.

Body weight

Body weight is easily measured and can indicate acute fluid losses but is a useless parameter unless regular recordings have previously been made for the animal.

Summary of aims of fluid therapy

- Corrects life-threatening hypovalaemia
- Restores accumulated deficits of fluids and corrects electrolyte and acid–base disturbances
- Provides sufficient fluids and electrolytes to meet continuing losses each day
- Meets normal body requirements, i.e. urinary and inevitable losses.

Causes of dehydration

The route of choice for a severely dehydrated animal would be intravenously due to the large volumes that can be administered and the speed of delivery.

Dehydration may be caused by primary water depletion due to one of the following factors:

- Prolonged inappetance
- Water is unavailable
- Unconsciousness
- Pyrexia
- Diabetes insipidus.

It may also be due to water and electrolyte depletion caused by:

- Vomiting
- Diarrhoea
- Third-space losses such as an intestinal obstruction
- Pyometra
- Wound drainage
- Potassium depletion:
  - Prolonged inappetance
  - Vomiting
  - Prolonged diarrhoea
  - Prolonged diuretic therapy
- Potassium accumulation:
  - Ruptured bladder
  - Urethral obstruction
  - Acute renal failure
  - Addison's disease.

Advantages of intravenous fluid therapy

- Rapid administration of fluid into vascular space
- Large volumes may be given
- Hypertonic solutions can be given, in addition to plasma expanders and blood products.

Disadvantages of intravenous fluid therapy

- Greater risk of side-effects, e.g. bacteraemia, septicaemia

- Specialised equipment is required
- Time-consuming
- Animal requires constant monitoring
- Risk of overhydrating, which puts pressure on the kidneys and heart.

Equipment required for intravenous fluid therapy

Figure 27.1 shows a selection of IV catheters and fluid administration sets.

- Suitable fluid solution: choice will depend upon animal's medical condition
- IV cannula/catheter: suitable size for animal:
  - Rabbits, cats, small dogs: 24 G or 22 G
  - Medium dogs: 22 G or 20 G
  - Large dog: 20 G or 18 G
  - Horses: 10 G to 16 G
- Catheters are also available in different lengths for different uses, e.g. for placement in the cephalic vein or the jugular vein. Table 27.3 shows the problems with different types of catheters
- Equipment required:
  - Giving set
  - Swabs and scrub materials – Hibiscrub, spirit
  - Clippers
  - Scalpel blade to cut down on to vein
  - Bandaging materials
  - Tape – Omnipore, zinc oxide tape
  - 2 ml syringe + needle
  - Dilute heparinised saline to flush cannula
  - Scissors
  - Buster collar
  - Three-way tap
  - Kink inhibitors
  - Glue or suture material (large animals).

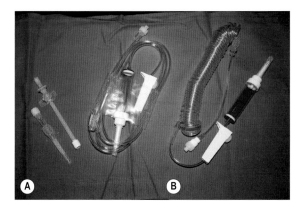

Figure 27.1 Selection of intravenous catheters and fluid administration (giving) sets. (a) non-coiled; (b) coiled.

Table 27.3 Types of catheter/cannula

Hypodermic needle	Can cause damage to veins Dislodges easily
Butterfly needles	Can cause damage to vein Can suture in place
Over-the-needle catheter	Can damage or dislodge catheter as needle is withdrawn
Through-the-needle catheter	Catheter of choice Remove needle when catheter is a third of the way in the vein, then introduce the rest

Procedure for catheterisation of small animals

1. Prepare equipment
2. Warm fluids to body temperature
3. Connect administration set (giving set) to fluids, ensuring the maintenance of sterility by pushing spike through the appropriate port of the fluid bag
4. Close the giving set, fill the chamber to the fill line then run fluids through the drip line ensuring there are no air bubbles; this should be possible without running off any fluid but it is more important to remove air bubbles than not lose fluid!
5. An assistant should restrain the patient in an appropriate position for the vein selected
6. Clip area around the injection site
7. Scrub as per preoperative routine using swabs, not cotton wool as it leaves fibres behind
8. Scrub skin using chlorhexidine solution followed by a spirit swab
9. The assistant raises the vein: some people prefer to cut down/back for the cephalic vein or the catheter can be directly inserted through the skin
10. When in place the catheter should be flushed with heparinised saline and secured
11. Connect the fluid and secure in place, loop the drip line and secure
12. Bandage in place
13. Check the fluid is flowing freely and monitor
14. Cannulas should be changed every 24–48 hours.

Catheterisation technique for large animals

In large animals, particularly in the equine, catheters are usually placed in jugular veins but the cephalic or saphenous vein can be utilised. Advantages of using jugular catheterisation include the fact that the jugular is a large vein which has easy access and its use may reduce the potential for injury as fewer repeat injections are required. Disadvantages of jugular catheterisation include infection, thrombosis, which in the jugular can be life-threatening, thrombophlebitis and injury to the handler or horse.

Method

1. Aseptic technique is required
2. Clip/aseptic prep of the area; the catheter is placed in the distal third of the neck to avoid the carotid artery
3. Apply local anaesthetic subcutaneously over the jugular vein
4. A small incision is made over the catheterisation site
5. Retrograde placement: against flow of blood to reduce chance air embolism
6. Antegrade placement: with flow – there is less irritation/increased flow rates
7. Advance the catheter at an angle of 70° until blood is seen in the hub
8. Reduce the angle to 20–30°, advance it till the hub is at skin level then remove the stylet to reduce the risk of kinking, although some people prefer to remove the stylet halfway through insertion
9. Secure the hub to the skin using sutures or tissue glue
10. Attach the extension piece and injection port and secure to the skin
11. A protective bandage can be applied to prevent contamination.

Monitoring and maintenance of indwelling catheters are essential. They should be checked several times a day for heat, swelling, pain and discharge. Whenever the catheter is used it should be flushed afterwards with heparinised saline to ensure all the drug goes into the vein and also prevent occlusion. 10/12 G catheters can remain in situ for up to 3 days and 16 G up to 30 days.

Administration sets

A number of different administration or giving sets are available depending on the volume of fluid to be delivered. They come with straight tubing and coiled tubing and some have inbuilt ports for drug administration.

A standard giving set delivers 15–20 drops/ml, a paediatric giving set delivers 60 drops/ml and smaller volumes can be administered using burettes. Blood giving sets are specialised units fitted with a net filter to stop coagulated proteins entering the circulation. Infusion pumps can be used in conjunction with giving sets to produce an accurate method to preset fluid administration.

Types of fluid

There are three types of fluid commonly used: colloids, crystalloids and blood. A colloid is a plasma replacer or expander; the product stays in the veins, increasing the circulatory volume. A crystalloid fluid passes readily through the cell membranes, therefore leaving the circulatory system and rehydrating the tissues. The presentation of a bag of fluids will identify whether or not the product is colloid or crystalloid, the expiry date and the osmotic potential of the fluid, i.e. isotonic (same concentration as plasma), hypertonic (more concentrated than plasma) or hypotonic (less concentrated than plasma), which will indicate the direction of fluid movement when administered. The choice of fluid should be based on the degree and nature of fluid loss, although availability may also be a determining factor.

The most common problem encountered during fluid therapy administration is a failure of the fluid to flow. This could be due to a number of reasons:

- The bag is finished
- The drip tubing is kinked
- The animal has pulled its leg back, kinking tubing
- The animal has chewed through drip tubing
- The catheter has become dislodged
- The catheter is blocked by a blood clot.

Solutions

- Change bag
- Can use kink resistors; wrap Elastoplast around the curve in the tube
- Pull out animal's leg/splints/bandaging
- Check tubing is intact; replace it if necessary
- Check location of catheter; replace it if necessary
- Remove blood clot (do not flush it into circulation!) then flush with heparinised saline and replace fluids.

Osmolality

This is based on the relationship to normal serum osmolality (300 mosmol/l).

Osmolality of solutions is usually determined by the sodium and glucose content.

Hypotonic fluids: osmolality < normal serum

- Use when you need to take fluid from vascular system into tissues
- Maintenance fluids to replace insensible losses.

Hypertonic fluids: osmolality > normal serum

- Use for replacement of intravascular fluids
- Indicated for hypovolaemic and endotoxic shock
- Small volume of hypertonic saline will immediately:
  - Increase cardiac output
  - Increase arterial blood pressure
  - Increase peripheral perfusion
- Then a secondary shift occurs in body fluid with fluid from the interstitial and intracellular fluid: intravascular component
- Administration of hypertonic fluids should be followed by the use of crystalloid fluids.

Isotonic fluids: osmolality = serum

- Crystalloids: replacement and maintenance solutions
- Examples include 0.9% sodium chloride.

Colloid solutions contain large molecules that will remain within intravascular space

- Used in shock and animals presenting with severe hypoalbulminaemia
- Plasma proteins play an important role in maintaining blood pressure
- Use commercial substances or colloids which have similar molecular weights and act in a similar manner in the circulation to plasma proteins
- Colloids remain intravascularly.

Fresh (fresh frozen) plasma

- Colloid
- Used for hypoproteinaemia, e.g. severe burns/coagulopathy, e.g. haemophilia
- Separated plasma is frozen within 6 hours of collection: this is fresh frozen plasma (FFP)
- Contains coagulation factors, von Willebrand's factor, plasma proteins
- Not really suitable as a resuscitation fluid.

Crystalloids

- Fluids that contain ionised substances capable of passing through semipermeable membranes
- Crystalloids will distribute to sites outside the circulatory system
- Therefore three times the volume of crystalloid compared to colloid must be administered to achieve effective plasma expansion
- Can be maintenance or replacement solutions.

Replacement solutions

- Contain lots of electrolytes
- Replace extracellular fluid deficits
- Electrolyte content restores the extracellular fluid balance
- Can be used to correct acid–base balance.

Maintenance solutions

- Contain electrolytes but in much smaller concentrations, particularly sodium ions
- Often hypotonic
- Maintain homeostasis by replacing insensible fluid losses and electrolytes lost in animals – nil by mouth, e.g. 0.18% NaCl in 4.5% dextrose
- Note that potassium supplementation may be required.

DISEASES

Conditions of the alimentary tract

Conditions of the alimentary tract are characterised by changes in dietary habits and often anorexia. Prolonged anorexia would lead to the following:

- Reduction of lean body mass
- Reduced immunological response
- Reduced rate of wound healing
- Generally reduced recovery time
- Increased metabolic load on liver and kidneys.

The underlying cause of anorexia needs to be established. The case history will be a valuable diagnostic tool in conjunction with diagnostic testing.

Patients who are anorexic will require a food that is palatable and easy to digest. Various methods can be employed to encourage animals to eat, including:

- Increase temperature of food
- Hand-feed
- Increase lipid content
- Establish individual preferences
- Select food with a strong odour
- Liquidise diet
- Moisten diet
- Pharmaceutical agents, e.g. diazepam (short-duration stimulant for cats when given at a dose rate of 0.5–1 mg/kg IV)
- Feeding tubes.

Refer to Table 27.4 for methods of assisted feeding.

Conditions of the oesophagus

These are characterised by vomiting or regurgitation. Vomiting is not always a true reflection of an animal's underlying disease. Ensure a complete history is obtained in addition to diagnostic methods prior to a final prognosis. Regurgitation is a passive process where food and fluid are passed up the oesophagus into the mouth. It is always undigested food and liquid and usually occurs postfeeding. There is no abdominal contraction (retching). Causes of regurgitation include:

- Oesophageal foreign bodies (FB)
- Megaoesophagus.

Table 27.4 Assisted feeding	
Hand-feeding	Method used to tempt fussy eaters Advisable to warm food With cats, placing food on the paw may stimulate grooming and then eating
Pharyngosotomy tube	Tube is surgically placed into the pharynx Food must be liquidised and specialised commercial preparations are available
Nasogastric tube	Tube is placed through the nostril and advanced into the stomach Food must be liquidised and specialised commercial preparations are available
Gastrotomy tube	Tube is surgically placed into the stomach Food must be liquidised and specialised commercial preparations are available
Naso-oesophageal tube	Tube is placed through the nostril and advanced into the oesophagus Food must be liquidised and specialised commercial preparations are available
Enterostomy tube (duodenostomy/ jejunostomy)	Tube is surgically placed into the small intestine Food must be liquidised and specialised commercial preparations are available
Nutrient enema	A specialised enema that can be administered via the rectum

Megaoesophagus

1. In the normal animal peristalsis occurs in the oesophagus
2. In megaoesophagus peristalsis ceases
3. The oesophagus becomes distended
4. The result is a large flaccid sac
5. Food becomes trapped before entering the cardiac sphincter, therefore no digestion occurs and food is regurgitated.

Vomiting is an active process where the following occurs:

* Apnoea
* Epiglottal closure
* Fixed diaphragm
* Fixed abdominal muscles
* Stomach squeezed
* Ejection of food.

Retching precedes vomiting. Vomiting can be further classified into primary vomiting, e.g. gastritis, and secondary vomiting, e.g. colitis, hepatitis and pyometra. Persistent vomiting or regurgitation can lead to aspiration pneumonia or metabolic acidosis.

Primary gastric disease is treated symptomatically:

* Complete dietary rest
* IV fluid therapy
* Treat underlying cause
* IV glucose
* Antiemetics
* Antacids
* Surgery (for a FB)
* Administration of gastrointestinal tract protectants
* Bland diet
* Small quantities of food, fed at increased frequency.

Conditions of the small intestine

There are four types of pathological conditions causing diarrhoea:

1. Increase in osmotic tension of the gut contents where water that should have been absorbed remains in the intestine and is drawn into the intestine from the vascular system
2. Diminished reabsorption of fluids and digestive end products. For example, in an average dog (lab-sized) 4 litres of fluid per day pass into the duodenum but only 75 ml is excreted. Disease conditions that can cause diminished reabsorption include enteritis
3. Excessive electrolyte secretion into the small intestine from the mesenteric blood vessels into the small intestine. This is often caused by irritants, e.g. poisons, decaying food

4. Increased peristalsis caused by irritation by microorganisms where the sensory nerve endings are affected and overstimulated.

Diarrhoea is the passage of unformed faeces of increased bulk or increased fluid. Blood will often be seen in the faeces and can give clues to the diagnosis. Fresh blood is often from the large intestines or rectum. Melaena is the presence of digested blood from the ileum or stomach or a diet of only red meat. Clinical signs of life-threatening diarrhoea include vomiting and diarrhoea, dehydration, anorexia and gastric pain. Treatment will include intensive fluid therapy, antibiotics, nil per os, antidiarrhoeal drugs, oral fluids and a low-fat diet introduced slowly. In acute diarrhoea animals often present as bright, alert and eating, dehydration is unlikely and the condition often rectifies spontaneously with dietary rest.

Chronic diarrhoea is usually due to malabsorption or maldigestion. Malabsorption is caused by damage to the small intestinal villi which prevents absorption of nutrients (often due to bacterial imbalance). Maldigestion is often the failure of the exocrine pancreas to produce sufficient enzymes.

Clinical signs of chronic diarrhoea include presence of chronic diarrhoea episodes, decreased weight, dehydration and polyphagia. Colitis is the most common cause of diarrhoea and is characterised by tenesmus, unproductive straining and the presence of blood and/or mucus in the faeces.

Foreign bodies

FB come in a variety of shapes and sizes, and can turn up all over the animal body. In the digestive tract oral FB results in excessive salivation, retching, pawing and gagging. Pharyngeal FB results in coughing, choking, pawing and dyspnoea. Oesophageal FBs result in regurgitation and can lead to aspiration pneumonia. Gastric FB can be asymptomatic if the pylorus is not a factor or may present with excessive vomiting or intermittent signs.

Small-intestine FB presents with excessive vomiting, dehydration and abdominal pain. Rectal FBs cause pain on defecation, tenesmus and blood. FBs usually require surgical intervention to remove them; common operations performed include enterotomy, gastrotomy and thoracotomy.

Gastric dilation/volvulus (gastric tympany or gastric torsion)

This is a true emergency condition which requires immediate veterinary treatment. Deep-chested dogs are more prone to be affected and it is thought that exercise before or after eating food could predispose animals to it. Clinical signs include a depressed animal, groaning, trying to vomit, listlessness, shock, pain and rapid abdominal distension. The animal must be seen by a vet and is treated for shock. It may be stomach-tubed to try to remove gastric contents but often surgery is required to empty the stomach and a gastropexy is performed, suturing the stomach to the abdominal wall to prevent recurrence. Gastric dilation describes the swelling of the stomach and it is said to be gastric volvulus when the stomach twists upon itself due to its expansion – this can often compromise the blood supply to the tissues.

Conditions of the liver

Hepatitis is inflammation of the liver and is characterised by icterus or jaundice, usually contributable to elevated bilirubin levels in the vascular system. There are three causes of icterus: prehepatic, due to an increase in the breakdown of erythrocytes; hepatic, due to primary liver disease, resulting in a static bile flow; and posthepatic from an obstructed bile duct. Cirrhosis describes the healing of liver tissue by fibrous tissue formation and not by regeneration of hepatic cells. Therefore the functional capacity of the liver is reduced. Bile flow is interrupted or interfered with, leading to portal hypertension which leads to ascites, accumulation of fluid in the abdominal cavity, which in turn leads to impaired liver function and ultimately liver failure.

Animals suffering from liver disease often exhibit vomiting and diarrhoea, abdominal pain, a decrease in weight, jaundice, pale faeces due to bile content and ascites. Remember that the liver has a massive functional reserve and can regenerate; a patient must lose 70% of functional liver capacity before signs of liver failure are observed.

Acute pancreatitis

The pancreas is a mixed exocrine and endocrine gland. Its exocrine function is to produce digestive enzymes, which are stored in the gallbladder as small granules called zymogens. Zymogens cannot become active in the pancreas, leading to self-digestion. If physiological mechanisms fail the animal can suffer from acute pancreatitis, resulting in self-digestion of the pancreatic tissue. Clinical signs include:

- Localised peritonitis (diagnosed by anterior abdominal radiograph)
- Leukocytosis (elevated white blood cell count)
- Occasional vomiting and diarrhoea
- Dehydration, leading to shock
- Anterior abdominal pain
- Anorexia
- Ascites/peritonitis.

Diseases of the nervous system

Diseases of the nervous system are characterised by neurological problems in the patient. These may be due to increased pressure within the brain or spinal cord resulting in paralysis or behavioural abnormalities. If the animal presents with cranial oedema, diuretics may be administered to reduce cerebral oedema in conjunction with steroids to reduce inflammation. If successful, symptoms may be reversed if the treatment is given before permanent damage to the brain cells in cases where the pressure is a result of concussion or trauma.

Spinal cord injury

Injury is often due to trauma, e.g. road traffic accident or intervertebral disc protrusion. The animal's prognosis is dependent upon the extent of the injury, the reversibility of the damage and the early initiation of therapy. Clinical signs will vary but important neurological signs to note are the loss of reflexes, loss of deep pain sensation and urinary or faecal incontinence. Remember that severe trauma can result in tissue shock which may dull reactions at the site of injury, therefore patients may need to be reassessed periodically. Once the patient is stabilised plain radiographs should be undertaken to enable a diagnosis. These may identify:

- Prolapsed, calcified discs
- Narrowing of the disc space
- Narrowing of the intervertebral foramen
- Opaque mass in the spinal cord above a normal/calcified disc.

A myelogram, which is a radiograph taken after a dye has been injected into the spinal tissues to enhance the image, may enable other conditions to be identified:

- Canine wobbler syndrome
- Canine degenerative radiculomyopathy
- Spinal tumours
- Thrombotic emboli (blood clots)
- Fractures/dislocations.

Seizures/epilepsy

Epilepsy is a medical condition where seizures will recur, not due to a short-term problem or an underlying disease. A seizure is a manifestation of a 'fit'. Usually these can be related to a short-term problem or underlying disease. The clinical symptoms of both are similar:

- Tonic spasms: extension spasm of limbs
- Clonic spasm: paddling spasms of the limbs
- Brief loss of consciousness
- Salivation/frothing

- Before and after the seizure the animal will often hallucinate, howl, bark or whine
- Ataxia (uncoordinated movement)
- Urination/defecation.

Seizures can be due to extracranial disturbances, e.g. hypoxia, hypoglycaemia or intracranial disturbances, e.g. neoplasia or head trauma. Young animals 6–10 months of age may suffer from idiopathic (unknown origin) or functional epilepsy; this is a condition where the animal has fits of a short duration with few residual side-effects and that occur at regular intervals. It is thought to be inherited in Keeshonds, German Shepherds, Toy Poodles and Cocker Spaniels. Treatment for all seizures varies according to the individual veterinary surgeon but common drugs utilised include phenytoin, Mysoline, phenobarbital and diazepam.

The nervous system functions by the production and propagation of electrical charges or nervous impulses. The release of these impulses is carefully controlled via interaction between excitatory and inhibitory neurotransmitters and normally occurs only at a frequency and amplitude to mediate normal sensory/motor neuronal activity. Seizure activity commences when the excitability of a group of neurones is increased. This can often be correlated to identifiable specific triggers such as flashing lights, sounds and drugs.

A grand mal is a classic long epileptic fit that has a sudden onset; a petit mal is an epileptic fit of short duration, which may present only as twitches.

Status epilepticus is continuous fits, one after another, which are difficult to treat successfully and often have a poor prognosis.

Diseases of the respiratory tract

The respiratory system is lined with ciliated, columnar epithelium which is interspersed with goblet cells producing mucus to provide a first line of defence against pathogens and foreign bodies. The tissues are prone to infection and inflammation, characterised by excessive mucus production and often accompanied by sneezing or coughing and discharges. The suffix 'itis' with the associated anatomical area of the respiratory tract describes the affected location, e.g. sinusitis is inflammation of the sinuses. The respiratory system can also have foreign bodies within it which may require surgical intervention and would often present with sneezing, coughing or epistaxis (haemorrhage from the nostrils).

Trauma can also result in physical damage to the respiratory tract; road traffic accidents may result in a ruptured diaphragm. Clinical signs are dependent upon the location and severity of the damage caused to the diaphragm. They include respiratory distress, dyspnoea, cyanosis, a mediastinal shift (displacement of heart sounds to the right-hand side of the thorax) and bowel sounds in the thorax on auscultation.

Acute pulmonary oedema

This is a condition caused by congestion of the lungs leading to the passage of serous fluid from the capillaries into the interstitial tissues and alveoli. It is caused by left ventricular heart failure, chest trauma, uraemia or inhalation of chemical irritants. Clinical signs include rales breathing on auscultation, rattling or abnormal lower respiratory tract sounds due to fluid accumulating in the interstitial spaces, hyperventilation, tachycardia, cyanosis, cardiac arrhythmias and, when the fluid moves into the bronchial tree, it leads to acute respiratory distress characterised by coarse bubbling rales, cardiac shock and metabolic and respiratory acidosis followed by death.

Skin diseases

Diseases of the skin are characterised by alopecia, a general term describing hair loss, and pruritus, irritation or inflammation of the skin. The skin may also suffer from seborrhoea or abnormal copious excretion of sebum, leading to oily skin or pyoderma where there is pyogenic (pus-forming) skin infection. Ectoparasites are common causes of dermatological problems and they are usually diagnosed using skin scrapings and microscopy.

Hormonal alopecia can be due to hypothyroidism, hyperadrenocorticism, Sertoli cell tumours or ovarian imbalance. Clinical signs are usually bisymmetrical alopecia present on the flanks, ventral abdomen and medial thigh, although it can involve the whole body and head. Pyoderma is often due to an imbalance in the commensal bacteria population of the skin, perhaps due to reduced immune status which allows the *Staphylococcus* or *Streptococcus* species to multiply, resulting in pustules. Treatment of skin conditions is often by medicated shampoos and associated antibiotics.

Dermatophytosis or ringworm is a fungal infection of the skin common in all animal species. It is transmitted by direct contact or indirect contact with fomites and is zoonotic. It presents as alopecia with scaling and can be diagnosed by laboratory cultures.

Animals may also present with allergic dermatitis which can have numerous causes. Clinical signs include urticaria, pruritus, erythema and alopecia.

Blood testing can be used to diagnose the cause via injection of allergens and blood serum allergen testing. Treatment is generally systemic but specially manufactured antiallergen formulas can be generated for injection.

Diseases of the reproductive tract

Endocrinological abnormalities include:

- Delayed puberty
- Prolonged anoestrus
- Silent oestrus (normal activity but no external signs)
- Split oestrus (signs of pro-oestrus followed 2 weeks later by normal cycle)
- Ovulation failure
- Pseudopregnancy (false pregnancy) or pseudocyesis – may require hormonal therapy.

Ovarian diseases

- Agenesis: no ovarian development
- Ovarian cysts: rare but can give symptoms of prolonged oestrus and can result in fertility problems
- Can be hermaphrodite, i.e. have ovarian and testicular tissue.

Diseases of the uterus

- Aplasia: abnormal development
- Agenesis: no development
- Intersex: uterus and vas deferens present
- Cystic endometrial hyperplasia: can develop into pyometra; hyperplasia occurs at the end of metoestrus due to levels of progesterone but no pregnancy.

Vaginitis

- Inflammation of the vagina
- Treat with antibiotics.

Tumours

A tumour is a solid swelling resulting from abnormal growth of tissue. The growth of this tissue exceeds that of normal tissue cells and is not mirrored by the surrounding normal tissue. Neoplasia means 'new growth' and is applied to tumours in general. Cancer is slang for a malignant growth. Metastasis (plural metastases) describes the spread of malignant tumour cells to other sites in the body, giving rise to secondary tumours which are similar to primary tumours.

Metastasis can occur as follows:

- In the circulation: fragmentation of the tumour gives rise to small portions which enter the blood stream and relocate in another area of tissue, commonly the lungs and liver
- In the lymphatic system: the tumour fragments lodge in the lymph nodes and continue to multiply, enlarging the nodes

- Through body cavities and via direct invasion: direct contact of the tumour cells with neighbouring viscera (extension) or by exfoliation of the tumour cells into a body cavity (transplantation).

Classification of tumours

Benign tumours

- Relatively slower multiplication growth rate
- Can be discrete or encapsulated
- Defined with the suffix '-oma'
- No infilitration
- No spread via vessels
- No secondaries
- If completely removed do not often recur
- Often located in the superficial tissues.

Benign tumours are generally mistakenly regarded as harmless but they may lead to:

- Haemorrhage
- Oedema
- Mobility problems
- Hormone production (oestrogens).

Malignant tumours

- Rapid growth
- Not well defined and usually not encapsulated
- Spread via lymphatic system and vascular system
- Tend to recur
- Tendency to be deep-rooted.

Malignant tumours are regarded as dangerous because they have the capacity to infiltrate and destroy somatic cells.

Mammary tumours The most common site for neoplasia in the bitch. Entire females suffer from a higher incidence and early neutering is regarded as an appropriate prophylactic measure. Growths can occur in any of the five mammary glands but the caudal pairs display a higher incidence. Mammary tumours in the bitch are commonly benign (50%) and complete resection is usually sufficient to remove the risk and save the patient. Malignant tumours, adenocarcinomas and sarcomas, will metastasise via the lymphatics and blood stream. In the queen mammary tumours usually present in any combination or all four pairs of mammary glands. Most mammary tumours of the queen are malignant and readily metastasise and a guarded prognosis is usually given.

Treatment for tumours includes surgical excision, diathermy (heat applied to tissues to cauterise the affected area), hyperthermia (heat therapy), radiotherapy, chemotherapy (cytotoxic drugs), hormones, radical surgery, e.g. amputation, steroids, cryosurgery, homeopathic remedies, analgesia and euthanasia.

To diagnose a tumour a biopsy is recommended. A biopsy is when a sample of tissue or other material is obtained for diagnosis and prognosis and to aid in the planning of appropriate therapy. An excision biopsy completely removes all the neoplastic tissue, whereas an incision biopsy only removes a small section of the mass, as does a punch biopsy or needle biopsy. The tissue sample is then preserved and sent for histopathology to determine the type of cancer present.

Diseases of the circulatory system

Heart or cardiac disease is the most common disease in the circulatory system. Clinical signs in patients with heart disease include:

- Cyanosis
- Tachypnoea
- Exercise intolerance
- Ascites/oedema
- Coughing, particularly after rest
- Obesity.

Heart disease may be congenital, i.e. the animal is born with the condition, or acquired.

Patent ductus arteriosus

In the fetus the circulation is from the pulmonary artery to the aorta and this condition represents the persistence of the normal fetal vessel connecting the aorta and the pulmonary artery. The vessel normally closes after birth and all that is left is the ligamentum arteriosus; in this case it fails to do so. Some blood is pumped directly from the aorta back into the lungs and therefore a pressure overload leads to left-side failure. There is evidence to suggest that this condition is inherited in the Miniature Poodle, German Shepherd Dog, Pomeranian and Sheltie. Diagnosis is via auscultation which gives a continuous machinery murmur.

Pulmonary stenosis

This is an abnormal narrowing of the main pulmonary artery as it leaves the right ventricle. The stenosis causes high pressure on the right side of the heart and thickening of the right ventricle wall (hypertrophy). Lung perfusion is usually adequate but the right ventricle has to work hard. If this mechanism fails it will lead to right-sided heart failure. Surgery is possible.

This condition is inherited in the Beagle.

Aortic stenosis

Aortic stenosis is a narrowing of the aorta as it leaves the left ventricle; therefore the ventricle has to work harder to pump the blood around the body. The narrowing of the aortic valve will in turn lead to high pressure in the left ventricle and poor cardiac output. The heart may be unable to maintain systemic blood pressure, which may lead to fainting or syncope. Sometimes sudden death may occur.

Ventricular septal defects

A defect may remain in the wall separating either the left from the right ventricle or the left from the right atrium, creating a so-called hole in the heart. Blood usually flows from left to right and results in right-hand heart failure.

Acquired heart disease

There are numerous acquired cardiac conditions, including:

- Endocarditis: inflammation of the valves of the heart
- Myocardial disease: primary (heart muscle dysfunction, common in giant breeds 2–7 years old) or secondary (heart is affected in the course of a systemic disease, e.g. taurine, hyperthyroidism)
- Cardiomyopathy: dilated in dogs (where the heart muscle is thin and there is poor contraction) or hypertrophic in cats (where the heart muscle has thickened so that the lumen is diminished and cardiac output is poor)
- Pericardial disease: inflammation of the pericardium usually secondary to other diseases
- Endocardiosis: this is chronic valve disease and involves the atrioventricular valves; as lesions increase in severity the valves become more inefficient. This is the commonest cause of congestive heart failure in the dog. Small breeds and male animals appear to be more prone.

Diagnosis of heart disease
Auscultation
- Soft blowing: mitral valve insufficiency heard over fifth/sixth intercostal space
- Soft blowing: tricuspid valve insufficiency as above but loudest over fourth intercostal space.

Radiography
- A degree of heart enlargement will be seen
- A normal heart is found 2–3 rib spaces laterally, three-quarters the depth of the thorax.

Electrocardiogram
- Changes will be detected, e.g. heart hypertrophy.

Congestive heart failure

This occurs when the heart's ability to compensate does not meet the requirements of the animal. The result is pooling of blood of one or more of the vascular beds behind the right or left sides of the heart. Right heart failure causes a poor venous return, congestion of liver/spleen/viscera and ascites. In right heart failure animals display exercise intolerance, tachypnoea, venous enlargement and ascites/oedema and lose weight. It may be the result of cardiomyopathy, pulmonic stenosis, tricuspid valve insufficiency or arrhythmias.

Left heart failure causes poor venous return from lungs, oedema, tachypnoea and coughing. It is characterised by exercise intolerance, nocturnal restlessness, lethargy, dyspnoea, wet pulmonary rales and coughing after rest. It may be the result of mitral valve insufficiency or cardiomyopathy. Animals with a lowered cardiac output suffer from water retention, sodium retention and an increase in extracellular fluid, hence the oedema, ascites and coughing (due to pulmonary oedema).

Endocrine disorders

These affect the rate of secretion of hormones. Hyposecretion is reduced output and occurs if target cells are deprived of needed stimulation. Hypersecretion is an abnormal increase in output and occurs if target cells are overstimulated. A normal amount of hormone could be secreted but the target cells may lack receptors or have faulty receptors and therefore cannot take up the hormone. Any abnormality will lead to predictable metabolic malfunctions and clinical symptoms.

Diabetes insipidus

This occurs due to failure of ADH from the pituitary gland or poor renal response to ADH. Central diabetes insipidus arises from a pituitary source and nephrogenic diabetes inspidus from a renal source.

ADH increases the permeability of the renal nephron to conserve the body's fluid balance. If ADH is low then more urine is produced. Clinical signs are polyuria (frequent urination) and polydipsia (frequent drinking) and a very low specific gravity of 1.000–1.007. Diagnosis is via a water deprivation test, where the water supply is withheld to see if urine concentrates. If it does not, the diagnosis of diabetes insipidus can be made. Treatment is lifelong drug therapy.

Canine hyperadrenocorticism

Also known as Cushing's disease, hyperadrenocorticism is an excessive production of glucocorticoids and is common in the horse and the dog but rare in the cat,

It is caused by inappropriate secretion of adrenocorticotrophic hormone (ACTH) which is pituitary-dependent. Pituitary tumours, e.g. microadenomas and macroadenomas, give false readings of levels of ACTH; tumours in adrenals, e.g. carcinomas and adenomas, may stop the action of ACTH on the adrenal glands, resulting in primary failure of the feedback response.

Cushing's disease can be spontaneous or iatrogenic. Spontaneous disease is due to inappropriate secretion of ACTH by the pituitary or because of a primary adrenal disorder. Primary pituitary-dependent hyperadrenocorticism accounts for 80% of the condition in dogs. Excessive ACTH causes hyperplasia in the adrenal cortex, leading to excess cortisol production; these levels can fluctuate (they require urine excreted over a 24-hour period to be tested for diagnosis). Ninety per cent of dogs suffering from the pituitary-dependent form are believed to have a pituitary tumour, e.g. microadenomas (< 10 mm) or macroadenomas (> 10 mm). The adrenal-dependent form accounts for the remaining 15–20% of cases which are usually caused by unilateral or bilateral tumours of the adrenal glands (may be benign or malignant). Certain breeds appear predisposed, including Poodles, Dachshunds and small terriers, e.g. Yorkshire Terriers and Jack Russell Terriers.

Adrenocortical tumours occur more frequently in large breeds; middle-aged and older dogs are more commonly affected.

Clinical signs are akin to the normal ageing processes. Symptoms include polyphagia, polyuria, polydipsia, abdominal distension, liver enlargement, muscle wasting/weakness, lethargy, poor exercise tolerance, skin changes, with the skin becoming thin and inelastic, alopecia, persistent anoestrus or testicular atrophy due to suppression of gondatrophins and negative feedback of cortisol, and neurological signs, e.g. dullness, depression, anorexia, ataxia, aimless wandering and circling. Diagnosis is from the clinical signs and haematology. Treatment is lifelong mitotane therapy: regular monitoring of dosage is required.

Hypoadrenocorticism

This is also known as Addison's disease. It is due to an insufficient secretion of mineralocorticoid and/or glucocorticoid from the adrenal cortices. Aldosterone is a mineralocorticoid whose function is to protect against hypotension and potassium intoxication (promotes reabsorption in the renal tubule and other tissues). It is produced in the adrenal cortices and destruction of over 90% of both adrenal cortices will result in primary adrenocorticism or Addison's disease. Secondary adrenocorticism is due to a deficiency of ACTH. Primary hypoadrenocorticism is relatively rare, although the following breeds are thought to be predisposed to it:

- Great Danes, Rottweilers, Westies, Standard Poodles, Portuguese Water Dogs and Wheaten terriers
- Evidence suggests there may be a hereditary factor in Poodles, Collies and Chinese crested dogs.

Clinical signs vary from mild to severe symptoms, including anorexia, lethargy/depression, weakness, vomiting, weight loss or failure to gain weight, dehydration, diarrhoea, polyuria and polydipsia, collapse, restlessness, melaena, weak pulse, bradycardia and abdominal pain.

The acute form will present with hypovolaemic shock. The animal will often be collapsed and there is rapid progression to death. The signs of the chronic form are often vague and may present as a general malaise. Diagnosis is by haematology, clinical examination and diagnostic tests such as electrocardiogram and radiography. Treatment includes fluid therapy for acute cases and steroids for chronic cases.

Diabetes mellitus

Diabetes mellitus is the failure of insulin transport, failure of insulin production or failure of tissue sensitivity to insulin. In dogs, animals over 7 years of age and females are more prone; in cats, older male animals are more likely to present with the condition. Clinical signs include polyuria, polydipsia, polyphagia, weight loss, exercise intolerance, ketotic breath, recurrent infections and hepatomegaly. Diagnosis is made when there has been persistent fasting hyperglycaemia and glucosuria by blood testing and urine analysis. Treatment is insulin stabilisation and continued therapy which will include nutritional changes to diet and frequency of feeding. Diabetic animals should have a diet which provides slow release of glucose and usually consists of a high-fibre and high-complex-carbohydrate food with feeding times depending on insulin administration regimes. Ketoacidosis is a life-threatening complication of diabetes where the body has undertaken lipid metabolism to provide energy, resulting in toxic levels of ketones being produced in the blood as a byproduct. Hypoglycaemia and hyperglycaemia can also compromise the animal and potentially result in death.

Hypothyroidism

Hypothyroidism occurs more in the dog and is due to the destruction of the thyroid gland or inappropriate secretion of thyroid-stimulating hormone (TSH) from the pituitary gland. Primary hypothyroidism relates to the destruction of thyroid gland whereas secondary hypothyroidism is due to an inappropriate secretion of TSH. In all, 95% cases are primary and 50% of these can be attributed to immune-mediated destruction (autoimmune disease); the remaining 50% are due to atrophy of the thyroid gland (idiopathic). Incidence is increased in middle-aged pedigree dogs and intact males and neutered females are overrepresented.

Clinical signs include dermatological abnormalities, e.g. seborrhoea, alopecia, pyoderma, reduced metabolic rate resulting in obesity, lethargy, cold intolerance, cardiovascular abnormalities, e.g. bradycardia, neuromuscular abnormalities, e.g. weakness, reproductive features, e.g. infertility in females, skeletal features such as dwarfism (congenital) and ocular features, e.g. uveitis. Diagnosis is via examination and blood testing (for thyroxine and triiodothyronine). Treatment is lifelong thyroxine supplementation.

Hyperthyroidism

Hyperthyroidism is due to excessive circulating levels of active thyroid hormones and is most common in middle-aged to old cats. The cause is idiopathic or a benign adenomatous hyperplasia of one or both thyroid lobes.

Clinical signs vary from mild to severe; the disease is insidiously progressive and early symptoms are often mistaken for normal ageing. Classically cats are ravenously hungry but still lose weight; they exhibit polyuria, polydipsia, tachycardia, hyperactivity and diarrhoea due to their increased metabolism. The tumour of the thyroid gland may present as a palpable goitre on the ventral aspect of the neck and bilateral alopecia may be present. Diagnosis is via blood testing (for thyroxine), examination and further diagnostic testing such as urine analysis, radiography and TSH-stimulating test. Treatment is clinical management followed by thyroidectomy and lifelong thyroxine supplementation.

Renal disease

Renal disease is due to damage or functional impairment of the kidneys. Renal insufficiency describes renal impairment that is not severe enough to cause azotaemia (increased blood levels of nitrogenous waste) but that is sufficient to cause a loss in the renal reserve and affect the urine concentration ability. There are two types of renal failure: acute and chronic. Chronic renal failure is the most common cause of uraemia (presence of urea in the blood).

Acute renal failure

This is defined as the complete or almost complete cessation of renal function with sudden dramatic clinical signs. It can be caused by acute glomerulonephritis, hyperkalaemia, severe dehydration, circulatory failure or renal trauma. Clinical signs include:

- Sudden onset of illness
- Oliguria or anuria
- Vomiting
- Lethargy, confusion and disorientation
- Halitosis – uraemic breath
- Neurological disturbances
- Diarrhoea.

All these symptoms will intensify as the levels of nitrogenous waste elevate within the vascular system. Acute renal failure can be categorised into three phases: oliguria phase, diuresis phase and recovery phase. Treatment involves close monitoring of the animal's vital signs, hydration via fluid therapy, diuretics, peritoneal dialysis if required, dietary changes and treatment of the underlying disease or trauma. If the patient fails to recover from acute renal failure the condition will progress to chronic renal failure.

Chronic renal failure

This is an insidious disease involving progressive renal deterioration and can be undetected for long periods of time. There are four main causes:

1. Congenital abnormalities of the kidney
2. Glomerulonephritis
3. Interstitial nephritis
4. Metabolic disorders.

The renal nephrons cannot be repaired or replaced, therefore damage to the nephrons results in irreparable loss of kidney function and efficacy. Recovery therefore depends upon the ability of the remaining healthy nephrons to function under the increased workload that in turn will put these nephrons under high stress, leading to renal compensation. If an underlying disease factor then causes the renal impairment to progress, the animal has decompensated its renal function. Clinical signs of chronic renal failure include anorexia, polyuria, polydipsia, vomiting, lethargy, halitosis, weight loss and anaemia. Treatment should involve rectifying the underlying cause, introduction of a low-protein diet, control of vomiting and correction of any fluid imbalances with simultaneous vitamin B supplementation.

Osteoarthritis

Osteoarthritis is a condition characterised by osteopathic changes in the articular surfaces of synovial joints and is often due to deterioration in the viscosity of the synovial fluid. This results in erosions of the articular surface around which bony changes occur, resulting in pain, inflammation and stiffness. There is evidence to suggest that canine osteoarthritis has an inheritable factor in certain breeds, e.g. Labrador. Diagnosis is from radiography and clinical examination; treatment includes anti-

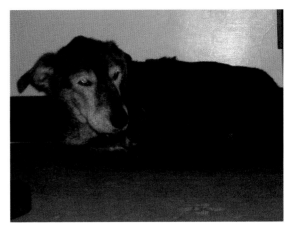

Figure 27.2 Typical appearance of geriatric canine.

inflammatory drugs, weight loss, exercise restriction and in some cases surgical intervention. Figure 27.2 shows the typical appearance of a geriatric canine.

Bibliography

Aspinall V 2006 The complete textbook of veterinary nursing. Butterworth Heinemann, London

Bacha W J Jr, Wood L M 1990 Color atlas of veterinary histology. Lea & Febiger, Philadelphia

Blood D C, Studdart V P 1988 Baillière's comprehensive veterinary dictionary. Baillière Tindall, Oxford

Chandler E A, Gaskell C J, Gaskell R M 1994 Feline medicine and therapeutics, 2nd edition. Blackwell Sciences/ BSAVA, Oxford

Coughlan A, Miller A 1998 Manual of small animal fracture repair and management. BSAVA, Oxford

Gaskell R M, Bennett M 1996 Feline and canine infectious disease. Blackwell Sciences, Oxford

Gorman N 1998 Canine medicine and therapeutics, 4th edn. Blackwell Sciences/BSAVA, Oxford

Lane D R, Cooper B, Turner L 2007 Textbook of veterinary nursing, 3rd edn. Butterworth Heinemann/ BSAVA, Oxford

McCurnin D, Bassett J 2005 Clinical textbook for veterinary technicians, 6th edn. W B Saunders, Philadelphia

Moore M 2000 Manual of veterinary nursing. BSAVA, Oxford

Moore A H, Simpson G 1999 Manual of advanced veterinary nursing. BSAVA, Oxford

Pratt P W 1998 Principles and practice of veterinary technology. Mosby, Philadelphia

Ramsey I, Tennant B 2001 Manual of canine and feline infectious diseases. BSAVA, Oxford

Simpson G 1994 Practical veterinary nursing, 3rd edn. BSAVA, Oxford

Torrance A G, Mooney C T 1998 Manual of small animal endocrinology, 2nd edn. BSAVA, Oxford

Tracy D L 1994 Small animal surgical nursing, 2nd edn. Mosby-Year Book, Philadelphia

Chapter | **28** | *Jane Williams*

Anaesthesia and radiography

This chapter continues the evaluation of the processes used in modern veterinary practices to facilitate therapeutic care of animals. The basic principles of anaesthesia and radiography are described in relation to companion animal species.

RADIOGRAPHY

Basic principles

Radiography is an essential tool in veterinary practice. It enables the veterinary surgeon to diagnose diseases, fractures and foreign bodies.

The radiograph or X-ray is produced by converting electricity into X-ray energy and firing this at the patient. The patient will absorb varying amounts of the X-ray energy depending upon the thickness and constituent of the tissue affected. The X-rays that are not absorbed pass through to a plate beneath and are detected by a photographic plate, producing an image that is revealed upon development by chemicals.

X-rays are high-frequency, short-wavelength radiation. They are high-energy particles that make them suitable for use in the production of an image. However they are an ionising radiation and they will affect living tissue; therefore a strict code of conduct and series of rules and regulations govern their use in veterinary practice. Radiography is an electromagnetic radiation of high energy and low wavelength. Radiation comes in many different forms, which have differing wavelengths but similar properties – they are on the electromagnetic spectrum. The higher the frequency and shorter the wavelength, the more penetrating the form of radiation. In veterinary practice, the generation of radiographs or X-rays uses electricity.

An electric current from the mains supply is transformed by the X-ray machine into a high-voltage current that is applied to an X-ray tube head to produce X-rays. Electricity consists of particles known as electrons, which have a negative charge and a small mass number – this enables them to travel at great speeds. The faster the electrons travel or the greater the kinetic (moving) energy they possess, the more penetrating the X-rays produced will be. High voltages equate to electrons that have a high velocity.

An electron is a negatively charged particle that produces electricity (Table 28.1). To produce the X-rays the electric current passes into the X-ray machine tube head. Here there are two terminals: one is positive, the anode, and the other is negative, the cathode. The current consists of electrons which as we know are negative particles; therefore the negative terminal repels the like charge. The cathode fires the electrons away from it. The electron beam is also concentrated using a focusing cup, which will increase their velocity.

Table 28.1 Recap of atomic theory

Electron	Negative charge	Minimal atomic mass
Proton	Positive charge	1 atomic mass unit
Neutron	Neutral charge	1 atomic mass unit

Negative particles will be attracted to positivity so the electrons will travel towards the positive anode. Remember that the electrons are travelling at a great speed or with lots of kinetic energy so when they collide with the positive anode the energy they contain cannot be destroyed and it is changed into another format.

When the electrons hit the anode the kinetic energy has to change as the electrons are brought to an abrupt stop. The kinetic energy changes into heat and X-rays (99% heat and 1% X-rays). The X-rays produced are fired from the anode down towards the target area.

Properties of X-rays

- They penetrate all materials
- They travel in straight lines
- They are not reflected
- They blacken certain materials, e.g. photographic film
- They cause fluorescence (inside plates)
- They have a biological effect:
  - Carcinogenic
  - Teratogenic
  - Mutagenic.

Health risks

X-rays are invisible and painless and their effects are latent and cumulative. This means that exposure to X-rays will not necessarily be known until a later date or after an individual has been exposed to lots of X-rays. In veterinary practice the strengths of X-rays used are not great; however, repeated low-dose exposure can prove to be a potentially contaminating factor.

Biological risks

- X-rays produce biological changes in living tissue by altering the atomic structure
- Somatic effects:
  - Direct changes in body tissues soon after exposure, e.g. skin reddening, baldness, blood disorders, digestive upsets
  - Different tissues are affected by radiation in different ways

- Carcinogenic effects:
  - Induction of tumours in exposed tissues
  - Can be many years after exposure
- Genetic effects:
  - Occur when gonads are irradiated
  - Cause mutations in chromosomes of germ cells, which may go on to develop into gametes, then give rise to mutated offspring.

Principles of radiographic protection

Radiography should only be undertaken if there is definite clinical justification for its use. Any exposure of personnel should be kept to a minimum and no dose limit should be exceeded. All practices that use X-ray machines have to conform to strict legislation. Conscious radiography of patients should only be undertaken if anaesthesia or sedation is contraindicated by the animal's condition.

Ionising radiation regulations act 1988

This is the law that governs the use of radiation and radioactive materials. It covers premises, equipment, personnel and procedures. Its aim is to minimise radiation doses.

Checklist of principles of radiographic protection

- Radiography should only be undertaken if there is definite clinical justification for its use
- Any exposure of personnel should be kept to a minimum
- No dose limit should be exceeded.

All practices that use X-ray machines have to notify the Health and Safety Executive and will be visited by them on regular occasions.

Radiation protection supervisor (RPS)

- Must be appointed within the practice
- Usually the practice principal or senior partner
- Responsible for ensuring local rules are adhered to in the practice
- Does not need to be present for every radiograph.

Radiation protection advisor (RPA)

- Usually an external appointee
- Strict qualification is needed to qualify
- Vets with diploma in radiography
- RPA gives advice on all aspects of radiation protection.

Controls in the veterinary practice

The controlled area

- A specific room should be identified for radiography
- Walls should be sufficiently thick so that no part of the controlled area is outside them (one brick thick or may be lead-lined)
- Room should be large enough to allow two people to stay in the room when X-raying at a distance of at least 2 metres from the primary beam
- Alternatively a lead screen can be used
- The controlled area is the area around the primary beam to a minimum radius of 2 metres but needs to be defined by the RPA (it is usually easier to designate a room as the controlled area)
- The controlled area must be clearly marked to highlight its presence to other users
- Use a radiation warning triangle/signs/lights
- If the X-ray machine is permanently installed, lights are required that come on when it is being fired for use – the lights are usually red or state 'X-ray'
- The X-ray machine must be disconnected from the mains supply when not in use
- All X-ray machines should have lights on the control panel indicating whether they are on and when an exposure is taking place
- Only designated persons over 16 years of age may enter the controlled area.

X-ray equipment

- X-ray machines should be regularly serviced by a qualified engineer to check for faults
- The X-ray table must be lead-lined or a sheet of lead 1 mm thick and larger than the maximum size of beam must be placed on the table beneath the X-ray cassette to reduce scatter
- The operator should select the appropriate exposures and use the fastest film to reduce length of time exposed to radiation
- Area to be radiographed should be only as big as necessary
- Patients should be anaesthetised or heavily sedated
- Restraint equipment should be used
- Protective equipment should be used.

Restraint equipment

- Drugs
- Troughs
- Sandbags
- Ties
- Foam wedges
- Weights.

Protective equipment

- Usually aprons, gloves, sleeves made of a material containing lead
- Only designed to protect against scatter
- Should be worn by any person who has to stay in the controlled area during exposure
- Lead aprons should be mid-length to protect gonads and have a minimum of 0.25 mm lead (most have 0.5 mm)
- Lead aprons should be stored flat and never folded as the lead cracks and this effects efficiency
- Lead gloves or hand shields are for use in manual restraint radiography
- They should only be used in extreme cases (with the exception of equine radiography)
- Gloves should have at least 0.35 mm thickness of lead and must never be put under the primary beam
- All protective clothing should be regularly checked for signs of perishing – to check you can X-ray the garment to see if any X-rays penetrate it
- Dosimeters:
  - should be worn by all personnel regularly involved in X-rays
  - should be worn on the trunk under the lead apron
  - should not be exposed to heat or sunlight (other types of radiation)
  - should only be worn by the designated wearer
  - are of two types – one containing radiographic film and the other radiation-sensitive crystals
  - can be acquired from the National Radiological Protection Board and should be read every 1–3 months.

Maximum permissible dose

This is the maximum dose considered not to constitute a health risk greater than that encountered in normal life.

Staff involved

- There should be a list of designated staff in the local rules
- Maximum permissible doses for 16/17-year-olds are significantly lower than staff over 18 years
- Owners should never be present
- Pregnant women are best to avoid any involvement with radiography
- As a general rule, there should be the minimum number of people present
- If possible everybody should leave when the exposure is being taken.

Records of radiographs

- All X-rays should be permanently identified
- Lead letters or x-rite tape can be used on film before exposure
- Alternatively in the dark room light markers can be used
- Left and right should be identified
- The date should be recorded and an identification number given
- It is a good idea also to record the animal's or owner's name
- If hip score, need Kennel Club registration number, date and whether left or right
- Every practice should have a radiography record book (Figure 28.1).

Processing chemicals

- There are health and safety implications
- Appropriate guidelines should be followed
- Apron, gloves and mask should be worn
- Cross-contamination must be avoided as this exhausts chemicals
- Follow manufacturer's instructions for dilutions
- Used chemicals should be disposed of in an approved container in clinical waste except if the processor has a silver trap, in which case the chemicals can be flushed down the drain
- Chemicals involved – developer, fixer – are strong acid and alkali.

Penetration and absorption

The final radiograph or X-ray depends on the penetrating power and the absorption of the manufactured X-rays within the different tissues. The final result is the equivalent of a photographic negative. All tissues react in different ways to X-rays. Radiolucent tissues, e.g. air, are displayed as dark areas and radiopaque tissues, such as bone and metal, are displayed as white. The tissues in between show up as varying shades of grey. Therefore the different shades seen on an X-ray relate to the absorption of X-rays within that animal.

Penetrating power

Atoms of tissues will only absorb X-ray particles of a certain velocity or energy. If the energy is greater than the resting or specific energy of the atom the X-ray will pass right through it. Density describes the specific gravity or concentration of a tissue or mass per unit volume. The absorption of X-rays will depend upon the varying densities of the tissue being examined – this can have an important effect, especially during contrast media studies. Air has a very low specific gravity (black on an X-ray), water and soft tissue are similar (grey on an X-ray), fat is denser (dark grey on an X-ray) and metal is most dense (white on an X-ray).

The lower the specific gravity of a tissue the easier X-rays will penetrate it and so more X-rays will pass through it and a black image will be produced. Thickness of tissue will also influence the final outcome. The greater the thickness, the more atoms are present and therefore more X-rays will be absorbed.

X-ray machine design

The purpose of the X-ray tube is to produce, in the shortest time possible, a beam of electrons and X-ray photons. The generating power and number of X-rays produced must be controllable so that it can be used for radiographic examinations. X-rays are produced when electrons travelling at a high velocity convert kinetic energy to heat and X-rays on contact with a stationary target.

X-ray machines are available as stationary or fixed anode machines. The anode is the positive terminal where the electrons hit and the cathode is the negative terminal, which fires the electrons.

Figures 28.2 and 28.3 show the parts of a radiography machine and Table 28.2 explains the parts of the machine.

How are electrons produced?

The machine is turned on at the mains, then:

- Electrons gather at the cathode
- The filament is heated up to incandescence (white heat)

ID number	Owner	Animal	Weight	Exposure MAS KV	Grid used	View	Quality	Staff initials

Figure 28.1 Radiography record.

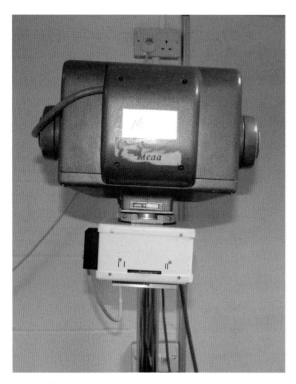

Figure 28.2 Radiography machine tube head.

Table 28.2 Parts of an X-ray machine

Filament wire	Constructed of tungsten wire 1/8th inch in diameter Set into copper as this is an excellent conductor and absorbs the heat produced at the anode
Anode	Electrons hit the anode and an X-ray is created
Cathode	Creates the electron cloud which is fired across to the anode
Vacuum	Increases the speed of electrons
Oil	'Heat sink' and acts as an insulator
Tungsten filament	High atomic number: lots of electrons will be produced
Tungsten target	High melting point Electrons hit this target
Copper shield	Absorbs heat
Lead encasement	Absorbs stray X-rays
Lead lining	Absorbs stray X-rays
Cooling fins	Cool the very hot copper down
Evacuated glass tube	Creates a vacuum and encases the area

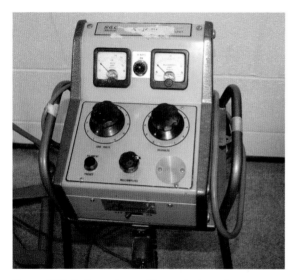

Figure 28.3 Radiography machine control panel.

- The electrons sit in a cloud around the tungsten wire; this is called thermionic emission
- The current required to heat the filament is small so the mains power is reduced by a step-down transformer or a filament transformer

- When the exposure button is depressed a large voltage is passed across the glass tube and the machine produces a voltage within the range of 40–100 kV
- The negative particles assemble around the wire
- Negative particles become very negative and are repelled by the negative electrode (cathode)
- Positive particles become very positive and the negative particles are attracted to the anode
- The kinetic (moving) energy of the electrons is converted to heat and X-rays
- A narrow beam of electrons is emitted from the X-ray tube head because the filament sits within a nickel-focusing cup. This has extra negative potential which helps to repel the electrons and focuses them into a narrow beam towards the anode
- The target is set at 20° to the vertical so that the area of the target with which the electrons make contact is the maximum possible
- This area is known as the actual focal spot
- Where the X-ray beams originate within the actual focal spot appears to be a very small area and this is known as the effective focal spot.

Certain machines allow for a choice of focal spot size by using two tungsten filaments of differing sizes. The smaller size or fine focus produces a narrow electron beam; therefore it has a smaller actual and effective focal spot. The emerging X-ray beam arises from a tiny hole and produces very fine radiographic detail. The heat generated is concentrated over a small area of target, which allows the exposure factors to be limited. The larger or coarse or broad focus produces X-ray beams with a larger actual focal spot allowing higher exposure factors to be used. The film detail using the broad focus is poor in detail due to the penumbra effect. The X-ray beam is allowed to escape the glass envelope by a hole, which is encased within an aluminium filter and then passes to the light beam diaphragm which collimates the primary beam. The penumbra effect produces a blurred image. A general rule is that fine focus is used for small detailed areas and coarse focus is used for thicker areas.

Exposure factors

Kilovoltage

This controls the quality or penetrating power of X-rays; a higher kV will be required for tissues of high atomic mass and for thick tissues. The nature and depth of the tissue must be considered before values are set for the exposure.

Milliamperage

This determines the tube current and the quantity of X-rays produced (the intensity of the electron beam produced). Altering the mA will affect and change the degree of blackening of the film under the areas penetrated.

Time

This is a product of mA and the length of exposure to give a composite value, the mAs or milliamperage per second. It represents the total quantity of X-rays used for that exposure. The longer the time, the greater the potential for movement blur to occur during the exposure.

Exposure charts

It is recommended that charts for individual machines are produced. The exposure values and patient details should be recorded in addition to the view and quality of the image produced. External influencing factors, e.g. the film focal distance, should remain consistent.

Scatter

Scatter is a phenomenon that occurs at settings of over 70 kV and in tissues over 15 cm in depth. Scatter is produced by a second kind of radiation produced within the tissue being X-rayed. The Compton effect produces this second kind of radiation. Remember that tissues are constructed from individual atoms packed together. An individual atom within the tissue is entered by an X-ray photon. The X-ray photon collides with particles within the atom and hits an electron, resulting in the electron moving out of the inner orbit or K-band of the atom. The X-ray photon transfers energy as kinetic energy to this electron to enable it to be released. The remaining energy of the X-ray photon produces a second X-ray within the atom. This resulting secondary X-ray has a longer wavelength and is therefore less penetrating and travelling at a lower energy. X-ray particles produced in this manner do not necessarily move in the same direction as the original incoming X-ray did.

Disadvantages of scatter

- It is dangerous to personnel as it can be produced in all directions
- It causes blurring as many X-rays do not reach the film and also a double exposure effect as many X-ray photons will hit the film in the same place, causing fogging
- It causes blackening of the emulsion as X-ray photons hit the film again in the same place
- It has a biological effect within the patient.

Back scatter

Back scatter occurs when X-ray particles react with atoms below the patient, e.g. the table, the floor. To reduce the risk of back scatter the following items are utilised:

- Lead-lined table: do not assume that tables will be lead-lined
- Lead sheets are used behind or underneath the cassette
- Restrict beam: collimation of the primary beam.

Prevention of scatter

Beam collimation

- Light beam diaphragm
- Tube head cone
- The result is that the primary beam covers the area of interest only.

Compression bands

- Used for fat dogs to obtain abdominal X-rays
- Restriction of the beam in a fat animal will result in X-ray photons passing over the edge of the animal; also the kV required to penetrate the tissue depth would need to be great
- Compression bands work via ties/winches to compress the abdomen and reduce the tissue depth, thus reducing the strength of the primary beam required to penetrate the tissues

459

- Do not use in animals with suspected abdominal/uterine/bladder distension!

Reduction of kV factor

- Use the lowest kV value possible to produce a diagnostic image.

Sheets of lead

- These are placed between the cassette and table top to absorb scatter X-ray photons produced.

Grids

- These are flat plates manufactured to match the size of the X-ray cassettes
- The grid is made of very fine strips of lead alternated with aluminium or acetate or plastic strips
- The grid is placed or fitted on top of the X-ray cassette in a holder (in most cases)
- The grid acts as a filter allowing only the X-rays which are travelling in the same direction as the primary beam to penetrate through it
- The lead strips will absorb all the X-rays that are travelling at an abnormal angle
- The grid image will show on the film.

Film quality

The quality of the radiographs produced is important in veterinary practice as if it is poor it will affect diagnostic ability. X-ray film is sensitive to:

- White light: store in a light-proof container
- Excessive temperatures
- Accidental exposure to radiation: store in a lead-lined cupboard, not in the X-ray room next to the table!
- High humidity: keep clean and dry
- Gases and vapours: store away from chemicals such as ammonium and formaldehyde
- Pressure which can lead to fading: store upright

Most X-ray film manufacturers produce a container which should meet most of the above criteria but remember these are only as efficient as the operator.

Intensifying screens

X-ray film is surprisingly not very sensitive to direct X-ray exposure. Therefore to produce a good, detailed diagnostic image long exposure times are required. Long exposure times lead to increased health and safety risks to operator and patients. Intensifying screens convert X-rays into visible light (this can be demonstrated by exposing an open cassette). This change amplifies the signal and reduces the amount of X-rays required to produce a quality image, thus decreasing the risk to operator and patient. Table 28.3 contains a quick reference guide to film faults.

Radiography: processing

When the radiograph has been exposed the film needs to undergo a developing process to give a latent image. Processing can be done manually or using an automatic processor: both systems utilise the same chemical processes to achieve the final result. Processing should occur in a dark room to prevent contamination of the image. The X-ray film is passed through a developer solution, then water, then a fixer solution, then water, and then needs to be dried. Developer is an alkaline solution containing the active ingredient phenidone or metol hydroquinone and it reduces the molecules in the X-ray film, causing the image to darken. Fixer is an acidic solution containing sodium or ammonium thiosulphate which removes unexposed silver halide crystals to clear the image on the film. Fixing also includes a process called tanning which fixes the image permanently on to the radiograph.

Radiographic positioning

The radiograph position for an animal is described in two ways:

1. The first word describes the direction in which the central ray of the primary beam penetrates the patient
2. The second word describes where the central ray of the primary beam exits the patient.

Figure 28.4 illustrates radiographic terminology used in the limbs above the carpus and tarsus. Refer to Boxes 28.1 and 28.2 for terminology relating to radiographic positions.

Patient preparation

To try and ensure an accurate radiograph:

- Remove any radiopaque objects from the vicinity
- Be careful with contrast media and the patient's coat – try and keep the coat clean!

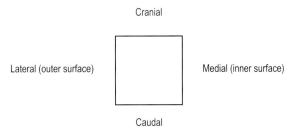

Figure 28.4 Radiographic positioning.

Table 28.3 Quick reference guide to film faults

Film fault	Appearance	Reason
High-density film	Very dark	Overexposure Overdevelopment Too long/too hot
Low-density film	Very grey/white	Underexposure Underdevelopment
High contrast	Soot and whitewash	kV too low
Low contrast	Grey/flat film	kV too high Scatter (fogging) Poor processing
Fogging	Blurred film	Patient movement Exposure to light Faulty cassette Scatter development, storage or chemical
White marks	Seen on developed film	Greasy fingers Fingernail marks on screens Dirt in cassettes Developer/fixer on screens
Dark marks	Seen on developed film	Fingerprints or nail marks on the film
Uneven development	Marks on film	Air bubbles Films in contact (touching) in developer Non-agitation of developer Developer not stirred
Yellow-stained film	Appears as aged	Film not properly fixed Film not washed properly Exhausted developer used
Double exposure	Duplicate image	Exposed twice
Border around film	Visible on film	Not agitated in developer Dirty channel hanger Dried in channel hanger
Dichroic fog	Pink/green tinge	Exhausted fixer Insufficient washing
Grid lines too coarse	Grid lines visible on film	X-ray beam not perpendicular to grid Focused or pseudofocused grid used upside down
Static lines	Branching black lines	Use antistatic cleaner Handle films carefully – you may be the cause!

- Starve the patient before the procedure or administer an enema to prevent faeces and gas shadows on the radiograph
- Consider sedation in all cases – conscious radiography should only be undertaken if the anaesthetic/sedation would prove detrimental to the animal's health.

Positioning aids

Positioning aids should be utilised for all patients to achieve optimum results and prevent rotation about the longitudinal axis of the patient and superimposition of anatomical areas and to maintain a parallel, close contact with the cassette. A variety of aids are available to achieve this (Figure 28.5):

Box 28.1

RADIOGRAPH POSITIONING TERMINOLOGY

Cranial – torso

Towards the head

Caudal – torso

Towards the tail

Rostral

Within the head and toward the muzzle

Medial

Nearer to or toward the midline

Lateral

Farther from the midline or toward the side

Dorsal (D)

Toward the dorsum (back)

Ventral (V)

Toward the ventrum (belly)

Proximal

Nearer to the point of origin or closer to the body

Distal

Farther from the point of origin or away from the body

Palmar (Pa)

Caudal surface (bottom) of the forelimb below the carpus

Plantar (Pl)

Caudal surface (bottom) of the hindlimb below the tarsus

Caudal – limb (Ca)

Lower (posterior) surface of the forelimb and hindlimb above the carpus and tarsus

Cranial – limb (Cr)

Top (anterior) surface of the forelimb and hindlimb above the carpus and tarsus

Internal

Inside – deep

External

Outside – superficial

- Radiolucent foam pads – can be purchased from suppliers or easily made
- Sandbags – can be purchased from suppliers or easily made from old intravenous fluid bags or body bags
- Ties – commercially produced or old shoelaces!

Box 28.2

COMMON RADIOGRAPHIC POSITIONS

Dorsoventral (DV): thorax/abdomen/pelvis/head
Ventrodorsal (VD): thorax/abdomen/pelvis/head/spine
Lateral
  (lat): thorax/abdomen/pelvis/head/spine/shoulder/limbs
Craniocaudal (CrCa): limbs above tarsus and carpus
Caudocranial (CaCr): limbs above tarsus and carpus
Dorsopalmar (Dpa) and palmarodorsal (PaD): front legs below carpus (wrist)
Dorsoplantar (DPl) and plantarodorsal (PlD): back legs below tarsus (hock)

- Compression bands – used more in human field
- Non-slip surfaces – rubber mats on top of table/lead sheets
- Sellotape/Micropore/Omnipore for securing small mammals, birds, reptiles and digits
- Cradles – can be radiopaque or radiolucent – beware!
- Inflatable supports – can be commercially produced or blown-up gloves
- Wooden blocks – utilised more in equine radiography.

Important considerations when positioning animals for radiograph include:

- The exposure factors employed
- Centre the main beam on the cassette (use the cross to guide and collimate to include the whole plate)
- Consider the most suitable position for the animal on the X-ray table, e.g. dorsal recumbency, sternal recumbency
- Make sure the area of interest is over the middle of the cassette and as near to it as possible
- Extend and tie the limbs if appropriate or use sandbags – do not tie conscious patients: use sandbags instead
- Use plenty of radiolucent foam pads to avoid rotation of the animal's body – aim to keep the animal straight with no longitudinal rotation of the spine
- Centre and collimate the main beam to include just the area of interest – you will need to know anatomical landmarks to achieve this!

Summary of radiography

- Always consider the welfare of your patient
- Think about restraint – is the animal conscious?
- Think health and safety – wear appropriate gowns and gloves (Figure 28.6)

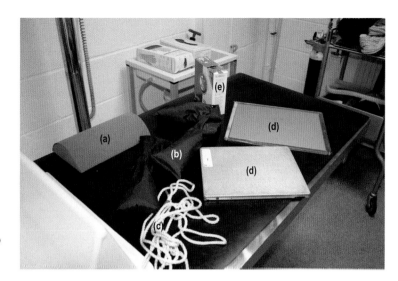

Figure 28.5 Radiography equipment. (a) Foam wedges; (b) sandbags; (c) ties; (d) X-ray plates, (e) x-rite tape.

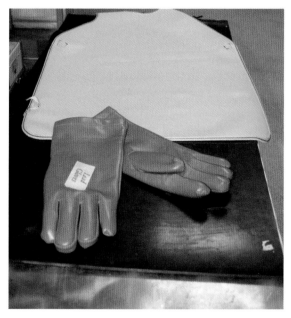

Figure 28.6 Radiographic personal protective equipment: lead gloves and apron.

- Pad, pad and pad some more – don't let your patient sag, droop or twist unless you desire it!
- Label left and right and identify X-rays with x-rite tape or light marker
- Keep records of exposure factors and adjust future X-rays accordingly
- Keep calm! Think logically – if you can't remember the anatomical nomenclature, use lay terms or point!
- Practice makes perfect – have a go.

ADVANCED DIAGNOSTIC TECHNIQUES

Diagnostic imaging methodology is ever advancing in both the human and veterinary fields. Veterinary medicine has successfully adapted many human techniques for diagnostic interpretation, although these techniques are invariably only available in specialised practices.

Advanced diagnostic techniques include:

- Fluoroscopy
- Computed tomography (CT scan)
- Magnetic resonance imaging (MRI)
- Diagnostic ultrasonography
- Nuclear scintigraphy.

All of these techniques enable the veterinary surgeon to obtain diagnostic images of body parts essential for accurate diagnoses.

Fluoroscopy

Fluoroscopy is real-time or live X-ray images of an organ. These images are viewed as motion pictures on a video monitor. Fluoroscopy is suitable for:

- Upper gastrointestinal tract – in dogs, but not viable in feline patients due to restraint required and superimposition of view
- Barium enema – lower digestive tract
- Arthrogram – iodine will be injected into joint space and the flow visualised in real time to determine if any injury is present
- Hysterosalpingogram – iodine dye is injected into the uterus – useful in infertility problems.

463

The results are present immediately for the radiologist to observe and prove extremely useful in dysphagia cases and megaoesophagus.

Computed tomography

CT scans are a form of X-ray examination that uses computer technology and X-rays to produce a sectional image of the body. CT produces a 'shadow graph' of the various body tissues due to the differential absorption of the tissues present on a detector placed on the opposite side of the patient.

The CT tube rotates rapidly around the patient and a series of electronic detectors arranged in a circle pick up the X-ray beam. The electronic signal being produced is analysed at varying sections of tissue and each scan is allocated a number reference. Tissues are graded with a numerical value, which will relate to what shade of black, grey or white the tissue will show on the final image produced. The result is a cross-sectional image or slice of the tissue. Bone and gas appear as on normal radiographs. The table on which the patient is anaesthetised is slowly advanced, allowing each cross-section to be pictured to build up a complete body scan. CT scans produce optimal images in the transverse plane, although sagittal and dorsal planes are available via computer reformatting (with a reduction in accuracy). Contrast studies can easily be incorporated into CT scanning. CT is a non-invasive, rapid study technique but the use of ionising radiation requires the same health and safety considerations as for conventional radiography.

In veterinary medicine CT scans are used:

- To diagnose brain lesions, e.g. neoplasia, hydrocephalus, trauma
- In critical care patients (unlike MRI)
- For the investigation of skeletal disease
- In plain and myelography spinal CT.

Magnetic resonance imaging

MRI is a way to visualise normal and abnormal tissues in the body that cannot be picked up by simple X-rays. MRI uses magnetic field and radiowaves instead of radiation to create a clear picture of the internal body structures.

MRI is not the best technique for imaging of bone but comes into its own for visualisation of soft-tissue structures, where it can create images that can differentiate between healthy and diseased tissue. MRI maps out the location of protons present in hydrogen nuclei within the body tissues. The body is placed within a strong magnetic field, which makes the protons align and spin at a predetermined frequency (by strength of the field). The protons are then bombarded with radiowaves at a similar frequency, which disorientates the protons and causes them to realign accompanied by a short pulse or radio signal being emitted from them. The radio signals are collected and interpreted by the computer into a two- or three-dimensional image. The MRI scanner is usually a long, cylindrical magnet into which the patient is positioned by lying on a movable tabletop.

Scanning times are longer than with CT, therefore patients must be anaesthetised. No metallic objects should be within the near vicinity due to magnetic interference so specialist monitoring and anaesthetic equipment must be used. MRI images are of a much better diagnostic quality than CT imaging, with much improved soft-tissue definition and all planes being accurate. Different types of scan and paracontrast studies can be incorporated to achieve superior images. In veterinary MRI, as in CT, the brain is the primary organ of study for both congenital defects and for neoplasia. Spinal evaluation using MRI negates the requirement for contrast media so is much less invasive and produces better tissue definition.

Diagnostic ultrasonography

Ultrasound is now widely available to general practitioners. It uses high-frequency sound waves (2–10 MHz) via an ultrasound transducer containing a crystal which produces sound waves when a current is passed through it, generating short, regular pulses of sound. The transducer is placed on to the body surface and the sound waves travel through the body tissues. Different tissues respond to the sound with differing resistances or acoustic impedance.

At junctions between tissue types some of the sound will be reflected and some will travel on; the greater the difference in acoustic impedance, then the higher the quantity of sound that will be reflected. The sound that returns or the echoes produced are detected by the transducer. The sound being produced by the crystal is occurring in pulses so the echoes can return in between these. If the echo lasts longer than the interval between pulses being generated then a small electrical current is produced. It is these electrical signals that are analysed to produce the image according to their strength and site or origin. Linear array transducers are used for superficial tissues and often for the diagnosis of tendon lesions. Sector transducers produce a fan of sound waves and tend to be used for deeper tissues and pregnancy diagnosis. A Doppler ultrasound system is more advanced and can be used to show blood flow in the heart in real time and can be used to diagnose valvular defects.

Nuclear scintigraphy

This is known in lay terms as bone scanning; it is a common diagnostic tool employed in lameness evaluation in the equine. A radioactive isotope is injected in the horse; the isotope is taken up by cells that are active due to bony metabolism changes and these show up when scanned as 'hot spots' of activity, indicating bony changes occurring in the animal. Nuclear scintigraphy is much more sensitive than radiography and can diagnose changes at a very early stage. The gamma camera measures the radioactivity and the associated computer creates an image or scintigram which can be recorded.

Health and safety considerations are paramount as the horses are technically radioactive during the active phase of the isotope. The product used has a quick half-life and it has dropped to normal background radiation levels within 48 hours. All equipment used for administration should be lead-lined and appropriate personal protective equipment should be worn. Once injected and scanned horses remain stabled during the active period of the isotope; waste must be specially disposed of.

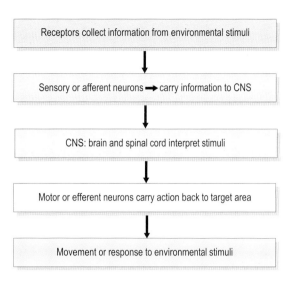

Figure 28.7 Recap of nervous system. CNS, central nervous system.

Box 28.3

DEFINITIONS

Local anaesthesia

Temporary interruption in nerve conduction in both the sensory and motor nerves

General anaesthesia

State of unconsciousness produced by a process of controlled, reversible intoxication of the central nervous system in which there is decreased sensitivity to environmental stimuli and a diminished motor response to such stimuli

---

ANAESTHESIA

Anaesthesia is a state of unconsciousness produced by a process of controlled, reversible drug-induced intoxication of the central nervous system in which the patient neither perceives nor recalls noxious stimuli (Box 28.3 and Figure 28.7).

Veterinary anaesthesia is required for:

- Humanitarian reasons: to minimise struggling, apprehension and restraint

- Technical efficiency: facilitation of procedure on animal and handler safety and protection from potentially dangerous agents, e.g. gases, self-injection.

It is essential to have satisfactory anaesthesia for the performance of painful surgical interference. Very few operations are allowed without anaesthesia, e.g. castration of calves, sheep and goats, disbudding calves (age-dependent) and docking tails or dew claw removal. Two main bodies of legislation govern veterinary anaesthesia:

- Veterinary Surgeons Act 1966 (plus amendments)
- Protection of Animals (Anaesthetics) Act 1964 (plus amendments).

Local anaesthetic agents tend to be non-volatile pharmaceuticals. General anaesthetic agents can be non-volatile pharmaceuticals but are often volatile agents or gaseous substances which are inhaled into the lungs. A volatile substance is a liquid or solid that can easily change into a gas, i.e. it evaporates quickly, often at room temperature. Types of anaesthesia are explained in Table 28.4.

Patient monitoring during anaesthesia

There are lots of different types of equipment available for use during perianaesthetic monitoring; however, the veterinary nurse should always use the following in addition or if the electronic equipment fails.

Table 28.4 Types of anaesthesia

Type	Indications
General	By inhalation By intravenous, intraperitoneal or intramuscular administration of non-gaseous anaesthetic agents By a combination of the above Elective/emergency surgery
Local	By surface application By intra- and subdermal infiltration Field blocking – linear infiltration of margins of surgical area Intravenous cannula placement, caesarean (local anaesthetic)
Spinal	Injection of local analgesic into spinal canal which causes temporary paralysis in spinal nerves Subarachnoid or epidural injection Spinal surgery
Regional	Local anaesthesia into a specific area to provide analgesia Caesarean (local anaesthetic)
Topical	Application of local anaesthetic Prior to intravenous cannula placement

Table 28.5 Reflexes that should be considered during anaesthesia

Reflex	How to test
Corneal	Eyelids close when the cornea is touched
Palpebral	Eyelids close when the eyelids are touched
Pupillary	Constriction of dilated pupil in response to increase in light Dilation in constricted pupil in response to increase in light intensity
Pedal	Pain reflex – measurement of pain response by pinching toes
Pharyngeal	Swallow when pharynx is touched
Laryngeal	Cough when larynx is touched
Jaw tone	Resistance to opening, yawn, tongue curls

- For general anaesthetic monitoring just two leads can be used, RA and LA, with them located on the brisket and between the xiphisternum and umbilicus respectively.

An ECG can be a useful diagnostic aid in the high-risk anaesthetised patient.

Manual monitoring

- Respiration
- Circulation
- Reflexes (Table 28.5)
- Temperature
- Depth of anaesthesia
- Equipment function
- The procedure
- Fluid output.

Electrocardiography (ECG)

- Place the patient in right lateral recumbency (the patient should be on an insulated surface)
- Clip the area where you plan to attach electrodes
- Attach electrodes to loose skin on the limbs – proprietary gels or surgical spirit can improve the connection by ensuring good conductivity:
  - Right arm (RA) red: right forelimb
  - Left arm (LA) yellow: left forelimb
  - Left foot (LF) green: left hindlimb
  - Right foot (RF) black: right hindlimb
- Record calibration mark
- Record multiple complexes at 50 mm/s, then a longer strip at 25 mm/s (second lead)

Pulse oximetry

This measures how much oxygen is delivered to the tissues. The oximeter probe passes light through the tissues of an extremity and detects how much light is absorbed by haemoglobin in the tissues at two different wavelengths.

Each wavelength corresponds to the wavelength light is best absorbed by oxygenated and deoxygenated haemoglobin. The comparison is used to calculate the proportion of haemoglobin that is saturated, the Spo_2: this is expressed as a percentage. The pulse rate is also usually displayed for the patient. Normal Spo_2 should be 99% (at least > 97%); if Spo_2 is < 93% supplementation should be considered and it is essential under 90%.

Probes should be connected to hairless, unpigmented skin or on a mucous membrane, e.g. pinna, nipple, vulva or tongue to facilitate readings.

Capnography/capnometry

The capnograph measures carbon dioxide levels in the airway which mirror carbon dioxide levels in arterial blood, if the animal has healthy lungs. This is measured in the exhaled gas either from the proximal or distal end of an endotracheal tube, the Y-connector or via nasal cannulae or masks. More accurate results come from using the endotracheal tube or Y-connector. It can detect circulatory changes, respiratory changes, metabolic changes and equipment failure or faults which show as abnormalities in the readings. The capnometer records a permanent reading, with the carbon dioxide level expressed as tension (mmHg) or as a concentration percentage. Normal carbon dioxide at end of expiration or $Petco_2$ should be 35–40 mmHg. It is a useful tool for anaesthetised patients undergoing artificial ventilation.

Respiratory monitors

Respiratory rate monitors and apnoea alarms are available. These use thermistors placed in the patient's airway or connected to the endotracheal tube to detect the difference in the temperature of inspired and exhaled gases and the result is a reassuring beep on your machine. An alarm sounds when the temperature difference is too low to be read, i.e. the patient's breathing has stopped. The respiratory rates of small mammals, reptiles and birds are too fast for accurate monitoring in some cases.

Oesophageal stethoscope

This is a useful device: it is easy to use, and provides information on cardiac and respiratory output via auscultation. The amplifier sits within the end of a flexible tube and is placed at the level of the patient's heart via the oesophagus. Prior to placement the tube is measured from the canine teeth to the level of the heart (approximately ribs 7–9 or at the point of flexion of the elbow joint) along the line of the oesophagus then marked to give the operator an idea of the correct location. It is lubricated and then passed into the oesophagus whilst the operator listens via ear pieces.

Other monitoring equipment available includes:

- Pulse monitors
- Heart rate monitors
- Central venous pressure monitors
- Blood pressure monitors (sphygmomanometers)
- Digital temperature monitors
- External temperature thermostats for use with heat pads.

PREOPERATIVE CARE, OWNER INSTRUCTIONS AND RISK BANDING

Most operations performed are elective procedures upon reasonably healthy, normal animals. Therefore it is important to ascertain that such animals are healthy and normal. A system can be used to describe a patient's preoperative condition and rate it according to risk but

individuality must be considered. Preoperative assessments should be made from the history and clinical examination.

Preoperative examination

The following should be checked for:

- Deformities
- Severe dental disease
- Colour of mucous membranes
- Brightness/dullness of eyes
- Degree of mental alertness
- Respiratory distress
- Obesity
- Enlargement of lymph nodes
- Dehydration levels
- Temperature
- Pulse
- Auscultation – respiratory and cardiovascular system
- Blood profile
- X-rays if applicable.

A range of normal values for vital parameters should be noted.

The consent form

The consent form is a legal document, and as such, should be kept for a minimum of 7 years. The consent form should contain the owner's name, address and contact numbers, the animal's signalment, the procedure to be undertaken, a statement of risk for the anaesthetic and procedure and the signature and date of the owner to provide permission to operate on the animal.

Additional tips

- As much history as possible should be written on the card or a separate form
- Ask the owner to walk the dog before coming into surgery –this allows the animal the opportunity to urinate and defecate
- Always try to explain what is going to happen to the animal before the day of the operation, as on the day itself the owner is often too worried to take in information.

Instructions to give to the owner before surgery

Most operations are elective; therefore there is generally enough time to prepare the owner for surgery. Ideally any instructions that are given should be written down on paper. Most people are good at forgetting what they

467

are told, especially when told by the veterinary surgeon!

Always note:

- Day and date of operation
- Time you would like them to arrive for surgery
- Which surgery you would like them to come to
- The time they should fast their animal for – explain the reasons why
- The time they should give medication – if any and if applicable
- Inform them to keep their cat in the night before the operation.

Food

Regurgitation is a passive process involving the expulsion of undigested food from the distal oesophagus. Passive regurgitation (reflux) is more likely to occur in deep anaesthesia due to relaxation of the stomach muscles. Vomiting is an active process, which results in the expulsion of vomitus, i.e. the contents of the stomach. Vomiting is most common at induction/recovery whilst under light anaesthesia. Inhalation of foreign material may result in inhalation pneumonia over a few days. Small mammals should be fed continually prior to anaesthesia but dogs, cats and ruminants should undergo a period of starvation.

Water

Water should not be withdrawn for more than 2 hours before anaesthesia and never for small mammals or exotics. Remember, dehydration can reduce the clearance of anaesthetic drugs and reduce blood pressure.

Additional notes for exotics

Exotic species often do not show clear signs of ill health and you should be suspicious even when they appear healthy. They are more prone to suffer from stress, which can affect physiological processes. Histories are often lacking or inaccurate due to owners often being children. All should be considered high-risk, according to experts in this field. Normal monitoring signs may vary with species: read up or ask what to expect, e.g. rodents' eyes are often fixed continuously whilst under general anaesthesia. Remember these animals have a greater ratio of surface area to body weight than dogs and cats so are more prone to metabolic and physiological problems.

Signs and stages of anaesthesia

The signs and stages of anaesthesia are descriptions of the physiological effects of anaesthetic agents upon the mammalian body. Surgical anaesthesia is subdivided into a number of stages and planes to allow accurate description of the physiological effects present or absent.

Classically, signs of anaesthesia and its depth are provided by the presence or absence of certain reflexes.

Reflex assessment should be undertaken at least every 5 minutes during anaesthetic monitoring. Simultaneously the patient's vital signs should be monitored:

- Respiration – rate, depth, rhythm
- Pulse – rate, character, strength
- Eye position
- Dilation of pupil
- Capillary refill time
- Mucous membrane assessment
- Muscle tone
- Temperature
- Heart rate – including comparison with peripheral pulse.

During veterinary anaesthesia the physiological characteristics displayed by the patient are dependent upon the agent utilised.

Physiology of anaesthesia

When considering anaesthetic physiology the effects of pharmaceutical agents upon the cardiovascular and respiratory systems of the patient are being considered. Anaesthetic agents have numerous effects on respiratory rate and spontaneous breathing. Expiratory tone becomes enhanced whilst inspiratory tone decreases, leading to irregularities in breathing patterns, periodic breathing or cessation of breathing in some cases. Anaesthetic agents are known to depress the effectiveness of carbon dioxide receptors, subsequently affecting ventilation patterns.

The respiratory changes can contribute to cardiovascular changes to compensate for lowered/high partial pressures of oxygen and carbon dioxide respectively. In addition individual agents may directly affect the cardiovascular system, causing mainly hypotension or reducing stroke volume.

Anaesthesia also produces a decrease in renal perfusion rates and glomerular filtration rate due to hypotension associated with the majority of anaesthetic drugs. In addition levels of antidiuretic hormone increase, leading to a tendency for water retention in the body for 24 hours (or in some cases more) postanaesthesia. It is thought that liver physiology is affected by anaesthesia.

The overall classification of the physiological characteristics exhibited is known as the Guedel classification. Remember that the skilled anaesthetist will consider respiration and cardiovascular performance in the patient before, during and after surgical anaesthesia.

Guedel classification

Stage 1: induction stage/stage of voluntary excitement

- Duration is from beginning of induction until the loss of consciousness
- Animal may make forcible attempts to resist anaesthesia
- Fear and apprehension may be exhibited
- Usually accompanied by an increase in respiration, heart and pulse rates
- Observe dilation of pupils
- Respiration is under voluntary control but periods of apnoea may be observed as a reaction to gaseous agents/drugs used
- Evacuation of urine and/or faeces may occur.

Stage 2: stage of involuntary excitement

- Duration – from when animal loses consciousness until the onset of automatic respiration
- Reflex response is exaggerated and subsequently limb movement may necessitate patient restraint
- Vocalisation often occurs
- Violence may be exhibited: the degree of violence is unpredictable and not related to the animal's normal temperament
- Respiration is irregular and apnoea may be seen
- Pharyngeal reflexes are present but become depressed as stage progresses
- Laryngeal reflex persists.

Stage 3: subdivided into planes

- Duration – begins with the onset of automatic respiration and finishes with the cessation of respiration
- Stage 3 is subdivided into three planes.

Stage 3 plane 1: light anaesthesia

- Begins with the onset of automatic respiration
- Cessation of all limb movement
- Eyeballs exhibit nystagmus, which becomes sluggish as the depth of anaesthesia increases
- Palpebral and corneal reflexes are reducing in intensity
- Pedal reflex is brisk
- Suitable for minor surgical procedures and diagnostic investigations.

Stage 3 plane 2: medium anaesthesia

- Little change in respiratory pattern until nearing the end of the stage when the amplitude and rate increase

- Eyeballs are fixed and begin to rotate downwards in cats and dogs
- Laryngeal reflex persists until approximately midway into the second plane
- Palpebral and corneal reflexes are absent
- Muscular relaxation becomes progressively more pronounced towards flaccidity until eventually muscle tone is lost
- Pedal reflex is sluggish
- Suitable for the majority of surgical procedures.

Stage 3 plane 3: deep anaesthesia

- Respiration is involuntary but rate has increased whilst the depth decreases
- Exhibit intercostal lag – a noticeable pause between inspiration and expiration
- Eyeballs become central and fixed
- Pedal reflex absent
- Abdominal muscle tone absent.

Stage 4

- Duration – onset at thoracic muscle paralysis and finishes with death
- Diaphragmatic activity remains but becomes jerky and respiration appears gasping – Cheyne–Stokes respiration
- Rapid pulse
- Pupils dilate and eyeballs present with 'fish-eye' or glassy appearance due to cessation of lacrimal secretions
- Intervention must occur to prevent imminent death
- Respiration gasps lose amplitude until they cease completely
- Cyanosis exhibited
- Respiratory and cardiac failure occur – and then the animal is dead.

Remember, not all stages or planes will be exhibited in all anaesthetics. Research studies for individual agents may over- or underemphasise respiratory and circulatory effect – they are no substitute for a skilled anaesthetist as individual animals may greatly influence the effect of drugs. Premedication agents can influence all stages of anaesthesia, e.g. certain agents can have a mydriatic or miotic effect on the pupi, which could give false observational evidence.

Endotracheal tubes

These connect the patient to the anaesthetic circuit and thus the breathing system (Figure 28.8). Two types are used:

1. Red rubber Magill's tubes, which provide poor resistance to kinking and conform poorly to airway contours

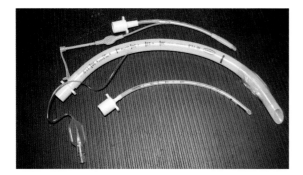

Figure 28.8 Selection of endotracheal tubes.

2. Polyvinylchloride tubes, which are softest and least irritating to tracheal mucosa. They have little tendency to kink and mould to the curve of the airway at body temperature.

The size of the tube is a measurement of its internal diameter in millimetres. The tube should extend from the incisor table to a point level with the spine of the scapula. Surplus dead space can be minimised by cutting off the end of the projecting tube.

Before use, endotracheal tubes must be checked for:

- Patency
- Roughened edges
- Bite holes in tube
- The cuff's ability to hold pressure – no weaknesses
- Absence or perishing of the cuff/tube.

Scavenging or minimising anaesthetic pollution

Scavenging is the removal of expired waste gas to a site distant from the working environment. All anaesthetic circuits must have an expiratory valve that can connect easily to a scavenging system. The purchase of an approved scavenging system does not itself guarantee low levels of waste anaesthetic gases.

Anaesthesia physiological control

The physiology of anaesthesia is still not fully understood but relates closely to the physiological control of respiration.

Hypoventilation

This can be caused by:

- Decreased respiratory rate
- Reduced (impaired) tidal volume

- Increased dead space
- A combination of the above.

The result of hypoventilation is hypercapnia and this in turn can facilitate respiratory acidosis due to a build-up of hydrogen ions in the blood as the increased levels of carbon dioxide dissociate into carbonic acid. Care should be taken during anaesthesia as most anaesthetic agents reduce the sensitivity of chemoreceptors to partial pressure of carbon dioxide.

Hyperventilation

Excessive ventilation results in hypocapnia, which in turn results in respiratory alkalosis. This can be seen during light anaesthetics or painful procedures or with incorrectly executed mechanical or manual ventilation. The resultant low partial pressure of carbon dioxide is insufficient to trigger the respiratory centres of the brain to breathe slower and deeper to return the respiratory pattern to normal. Administration of carbon dioxide can be useful in these scenarios – humans can breathe into a paper bag to increase the concentration of carbon dioxide in the blood.

Hypoxia

Hypoxia is abnormally low partial pressures or concentration of oxygen within the blood. If allowed to continue unresolved it will cause tissue hypoxia and cardiac arrest can occur. It is caused by:

- Reduced oxygen input
- Reduced alveolar ventilation
- Lung pathology
- Insufficient cardiac output
- Increased tissue demand for oxygen.

Perfusion

Perfusion is the movement of fluid through vessels and/or organs. In anaesthetic physiology it concerns the velocity of blood flow primarily through the capillary network, as this is where gaseous exchange occurs at tissue level. The velocity of blood in the capillaries will be affected by blood pressure in both arterial and venous pressure and resistance of the vessels within the tissues. When oxygen levels fall, carbon dioxide levels should also increase, bringing about an increased respiratory rate and heart rate to distribute the fresh intake of oxygen. When this occurs arterial blood pressure has increased and the precapillary sphincters relax, allowing maximal blood to flow through the tissues to provide oxygen and remove carbon dioxide.

Cardiovascular physiology

Systemic vascular resistance (SVR)

This describes the effective state of the precapillary sphincters throughout the body. If these were closed the cardiovascular system would be shut off or vasoconstriction would have occurred and this would reduce the diameter of the vessels and therefore increase SVR and blood pressure. If the precapillary sphincters were open, the cardiovascular system would be free-flowing and vasodilation would have occurred. The precapillary sphincters respond to:

- Metabolic factors, e.g. partial pressures of carbon dioxide and oxygen as above
- Tonic vasoconstrictor nerve discharge
- Hormones and drugs.

The heart rate itself is governed by the autonomic nervous system – parasympathetic slows it down and sympathetic quickens the rate. The pathology of the heart itself will be another variable that should be considered. This can affect the rhythm of the heart and the cardiac output or the volume of blood ejected by the heart per minute (l/min).

Blood pressure

This is a measure of the pressure exerted by the circulatory volume, i.e. the blood upon the walls of the blood vessels. Readings could be taken for arteries, veins and capillaries but in veterinary medicine we usually consider arterial blood pressure. Arterial blood pressure is detected by baroreceptors which are mainly located in the carotid artery at the carotid sinus. These detect stretching of the elastic muscle due to increased volume of blood present, which would translate to an increase in blood pressure. The baroreceptors initiate neural impulses which:

- Reduce heart rate and the force of contraction
- Increase parasympathetic vagal activity – slowing heart
- Suppress vasomotor centre activity, causing vasodilation in mesenteric and cutaneous vascular beds to reduce blood pressure and SVR.

Hypotension

This is low blood pressure and results from:

- Reduced cardiac output
- Reduced SVR
- Or both.

Hypertension

This is high blood pressure and results from:

- Increased cardiac output
- Increased SVR
- Or both.

Anaesthetic circuits

The anaesthetic circuit carries respiratory gases between the patient and the anaesthetic machine. It has three main functions:

1. Removal of carbon dioxide
2. Supply of oxygen to the patient
3. Supply of anaesthetics to the patient.

Removal of carbon dioxide is achieved by:

- Replacing expired air with fresh gas
- Removing carbon dioxide from the circuit before the air is rebreathed.

Oxygen is supplied via the anaesthetic machine and at a rate which suits both the individual animal and the circuit being used. Inhalant anaesthetics are supplied to the patient by the carrier gas (oxygen) through the anaesthetic circuit. The amount of volatile agent is controllable and a calibrated vaporiser is used. Refer to Box 28.4 for a classification of anaesthetic circuits.

Rebreathing circuits

These are where expired gases are passed through an absorber which contains soda lime to remove carbon dioxide. Gases are inhaled more than once by the patient. Examples include the circle (Figure 28.9) and Waters (to and fro).

Box 28.4

CLASSIFICATION OF ANAESTHETIC CIRCUITS

Open

An agent on a swab held close to the airway

Semi-open

Agent on a swab held over airway, e.g. in a mask

Semi-closed

Enclosed system without carbon dioxide absorption, e.g. non-rebreathing circuits

Closed

Enclosed system with carbon dioxide absorption, e.g. rebreathing systems

---

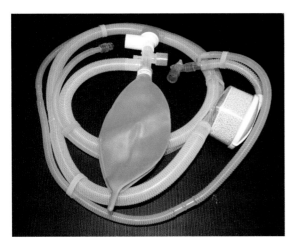

Figure 28.9 Small-animal rebreathing circuit: circle.

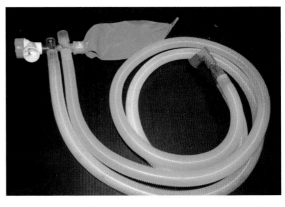

Figure 28.10 Small-animal non-rebreathing circuit: parallel Lack.

Rebreathing circuits are intended for use in larger dogs and other large animals and should not be used in animals under 10 kg due to the resistance to respiration provided by the inclusion of soda lime (some modern versions can be used in animals of 5 kg and above). They necessitate the animal to rebreathe anaesthetic gases, which contain:

- Low levels of volatile agent
- Some oxygen
- Carbon dioxide.

The carbon dioxide is eliminated from the circuit by a chemical absorber, i.e. soda lime, rather than the use of high gas flow rates, whilst the remaining gases and volatile agent pass to the reservoir bag to mix with the fresh gas.

Expired breath, in comparison to inspired gas, is low in oxygen and anaesthetic but high in carbon dioxide, contains water vapour and is warm. The carbon dioxide is removed by the soda lime, leaving warm, moist gas to be recirculated to the patient. Fresh gas flow rates are based on the oxygen and anaesthetic requirements of the patient.

Denitrogenation

At the onset of anaesthesia patients expire considerable amounts of nitrogen. This is not a problem in non-rebreathing systems due to the high fresh gas flow rates, but in rebreathing systems the volume of nitrogen can displace oxygen in the circuit, leading to hypoxic levels. To counteract this effect, high flow rates are required initially (for approximately 10–15 minutes) to purge the nitrogen through the pressure relief valve. If this is not done then regular dumping or emptying of the reservoir

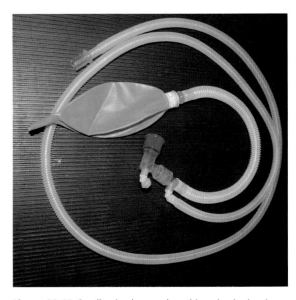

Figure 28.11 Small-animal non-rebreathing circuit: Ayre's T-piece.

bag is required (every 3 minutes for the first 15 minutes, then every 30 minutes thereafter).

Non-rebreathing circuits

These are where expired gases are ventilated to the environment or atmosphere and cannot be rebreathed (Figures 28.10 and 28.11). Examples include the Bain, Magill, Lack and T-piece.

Remember that the anaesthetist can vary how individual circuits operate by manipulating the patient's flow rates. If a flow rate is too low for a patient on a non-rebreathing system, gas will be breathed more than once by the patient. If flow rates are too high in a closed system, fresh gas will only be inhaled once before it is discarded. Average flow rates are available for animals but these can vary for individual cases according to lung capacity, systemic diseases and lung pathology.

ANALGESIA

Reasons for treating pain:

- It causes stress and suffering to the patient
- It leads to catabolism and decreased food intake
- It causes delayed healing
- It can impair respiration if it is thoracic or cranial abdominal in origin
- It can lead to self-mutilation
- It causes hypersensitisation leading to chronic pain.

Remember that analgesics work best when there is no pain – therefore it important to prevent pain, rather than treat it.

Nursing considerations in pain control

- Tender loving care – attention will help to decrease the distress associated with pain and an unfamiliar environment. In humans a cycle of pain/distress/ sleeplessness can develop and lead to a demoralised, psychologically depressed patient who heals more slowly – there is no reason to assume that this does not happen in animals!
- Environment – must be warm, dry and comfortable
- Wound care – prevent further infection and pain
- Immobilise fracture sites – this reduces pain and self-mutilation
- Nutrition – animals with a positive energy/protein balance heal quicker
- Adjunctive therapy – physiotherapy.

Drugs used in veterinary analgesia

- Opioid analgesics
- Non-steroidal anti-inflammatory drugs (NSAIDs)
- Alpha-2-agonist (though technically a sedative)
- Ketamine (also technically a sedative).

Opioid analgesics

These drugs are potent analgesics used in the treatment of severe pain, such as that following surgery or other trauma. They are also commonly used in premedication. They can be divided into groups depending upon their

activity on the various classes of opioid receptors (mu, kappa, delta, epsilon, sigma).

Neuroleptanalgesia

Sedative–opioid combinations can be used to provide premedication and chemical restraint: their effects are synergistic. Neuroleptanalgesia is a term used to describe the state of produced by the administration of a potent opioid with a neuroleptic (antipsychotic such as ACP). Depending upon the agents used the effect ranges from moderate sedation to unconsciousness with analgesia sufficient to tolerate moderate surgery. These combinations tend to produce marked respiratory depression and cardiovascular effects. It is wise to have a reversal agent to hand plus facilities for respiratory and circulatory support.

Non-steroidal anti-inflammatory drugs

The action of NSAIDs is to diminish the vascular and cellular components of the inflammatory response at the site of tissue injury. Therefore the acute phase of inflammation is reduced and the chronic phase is not initiated.

The use of NSAIDs is contraindicated for the perioperative period and in shocked, hypovolaemic animals. Their use should be delayed until the postoperative period or until the patient is normovolaemic. Carprofen is the exception to the rule and can be administered safely in both these categories of patient.

Dissociative anaesthesia

In this type of anaesthesia, patients are unconscious but certain muscle reflexes are still present and no muscle relaxation is achieved. The patient is unaware of surroundings and dissociated from the external environment. Dissociative anaesthesia is a state whereby somatic (body tissue) analgesia is combined with a light plane of unconsciousness but the animal appears dissociated from its environment:

- Eyes remain open
- Laryngeal and swallowing reflexes remain
- Muscle tone remains and may even be enhanced.

Local anaesthesia

Remember that local anaesthesia is technically local analgesia used to facilitate a surgical procedure. Sedative agents may or may not be used depending upon:

- Temperament
- Health
- Procedure.

Local anaesthesia is often employed in large-animal medicine where prolonged recumbency would be detrimental, to evaluate chronic pain problems, or to facilitate intubation.

Local analgesia works by blocking the nervous impulses from the operative site. The animal feels no pain and no muscle stimulation, therefore does not move or moves as it would without the pain. These agents can cause cardiovascular (arrhythmias), respiratory (depression) and central nervous system effects, and occasionally allergic reactions are exhibited. Methods used in veterinary practice include:

- Surface analgesia – freezing of the skin
- Intrasynovial analgesia – for a diagnosis of lameness
- Infiltration analgesia – field blocks
- Regional analgesia – nerve blocks
- Spinal analgesia – this is an epidural which blocks nerves caudal to the block site and will affect those parts of the animal they innervate.

Inhalant anaesthesia

The anaesthetic machine is the most important piece of equipment in the theatre. Even if injectable anaesthesia is being used the anaesthetic machine should be ready for use in case of an emergency. There are a wide range of machines available. Some are designed specifically for veterinary use whereas others have been adapted from human medicine. The latter may incorporate additional features not necessary within the field of veterinary anaesthesia (Figure 28.12).

Functions of the anaesthetic machine

- It produces and delivers safe concentrations of anaesthetic vapour
- It provides a means of giving oxygen and allowing intermittent positive-pressure ventilation during apnoea and cardiopulmonary arrest.

Gas cylinders

Anaesthetic gases are supplied under pressure in steel cylinders, which are classified in order of increasing size by letter, from AA to J.

The smaller cylinders are mounted directly on to the machine, whilst the larger cylinders are usually held in storage rooms and the gas is piped to the machine via reinforced, colour-coded tubes. Oxygen comes in black cylinders with white shoulders.

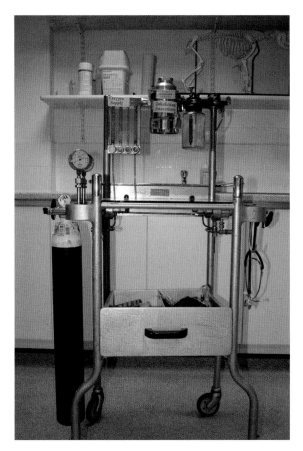

Figure 28.12 Small-animal anaesthetic machine.

The administration of inhalant anaesthesia requires:

- A source of oxygen
- A vaporiser or source of anaesthetic gas
- A patient or breathing circuit.

The components of the anaesthetic machine

Cylinders

- Label: empty, in use, full
- Attached to machine by pin index system – this ensures that only the correct category of gas fits on to the correct port on the machine, i.e. oxygen cylinders only attach to the oxygen port. It is a system of pins that works like a key and lock mechanism.

Port

- Where the cylinder attaches to machine
- Should have a Bocock seal present – this is a small rubber washer that prevents leaks between cylinder and port attachment

- The port can have a metal yoke which is placed over the attached cylinder to hold it in place
- Other types of cylinder screw on to the port and do not require a washer.

Pressure gauges

- Enable the anaesthetist to ascertain if any gas, particularly oxygen, is left in the cylinder
- Most common type used are Bourdon gauges.

Reducing valves or regulators

- Located between the source of compressed gas and the flowmeter
- Usually found either within the hanger yoke or just below it
- Used to:
  - ○ Regulate or prevent variations in gas delivery due to pressure/temperature changes
  - ○ Allow small alterations in quantities of gas being delivered
  - ○ Reduce the pressure within the connecting tubing (and to the patient), preventing damage
- Commonest type in use are the Medishield valves.

Flowmeters

- These control the flow of gas and give an indication of the amount of gas passing to the patient
- Most common type in use is the rotameter
- Rotameter consists of a glass tube inside which a rotating bobbin is free to move. The bore of the tube gradually increases from below upwards and the bobbin has channels cut in it which allow the bobbin to ride on the cushion of gas and effectively eliminate errors due to frictional force
- Tubes must be vertical for accurate readings
- Rotameters are calibrated to incorporate the viscosity and density of the gas it is designed to be used with so they should not be swapped between gas types
- They are calibrated for normal atmospheric pressure, therefore show inaccuracies at high altitudes.

Vaporisers

- Used in conjunction with volatile liquids
- Lots of types available
- Ball float meters also have a tapered bore and are variable orifice meters
- With ball floats the reading is taken from the point of maximum circumference or equator, not the top of the float, as with the bobbin

- Out of circuit vaporisers or Tec vaporisers are more commonly used in veterinary medicine, examples include:
  - ○ Fluotec – halothane
  - ○ Isotec – isoflurane
  - ○ Pentec – methoxyflurane
- Tecs incorporate a bimetallic strip as a temperature compensator
- When the gas enters the vaporiser it splits into two streams: one bypasses the volatile agent and the other goes through it
- The one which enters the liquid becomes saturated with vapour
- Concentrations of vapour leaving can be calculated if the saturated vapour pressure of the volatile anaesthetic agent and the splitting ratio are known
- Tecs remain constant despite changes in variables, e.g. temperature, time, liquid amount, gas flow
- Vaporisers should be filled before use with the minimal amount of vapours being inhaled
- Vaporisers should be checked daily for wear and tear of dial as well as liquid levels
- Tec vaporisers can be disconnected and are pin-coded to prevent them being attached to the wrong port.

Pipe lines

- Transport gases from cylinders through machine workings to patient.

Oxygen flush/purge

- Piping that runs from the oxygen cylinder to the patient, bypassing the vaporiser
- Used in emergencies and to purge systems postanaesthesia.

Oxygen warning

- Some machines have a valve that opens as oxygen pressure falls, diverting the remaining gas through a whistle, which sounds loudly then decreases in volume as the oxygen pressure falls to atmospheric pressure.

Bosun's whistle

- Warning system which operates in circuits incorporating nitrous oxide and oxygen
- Nitrous oxide must be turned on for it to work
- When both nitrous oxide and oxygen cylinders are on, the whistle sounds if the oxygen cylinder runs out
- Should be checked daily by turning the oxygen cylinder off to hear the audible alarm.

475

Common gas outlet

- Port where the anaesthetic circuit attaches to the machine
- Delivers all gases to the patient.

Bibliography

Aspinall V 2006 The complete textbook of veterinary nursing. Butterworth Heinemann, London

Bacha W J Jr, Wood L M 1990 Color atlas of veterinary histology. Lea & Febiger, Philadelphia

Lane D R, Cooper B, Turner L 2007 Textbook of veterinary nursing, 3rd edn. Butterworth Heinemann/BSAVA, Oxford

Lavin L M 1994 Radiography in veterinary technology. Harcourt-Brace, London

McCurnin D, Bassett J 2005 Clinical textbook for veterinary technicians, 6th edn. W B Saunders, Philadelphia

Moore M 2000 Manual of veterinary nursing. BSAVA, Oxford

Moore A H, Simpson G 1999 Manual of advanced veterinary nursing. BSAVA, Oxford

Morgan J P 1993 Techniques in veterinary radiography, 5th edn. Iowa State University Press, Iowa

Paddleford R P 1998 Manual of small animal anaesthesia, 2nd edn. W B Saunders, Philadelphia

Pratt P W 1998 Principles and practice of veterinary technology. Mosby, Philadelphia

Simpson G 1994 Practical veterinary nursing, 3rd edn. BSAVA, Oxford

Appendix

Normal clinical parameters of companion animals

Species	Body temperature (°C)	Pulse rate (beats/min)	Respiratory rate (breaths/min)	Lifespan
Dog	38.3–38.7	60–180	10–30	10–15 years
Cat	38–38.5	110–180	20–30	15–20 years
Horse	38–38.2	32–44	8–12	25–30 years
Rabbit	37–39.4	198–330	35–60	7 years
Guinea pig	37.2–39.5	240–310	40–80	5–6 years
Ferret	37.8–40	200–300	33–36	5–11 years
Gerbil	38.2	85–160	85–160	24–39 months
Mouse	37.1	427–697	91–216	12–36 months
Rat	37.7	313–493	71–146	26–40 months
Hamster	37.6	310–471	38–110	18–36 months

Index

NB: Page numbers in **bold** refer to boxes, figures and tables